Guide to Diagnostic Tests

Seventh edition

Diana Nicoll, MD, PhD, MPA
Clinical Professor and Vice Chair
Department of Laboratory Medicine
University of California, San Francisco
Associate Dean
University of California, San Francisco School of Medicine
Chief of Staff and Chief, Laboratory Medicine Service
Veterans Affairs Medical Center, San Francisco

Chuanyi Mark Lu, MD
Professor of Laboratory Medicine
University of California, San Francisco
Chief, Hematology and Hematopathology
Laboratory Medicine Service
Veterans Affairs Medical Center, San Francisco

Stephen J. McPhee, MD
Professor of Medicine, Emeritus
Division of General Internal Medicine
Department of Medicine
University of California, San Francisco

With Associate Authors

Mc Graw Hill Education

New York   Chicago   San Francisco   Athens   London   Madrid   Mexico City
Milan   New Delhi   Singapore   Sydney   Toronto

Guide to Diagnostic Tests, Seventh Edition

4 5 6 7 8 9   LCR   22 21 20 19

ISBN 978-1-259-64089-6
MHID 1-259-64089-2
ISSN 1061-3463

Notice

This book was set in Times LT Std by Cenveo® Publisher Services.
The editors were Amanda Fielding and Harriet Lebowitz.
The production supervisor was Catherine Saggese.
Project management was provided by Revathi Viswanathan at Cenveo Publisher Services.

This book was printed on acid-free paper.

International Edition. ISBN 978-1-260-08433-7; MHID 1-260-08433-7. Copyright ©2017 by McGraw-Hill Education. Exclusive rights by McGraw-Hill Education for manufacture and export. This book cannot be re-exported from the country to which it is consigned by McGraw-Hill Education. The International Edition is not available in North America.

McGraw-Hill books are available at special quantity discounts to use as premiums and sales promotions, or for use in corporate training programs. To contact a representative, please visit the Contact Us pages at www.mhprofessional.com.

Contents

Associate Authors

Barbara L. Haller, MD, PhD
Clinical Professor of Laboratory Medicine
Chief of Microbiology
Department of Laboratory Medicine
University of California, San Francisco
Zuckerberg San Francisco General Hospital & Trauma Center, San Francisco
Microbiology: Test Selection

Fred M. Kusumoto, MD
Professor of Medicine
Department of Medicine
Division of Cardiovascular Diseases
Director of Electrophysiology and Pacing
Mayo Clinic Jacksonville, FL
Basic Electrocardiography & Echocardiography

Zhen Jane Wang, MD
Associate Professor of Radiology
Department of Radiology
University of California, San Francisco
Diagnostic Imaging: Test Selection & Interpretation

Benjamin M. Yeh, MD
Professor of Radiology
Department of Radiology
University of California, San Francisco
Diagnostic Imaging: Test Selection & Interpretation

Phil Tiso
UCSF Principal Editor
Division of General Internal Medicine
Department of Medicine
University of California, San Francisco

Preface

Purpose

The *Guide to Diagnostic Tests, Seventh edition*, is intended to serve as a reference manual for medical, nursing, and other health professional students, house officers, and practicing physicians, physician assistants, and nurses. It is a quick reference guide to the selection and interpretation of commonly used diagnostic tests, including laboratory procedures in the clinical setting, common laboratory tests (chemistry, hematology, coagulation, immunology, microbiology, drug monitoring, pharmacogenetic, and molecular and genetic testing), diagnostic imaging tests (plain radiography, CT, MRI, and ultrasonography), electrocardiography, echocardiography, and the use of tests in differential diagnosis, helpful diagnostic algorithms, and nomograms and reference material.

This book enables readers to understand frequently used diagnostic tests and diagnostic approaches to common disease states.

Outstanding Features

- Over 350 tests presented in a concise, consistent, and readable format.
- Full coverage of more than two dozen new laboratory tests and diagnostic algorithms.
- Expanded content regarding molecular and genetic tests, including pharmacogenetic tests.
- Full section on diagnostic imaging.
- Sections on basic electrocardiography and echocardiography.
- Updated and additional microbiologic coverage of emerging (new) and reemerging pathogens and infectious agents.
- Fields covered: internal medicine, pediatrics, surgery, neurology, and obstetrics and gynecology.
- Costs and risks of various procedures and tests.
- Full literature citations with PubMed (PMID) numbers included for each reference.
- An index for quick reference on the back cover.

Organization

This pocket reference manual is not intended to include all diagnostic tests or disease states. The authors have selected the tests and diseases that are most common and relevant to the general practice of medicine.

Guide to Diagnostic Tests is divided into 10 sections:

1. Diagnostic Testing & Medical Decision Making
2. Point-of-Care Testing & Provider-Performed Microscopy
3. Common Laboratory Tests: Selection & Interpretation
4. Therapeutic Drug Monitoring & Pharmacogenetic Testing: Principles & Test Interpretation
5. Microbiology: Test Selection
6. Diagnostic Imaging: Test Selection & Interpretation
7. Basic Electrocardiography & Echocardiography
8. Diagnostic Tests in Differential Diagnosis
9. Diagnostic Algorithms
10. Nomograms & Reference Material

New to This Edition

1. More than two dozen new or substantially revised clinical laboratory test entries, including: beta-D-glucan, *BRCA1/BRCA2* genotyping, *calreticulin (CALR)* mutation, cystatin C, D-dimer, heparin anti-Xa assay, hepatitis B e antigen/antibody (HBeAg/Ab), hepatitis C virus genotyping, hepatitis C viral load, new HIV screening algorithm, HLA-B51 typing, IgG subclasses, kappa and lambda free light chains with ratio, lipoprotein(a), lipoprotein-associated phospholipase A2 (Lp-PLA2), procollagen type-1 intact N-terminal propeptide (PINP), ribosomal DNA (16S rDNA) sequencing, and syphilis tests (new algorithm).
2. Microbiologic tests for emerging (new) and reemerging pathogens and infectious agents, including Chikungunya virus, *Cryptococcus gattii*, dengue virus, Ebola virus, Middle East respiratory syndrome (MERS) coronavirus, human granulocytic anaplasmosis, carbapenem-resistant Enterobacteriaceae (CRE), and Zika virus.
3. More than one dozen new or substantially revised tables or algorithms concerning diagnostic approaches to genetic diseases (molecular diagnostic testing), prenatal diagnostic testing, blood component therapy, adrenocortical insufficiency, inherited bleeding disorders, jaundice, lymphocytosis, monoarthritis, pulmonary embolism, syphilis testing, and thrombocytosis.
4. New reference materials displaying the complement system and steroidogenesis pathways.

Intended Audience

Medical students will find the concise summary of diagnostic laboratory, microbiologic, and imaging studies, and of electrocardiography and echocardiography in this convenient reference book of great help during clinical ward rotations. Busy house officers, physicians' assistants, nurse practitioners, and physicians (internal medicine and family medicine, etc.) will find the clear organization and current literature references useful in devising proper patient management. Nurses and other health practitioners will find the format and scope of the *Guide to Diagnostic Tests* valuable for understanding the use of laboratory tests in patient management.

Acknowledgments

The editors acknowledge the invaluable editorial contributions of William M. Detmer, MD, and Tony M. Chou, MD, to the first through third editions, and Michael Pignone, MD, to the third through sixth editions of this book.

In addition, the late G. Thomas Evans, Jr., MD, contributed the electrocardiography section of Chapter 7 for the second and third editions. In the fourth, fifth, sixth, and this seventh edition, this section has been revised by Fred M. Kusumoto, MD.

We thank Jane Jang, BS, MT (ASCP) SM, for her revision of the microbiology chapter in the fifth edition. In the sixth and seventh editions, the chapter has been substantially revised by Barbara Haller, MD, PhD.

We thank our associate authors for their contributions to this book and are grateful to the many clinicians, residents, and students who have made useful suggestions. We welcome comments and recommendations from our readers for future editions.

Diana Nicoll, MD, PhD, MPA
Chuanyi Mark Lu, MD
Stephen J. McPhee, MD

Diagnostic Testing & Medical Decision Making

C. Diana Nicoll, MD, PhD, MPA, and Chuanyi Mark Lu, MD

The clinician's main task is to make reasoned decisions about patient care based on available clinical information and estimated clinical outcomes. Although data elicited from the history and physical examination may be sufficient for making a diagnosis or for guiding therapy, more information is often required. Today's clinicians rely increasingly on diagnostic tests and face challenges in selecting which tests to order and in interpreting test results. This chapter aims to help clinicians understand the utility as well as the limitations of diagnostic testing in clinical diagnosis and management.

BENEFITS, COSTS & RISKS

When used appropriately, diagnostic tests can be of great assistance to the clinician. Tests can be used for **screening**, ie, to identify risk factors for disease and to detect occult disease in asymptomatic persons. Identification of risk factors may allow early intervention to prevent disease occurrence, and early detection of occult disease may reduce disease morbidity and mortality through early treatment. Blood pressure measurement is recommended for preventive care of asymptomatic low risk adults. Screening for breast, cervix, colon, and lung cancer is also recommended, whereas screening for prostate cancer remains controversial. Screening without demonstrated benefits should be avoided. Optimal screening tests should meet the criteria listed in Table 1–1. Some screening test results (eg, rapid HIV Ab tests) require confirmatory testing.

Tests can be used for **diagnosis**, ie, to help establish or exclude the presence of disease in symptomatic persons. Some tests assist in early diagnosis after onset of symptoms and signs; others assist in developing a differential diagnosis; others help determine the stage or activity of disease.

Tests can also be used in **patient management**. They can help (1) evaluate the severity of disease, (2) estimate prognosis, (3) monitor the course of disease (progression, stability, or resolution), (4) detect disease recurrence, and (5) select drugs and adjust therapy.

One evolving field of medicine is personalized medicine, which involves tailoring treatment to the individual patient. A companion diagnostic test may be used to identify which patients could benefit from a drug and which patients would not benefit or even be harmed. As an example, only patients with breast cancer that shows overexpression of HER2 protein or extra copies of the *HER2* gene or both could benefit from trastuzumab treatment.

When ordering diagnostic tests, clinicians should weigh the potential benefits against the potential costs and adverse effects. Some tests carry a risk of morbidity or mortality—eg, cerebral angiogram leads to stroke in 0.5% of cases. The potential discomfort associated with tests such as colonoscopy may deter some patients from completing a diagnostic workup. The result of a diagnostic test may mandate additional testing or frequent follow-up, and the patient may incur significant cost, risk, and discomfort during follow-up procedures.

TABLE 1–1.   CRITERIA FOR USE OF SCREENING PROCEDURES.

Characteristics of Population
  1. Sufficiently high prevalence of disease.
  2. Likely to be compliant with subsequent tests and treatments.

Characteristics of Disease
  1. Significant morbidity and mortality.
  2. Effective and acceptable treatment available.
  3. Presymptomatic period detectable.
  4. Improved outcome from early treatment.

Characteristics of Test
  1. Good sensitivity and specificity.
  2. Low cost and risk.
  3. Confirmatory test available and practical.

Furthermore, a false-positive test may lead to incorrect diagnosis or further unnecessary testing. Classifying a healthy patient as diseased based on a falsely positive diagnostic test can cause psychological distress and may lead to risks from unnecessary or inappropriate therapy. A screening test may identify disease that would not otherwise have been recognized and that would not have affected the patient. For example, early-stage prostate cancer detected by prostate-specific antigen (PSA) screening in a 76-year-old man with known heart failure will probably not become symptomatic during his lifetime, and aggressive treatment may result in net harm.

The costs of diagnostic testing must also be understood and considered. Total costs may be high, patient out-of-pocket costs may be prohibitive, or cost-effectiveness may be unfavorable. Even relatively inexpensive tests may have poor cost-effectiveness if they produce very small health benefits. Factors adversely affecting cost-effectiveness include ordering a panel of tests when one test would suffice, ordering a test more frequently than necessary, ordering an inappropriate test, and ordering tests for medical record documentation only. The value-based, operative question for test ordering is, "Will the test result help establish a diagnosis, affect a treatment decision, or help predict a prognosis?" If the answer is "no," then the test is not justified. Unnecessary tests generate unnecessary labor, reagent and equipment costs, and lead to high health care expenditures.

Molecular and genetic testing is readily available, and genome-scale and high-throughput DNA sequencing technology is increasingly being applied in the clinical diagnostic realm. However, their cost-effectiveness and health outcome benefits need to be carefully examined. Diagnostic genetic testing based on symptoms (eg, testing for fragile X in a boy with mental retardation) differs from predictive genetic testing (eg, evaluating a healthy person with a family history of Huntington disease) and from predisposition genetic testing, which may indicate relative susceptibility to certain conditions or response to certain drug treatment (eg, *BRCA1/BRCA2* or *HER2* testing for breast cancer). The outcome benefits of many new pharmacogenetic tests have not yet been established by prospective clinical studies; eg, there is insufficient evidence that genotypic testing for warfarin dosing leads to outcomes that are superior to those using conventional dosing algorithms, in terms of reduction of out-of-range INRs. Other testing (eg, testing for inherited causes of thrombophilia, such as factor V Leiden, prothrombin gene mutation, etc) has only limited value for treating patients, since knowing whether a patient has inherited thrombophilia generally does not change the intensity or duration of anticoagulation treatment. Carrier testing (eg, for cystic fibrosis) and prenatal fetal testing (eg, for Down syndrome) often requires counseling of patients so that there is adequate understanding of the clinical, social, ethical, and sometimes legal impact of the results.

Clinicians order and interpret large numbers of laboratory tests every day, and the complexity of these tests continues to increase. The large and growing test menu and the inconsistencies in nomenclature for many tests have introduced significant challenges for clinicians, eg, selecting the correct laboratory test and correctly interpreting the test results. Errors in test selection and test results interpretation are common and could impact patient safety but are often difficult to detect. Using evidence-based testing algorithms that provide guidance for test selection in specific disorders and expert-driven test interpretation (eg, reports and interpretative comments generated by clinical pathologists) can help decrease such errors. Consultation and collaboration with laboratory professionals (ie, pathologists, medical technologists) can also help improve the timeliness of diagnostic testing and optimize laboratory test utilization.

PERFORMANCE OF DIAGNOSTIC TESTS

Factors affecting both the patient and the specimen are important. The most crucial element in a properly conducted laboratory test is an appropriate specimen.

Patient Preparation

Preparation of the patient is important for certain tests—eg, a fasting state is needed for optimal glucose and triglyceride measurements; posture and sodium intake should be strictly controlled when measuring renin and aldosterone levels; and strenuous exercise should be avoided before taking samples for creatine kinase determinations, since vigorous muscle activity can lead to falsely abnormal results.

Specimen Collection

Careful attention must be paid to patient identification and specimen labeling—eg, two patient identifiers (name and birth date, or name and unique institutional identifier) must be used. Knowing when the specimen was collected may be important. Correct timing is particularly important in therapeutic drug monitoring. For instance, aminoglycoside levels cannot be interpreted appropriately without knowing whether the specimen was drawn just before ("trough" level) or after ("peak" level) drug administration. Drug levels cannot be interpreted if they are drawn during the drug's distribution phase (eg, digoxin levels drawn during the first 6 hours after an oral dose). Substances that have a circadian variation (eg, cortisol) can be interpreted only in the context of the time of day the sample was drawn.

During specimen collection, certain principles should be remembered. Standard blood collection devices and appropriate vacuum tubes (ie, those containing appropriate anticoagulant or gel separator or both for serum or plasma preparation) should be used. Specimens should not be drawn above an intravenous line because this may contaminate the sample with intravenous fluid and drug (eg, heparin). Excessive tourniquet time leads to hemoconcentration and an increased concentration of protein-bound substances such as calcium. Lysis of cells during collection of a blood specimen results in spuriously increased serum levels of substances concentrated in cells (eg, lactate dehydrogenase and potassium). Certain test specimens may require special handling or storage (eg, specimens for blood gas and serum cryoglobulin). Delay in delivery of specimens to the laboratory can result in ongoing cellular metabolism and therefore spurious results for some studies (eg, low serum glucose). Pre-analytical errors have been reported to account for 75% of testing errors, and they can be costly.

There is growing interest in point-of-care testing, for which specimen collection and handling are equally important. Point-of-care testing involves extensive training and competency evaluation of those at the site of care delivery (eg, emergency department, intensive care unit staff). The unit cost per test is large, through loss of economy of scale offered by automation, but there are potential benefits to patient care because of rapid delivery of results and also potential reduction of other facility costs.

TABLE 1–2. PROPERTIES OF USEFUL DIAGNOSTIC TESTS.

1. Test methodology has been described in detail so that it can be accurately and reliably reproduced.
2. Test accuracy and precision have been determined.
3. The reference interval has been established appropriately.
4. Sensitivity and specificity have been reliably established by comparison with a gold standard. The evaluation has used a range of patients, including those who have different but commonly confused disorders and those with a spectrum of mild and severe, treated and untreated disease. The patient selection process has been adequately described so that results will not be generalized inappropriately.
5. Independent contribution to overall performance of a test panel has been confirmed if a test is advocated as part of a panel of tests.

TEST CHARACTERISTICS

Table 1–2 lists the general characteristics of useful diagnostic tests. Most of the principles detailed in this section can be applied not only to laboratory and radiologic tests but also to elements of the history and physical examination. An understanding of these characteristics is very helpful to the clinician when ordering and interpreting diagnostic tests.

Accuracy

The accuracy of a laboratory test is its correspondence with the true value. A test is deemed inaccurate when the result differs from the true value even though the results may be reproducible (Figure 1–1A), also called systematic error (or bias). For example, serum creatinine is commonly measured by a kinetic Jaffe method, which has a systematic error as large as 0.23 mg/dL (20.33 mcmol/L) when compared with the gold standard gas chromatography-isotope dilution mass spectrometry method. In the clinical laboratory, accuracy of tests is maximized by calibrating laboratory equipment with standard reference material and by participation in external proficiency testing programs (eg, proficiency testing program offered by the College of American Pathologists).

Precision

Test precision is a measure of a test's reproducibility when repeated on the same sample. If the same specimen is analyzed many times, some variation in results (random error) is expected; this variability is expressed as a coefficient of variation (CV: the standard deviation divided by the mean, often expressed as a percentage). For example, when the laboratory reports a CV of 5% for serum creatinine and accepts results within ± 2 standard deviations, it denotes that, for a sample with serum creatinine of 1.0 mg/dL (88.4 mcmol/L),

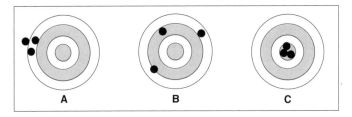

Figure 1–1. Relationship between accuracy and precision in diagnostic tests. The center of the target represents the true value of the substance being tested. **A:** A diagnostic test that is precise but inaccurate; repeated measurements yield very similar results, but all results are far from the true value. **B:** A test that is imprecise and inaccurate; repeated measurements yield widely different results, and the results are far from the true value. **C:** An ideal test that is both precise and accurate.

the laboratory may report the result as anywhere from 0.90 (79.56 mcmol/L) to 1.10 mg/dL (97.24 mcmol/L) on repeated measurements from the same sample.

An imprecise test is one that yields widely varying results on repeated measurements (Figure 1–1B). The precision of diagnostic tests, which is monitored in clinical laboratories by using quality control material, must be good enough to distinguish clinically relevant changes in a patient's status from the analytic variability (imprecision) of the test. For instance, the manual peripheral blood white blood cell differential count may not be precise enough to detect important changes in the distribution of cell types, because it is calculated by subjective evaluation of a small sample (eg, 100 cells). Repeated measurements by different technologists on the same sample result in widely differing results. Automated differential counts are more precise because they are obtained from machines that use objective physical characteristics to classify a much larger sample (eg, 10,000 cells).

An ideal test is both precise and accurate (Figure 1–1C).

Sigma Metrics

The Sigma metric is used to measure the overall quality of a laboratory test. A single numeric value that is calculated based on three traditional elements used to evaluate test performance: accuracy (bias), precision (CV), and allowable total error (TEa) (or tolerance limit of a test), the Sigma metric = (TEa – Bias)/CV (with all values expressed as percents). On a scale of 0 to 6, a higher Sigma metric value means fewer analytical errors, ie, fewer questionable test results are accepted and reported and fewer acceptable test results are falsely rejected and not reported. A Sigma metric of 6 for a test indicates that it can be considered "world class," meaning more than 99% of test results are error free. On the other hand, a test with a Sigma metric of 3 or less is generally considered unreliable and should not be used.

Reference Interval

Some diagnostic tests are reported as positive or negative, but most are reported quantitatively. Use of reference intervals is a technique for interpreting quantitative results. Reference intervals are often method- and laboratory-specific. In practice, they often represent test results found in 95% of a small population presumed to be healthy; by definition, then, 5% of healthy patients will have an abnormal test result (Figure 1–2). Slightly abnormal results should be interpreted critically—they may be either truly abnormal or falsely abnormal.

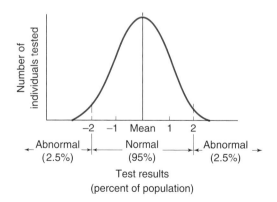

Figure 1–2. The reference interval is usually defined as within 2 SD of the mean test result (shown as –2 and 2) in a small population of healthy volunteers. Note that in this example, test results are normally distributed; however, many biologic substances have distributions that are skewed.

TABLE 1–3. RELATIONSHIP BETWEEN THE NUMBER OF TESTS AND THE PROBABILITY THAT A HEALTHY PERSON WILL HAVE ONE OR MORE ABNORMAL RESULTS.

Number of Tests	Probability That One or More Results Will Be Abnormal
1	5%
6	26%
12	46%
20	64%

Statistically, the probability that a healthy person will have 2 separate test results within the reference interval is $0.95 \times 0.95 = 0.9025$, or 90.25%; for 5 separate tests, it is 77.4%; for 10 tests, 59.9%; and for 20 tests, 35.8%. The larger the number of tests ordered, the greater the probability that one or more of the test results will fall outside the reference interval (Table 1–3). Conversely, values within the reference interval may not rule out the actual presence of disease since the reference interval does not establish the distribution of results in patients with disease. As such, reference intervals must be used within the context of medical knowledge about the disorder in question.

It is important to consider also whether published reference intervals are appropriate for the particular patient being evaluated, since some intervals depend on age, sex, weight, diet, time of day, activity status, posture, or even season. Biologic variability occurs among individuals as well as within the same individual. For instance, serum estrogen levels in women vary from day to day depending on the menstrual cycle; serum cortisol shows diurnal variation, being highest in the morning and decreasing later in the day; and vitamin D shows seasonal variation with lower values in winter.

Chapter 3 contains the reference intervals for commonly used chemistry and hematology tests. Test performance characteristics such as sensitivity and specificity are needed to interpret results and are discussed below.

Interfering Factors

The results of diagnostic tests can be altered by external factors, such as ingestion of drugs and use of contrast media, and internal factors, such as abnormal physiologic states. These factors contribute to the biologic variability and must be considered in the interpretation of test results.

External interferences can affect test results in vivo or in vitro. In vivo, alcohol increases gamma-glutamyl transpeptidase, and diuretics can affect sodium and potassium concentrations. Cigarette smoking can induce hepatic enzymes and thus reduce levels of substances such as theophylline that are metabolized by the liver. In vitro, cephalosporins may produce spurious serum creatinine levels due to interference with a common laboratory method of analysis.

Internal interferences result from abnormal physiologic states interfering with the test measurement. For example, patients with gross lipemia may have spuriously low serum sodium levels if the test methodology includes a step in which serum is diluted before sodium is measured, and patients with endogenous antibodies (eg, human anti-mouse antibodies) may have falsely high or low results in automated immunoassays for various analytes. Therapeutic monoclonal antibodies (eg, daratumumab) can interfere with blood bank testing (eg, indirect antiglobulin test) and impact the interpretation of serum protein electrophoresis. Because of the potential for test interference, clinicians should be wary of unexpected test results and should investigate reasons other than disease that may explain abnormal results, including pre-analytical and analytical laboratory error.

Sensitivity & Specificity

Clinicians should use measures of test performance such as sensitivity and specificity to judge the quality of a diagnostic test for a particular disease.

Test **sensitivity** is the ability of a test to detect disease and is expressed as the percentage of patients with disease in whom the test is positive. Thus, a test that is 90% sensitive gives positive results in 90% of diseased patients and negative results in 10% of diseased patients (false negatives). Generally, a test with high sensitivity is useful to exclude a diagnosis because a highly sensitive test renders few results that are falsely negative. To exclude infection with the virus that causes AIDS, for instance, a clinician might choose a highly sensitive test, such as the HIV p24 antigen and HIV antibody combination test.

A test's **specificity** is the ability to detect absence of disease and is expressed as the percentage of patients without disease in whom the test is negative. Thus, a test that is 90% specific gives negative results in 90% of patients without disease and positive results in 10% of patients without disease (false positives). A test with high specificity is useful to confirm a diagnosis, because a highly specific test has few results that are falsely positive. For instance, to make the diagnosis of gouty arthritis, a clinician might choose a highly specific test, such as the presence of negatively birefringent needle-shaped urate crystals on microscopic evaluation of joint fluid.

To determine test sensitivity and specificity for a particular disease, the test must be compared against an independent "gold standard" test or established standard diagnostic criteria that define the true disease state of the patient. For instance, the sensitivity and specificity of rapid antigen detection testing in diagnosing group A beta-hemolytic streptococcal pharyngitis are obtained by comparing the results of rapid antigen testing with the gold standard test, throat swab culture. Application of the gold standard test to patients with positive rapid antigen testing establishes specificity. Failure to apply the gold standard test following negative rapid tests may result in an overestimation of sensitivity, since false negatives will not be identified. However, for many disease states (eg, pancreatitis), an independent gold standard test either does not exist or is very difficult or expensive to apply—and in such cases reliable estimates of test sensitivity and specificity are sometimes difficult to obtain.

Sensitivity and specificity can also be affected by the population from which these values are derived. For instance, many diagnostic tests are evaluated first using patients who have severe disease and control groups who are young and well. Compared with the general population, this study group will have more results that are truly positive (because patients have more advanced disease) and more results that are truly negative (because the control group is healthy). Thus, test sensitivity and specificity will be higher than would be expected in the general population, where more of a spectrum of health and disease is found. Clinicians should be aware of this **spectrum bias** when generalizing published test results to their own practice. To minimize spectrum bias, the control group should include individuals who have diseases related to the disease in question, but who lack this principal disease. For example, to establish the sensitivity and specificity of the anti-cyclic citrullinated peptide test for rheumatoid arthritis, the control group should include patients with rheumatic diseases other than rheumatoid arthritis. Other biases, including spectrum composition, population recruitment, absent or inappropriate reference standard, and verification bias, should also be considered in certain situations, where critical appraisal of published articles may be necessary.

It is important to remember that the reported sensitivity and specificity of a test depend on the analyte level (threshold) used to distinguish a normal from an abnormal test result. If the threshold is lowered, sensitivity is increased at the expense of decreased specificity. If the threshold is raised, sensitivity is decreased while specificity is increased (Figure 1–3).

Figure 1–4 shows how test sensitivity and specificity can be calculated using test results from patients previously classified by the gold standard test as diseased or nondiseased.

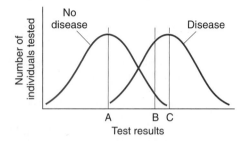

Figure 1–3. Hypothetical distribution of test results for healthy and diseased individuals. The position of the "cutoff point" between "normal" and "abnormal" (or "negative" and "positive") test results determines the test's sensitivity and specificity. If point A is the cutoff point, the test would have 100% sensitivity but low specificity. If point C is the cutoff point, the test would have 100% specificity but low sensitivity. For many tests, the cutoff point is determined by the reference interval, ie, the range of test results that is within 2 SD of the mean of test results for healthy No disease individuals (point B). In some situations, the cutoff is altered to enhance either sensitivity or specificity.

The performance of two different tests can be compared by plotting the receiver operator characteristic (ROC) curves at various reference interval cutoff values. The resulting curve for each test, obtained by plotting the sensitivity against (1–specificity), often shows which test is more accurate; a clearly superior test will have an ROC curve that always lies above and to the left of the inferior test curve, and, in general, the better test will have a

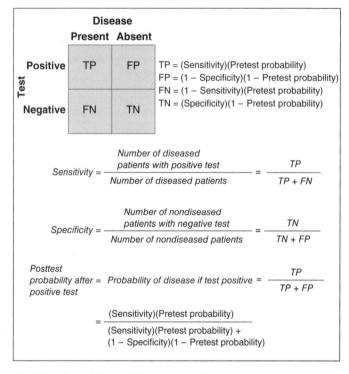

Figure 1–4. Calculation of sensitivity, specificity, and probability of disease after a positive test (posttest probability). TP, true positive; FP, false positive; FN, false negative; TN, true negative.

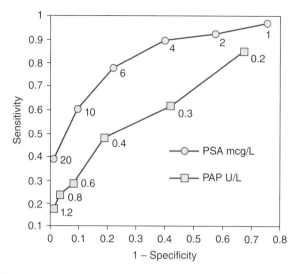

Figure 1–5. Receiver operator characteristic (ROC) curves for prostate-specific antigen (PSA) and prostatic acid phosphatase (PAP) in the diagnosis of prostate cancer. For all cutoff values, PSA has higher sensitivity and specificity; therefore, it is a better test based on these performance characteristics. (*Modified and reproduced with permission from Nicoll D et al. Routine acid phosphatase testing for screening and monitoring prostate cancer no longer justified. Clin Chem. 1993 Dec;39(12):2540–1.*)

larger area under the ROC curve. For instance, Figure 1–5 shows the ROC curves for PSA and prostatic acid phosphatase in the diagnosis of prostate cancer. PSA is a superior test because it has higher sensitivity and specificity for all cutoff values.

Note that, for a given test, the ROC curve also allows one to identify the cut-off value that minimizes both false-positive and false-negative results, which is located at the point closest to the upper-left corner of the curve. The optimal clinical cut-off value, however, depends on the condition being detected and the relative importance of false-positive versus false-negative results.

USE OF TESTS IN DIAGNOSIS & MANAGEMENT

The usefulness of a test in a particular clinical situation depends not only on the test's characteristics (eg, sensitivity and specificity, which are not predictive measures) but also on the probability that the patient has the disease before the test result is known (pretest probability). The results of a useful test substantially change the probability that the patient has the disease (posttest probability). Figure 1–4 shows how posttest probability can be calculated from the known sensitivity and specificity of the test and the estimated pretest probability of disease (or disease prevalence), based on Bayes theorem.

The pretest probability, or prevalence, of disease has a profound effect on the posttest probability of disease. As demonstrated in Table 1–4, when a test with 90% sensitivity and specificity is used, the posttest probability can vary from 8% to 99% depending on the pretest probability of disease. Furthermore, as the pretest probability of disease decreases, it becomes more likely that a positive test result represents a false positive.

As an example, suppose the clinician wishes to calculate the posttest probability of prostate cancer using the PSA test and a cutoff value of 4 ng/mL (4 mcg/L). Using the data shown in Figure 1–5, sensitivity is 90% and specificity is 60%. The clinician estimates the pretest probability of disease given all the evidence and then calculates the posttest probability using the approach shown in Figure 1–4. The pretest probability that an otherwise

TABLE 1–4. INFLUENCE OF PRETEST PROBABILITY ON
THE POSTTEST PROBABILITY OF DISEASE WHEN A TEST
WITH 90% SENSITIVITY AND 90% SPECIFICITY IS USED.

Pretest Probability	Posttest Probability
0.01	0.08
0.50	0.90
0.99	0.999

healthy 50-year-old man has prostate cancer is equal to the prevalence of prostate cancer in that age group (probability = 10%) and the posttest probability after a positive test is only 20%. Even though the test is positive, there is still an 80% chance that the patient does not have prostate cancer (Figure 1–6A). If the clinician finds a prostate nodule on rectal examination, the pretest probability of prostate cancer rises to 50% and the posttest probability using the same test is 69% (Figure 1–6B). Finally, if the clinician estimates the pretest probability to be 98% based on a prostate nodule, bone pain, and lytic lesions on spine radiographs, the posttest probability using PSA is 99% (Figure 1–6C). This example illustrates that pretest probability has a profound effect on posttest probability and that tests provide more information when the diagnosis is truly uncertain (pretest probability about 50%) than when the diagnosis is either unlikely or nearly certain.

ODDS-LIKELIHOOD RATIOS

Another way to calculate the posttest probability of disease is to use the odds-likelihood (or odds-probability) approach. Sensitivity and specificity are combined into one entity called the **likelihood** ratio (LR):

$$LR = \frac{\text{Probability of result in diseased persons}}{\text{Probability of result in nondiseased persons}}$$

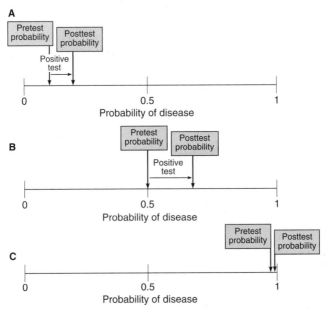

Figure 1–6. Effect of pretest probability and test sensitivity and specificity on the posttest probability of disease. (See text for explanation.)

When test results are dichotomized, every test has two likelihood ratios, one corresponding to a positive test (LR^+) and one corresponding to a negative test (LR^-):

$$LR^+ = \frac{\text{Probability that test is positive in diseased persons}}{\text{Probability that test is positive in nondiseased persons}}$$

$$= \frac{\text{Sensitivity}}{1 - \text{Specificity}}$$

$$LR^- = \frac{\text{Probability that test is negative in diseased persons}}{\text{Probability that test is negative in nondiseased persons}}$$

$$= \frac{1 - \text{Sensitivity}}{\text{Specificity}}$$

For continuous measures, multiple likelihood ratios can be defined to correspond to ranges or intervals of test results. (See Table 1–5 for an example.)

Likelihood ratios can be calculated using the above formulas. They can also be found in some textbooks, journal articles, and online programs (see Table 1–6 for sample values). Likelihood ratios provide an estimation of whether there will be significant change in pretest to posttest probability of a disease given the test result, and thus can be used to make quick estimates of the usefulness of contemplated diagnostic tests in particular situations. A likelihood ratio of 1 implies that there will be no difference between pretest and posttest probabilities. Likelihood ratios of > 10 or < 0.1 indicate large, often clinically significant differences. Likelihood ratios between 1 and 2 and between 0.5 and 1 indicate small differences (rarely clinically significant).

TABLE 1–5. LIKELIHOOD RATIOS OF SERUM FERRITIN IN THE DIAGNOSIS OF IRON DEFICIENCY ANEMIA.

Serum Ferritin (mcg/L)	Likelihood Ratios for Iron Deficiency Anemia
≥ 100	0.08
45–99	0.54
35–44	1.83
25–34	2.54
15–24	8.83
≤ 15	51.85

Data from Guyatt G et al. Laboratory diagnosis of iron deficiency anemia. J Gen Intern Med. 1992 Mar–Apr;7(2):145–53.

TABLE 1–6. EXAMPLES OF LIKELIHOOD RATIOS (LR).

Target Disease	Test	LR⁺	LR⁻
Abscess	Abdominal CT scanning	9.5	0.06
Coronary artery disease	Exercise electrocardiogram (1 mm depression)	3.5	0.45
Lung cancer	Chest radiograph	15	0.42
Left ventricular hypertrophy	Echocardiography	18.4	0.08
Myocardial infarction	Troponin I	24	0.01
Prostate cancer	Digital rectal examination	21.3	0.37

The simplest method for calculating posttest probability from pretest probability and likelihood ratios is to use a nomogram (Figure 1–7). The clinician places a straightedge through the points that represent the pretest probability and the likelihood ratio and then reads the posttest probability where the straightedge crosses the posttest probability line.

A more formal way of calculating posttest probabilities uses the likelihood ratio as follows:

$$\text{Pretest odds} \times \text{Likelihood ratio} = \text{Posttest odds}$$

To use this formulation, probabilities must be converted to odds, where the odds of having a disease are expressed as the chance of having the disease divided by the chance of not having the disease. For instance, a probability of 0.75 is the same as 3:1 odds (Figure 1–8).

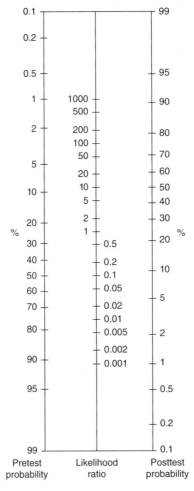

Figure 1–7. Nomogram for determining posttest probability from pretest probability and likelihood ratios. To figure the posttest probability, place a straightedge between the pretest probability and the likelihood ratio for the particular test. The posttest probability will be where the straightedge crosses the posttest probability line. (*Adapted and reproduced, with permission, from Fagan TJ. Nomogram for Bayes theorem.* [*Letter.*] N Engl J Med. *1975 Jul 31;293(5):257.*)

$$\textbf{Odds} = \frac{\textbf{Probability}}{\textbf{1 - Probability}}$$

Example: If probability = 0.75, then

$$\text{Odds} = \frac{0.75}{1-0.75} = \frac{0.75}{0.25} = \frac{3}{1} = 3{:}1$$

$$\textbf{Probability} = \frac{\textbf{Odds}}{\textbf{Odds + 1}}$$

Example: If odds = 3:1, then

$$\text{Probability} = \frac{3/1}{3/1+1} = \frac{3}{3+1} = 0.75$$

Figure 1–8. Formulas for converting between probability and odds.

To estimate the potential benefit of a diagnostic test, the clinician first estimates the pretest odds of disease given all available clinical information and then multiplies the pretest odds by the positive and negative likelihood ratios. The results are the **posttest odds**, or the odds that the patient has the disease if the test is positive or negative. To obtain the posttest probability, the odds are converted to a probability (Figure 1–8).

For example, if the clinician believes that the patient has a 60% chance of having a myocardial infarction (pretest odds of 3:2) and the troponin I test is positive ($LR^+ = 24$), then the posttest odds of having a myocardial infarction are

$$\frac{3}{2} \times 24 = \frac{72}{2} \text{ or } 36{:}1 \text{ odds} \left(\frac{36/1}{(36/1)+1} = \frac{36}{37} = 97\% \text{ probability} \right)$$

If the troponin I test is negative ($LR^- = 0.01$), then the posttest odds of having a myocardial infarction are

$$\frac{3}{2} \times 0.01 = \frac{0.03}{2} \text{ or } 0.015{:}1 \text{ odds} \left(\frac{0.015/1}{(0.015/1)+1} = \frac{0.015}{1.015} = 1.5\% \text{ probability} \right)$$

Sequential Testing

To this point, the impact of only one test on the probability of disease has been discussed, whereas during most diagnostic workups, clinicians obtain clinical information in a sequential fashion. To calculate the posttest odds after three tests, for example, the clinician might estimate the pretest odds and use the appropriate likelihood ratio for each test:

$$\text{Pretest odds} \times LR_1 \times LR_2 \times LR_3 = \text{Posttest odds}$$

When using this approach, however, the clinician should be aware of a major assumption: the chosen tests or findings must be **conditionally independent**. For instance, with liver cell damage, the aspartate aminotransferase (AST) and alanine aminotransferase (ALT) enzymes may be released by the same process and are thus not conditionally independent. If conditionally dependent tests are used in this sequential approach, an inaccurate posttest probability will result.

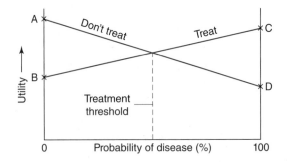

Figure 1–9. The "treat/don't treat" threshold. **A:** Patient does not have disease and is not treated (highest utility). **B:** Patient does not have disease and is treated (lower utility than A). **C:** Patient has disease and is treated (lower utility than A). **D:** Patient has disease and is not treated (lower utility than C).

Threshold Approach to Decision Making

A key aspect of medical decision making is the selection of a treatment threshold, ie, the probability of disease at which treatment is indicated. The treatment threshold is determined by the relative consequences of different actions: treating when the disease is present; not treating when the disease is absent; treating when the disease is actually absent; or failing to treat when the disease is actually present. Figure 1–9 shows a possible way of identifying a treatment threshold by considering the value (utility) of these four possible outcomes.

Use of a diagnostic test is warranted when its result could shift the probability of disease across the treatment threshold. For example, a clinician might decide to treat with antibiotics if the probability of streptococcal pharyngitis in a patient with a sore throat is > 25% (Figure 1–10A).

If, after reviewing evidence from the history and physical examination, the clinician estimates the pretest probability of strep throat to be 15%, then a diagnostic test such as throat culture ($LR^+ = 7$) would be useful only if a positive test would shift the posttest probability above 25%. Use of the nomogram shown in Figure 1–7 indicates that the posttest probability would be 55% (Figure 1–10B); thus, ordering the test would be justified since it affects patient management. On the other hand, if the history and physical examination had suggested that the pretest probability of strep throat was 60%, the throat culture ($LR^- = 0.33$) would be indicated only if a negative test would lower the posttest probability below 25%. Using the same nomogram, the posttest probability after a negative test would be 33% (Figure 1–10C). Therefore, ordering the throat culture would not be justified because it does not affect patient management.

This approach to decision making is now being applied in the clinical literature.

Decision Analysis

Up to this point, the discussion of diagnostic testing has focused on test characteristics and methods for using these characteristics to calculate the probability of disease in different clinical situations. Although useful, these methods are limited because they do not incorporate the many outcomes that may occur in clinical medicine or the values that patients and clinicians place on those outcomes. To incorporate outcomes and values with characteristics of tests, decision analysis can be used. Decision analysis is a quantitative evaluation of the outcomes that result from a set of choices in a specific clinical situation. Although it is infrequently used in routine clinical practice, the decision analysis approach can be helpful to address questions relating to clinical decisions that cannot easily be answered through clinical trials.

The basic idea of decision analysis is to model the options in a medical decision, assign probabilities to the alternative actions, assign values (utilities) (eg, survival rates,

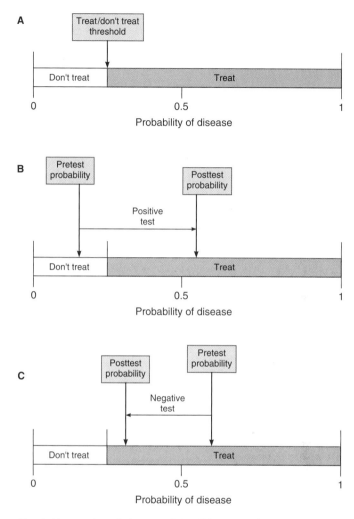

Figure 1–10. Threshold approach applied to test ordering. If the contemplated test will not change patient management (as in scenario C), the test should not be ordered. (See text for explanation.)

quality-adjusted life years, or costs) to the various outcomes, and then calculate which decision gives the greatest expected value (expected utility). To complete a decision analysis, the clinician would proceed as follows:

(1) Draw a decision tree showing the elements of the medical decision;
(2) Assign probabilities to the various branches;
(3) Assign values (utilities) to the outcomes;
(4) Determine the expected value (expected utility) (the product of probability and value [utility]) of each branch;
(5) Select the decision with the highest expected value (expected utility).

The results obtained from a decision analysis depend on the accuracy of the data used to estimate the probabilities and values of outcomes.

Figure 1–11 shows a decision tree in which the decision to be made is whether to treat without testing, perform a test and then treat based on the test result, or perform no tests and give no treatment. The clinician begins the analysis by building a decision tree showing the important elements of the decision. Once the tree is built, the clinician assigns probabilities to all the branches. In this case, all the branch probabilities can be calculated from: (1) the probability of disease before the test (pretest probability), (2) the chance of a positive test result if the disease is present (sensitivity), and (3) the chance of a negative test result if the disease is absent (specificity). Next, the clinician assigns value (utility) to each of the outcomes.

After the expected value (expected utility) is calculated for each branch of the decision tree, by multiplying the value (utility) of the outcome by the probability of the outcome, the clinician can identify the alternative with the highest expected value (expected utility). When costs are included, it is possible to determine the cost per unit of health gained for one approach compared with an alternative (cost-effectiveness analysis). This information can help evaluate the efficiency of different testing or treatment strategies.

Although time-consuming, decision analysis can help structure complex clinical problems, assist in difficult clinical decision-making, and improve the quality of clinical decisions.

Evidence-Based Medicine

Vast resources are being spent on diagnostic testing. New laboratory tests are being developed and marketed all the time. Clinicians need to know how to appraise published studies on new diagnostic tests (eg, performance characteristics) and how to determine whether

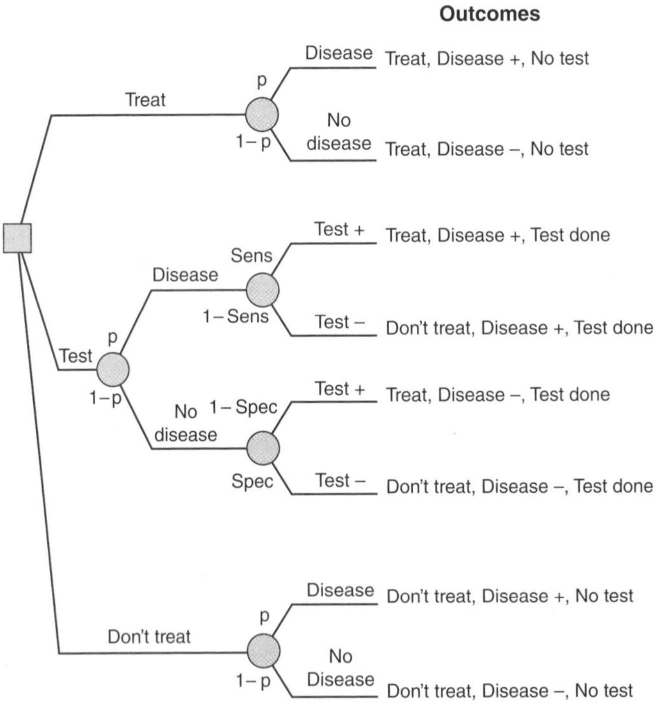

Figure 1–11. Generic tree for a clinical decision where the choices are: (1) to treat the patient empirically, (2) to do the test and then treat only if the test is positive, or (3) to withhold therapy. The square node is called a decision node, and the circular nodes are called chance nodes. p, pretest probability of disease; Sens, sensitivity; Spec, specificity.

a new test is superior to existing test(s) in terms of clinical utility and cost-effectiveness. Careful examination of the best available evidence is essential.

Evidence-based medicine is the care of patients using the best available research evidence to guide clinical decision making. It relies on the identification of methodologically sound evidence, critical appraisal of research studies for both internal validity (freedom from bias) and external validity (applicability and generalizability), and the dissemination of accurate and useful summaries of evidence to inform clinical decision making. Systematic reviews can be used to summarize evidence for dissemination, as can evidence-based synopses of current research. Systematic reviews often use meta-analysis: statistical techniques to combine evidence from different studies to produce a more precise estimate of the effect of an intervention or the accuracy of a test. The concept of evidence-based medicine can be readily applied to diagnostic testing, since appropriate use of a diagnostic test is part of the decision-making process.

The *Choosing Wisely* campaign, launched by the American Board of Internal Medicine in 2012, encourages clinicians and their patients to examine the usefulness of certain laboratory tests and medical procedures, and promotes choosing care that is necessary, evidence-based, and not harmful. More than 50 specialty societies have joined the campaign, and identified tests and procedures commonly used in their respective field that either are considered unnecessary or that should be questioned. Those unnecessary tests and procedures are available online at the *Choosing Wisely* website (www.choosingwisely.org).

Clinical practice guidelines are systematically developed statements intended to assist practitioners in making decisions about health care. Clinical algorithms and practice guidelines are now ubiquitous in medicine, developed by various professional societies or independent expert panels. Diagnostic testing is an integral part of such algorithms and guidelines. Their utility and validity depend on the quality of the evidence that shaped the recommendations, on their being kept current, and on their acceptance and appropriate application by clinicians. Although some clinicians are concerned about the effect of guidelines on professional autonomy and individual decision making, many organizations are trying to use compliance with practice guidelines as a measure of quality of care. It is important to note, however, that evidence-based guidelines are used to complement, not replace, clinical judgment tailored to individual patients. Furthermore, personalized treatment (ie, using advanced diagnostic or prognostic tools and incorporating patient preferences to guide an individual patient's treatment) is increasingly recommended as part of practice guidelines. The approach is in keeping with the rapidly evolving field of personalized medicine, in which diagnostic testing plays an important role in selecting the best possible therapies that are tailored to the individual characteristics of each patient.

Computerized and mobile information technologies provide clinicians with information from laboratory, imaging, physiologic monitoring systems, and many other sources. Computerized clinical decision support systems, along with test order communication systems, have been increasingly used to develop, implement, and refine computerized protocols for specific processes of care derived from evidence-based practice guidelines. It is important that clinicians use modern information technology to deliver standard medical care in their practice.

REFERENCES

Benefits, Costs, and Risks

Chiolero A et al. How to prevent overdiagnosis. Swiss Med Wkly. 2015;145:w14060. [PMID: 25612105]

Cuzick J et al. Prevention and early detection of prostate cancer. Lancet Oncol. 2014;15:e484. [PMID: 25281467]

Horvath AR. From evidence to best practice in laboratory medicine. Clin Biochem Rev. 2013;34:47. [PMID: 24151341]

Kimmel SE et al; COAG Investigators. A pharmacogenetic versus a clinical algorithm for warfarin dosing. N Engl J Med. 2013;369:2283. [PMID: 24251361]

Klarkowski D et al. Causes of false positive HIV rapid diagnostic test results. Expert Rev Anti Infect Ther. 2014;12:49. [PMID: 24404993]

Kobewka DM et al. Influence of educational, audit and feedback, system based, and incentive and penalty interventions to reduce laboratory test utilization: a systematic review. Clin Chem Lab Med. 2015;53:157. [PMID: 25263310]

Nanavaty P et al. Lung cancer screening: advantages, controversies, and applications. Cancer Control. 2014;21:9. [PMID: 24357736]

Pace LE et al. A systematic assessment of benefits and risks to guide breast cancer screening decisions. JAMA. 2014;311:1327. [PMID: 24691608]

Siebert U et al. When is enough evidence enough? Using systematic decision analysis and value of information analysis to determine the need for further evidence. Z Evid Fortbild Qual Gesundhwes. 2013;107:575. [PMID: 24315327]

Siontis KC et al. Diagnostic tests often fail to lead to changes in patient outcomes. J Clin Epidemiol. 2014;67:612. [PMID: 24679598]

Smith RA et al. Cancer screening in the United States, 2015: a review of current American cancer society guidelines and current issues in cancer screening. CA Cancer J Clin. 2015;65:30. [PMID: 25581023]

Yoo C et al. Companion diagnostics for the targeted therapy of gastric cancer. World J Gastroenterol. 2015;21:10948. [PMID: 26494953]

Zhi M et al. The landscape of inappropriate laboratory testing: a 15-year meta-analysis. PLoS One. 2013;8:e78962. [PMID: 24260139]

Performance of Diagnostic Tests

Baird G. Preanalytical considerations in blood gas analysis. Biochem Med (Zagreb). 2013;23:19. [PMID: 23457763]

Bowen RA et al. Interferences from blood collection tube components on clinical chemistry assays. Biochem Med (Zagreb). 2014;24:31. [PMID: 24627713]

Green SF. The cost of poor blood specimen quality and errors in preanalytical processes. Clin Biochem. 2013;46:1175. [PMID: 23769816]

Larsson A et al. The state of point-of-care testing: a European perspective. Ups J Med Sci. 2015;120:1. [PMID: 25622619]

Naugler C et al. Break the fast? Update on patient preparation for cholesterol testing. Can Fam Physician. 2014;60(10):895–7, e471–4. [PMID: 25316740]

Sanchis-Gomar F et al. Physical activity—an important preanalytical variable. Biochem Med (Zagreb). 2014;24(1):6–79. [PMID: 24627716]

Test Characteristics

Dalenberg DA et al. Analytical performance specifications: relating laboratory performance to quality required for intended clinical use. Clin Lab Med. 2013;33:55. [PMID: 23331729]

Hens K et al. Sigma metrics used to assess analytical quality of clinical chemistry assays: importance of the allowable total error (TEa) target. Clin Chem Lab Med. 2014;52:973. [PMID: 24615486]

Lakos G. Interference in antiphospholipid antibody assays. Semin Thromb Hemost. 2012;38:353. [PMID: 22618529]

Lippi G et al. Interference of medical contrast media on laboratory testing. Biochem Med (Zagreb). 2014;24:80. [PMID: 24627717]

Wacker C et al. Procalcitonin as a diagnostic marker for sepsis: a systematic review and meta-analysis. Lancet Infect Dis. 2013;13:426. [PMID: 23375419]

Wang Y et al. Meta-analysis: diagnostic accuracy of anti-cyclic citrullinated peptide antibody for juvenile idiopathic arthritis. J Immunol Res. 2015;2015:915276. [PMID: 25789331]

Whiting PF et al. A systematic review classifies sources of bias and variation in diagnostic test accuracy studies. J Clin Epidemiol. 2013;66:1093. [PMID: 23958378]

Use of Tests in Diagnosis & Management

Eusebi P. Diagnostic accuracy measures. Cerebrovasc Dis. 2013;36:267. [PMID: 24135733]

Leeflang MM et al. Variation of a test's sensitivity and specificity with disease prevalence. CMAJ. 2013;185:E537. [PMID: 23798453]

Roberts E et al; NICE Guideline Development Group for Acute Heart Failure. The diagnostic accuracy of the natriuretic peptides in heart failure: systematic review and diagnostic meta-analysis in the acute care setting. BMJ. 2015;350:h910. [PMID: 25740799]

Decision Analysis & Evidence Based Medicine

Bossuyt PM et al. Beyond diagnostic accuracy: the clinical utility of diagnostic tests. Clin Chem. 2012;58:1636. [PMID: 22730450]

Bright TJ et al. Effect of clinical decision-support systems: a systematic review. Ann Intern Med. 2012;157:29. [PMID: 22751758]

Cox CE et al. A universal decision support system. Addressing the decision-making needs of patients, families, and clinicians in the setting of critical illness. Am J Respir Crit Care Med. 2014;190:366. [PMID: 25019639]

Joaquim AF et al. Thoracolumbar spine trauma: evaluation and surgical decision-making. J Craniovertebr Junction Spine. 2013;4:3. [PMID: 24381449]

Linnet K et al. Quantifying the accuracy of a diagnostic test or marker. Clin Chem. 2012;58:1292. [PMID: 22829313]

Mickan S et al. Use of handheld computers in clinical practice: a systematic review. BMC Med Inform Decis Mak. 2014;14:56. [PMID: 24998515]

Rouster-Stevens KA et al. Choosing Wisely: the American College of Rheumatology's Top 5 for pediatric rheumatology. Arthritis Care Res (Hoboken). 2014;66:649. [PMID: 24756998]

Savel TG et al. PTT Advisor: a CDC-supported initiative to develop a mobile clinical laboratory decision support application for the iOS platform. Online J Public Health Inform. 2013;5:215. [PMID: 23923100]

Vikse J et al. The role of serum procalcitonin in the diagnosis of bacterial meningitis in adults: a systematic review and meta-analysis. Int J Infect Dis. 2015;38:68. [PMID: 26188130]

2

Point-of-Care Testing & Provider-Performed Microscopy

Chuanyi Mark Lu, MD, and Stephen J. McPhee, MD

This chapter presents information on specimen collection, common point-of-care (POC) tests and provider-performed microscopy (PPM), and other procedures.

POC testing is defined as medical testing at or near the site of patient care. POC tests are performed outside a central clinical laboratory using portable and hand-held devices and test kits or cartridges. PPM procedures are microscopic examinations performed by a healthcare provider during the course of a patient visit. PPM procedures typically involve specimens that are labile and not easily transportable, or for which delay in performing the test could compromise the accuracy of the test result.

POC testing is considered an integral part of clinical laboratory service and is under the direction of the central laboratory. Physician interpretation of PPM findings (eg, direct wet-mount preparation and KOH preparation) requires appropriate clinical privileges and competency assessments.

In the United States, test results can be used for patient care only when the tests are performed according to the requirements of the Clinical Laboratory Improvement Amendments of 1988 (CLIA'88). These include personnel training and competence assessment before any test or procedure can be performed, following standard operating procedures and/or manufacturer instructions, performance and documentation of quality control for all tests, and participation in a proficiency testing program, if available.

Contents

1. OBTAINING & HANDLING SPECIMENS

Specimens should be collected and handled according to the institution's policies and procedures.

A. Safety Considerations

General Safety Considerations

All patient specimens are potentially infectious and are regarded as biohazardous materials, so precautions should be universally observed. The Blood Borne Pathogens Standard, developed by the Occupational Safety and Health Administration (OSHA), identifies standard precautions and protective equipment needed for the handling of biohazardous material. The Joint Commission and OSHA require training on the prevention of occupational exposure to blood (and tuberculosis) as part of initial and annual training of potentially exposed medical personnel.

a. Universal body fluid and needle stick precautions must be observed at all times. Safety needle devices should be used.

b. Disposable medical gloves, gown, and, if appropriate, mask, goggle, and face shield must be worn when collecting specimens.

c. Gloves must be changed and hands washed after contact with each patient.

d. Care should be taken not to spill or splash blood or other body fluids. Any spills should be cleaned up with a freshly made 10% bleach solution.

Handling and Disposing of Needles and Gloves

a. Do not resheath needles.

b. Discard needles in a sharps container and gloves in a designated biohazard container.

c. Do not remove a used needle from a syringe by hand. The entire assembly should be discarded as a unit into a designated sharps container. Accidental needle stick injuries should be immediately reported.

d. When obtaining blood cultures, it is unnecessary to change venipuncture needle when filling additional culture bottles.

B. Specimen Handling

Identification of Specimens

a. Identify the patient by having the patient state two identifiers (eg, full name plus date of birth or social security number) before obtaining any specimen.

b. Label each specimen tube or container with the patient's name and unique identification number (eg, medical record number), and document the time of specimen collection on the tube label.

Specimen Tubes: Standard specimen tubes that contain a vacuum (called evacuated tubes) are now widely available and are easily identified by the color of the stopper (see also p. 38 in Chapter 3). The following is a general guide:

a. Plain red-top tubes contain no anticoagulants or preservatives and are used for serum chemistry tests and certain serologic tests.

b. Serum separator tubes (SST) (red-gold top) contain gel material that allows separation of serum and clot by centrifugation and are used for serum chemistry tests.

c. Lavender-top (purple) and pink-top tubes contain K_2EDTA and are used for hematology tests (eg, blood cell counts, differentials), blood banking (plasma), flow cytometry, and molecular diagnostic tests (cell-based).

d. Green-top tubes contain heparin and are used for plasma chemistry tests and chromosome analysis. Green-gold plasma preparation tubes (PPT) contain heparin and gel material that allows separation of plasma from cells, and are used for plasma chemistry tests.

e. Blue-top tubes contain sodium citrate and are used for coagulation tests. Royal blue-top tubes contain clot activator (for serum) or K_2EDTA (for whole blood) and are used for trace metal elements.

   f. Gray-top tubes contain sodium fluoride and are used for some chemistry tests (eg, glucose or alcohol requiring inhibition of glycolysis) if the specimen cannot be analyzed immediately.

   g. Yellow-top tubes contain acid citrate dextrose (ACD) and are used for flow cytometry and HLA typing.

   h. Pearl-white plasma preparation tubes (PPT) contain K_2EDTA and gel material and are used for molecular tests (plasma-based), such as HIV and HCV viral loads.

Procedure

Venipuncture is typically performed to obtain blood samples for acid-base and electrolyte studies, metabolic studies, hematologic studies, and coagulation studies. Arterial punctures are performed to obtain blood samples to assess arterial blood gases. Some tests (eg, glucose, rapid HIV test) can be performed on capillary blood obtained by puncturing the fingertip or baby's heel using a lancet device.

   a. When collecting multiple blood specimens by venipuncture, follow the recommended order of filling evacuated tubes, ie, blood culture bottles, coagulation tube (blue), non-additive tube (eg, plain red glass tube), SST, heparin tube (green), EDTA tube (lavender/purple), sodium fluoride tube (gray), and ACD tube (yellow). When using a butterfly collection device and drawing blood for a coagulation test, prime the tubing with a discard tube prior to specimen collection.

   b. Fill each tube completely. Tilt each tube containing anticoagulant or preservative gently to mix thoroughly. Do not shake tube. Deliver specimens to the laboratory promptly.

   c. For each of the common body fluids, Table 2–1 summarizes commonly requested tests and requirements for specimen handling and provides cross-references to tables and figures elsewhere in this book for help in interpretation of the results.

TABLE 2–1. BODY FLUID TESTS, HANDLING, AND INTERPRETATION.

Body Fluid	Commonly Requested Tests	Specimen Tube and Handling	Interpretation Guide
Ascitic fluid	Cell count, differential Protein, amylase Gram stain, culture Cytology (if neoplasm suspected)	Lavender top Red top Sterile tube Lavender top	See ascitic fluid profiles, Table 8–6.
Cerebrospinal fluid (collect in sterile and numbered plastic tubes)	Cell count, differential Gram stain, culture Protein, glucose, LDH VDRL or other studies (oligoclonal bands, IgG index, paraneoplastic antibodies, flow cytometry) Cytology (if neoplasm suspected)	Tube #3 or #4 Tube #2 Tube #3 Tube #3 or #4 Any (#1-#4)	See cerebrospinal fluid profiles, Table 8–9.
Pleural fluid	Cell count, differential Protein, glucose, amylase Gram stain, culture Cytology (if neoplasm suspected)	Lavender top Red top Sterile tube Lavender top	See pleural fluid profiles, Table 8–16.
Synovial fluid	Cell count, differential Gram stain, culture Microscopic examination for crystals Cytology (if neoplasm [villonodular synovitis, metastatic disease] suspected)	Lavender top Sterile tube Lavender top Lavender top	See synovial fluid profiles, Table 8–4.

Urine (collect in clean and/or sterile plastic tube or container)	Urinalysis
	  Dipstick
	  Microscopic examination
	  Gram stain, culture
	Cytology (if neoplasm suspected)
		
		Clean tube or container
		Centrifuge tube
		Sterile tube or container
		Clean tube or container
			See Table 2–3.
			See Figure 2–1.

Time to Test

For most accurate results, samples should be tested immediately after collection. Samples are suitable for analysis for a limited time and thus should be tested within the time limits specified by the laboratory's standard operating procedures.

2. COMMONLY USED POINT-OF-CARE TESTS

POC testing is typically performed in a primary care clinic, physician office, emergency room, operating room, or intensive care unit. It is usually performed by non-laboratory personnel. Certain self-testing can also be performed by the patient at home.

Table 2–2 lists the commonly used POC tests, many of which are exempt from CLIA regulatory procedures (so-called waived tests).

Advantages of POC testing include:

a. Potential to improve patient outcome and/or workflow by having results immediately available for patient management.
b. Potential to expedite medical decision making.
c. Use of portable or hand-held devices, allowing laboratory testing in a variety of locations, sites, and circumstances.
d. Use of small sample volume (minimizes blood loss to patient).
e. Elimination of need to transport the specimen to a clinical laboratory.

Disadvantages of POC testing include:

a. Given the variable training levels and experience of staff performing the tests, quality of test results is difficult to assure.
b. Competency assessment can be challenging.
c. Test methods are often different from central laboratory methods and thus can have unique interferences and limitations (eg, interference of POC blood glucose by maltose and xylose; potential unreliability of fingerstick blood glucose levels in critically ill patients).
d. Results are not necessarily comparable to central laboratory results and may not be approved for all uses that a similar central laboratory test can be used for (eg, waived PT/INR is approved only for monitoring warfarin therapy and thus cannot be used for assessment of bleeding diathesis).
e. Interfacing results to the electronic patient record may be difficult or impossible. Manual recording and reporting are prone to clerical error, and results may not be immediately available in the medical record.
f. Per test cost is often significantly higher than the cost of central laboratory testing.

3. PROVIDER-PERFORMED MICROSCOPY PROCEDURES

A. **Urinalysis (Urine Dipstick and Sediment Examination)**
   Collection and Preparation of Specimen
   a. Obtain a midstream, clean-catch urine specimen in a clean container.
   b. Examine the specimen while fresh (within 2 hours; do not refrigerate specimen); otherwise, bacteria may proliferate, casts and crystals may dissolve, and particulate matter may settle out.
   c. Place 10 mL in a conical test tube and centrifuge at 2000–3000 rpm for 5 minutes. Do not apply brake at the end of centrifugation to avoid re-suspension of sediment.
   d. Invert the tube and drain off the supernatant without dislodging the sediment button. Return the tube to an upright position, and re-suspend the sediment by gently tapping the bottom of the tube.
   e. Place a drop of sediment on a glass slide, cover it with a coverslip, and examine under the microscope; no stain is needed.

TABLE 2–2. COMMONLY USED POINT-OF-CARE (POC) TESTS.

POC Test Systems	Menu of Tests	Comments

Abbott *i-STAT* System	Chemistry/electrolytes
	  Sodium (Na)
	  Potassium (K)
	  Chloride (Cl)
	  Total CO$_2$ (Tco$_2$)
	  Anion gap (calculated)
	  Ionized calcium (iCa)
	  Glucose (Glu)
	  Urea nitrogen (BUN)
	  Creatinine (Creat)
	  Lactate
	Hematology
	  Hematocrit (Hct)
	  Hemoglobin (Hgb)
	Blood gases
	  pH
	  Pco$_2$
	  Po$_2$
	  HCO$_3^-$
	Coagulation
	  Activated clotting time (ACT)
	  Prothrombin time (PT/INR)
	Cardiac markers
	  Cardiac troponin I (cTnl)
	  CK-MB
	  BNP (B-type natriuretic peptide)
		The *i-STAT* 1 Analyzer uses a hand-held device and various single-use test cartridges. It is intended for use in the quantification of various analytes in whole blood. Each test cartridge contains chemically sensitive biosensors on a silicon chip that are configured to perform specific tests. To perform a test or a test panel (eg, electrolytes), 2–3 drops whole blood are applied to a cartridge, which is then inserted into the hand-held device. Commonly used test cartridges include *i-STAT G*, Crea, E3+, EC4+, EC6+, and Chem8+. Tests performed on venous whole blood samples are categorized as waived testing by CLIA (see text). The system is interfaceable to an electronic laboratory information system, and a wireless device is also available.
		Use the *i-STAT* glucose test in critically ill patients with caution.

Roche CoaguChek Systems (XS, XS Plus, and XS Pro)	Prothrombin time (PT/INR)	Used for monitoring coumadin (warfarin) anticoagulation therapy. The XS system uses a hand-held meter and PT test strip. Test can be performed on fresh capillary (fingerstick) or on nonanticoagulated venous whole blood. The test strip is first inserted into the meter and warmed. After 1 drop of blood is applied to the strip, the result appears on the meter in about 1 minute. The XS Plus system has built-in quality control and data management. The XS Pro system is based on the XS Plus but with an added bar code scanner.
Roche Accu-Chek Inform System	Blood glucose	The system uses a hand-held meter and reagent test strips and is intended for use in the quantitative determination of glucose levels in whole blood samples. Capillary blood from a fingerstick is typically used. The GDH-PQQ (glucose dehydrogenase pyrroloquinoline quinone) test strips cannot distinguish between glucose and certain non-glucose sugars, including maltose, xylose, and galactose. Patients who are receiving therapeutic products containing these non-glucose sugars will have falsely elevated blood glucose results. Use the Accu-Chek glucose test in critically ill patients with caution.
Alere/Biosite Triage Meter Pro	BNP Cardiac panel (CK-MB, myoglobin, cTnl) D-dimer Drugs of abuse panel (urine)	The system is based on sensitive fluorescence immunoassay technology. It uses a portable Triage Meter and various triage test devices. After a test sample is added to a test device, the device is inserted in the Triage Meter, which measures an analyte of interest based on standards that have been preprogrammed into the meter. It provides quantitative results for blood BNP, cardiac markers, and D-dimer, and qualitative results for urine toxicology screen in about 15 minutes.

(Continued)

TABLE 2–2. COMMONLY USED POINT-OF-CARE (POC) TESTS. (*Continued*)

POC Test Systems	Menu of Tests	Comments
Nova Biomedical StatStrip and Stat-Sensor Systems	Blood glucose Lactate Creatinine+eGFR (whole blood)	The systems use hand-held meters and reagent test strips, and are intended for use in the quantitative determinations of glucose, lactate (for sepsis) and creatinine+eGFR (for kidney function) in whole blood samples. The StatStrip glucose hospital meter system has been FDA approved for use with all patients, including critically ill patients.
POC HIV Test (eg, OraQuick ADVANCE-HIV1/2, Uni-Gold Recombigen HIV, Alere HIV-1/2 Ag/Ab Combo)	Rapid HIV-1/2 test	These tests are approved for oral fluid, fingerstick, or venipuncture whole blood specimens. Each test provides results within 20 minutes, enabling patients to learn their status in a single visit. The Alere HIV Ag/Ab Combo test detects HIV sooner (12–26 days after infection) than conventional rapid HIV tests (20–45 days after infection).
Rapid Strep Test (eg, CLIA waived Inc., Inverness Medical Clearview, Alere-i Strep A)	Rapid group A streptococcal antigen test	The test is approved for throat/tonsil swab specimen, and result is generally available in 10–15 minutes. It is used to determine whether a patient has streptococcal pharyngitis. The test is typically used in physicians' offices and emergency rooms.
Reagent strips for urinalysis (eg, Siemens Combistix and Multistix SG strips, Iris iChem strips, Pro Advantage strips)	Urinalysis, nonautomated	Urine dipsticks (strips) are used to analyze urine specimens for various biochemical substances (eg, blood, glucose, protein, bilirubin, nitrite, leukocyte esterase, ketone), and results are available within a few minutes. Results are interpreted using visual comparison of reagent pads to the color chart guide or using a compatible dipstick reader. See Table 2–3 for more details.
Fecal occult blood test (FOBT) (eg, Hemoccult Sensa, Hemosure, Clearview ULTRA, InSure FIT, Polymedco FIT-CHEK)	Rapid FOBT	Test is used for rapid, qualitative detection of human blood (hemoglobin) in feces. It is mainly used for colorectal cancer (CRC) screening in the outpatient setting. If guaiac-based FOBT (gFOBT) is used, three specimens on three different days are recommended to improve sensitivity. The fecal immunochemical test (FIT) detects the globin protein of hemoglobin in stool and is specific for colorectal bleeding.
Urine pregnancy test (various over-the-counter FDA-approved, CLIA waived tests are available)	Urine beta-hCG (human chorionic gonadotropin), qualitative	Based on detection of the hormone hCG in urine. In healthy subjects of childbearing age, positive hCG in urine provides an early indication of pregnancy. The detection limit for pregnancy is the day of the first missed period. If negative, recommend repeat testing in 5–7 days if menses have not occurred.
Pulse oximetry	Oxygen saturation of hemoglobin (Sao_2) and pulse rate (PR) (finger, ear, foot)	Pulse oximetry allows for noninvasive and continuous monitoring of arterial blood oxygen saturation (Sao_2). Sao_2 is not directly proportional to oxygen partial pressure (Pao_2). A relatively small change in Sao_2 (eg, from 94% to 83%) can represent a large change in Pao_2 (eg, from 80 to 50 mm Hg). To ensure accurate assessment of oxygenation status, pulse oximetry should be correlated with arterial blood gas analysis, if available. A reduction in peripheral pulsatile blood flow causes inaccurate reading.

Procedural Technique
    a. While the urine is being centrifuged, examine the remainder of the specimen by inspection and reagent strip (dipstick) testing.
    b. Inspect the specimen for color and clarity. Normally, urine is light yellow (due to urochrome). Intense yellow urine is caused by urine concentration (dehydration) or B vitamin supplements; dark orange urine, by ingestion of the

urinary tract analgesic phenazopyridine; orange-reddish urine, by rifampin or rifabutin therapy; red urine, by erythrocytes, hemoglobinuria, myoglobinuria, porphyrins, senna, or beets; green urine, by *Pseudomonas* infection or iodochlorhydroxyquin or amitriptyline therapy; brown urine, by bilirubinuria or fecal contamination; black urine, by intravascular hemolysis, alkaptonuria, melanoma, or methyldopa therapy; and milky white urine, by pus, chyluria, or amorphous crystals (urates or phosphates). Turbidity of urine is caused by pus, red blood cells, or crystals.

   c. Reagent strips provide information about specific gravity, pH, protein, glucose, ketones, bilirubin, blood (heme), nitrite, and leukocyte esterase (Table 2–3). Dip a reagent strip in the urine and compare it with the interpretation guide chart on the bottle. Follow the timing instructions carefully. *Note:* Reagent strips cannot be relied on to detect some proteins (eg, globulins, light chains) or reducing sugars (other than glucose). Falsely positive protein results may be obtained with alkaline urine (eg, urine pH > 8.0); sulfosalicylic acid (SSA) test can be used to confirm the presence of protein. Positive bilirubin on a reagent strip should be confirmed by an Ictotest tablet. Substances that cause abnormal urine color may affect the readability of test pads on reagent strips (eg, visible levels of blood or bilirubinuria and drugs containing dyes, nitrofurantoin, rifampin or rifabutin).

   d. Record and report the results.

Manual Microscopic Urine Sediment Examination

   a. Examine the area under the coverslip under low-power (10×) and high-dry (40×) lenses for cells, casts, crystals, and bacteria.

   b. Cells may be red cells, white cells, squamous cells, transitional (bladder) or tubular epithelial cells, or atypical (tumor) cells. Red cells suggest upper or lower urinary tract infections (cystitis, prostatitis, pyelonephritis), glomerulonephritis, collagen vascular disease, renal calculi, tumors, drug reactions, and structural abnormalities (polycystic kidneys). White cells suggest inflammatory processes such as urinary tract infection (most common), collagen vascular disease (eg, lupus), or interstitial nephritis. Red cell casts are considered pathognomonic of glomerulonephritis; white cell casts, of pyelonephritis; and fatty (lipid) casts, of nephrotic syndrome.

   c. Presence of crystals is often of no clinical significance. Presence of casts, however, is associated with various pathologic conditions. For example, WBC (leukocyte) casts are seen in patients with pyelonephritis and interstitial nephritis; RBC (erythrocyte) casts in acute glomerulonephritis, lupus nephritis, Goodpasture syndrome, and subacute bacterial endocarditis; renal epithelial casts in toxic tubular necrosis; waxy casts in severe chronic renal disease and amyloidosis; and fatty casts in nephrotic syndrome and diabetes mellitus.

Comments

See Table 2–3 for a guide to interpretation of urinalysis, and Figure 2–1 for a guide to microscopic findings in urine.

NOTE: Fully automated urinalysis systems (either image- or flow cytometry-based) are now available in many clinical laboratories, so manual microscopy examination may not be performed routinely in a central laboratory.

B. Vaginal Fluid Wet-Mount Preparation

Preparation of Smear and Staining Technique

   a. Apply a small amount of vaginal discharge to a glass slide.

   b. Add 2 drops of sterile saline solution.

   c. Place a coverslip over the area to be examined.

Microscopic Examination

   a. Examine under the microscope, using the high-dry (40×) lens and a low light source.

TABLE 2–3. COMPONENTS OF THE URINE DIPSTICK.[a]

Test	Normal Values	Sensitivity	Comments
Specific gravity	1.001–1.035	1.000–1.030[b]	Highly buffered alkaline urine may cause low specific gravity readings. Moderate proteinuria (100–750 mg/dL) may cause high readings. Loss of concentrating or diluting capacity indicates renal dysfunction. If the specific gravity of a random urine specimen is ≥ 1.023, the concentrating ability of the kidneys can be considered normal.
pH	4.6–8.0	5.0–8.5 (visually)[b]	Excessive urine on strip may cause protein reagent to run over onto pH area, yielding falsely low pH reading. Bacterial growth by certain organisms (eg, *Proteus*) in a specimen may cause a marked alkaline shift (urine pH > 8), usually because of urea conversion to ammonia.
Protein	Negative <15 mg/dL	15–30 mg/dL albumin	Test is based on protein-error-of-indicators principle. False-positive readings can be caused by highly buffered alkaline urine. Reagent is more sensitive to albumin than other proteins. A negative result does not rule out the presence of globulins, hemoglobin, light chains (Bence Jones) proteins, or mucoprotein. 1+ = 30 mg/dL 3+ = 300 mg/dL 2+ = 100 mg/dL 4+ = ≥ 2000 mg/dL
Glucose	Negative (<15 mg/dL or <50 mg/day)	75–125 mg/dL	Test is based on a double sequential enzyme reaction (glucose oxidase and peroxidase), and is specific for glucose. False-negative results occur with urinary ascorbic acid concentrations ≥ 30 mg/dL and with ketone body levels ≥ 40 mg/dL. Test reagent reactivity also varies with specific gravity and temperature. Trace = 100 mg/dL 1 = 1000 mg/dL ¼ = 250 mg/dL 2 = ≥ 2000 mg/dL ½ = 500 mg/dL
Ketone	Negative	5–10 mg/dL acetoacetate	Test does not react with acetone or β-hydroxybutyric acid. False-positive (trace) results may occur with highly pigmented urines or those containing levodopa metabolites or sulfhydryl-containing compounds (eg, Mesna). Trace results may occur during physiological stress conditions (fasting, pregnancy, strenuous exercise). Trace = 5 mg/dL Moderate = 40 mg/dL Small = 15 mg/dL Large = 80–160 mg/dL
Bilirubin	Negative (≤ 0.02 mg/dL)	0.4–0.8 mg/dL	Positive (conjugated) bilirubin indicates hepatitis. False-negative readings can be caused by ascorbic acid concentrations ≥ 25 mg/dL. False-positive readings can be caused by metabolites of Iodine (etodolac). Test is based on the coupling of bilirubin with diazotized dichloroaniline in an acidic medium. Test is less sensitive and specific than Ictotest Reagent Tablets. A positive test may be confirmed by Ictotest Reagent Tablets. To detect very small amounts of bilirubin in urine (eg, in the earliest phase of viral hepatitis), Ictotest Reagent Tablets should be used.
Blood	Negative (<0.010 mg/dL hemoglobin or <3 RBC/mcL)[c]	0.015–0.062 mg/dL hemoglobin or 5–20 RBC/mcL	Test is equally sensitive to myoglobin and hemoglobin (including both intact RBC and free hemoglobin). Test is based on the peroxidase-like activity of hemoglobin. False-positive results can be caused by oxidizing contaminants (hypochlorite) and microbial peroxidase (urinary tract infection). Test sensitivity is reduced in urines with high specific gravity, captopril, or heavy proteinuria.
Nitrite	Negative	0.06–0.10 mg/dL nitrite ion	Test depends on the conversion of nitrate (derived from the diet) to nitrite by gram-negative bacteria in urine when their number is >10⁵/mL (≥ 0.075 mg/dL nitrite ion). Test is specific for nitrite. False-negative readings may occur with shortened urine time in the bladder (<4 hr) and can also be caused by ascorbic acid. Test sensitivity is reduced in urines with high specific gravity. A negative result does not rule out significant bacteriuria.

Leukocytes (esterase)	Negative[d]	5–15 WBCs/hpf	Indicator of urinary tract infection. Test detects esterases contained in granulocytic leukocytes. Test sensitivity is reduced in urines with elevated glucose concentrations ≥3 g/dL), or presence of cephalexin, cephalothin, tetracycline, or high concentrations of oxalate. False-positive results may occur with specimen contamination by vaginal discharge.

[a]*Package insert, revised 08/08. Bayer Diagnostics Reagent Strips for Urinalysis, Siemens Healthcare Diagnostics.*
[b]*Analytical measurement range (AMR) of the reagent strips.*
[c]*Except in menstruating females.*
[d]*Except in females with vaginitis.*

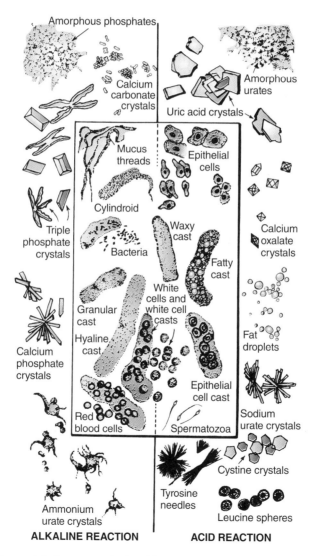

Figure 2–1. Microscopic findings on examination of the urine.

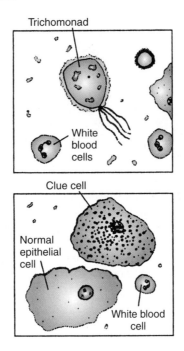

Figure 2–2. Wet-mount preparation showing trichomonads, white blood cells, and clue cells.

   b. Look for motile trichomonads (undulating protozoa propelled by four flagella). Look for clue cells (vaginal epithelial cells with a distinctive stippled appearance which have large numbers of organisms attached to their surface, obscuring cell borders). These are pathognomonic for vaginosis caused by *Gardnerella vaginalis.*

   c. See Figure 2–2 for an example of a positive wet prep (trichomonads, clue cells).

Comment

Rapid molecular tests using specific DNA probes (eg, BD Affirm VPIII) are now available for direct detection and identification of the three major causes of vaginitis: *Candida* species, *Gardnerella vaginalis* and *Trichomonas vaginalis*. Although the molecular tests are highly sensitive and specific, and are being used as a superior alternative to the conventional microscopic examination, they may not be available in community-based or rural outpatient clinics.

C. **Skin Scraping or Vaginal Fluid KOH Preparation**

   Preparation of Smear and Staining Technique

   a. Obtain a skin specimen by using a scalpel blade to scrape scales from the skin lesion onto a glass slide or to transfer the top of a vesicle to the slide, or, place a single drop of vaginal discharge on the slide.

   b. Place 1 or 2 drops of potassium hydroxide (KOH) (15%) on top of the specimen (skin scrapings or vaginal discharge) on the slide. Put a coverslip over the area to be examined.

   c. Allow the KOH prep to sit at room temperature until the material has been cleared. The slide may be warmed to speed the clearing process.

   Note: A fishy amine odor upon addition of KOH to a vaginal discharge is typical of bacterial vaginosis caused by *Gardnerella vaginalis.*

Microscopic Examination

  a. Examine the smear under low-power (10×) and high-dry (40×) lenses for mycelial forms. Branched, septate hyphae are typical of dermatophytosis (eg, trichophyton, epidermophyton, microsporum species); branched, septate pseudohyphae, with or without budding yeast forms, are seen with candidiasis (*Candida* species); and short, curved hyphae plus clumps of spores ("spaghetti and meatballs") are seen with tinea versicolor *(Malassezia furfur)*.

  b. Record and report any yeast, pseudohyphae, or hyphae, indicating budding and septation.

Comment

See Figure 2–3 for an example of a positive KOH prep.

D. Synovial Fluid Examination for Crystals

Preparation of Smear Technique

  a. Place a small amount of synovial fluid on a glass slide. No stain is necessary.

  b. Place a coverslip over the area to be examined.

Microscopic Examination

  a. Examine under a polarized light microscope with a red compensator, using the high-dry lens and a moderately bright light source.

  b. Look for needle-shaped, negatively birefringent urate crystals (crystals parallel to the axis of the compensator appear yellow) in gout, or rhomboidal, positively birefringent calcium pyrophosphate crystals (crystals parallel to the axis of the compensator appear blue) in pseudogout.

Comment

See Figure 2–4 for examples of positive synovial fluid examinations for these two types of crystals.

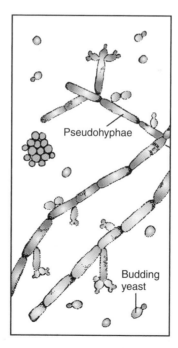

Figure 2–3. KOH preparation showing mycelial forms (pseudohyphae) and budding yeast typical of *Candida albicans*.

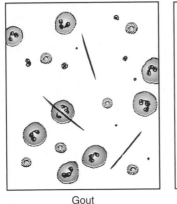
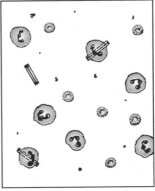

Gout   Pseudogout

Figure 2–4. Examination of synovial fluid for crystals using a compensated, polarized microscope. In gout, crystals are needle shaped, negatively birefringent, and composed of monosodium urate. In pseudogout, crystals are rhomboidal, positively birefringent, and composed of calcium pyrophosphate dihydrate. In both diseases, crystals can be found free-floating or within polymorphonuclear cells.

E. Fern Test of Amniotic Fluid

The Fern test, in conjunction with pH determination using pH paper (Nitrazine test), detects the leakage of amniotic fluid from the membrane surrounding the fetus during pregnancy.

Preparation of Smear Technique

a. Collect vaginal secretion from the posterior vaginal fornix with a sterile swab. Do not touch the mucus plug in the cervix.

b. Immediately rub the swab against a clean glass slide, creating a very thin smear.

c. Allow slide to dry. Do not cover with a coverslip.

Microscopic Examination

a. Examine the dried smear under the low-power (10×) lens.

b. If present, the amniotic fluid crystallizes to form a fern-like pattern (ferning) (Figure 2–5).

Comment

The Fern test should be performed together with the Nitrazine test (normal vaginal pH is 3.8–4.2, and amniotic fluid pH is 7.0–7.5). If both tests are positive (ferning present, pH 6.5–7.5), amniotic membrane rupture has occurred. If the Fern test is positive but the Nitrazine test is negative, there is probable rupture of membrane. If the Fern test is negative but the Nitrazine test is positive, a second specimen should be collected and examined using both tests. Premature rupture of the membranes may lead to fetal infection and subsequent morbidity. Induction of labor should be evaluated in this situation.

F. Pinworm Tape Test

This test is a method used to diagnose a pinworm infection by microscopic examination of specimens taken from the perianal region to identify *Enterobius vermicularis* eggs or adult female worms, if present.

Procedural Technique

a. Firmly press the sticky side of a 1-inch strip of transparent adhesive (Cellophane) tape over the right and left perianal folds for a few seconds.

b. Place the tape on a clean glass slide, sticky side down.

c. Using a microscope, examine the entire tape for eggs or worms under the low-power (10×) lens. The eggs are oval, elongated, and flattened on one side, with

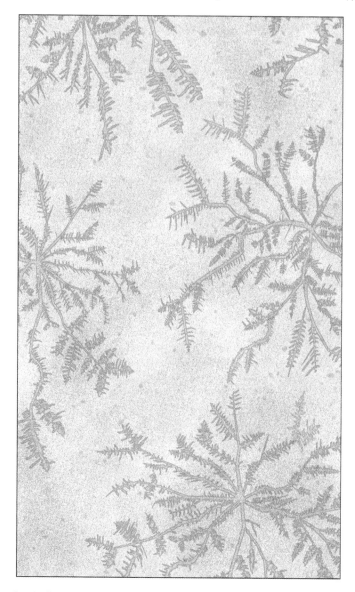

Figure 2–5. Positive Fern test showing crystallized amniotic fluid collected from the posterior vaginal fornix.

a thick colorless shell. The adult female worms are tiny, white, and threadlike, with a long, pointed tail.

d. Record and report findings.

e. See Figure 2–6 for an example of a positive Pinworm tape test.

Comments

Test should be done first thing in the morning before a bowel movement or bath. Note that specimen may also be collected at home with a collection paddle (eg, Becton-Dickinson SWUBE Paddle), and kept in a specimen tube until microscopic

A

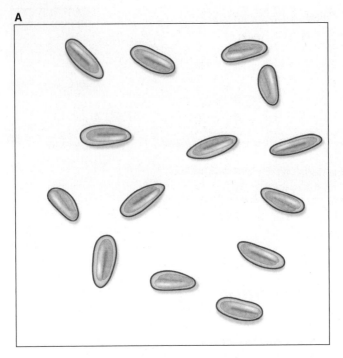

B

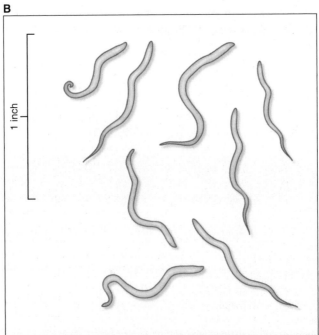

Figure 2–6. Positive Pinworm tape test showing *Enterobius vermicularis* eggs (**A**) and adult female worms (**B**).

examination. Female pinworms deposit eggs sporadically, so test must be done on at least 4 consecutive days to rule out the infection.

G. Qualitative Semen Analysis

Qualitative semen analysis is used to document the success of vasectomy. Semen samples should be examined for presence or absence of motile and/or nonmotile sperm at 8–12 weeks post-vasectomy.

Procedural Technique

    a. Ask patient to collect the entire ejaculate by masturbation into a clean container labeled with patient name and unique identification number.

    b. Keep the specimen at body temperature (37°C) to ensure proper liquefaction.

    c. Verify that the semen has liquefied before proceeding with the test. If not liquefied, check specimen at 10-minute intervals until it has liquefied.

    d. Place a small drop of liquefied semen on a clean glass slide and add a coverslip.

Microscopic Examination

    a. Immediately examine under the high-dry (40×) lens. Examine several fields before reporting the absence of sperm. If sperm are present, classify them according to their motility (motile versus nonmotile) in percentages.

    b. Record and report results.

Comments

Semen samples should be collected after an abstinence period of no less than 48 hours and no more than 7 days and maintained at body temperature. Specimen must be examined as soon as possible to ensure maximum accuracy of results. Specimens collected in condoms should be rejected. If sperm are present, the patient should be cautioned to continue temporary contraception and to resubmit a second specimen for reexamination after 4–6 additional weeks.

    For evaluation of infertility, full semen analysis should be performed at a central laboratory.

4. POINT-OF-CARE ULTRASOUND EXAMINATION

Point-of-care (POC) ultrasound is the use of compact and portable ultrasonography at a patient's bedside for a time-sensitive diagnostic or therapeutic purpose. Interpretation of the ultrasound images and immediate clinical decisions can be made by the clinicians conducting the examination, thereby enabling rapid assessment and intervention. To be used for POC examination, the technique should be easily learned and quickly performed, and be used for a well-defined purpose with easily recognizable findings.

POC ultrasound is commonly used in cardiology, obstetrics, anesthesiology, emergency medicine, intensive and critical care, pain management, and vascular surgery settings. Examples of POC ultrasound applications include:

    a. To determine whether an unresponsive patient is bleeding into the abdominal cavity or if a patient is having cardiac tamponade, pulmonary embolism or pneumothorax.

    b. To provide static or dynamic ultrasound-based procedural guidance (eg, vascular access, central venous catheter placement, regional nerve block, thoracentesis).

    c. To monitor pregnancy (status of fetus), intraoperative fluid status and cardiac function, or to diagnose acute synovitis, acute cholecystitis, perforated appendicitis, hemarthrosis, or aortic aneurysm.

    d. To assess the status of bleeding from kidneys, urinary bladder, or prostate and to evaluate a hematoma.

Comment

POC ultrasound examination requires adequate training, competency assessment, and quality assurance. Each institution must establish policies and procedures to govern the clinical uses of POC ultrasonography in various clinical settings.

REFERENCES

Point-of-Care Testing
Briggs C et al. Where are we at with point-of-care testing in haematology? Br J Haematol 2012;158:679. [PMID: 22765160]
Drain PK et al. Diagnostic point-of-care tests in resource-limited settings. Lancet Infect Dis 2014;14:239. [PMID: 24332389]
Liikanen E et al. Training of nurses in point-of-care testing: a systematic review of the literature. J Clin Nurs 2013;22:2244. [PMID: 23679832]
St John A et al. Existing and emerging technologies for point-of-care testing. Clin Biochem Rev 2014;35:155. [PMID: 25336761]

Urinalysis
Delanghe J et al. Preanalytical requirements of urinalysis. Biochem Med (Zagreb) 2014;24:89. [PMID: 24627718]
Kaplan BS et al. Urinalysis interpretation for pediatricians. Pediatr Ann 2013;42:45. [PMID: 23458861]
McFarlane PA. Testing for albuminuria in 2014. Canad J Diabetes 2014;38:372. [PMID: 25284700]

Vaginal Wet-Mount Preparation
Meites E. Trichomoniasis: the "neglected" sexually transmitted disease. Infect Dis Clin North Am 2013;27:755. [PMID: 24275268]
Mylonas I et al. Diagnosis of vaginal discharge by wet mount microscopy: a simple and underrated method. Obstet Gynecol Surv 2011;66:359. [PMID: 21851750]

Synovial Fluid Examination
Courtney P et al. Joint aspiration and injection and synovial fluid analysis. Best Pract Res Clin Rheumatol 2013;27:137. [PMID: 23731929]
Ea HK et al. Diagnosis and clinical manifestations of calcium pyrophosphate and basic calcium phosphate crystal deposition diseases. Rheum Dis Clin North Am 2014;40:207. [PMID: 24703344]
Graf SW et al. The accuracy of methods for urate crystal detection in synovial fluid and the effect of sample handling: a systematic review. Clin Rheumatol 2013;32:225. [PMID: 23138881]

Pinworm Tape Test
Nasseri YY et al. Pruritus ani: diagnosis and treatment. Gastroenterol Clin North Am 2013;42:801. [PMID: 24280401]
Van Onselen J. Childhood infestations: prevention and eradication. J Fam Health Care 2014;24:24. [PMID: 25112046]

Semen Analysis, Qualitative
Dohle GR et al. European Association of Urology guidelines on vasectomy. Eur Urol 2012;61:159. [PMID: 22033172]
Rayala BZ et al. Common questions about vasectomy. Am Fam Physician 2013;88:757. [PMID: 24364523]
Talwar P et al. Sperm function test. J Hum Reprod Sci 2015;8:61. [PMID: 26157295]

Point-of-Care Ultrasound
Moore CL et al. Point-of-care ultrasonography. N Engl J Med 2011;364:749. [PMID: 21345104]
Peterson D et al. Critical care ultrasonography. Emerg Med Clin North Am 2014;32:907. [PMID: 25441042]
Squizzato A et al. Point-of-care ultrasound in the diagnosis of pulmonary embolism. Crit Ultrasound J 2015;7:7. [PMID: 26034556]
Wiley B et al. Handheld ultrasound and diagnosis of cardiovascular disease at the bedside. J Am Coll Cardiol 2014;64:229. [PMID: 25011727]

3

Common Laboratory Tests: Selection & Interpretation

Diana Nicoll, MD, PhD, MPA, Chuanyi Mark Lu, MD, and Stephen J. McPhee, MD

HOW TO USE THIS SECTION

This section contains information about commonly used laboratory tests. It includes most of the blood, urine, and cerebrospinal fluid tests found in this book, with the exception of therapeutic drug monitoring and pharmacogenetic tests (see Chapter 4). Entries are arranged alphabetically.

Test/Reference Range/Collection

This first column lists the common test name, the specimen analyzed, and any test name abbreviation (in parentheses).

Below this is the reference range (also called reference interval) for each test. The first entry is in conventional units, and the second entry (in [brackets]) is in SI units (Système International d'Unités). Any panic values for a particular test are placed here after the word ***Panic.*** The reference ranges provided are from several large medical centers; consult your own clinical laboratory for those used in your institution.

This column also shows which tube to use for collecting blood and other body fluids, how much the test costs (using symbols; see below), and how to collect the specimen.

The scale used for the cost of each test is:

Approximate Cost	Symbol Used in Tables
$1–20	$
$21–50	$$
$51–100	$$$
> $100	$$$$

Listed below are the common specimen collection tubes and their contents:

Tube Top Color	Tube Contents	Typical Use
Lavender or Pink	K_2EDTA	Complete blood count; blood banking (plasma); molecular testing (cell-based); flow cytometry (immunophenotyping)
Gold SST	Clot activator and gel for serum separation	Serum chemistry tests
White PPT	K_2EDTA and gel for plasma separation	Molecular testing (plasma-based)
Red	None	Blood banking (serum); therapeutic drug monitoring
Blue	Sodium citrate	Coagulation studies
Green PPT, Light green PPT	Sodium heparin or lithium heparin (green PPT, without gel; light green PPT, with gel for plasma separation)	Plasma chemistry tests (light green PPT); chromosome analysis (sodium heparin) (green PPT)
Yellow	Acid citrate dextrose (ACD); sodium polyanethol sulfonate (SPS)	ACD: HLA typing; blood banking (plasma); flow cytometry (immunophenotyping) SPS: Blood culture (microbiology)
Dark blue	Clot activator (free of trace metal)	Trace metals (eg, lead, mercury, arsenic)
Orange RST	Thrombin and gel for serum separation	Serum chemistry tests
Navy	Trace metal-free	Trace metals (eg, lead, mercury, arsenic)
Gray	Inhibitor of glycolysis (sodium fluoride)	Lactic acid; glucose
Black	Sodium citrate; None (plain black screw top)	Erythrocyte sedimentation rate (sodium citrate); sterile body fluids for microbiology (plain black screw top)

ACD, acid citrate dextrose; EDTA, ethylenediamine tetraacetic acid; PPT, plasma preparation tube; RST, rapid serum tube; SPS, sodium polyanethol sulfonate; SST, serum separator tube.

Physiologic Basis

This column contains physiologic information about the substance being tested. Information on classification and biologic importance, as well as interactions with other biologic substances and processes, is included.

Interpretation

This column lists clinical conditions that affect the substance being tested. Generally, conditions with higher prevalence are listed first. When the sensitivity of the test for a particular disease is known, that information follows the disease name in parentheses, for example, "rheumatoid arthritis (83%)." Some common drugs that can affect the test *in vivo* are also included in this outline listing.

Comments

This column gives general information pertinent to the use and interpretation of the test and important *in vitro* interferences with the test procedure. Appropriate general references with PubMed ID (PMID) numbers are also listed.

Test Name

The test name is also placed as a page header to allow for quick referencing.

Test/Range/Collection	Physiologic Basis	Interpretation	Comments
ABO Typing			
ABO typing, serum or plasma and red cells (ABO) Red or lavender/pink $ Properly identified and labeled blood specimen is critical. A second "check" specimen is required.	The ABO antigen and antibodies remain the most significant for transfusion practice. The 4 blood groups A, B, O, and AB are determined by the presence of antigens A and B or their absence (O) on a patient's red blood cells. Individuals possess antibodies directed toward the A or B antigen absent from their own red cells. In the US white population, 45% are type O, 40% A, 11% B, 4% AB. In the US Hispanic population, 57% are type O, 30% A, 10% B, 3% AB. In the African American population, 49% are type O, 27% A, 20% B, 4% AB. In the US Asian population, 40% are type O, 28% A, 27% B, 5% AB. In the Native American population, 55% are type O, 35% A, 8% B, 2% AB.	Type O patients can receive only type O red cells, and type A, B, O, or AB plasma. Type A patients can receive type A or O red cells and type A or AB plasma. Type B patients can receive type B or O red cells and type B or AB plasma. Type AB patients can receive type AB, A, B, or O red cells but only type AB plasma. In an emergency situation, type O red cells and type AB plasma may be given to patients with any ABO blood type.	For both blood donors and recipients, routine ABO typing includes both red cell and serum testing, as checks on each other. Tube testing is as follows: patient's red cells are tested with anti-A and anti-B for the presence or absence of agglutination (forward or cell type), and patient's serum or plasma is tested against known A and B cells (reverse or serum/plasma type). *Technical Manual of the American Association of Blood Banks,* 18th ed. American Association of Blood Banks, 2014.
Acetaminophen			
Acetaminophen, serum (Tylenol; others) 10–20 mg/L [66–132 mcmol/L] ***Panic:*** >50 mg/L Red $$ For suspected overdose, draw 2 samples at least 4 hrs apart, at least 4 hrs after ingestion. Note time of ingestion, if known. Order test stat.	In overdose, liver and renal toxicity are produced by the hydroxylated metabolite if it is not conjugated with glutathione in the liver.	**Increased in:** Acetaminophen overdose. Interpretation of serum acetaminophen level depends on time since ingestion. Levels drawn < 4 hrs after ingestion cannot be interpreted, since the drug is still in the absorption and distribution phase. If needed, the widely available acetaminophen nomogram may help evaluate possible toxicity. Levels > 150 mg/L at 4 hrs or >50 mg/L at 12 hrs after ingestion are often associated with toxicity.	Acetaminophen overdose is potentially fatal and early recognition is critical. Do not delay acetylcysteine (Mucomyst) treatment (140 mg/kg orally) if stat levels are unavailable. A nomogram for prediction of acetaminophen hepatotoxicity following acute overdosage is available in the 1975 reference below. Hodgman MJ et al. A review of acetaminophen poisoning. Crit Care Clin 2012;28:499. [PMID: 22998987] Klein-Schwartz W et al. Intravenous acetylcysteine for the treatment of acetaminophen overdose. Expert Opin Pharmacother 2011;12:119. [PMID: 21126198] Rumack BH et al. Acetaminophen poisoning and toxicity. Pediatrics 1975;55: 871. [PMID: 1134886]

(Continued)

Test/Range/Collection	Physiologic Basis	Interpretation	Comments
Acetoacetate, urine 0 mg/dL [mcmol/L] Urine container $ Urine sample should be fresh.	Acetoacetate, acetone, and β-hydroxybutyrate contribute to ketoacidosis when oxidative hepatic metabolism of fatty acids occurs as a consequence of absolute or relative insulin deficiency. Proportions vary in the bloodstream but are generally ~20% acetoacetate, ~78% β-hydroxybutyrate, and ~2% acetone.	**Present in:** Diabetic ketoacidosis, alcoholic ketoacidosis, prolonged fasting, starvation, severe carbohydrate restriction with normal fat intake, prolonged exercise.	Urine nitroprusside test is semiquantitative; it detects acetoacetate and is sensitive down to 5–10 mg/dL. Trace = 5 mg/dL, small = 15 mg/dL, moderate = 40 mg/dL, large = 80 mg/dL [1 mg/dL = 100 mcmol/L]. β-Hydroxybutyrate has no ketone group; therefore, it is not detected by the nitroprusside test. Acetone is also not reliably detected by the urine nitroprusside test because its sensitivity for acetone is poor. Failure of the nitroprusside test to detect β-hydroxybutyrate in ketoacidosis may produce a seemingly paradoxical increase in ketones with clinical improvement as nondetectable β-hydroxybutyrate is replaced by detectable acetoacetate. Testing the blood for β-hydroxybutyrate is clinically more useful in this setting. Klocker AA et al. Blood β-hydroxybutyrate vs. urine acetoacetate testing for the prevention and management of ketoacidosis in type 1 diabetes: a systematic review. Diabet Med 2013;30:818. [PMID: 23330615]
Acetylcholine receptor antibodies, serum Negative SST, red $$	Most patients with myasthenia gravis have detectable antibodies to the acetylcholine receptor (AChR). The AChR autoantibodies can be divided into binding, blocking and modulating antibodies, all of which are involved in the pathogenesis of myasthenia gravis. The binding antibody is most commonly tested. A sensitive radioimmunoassay (RIA) or enzyme-linked immunosorbent assay (ELISA) is available.	**Positive in:** Myasthenia gravis (sensitivity 87–98%, specificity 98–100%).	Antibody levels correlate with severity of autonomic failure. Antibodies can also be associated with other neurologic disorders unrelated to the autonomic nervous system. Besides AChR antibodies, detection of autoantibodies targeting MuSK (muscle-specific kinase) and LRP4 (lipoprotein related protein 4) can also help diagnose myasthenia gravis, but with much lower sensitivity. Berrih-Aknin S et al. Diagnostic and clinical classification of autoimmune myasthenia gravis. J Autoimmun 2014;48-49:143. [PMID: 24530233] Leite MI et al. Diagnostic use of autoantibodies in myasthenia gravis. Autoimmunity 2010;43:371. [PMID: 20380582] Zisimopoulou P et al. Serological diagnostics in myasthenia gravis based on novel assays and recently identified antigens. Autoimmun Rev 2013;12:924. [PMID: 23537507]

(Continued)

Activated clotting time	Adrenocorticotropic hormone
Activated clotting time, whole blood (ACT) 70–180 sec (method-specific) $$ Obtain blood in a plastic syringe without anticoagulant. Test should be performed immediately at patient's bedside. A clean venipuncture is required. A special vacutainer tube containing activator (eg, celite, kaolin) is also available.	**Adrenocorticotropic hormone,** plasma (ACTH) 9–52 pg/mL [2–11 pmol/L] Lavender, pink $$$$ Separate plasma from cells and freeze ASAP. Send promptly to laboratory on ice. ACTH is unstable in plasma, is inactivated at room temperature, and adheres strongly to glass. Avoid all contact with glass.
ACT is a point-of-care test used to monitor high-dose heparin as an anticoagulant during cardiac surgery (extracorporeal circulation), angioplasty, and hemodialysis. It is also used to determine the dose of protamine sulfate to reverse the heparin effect on completion of the procedure. ACT is also used to monitor heparin or direct thrombin inhibitor in patients with lupus anticoagulant.	Pituitary ACTH (release stimulated by hypothalamic corticotropin-releasing factor) stimulates cortisol release from the adrenal gland. There is feedback regulation of the system by cortisol. ACTH is secreted episodically and shows circadian variation, with highest levels at 6:00–8:00 AM; lowest levels at 9:00–10:00 PM.
Prolonged in: Heparin therapy, direct thrombin inhibitor therapy, severe deficiency of clotting factors (except factors VII and XIII), functional platelet disorders. In general, the accepted goal during cardiopulmonary bypass surgery is 400–500 sec. For carotid artery stenting, the optimal ACT is 250–300 sec.	**Increased in:** Pituitary (40–200 pg/mL) and ectopic (200–71,000 pg/mL) Cushing syndrome, primary adrenal insufficiency (> 250 pg/mL), adrenogenital syndrome with impaired cortisol production. **Decreased in:** Adrenal Cushing syndrome (< 20 pg/mL), pituitary ACTH (secondary adrenal insufficiency (< 50 pg/mL).
ACT is the choice of test when heparin levels are too high (eg, > 1.0 U/mL heparin) to allow monitoring with PTT and/or when a rapid result is necessary to monitor treatment. Because different methodologies and a number of variables (eg, platelet count and function, hypothermia, hemodilution, and certain drugs like aprotinin) may affect the ACT, the ACT test is not yet standardized. Reproducibility of prolonged ACTs may be poor. Finley A et al. Review article: heparin sensitivity and resistance: management during cardiopulmonary bypass. Anesth Analg 2013;116:1210. [PMID: 23408671] McNair E et al. Bivalirudin as an adjunctive anticoagulant to heparin in the treatment of heparin resistance during cardiopulmonary bypass-assisted cardiac surgery. Perfusion 2016;31:189. [PMID: 25934498] Sniecinski RM et al. Anticoagulation management associated with extracorporeal circulation. Best Pract Res Clin Anaesthesiol 2015;29:189. [PMID: 26060030]	ACTH levels can be interpreted only when measured with cortisol after standardized stimulation or suppression tests (see Adrenocortical insufficiency algorithm, Figure 9–3, and Cushing syndrome algorithm, Figure 9–8). Lefebvre H. Corticotroph deficiency. Ann Endocrinol (Paris) 2012;73:135. [PMID: 22516763] Neary N et al. Adrenal insufficiency: etiology, diagnosis and treatment. Curr Opin Endocrinol Diabetes Obes 2010;17:217. [PMID: 20375886] Raff H. Cushing syndrome: update on testing. Endocrinol Metab Clin North Am 2015;44:43. [PMID: 25732641]

Test/Range/Collection	Physiologic Basis	Interpretation	Comments
Alanine aminotransferase, serum or plasma (ALT, SGPT, GPT) 0–35 U/L [0–0.58 mckat/L] (laboratory-specific) SST, red, PPT (light green) $	Intracellular enzyme involved in amino acid metabolism. Present in large concentrations in liver; in clinically negligible amounts in kidney, skeletal muscle and heart. Released with tissue damage, particularly liver injury.	**Increased in:** Acute viral hepatitis (ALT > AST), biliary tract obstruction (cholangitis, choledocholithiasis), alcoholic hepatitis and cirrhosis (AST > ALT), liver abscess, metastatic or primary liver cancer; nonalcoholic steatohepatitis; right heart failure, ischemia or hypoxia, injury to liver ("shock liver"), extensive muscle trauma; drugs that cause cholestasis or hepatotoxicity. **Decreased in:** Pyridoxine (vitamin B_6) deficiency.	ALT is the preferred enzyme for evaluation of liver injury since it is more sensitive than AST. Screening ALT in low-risk populations has a low (12%) positive predictive value and is not recommended. Lee TH et al. Evaluation of elevated liver enzymes. Clin Liver Dis 2012;16:183. [PMID: 22541694] Woreta TA et al. Evaluation of abnormal liver tests. Med Clin North Am 2014;98:1. [PMID: 24266911]
Albumin, serum or plasma 3.4–4.7 g/dL [34–47 g/L] SST, PPT (light green) $	Major component of plasma proteins; influenced by nutritional state, hepatic function, renal function, and various diseases. Major binding protein. Although there are more than 50 different genetic variants (alloalbumins), only occasionally does a mutation cause abnormal binding (eg, in familial dysalbuminemic hyperthyroxinemia).	**Increased in:** Dehydration, shock, hemoconcentration. **Decreased in:** Decreased hepatic synthesis (chronic liver disease, malnutrition, malabsorption, malignancy, congenital analbuminemia [rare]). Increased losses (nephrotic syndrome, burns, trauma, hemorrhage with fluid replacement, fistulas, enteropathy, acute or chronic glomerulonephritis). Hemodilution (pregnancy, HF). Drugs: estrogens.	Serum albumin indicates severity in chronic liver disease. Useful in nutritional assessment if there is no impairment in production or increased loss of albumin. Independent risk factor for all-cause mortality in the elderly (age >70) and for complications in hospitalized and post-surgical patients. There is a 10% reduction in serum albumin level in late pregnancy (related to hemodilution). See Child-Turcotte-Pugh and MELD scoring systems for staging cirrhosis (Table 8–10). Cross MB et al. Evaluation of malnutrition in orthopaedic surgery. J Am Acad Orthop Surg 2014;22:193. [PMID: 24603829] Lammers WJ et al. Predicting outcome in primary biliary cirrhosis. Ann Hepatol 2014;13:316. [PMID: 24927602] Woreta TA et al. Evaluation of abnormal liver tests. Med Clin North Am 2014;98:1. [PMID: 24266911]

Albumin, urine		
Albumin, urine <30 mg/24 hr <20 mcg/min (timed collection) $$$$	The normal urinary albumin excretion is less than 30 mg/24 hr. On random spot urine collection, the albumin-to-creatinine ratio (mcg/mg) should be less than 30. The term "microalbuminuria" is defined as a subtle increase in the urinary excretion of albumin that cannot be detected by conventional urinalysis. Specifically, the excretion of 30–300 mg albumin per 24 hrs or an albumin-to-creatinine ratio of 30–300 (mcg/mg) is considered microalbuminuria (urine albumin excretion is high). Albumin excretion of 300 mg or more per day or an albumin-to-creatinine ratio of 300 or higher indicates gross albuminuria (urine albumin very high or in nephrotic range).	**Increased in:** Diabetes mellitus, diabetic nephropathy.	Microalbuminuria is a useful indicator of early nephropathy in diabetic patients. Urine albumin measurement requires a sensitive immunochemical assay. Urine dipstick analysis is often insensitive to microalbuminuria. Screening for microalbuminuria is often performed by measurement of the albumin-to-creatinine ratio in a random spot collection (preferred method). Twenty-four-hour or timed urine collections are more burdensome. Johnson DW et al. Chronic kidney disease and measurement of albuminuria or proteinuria: a position statement. Med J Aust 2012;197:224. [PMID: 22900872] Kuritzky L et al. Identification and management of albuminuria in the primary care setting. J Clin Hypertens (Greenwich) 2011;13:438. [PMID: 21649844] Wu HY et al. Diagnostic performance of random urine samples using albumin concentration vs ratio of albumin to creatinine for microalbuminuria screening in patients with diabetes mellitus: a systematic review and meta-analysis. JAMA Intern Med 2014;174:1108. [PMID: 24798807]

(Continued)

Aldosterone, serum

Test/Range/Collection	Physiologic Basis	Interpretation	Comments
Aldosterone, serum *Salt-loaded* (120 meq Na⁺/d for 3–4 days): Supine: 3–10 ng/dL Upright: 5–30 ng/dL *Salt-depleted* (10 meq Na⁺/d for 3–4 days): Supine: 12–36 ng/dL Upright: 17–137 ng/dL SST, Red $$$$ Early AM fasting specimen. Separate immediately and freeze.	Aldosterone is the major mineralocorticoid hormone and is a major regulator of extracellular volume and serum potassium concentration. For evaluation of hypoaldosteronism (associated with hyperkalemia), patients should be salt-depleted and upright when specimen is drawn.	**Increased in:** Primary hyperaldosteronism (2/3 from adrenal hyperplasia, 1/3 from adrenal adenomas) may account for 5–10% of hypertension. **Aldosterone/PRA ratio >15** (mL/dL/hour) when aldosterone is expressed as ng/dL and plasma renin activity, as ng/mL/hour (sensitivity 73–87%, specificity 74–75%) **Decreased in:** Primary or secondary hypoaldosteronism.	Screening for hyperaldosteronism should use simultaneous determination of serum aldosterone and plasma renin activity (PRA) (see Figure 9–14). In primary aldosteronism, plasma aldosterone is usually elevated whereas PRA is low; in secondary hyperaldosteronism, both serum aldosterone and PRA are usually elevated. The aldosterone/PRA ratio (also known as aldosterone-to-renin ratio or ARR) is often used for diagnosis of hyperaldosteronism, but the cutoff value has not been well established and the specificity is low. Carey RM. Primary aldosteronism. J Surg Oncol 2012;106:575. [PMID: 22806599] Monticone S et al. Primary aldosteronism: who should be screened? Horm Metab Res 2012;44:163. [PMID: 22120135] Stowasser M et al. Factors affecting the aldosterone/renin ratio. Horm Metab Res 2012;44:170. [PMID: 22147655]

Aldosterone, urine		
Aldosterone, urine* *Salt-loaded* (120 meq Na+/d for 3–4 days): 1.5–12.5 mcg/24 hr *Salt-depleted* (10 meq Na+/d for 3–4 days): 18–85 mcg/24 hr [1 mcg/24 hr = 2.77 nmol/d] Bottle containing boric acid $$$$	Secretion of aldosterone is controlled by the renin-angiotensin system. Renin (synthesized and stored in juxtaglomerular cells of kidney) is released in response to both decreased perfusion pressure at the juxtaglomerular apparatus and negative sodium balance. Renin then hydrolyzes angiotensinogen to angiotensin I, which is converted to angiotensin II, which then stimulates the adrenal gland to produce aldosterone.	**Increased in:** Primary and secondary hyper-aldosteronism, some patients with essential hypertension. **Decreased in:** Primary hypoaldosteronism (eg, 18-hydroxylase deficiency), second-ary hypoaldosteronism (hyporeninemic hypoaldosteronism).	Urinary aldosterone is the most sensitive test for primary hyperaldo-steronism. Levels >14 mcg/24 hrs after 3 days of salt-loading have a 96% sensitivity and 93% specificity for primary hyperaldosteronism. Among patients with essential hypertension, 7% have urinary aldosterone levels >14 mcg/24 hr after salt-loading. Ceral J et al. The role of urinary aldosterone for the diagnosis of primary aldosteronism. Horm Metab Res 2014;46:663. [PMID: 24810470] Kerstens MN et al. Reference values for aldosterone-renin ratios in normotensive individuals and effect of changes in dietary sodium consumption. Clin Chem 2011;57:1607. [PMID: 21865483]

*To evaluate hyperaldosteronism, patient is salt-loaded and recumbent. Obtain 24-hour urine for aldosterone (and for sodium to check that sodium excretion is ≥ 250 meq/d). To evaluate hypoaldosteronism, patient is salt-depleted and upright; check patient for hypotension before 24-hour urine is collected.

	Alkaline phosphatase			Ammonia
Test/Range/Collection	**Physiologic Basis**	**Interpretation**	**Comments**	

Alkaline phosphatase, serum or plasma (ALP)

41–133 IU/L

[0.7–2.2 mckat/L] (method and age-dependent)

SST, PPT (light green)

$

Physiologic Basis: Alkaline phosphatases are primarily found in liver, bone, intestines, kidney, and placenta. Test is used to detect liver disease and bone disorders.

Interpretation: **Increased in:** Obstructive hepatobiliary disease, bone disease (physiologic bone growth, Paget disease, osteomalacia, osteogenic sarcoma, bone metastases), hyperparathyroidism, rickets, benign familial hyperphosphatasemia, pregnancy (third trimester), GI disease (perforated ulcer or bowel infarct), hepatotoxic drugs. **Decreased in:** Hypophosphatasia.

Comments: Alkaline phosphatase performs well in measuring the extent of bone metastases in prostate cancer. Normal in osteoporosis. Alkaline phosphatase isoenzyme separation by electrophoresis or differential heat inactivation is unreliable. Use γ-glutamyl transpeptidase, which increases in hepatobiliary disease but not in bone disease, to infer origin of increased alkaline phosphatase (ie, liver rather than bone).
Cundy T et al. Paget's disease of bone. Clin Biochem 2012;45:43. [PMID: 22024254]
Siddique A et al. Approach to a patient with elevated serum alkaline phosphatase. Clin Liver Dis 2012;16:199. [PMID: 22541695]
Woreta TA et al. Evaluation of abnormal liver tests. Med Clin North Am 2014;98:1. [PMID: 24266911]

Ammonia, plasma (NH₃)

11–35 mcmol/L

Green, lavender

$$

Place specimen on ice immediately. Separate plasma from cells ASAP or within 2 hrs. Analyze immediately, or freeze for storage or shipment.

Physiologic Basis: Ammonia is liberated by bacteria in the large intestine or by protein metabolism and is rapidly converted to urea in the liver. In liver disease or portal-systemic shunting, the blood ammonia concentration increases. In acute liver failure, elevation of blood ammonia may cause brain edema; in chronic liver failure, it may be responsible for hepatic encephalopathy.

Interpretation: **Increased in:** Liver failure, hepatic encephalopathy (especially if protein consumption is high or if there is GI bleeding), fulminant hepatic failure, Reye syndrome, portacaval shunting, cirrhosis, urea cycle metabolic defects, urea-splitting urinary tract infection with urinary diversion, and organic acidemias. Drugs: diuretics, acetazolamide, asparaginase, fluorouracil (transient), others. Spuriously increased by any ammonia-containing detergent on laboratory glassware. **Decreased in:** Decreased production by gut bacteria (kanamycin, neomycin). Decreased gut absorption (lactulose).

Comments: Plasma ammonia level correlates poorly with degree of hepatic encephalopathy in chronic liver disease. Test not useful in adults with known liver disease. Ammonia crosses the blood-brain barrier. Ammonia toxicity is probably mediated by glutamine, synthesized in excess from ammonia and glutamate in the brain. Ammonia reduction can be achieved by targeting its production, absorption or elimination.
Jover-Cobos M et al. Treatment of hyperammonemia in liver failure. Curr Opin Clin Nutr Metab Care 2014;17:105. [PMID: 24281376]
Romero-Gómez M et al. Hepatic encephalopathy in patients with acute decompensation of cirrhosis and acute-on-chronic liver failure. J Hepatol 2015;62:437. [PMID: 25218789]

(Continued)

	Amylase				Angiotensin-converting enzyme		

Amylase, serum or plasma

20–110 U/L

[0.33–1.83 mckat/L] (laboratory-specific)

Gold SST, PPT (light green)

$

Amylase hydrolyzes complex carbohydrates. Serum amylase is derived primarily from pancreas and salivary glands and is increased with inflammation or obstruction of these glands. Other tissues have some amylase activity, including ovaries, small and large intestine, and skeletal muscle.

Increased in: Acute pancreatitis (70–95%), pancreatic pseudocyst, pancreatic duct obstruction (cholecystitis, choledocholithiasis, pancreatic carcinoma, stone, stricture, duct sphincter spasm), trauma to the pancreas, bowel obstruction and infarction, mumps, parotitis, diabetic ketoacidosis, penetrating peptic ulcer, peritonitis, ruptured ectopic pregnancy, macroamylasemia. Drugs: azathioprine, hydrochlorothiazide. **Decreased in:** Pancreatic insufficiency, cystic fibrosis. Usually normal or low in chronic pancreatitis.

Macroamylasemia is indicated by high serum but low urine amylase. Serum or plasma lipase is an alternative test for acute pancreatitis. It has clinical sensitivity equivalent to that of amylase but with better specificity. There is no advantage to performing both tests in diagnosing acute pancreatitis. Amylase isoenzymes are not of practical use because of technical problems. Harper SJ et al. Acute pancreatitis. Ann Clin Biochem 2011;48:23. [PMID: 20926469] Lippi G et al. Laboratory diagnosis of acute pancreatitis: in search of the Holy Grail. Crit Rev Clin Lab Sci 2012;49:18. [PMID: 22339380] Mahajan A et al. Utility of serum pancreatic enzyme levels in diagnosing blunt trauma to the pancreas: a prospective study with systematic review. Injury 2014;45:1384. [PMID: 24702828]

Angiotensin-converting enzyme, serum (ACE)

8–65 U/L

(age-dependent)

Gold SST, red

$$

Separate serum from cells as soon as possible or within 2 hrs after collection.

ACE is part of the renin-angiotensin cascade. It is a dipeptidyl carboxypeptidase that converts angiotensin I to the vasopressor, angiotensin II. ACE is normally present in the kidneys and other peripheral tissues. Serum levels in healthy subjects are dependent on polymorphisms in ACE genes. In granulomatous disease, ACE levels increase, derived from epithelioid cells within granulomas. There is a high level of inter-individual variability in serum ACE due to genetic polymorphism.

Increased in: Sarcoidosis (~60%), hyperthyroidism, acute hepatitis, primary biliary cirrhosis, diabetes mellitus, multiple myeloma, osteoarthritis, amyloidosis, Gaucher disease, pneumoconiosis, histoplasmosis, miliary tuberculosis. Drugs: dexamethasone. **Decreased in:** Renal disease, obstructive pulmonary disease, hypothyroidism.

Serum ACE is elevated in most (~60%) patients with active sarcoidosis. Test is not useful as a screening test for sarcoidosis since the sensitivity is low. Specificity is compromised by positive tests in diseases more common than sarcoidosis. Result needs to be correlated with diagnostic imaging and tissue biopsy findings. Some advocate measurement of ACE to follow disease activity in sarcoidosis; there is a significant decrease in ACE activity in some patients receiving prednisone. Genotyping may increase the utility of ACE in sarcoidosis due to the large interindividual biological variation in ACE levels. Floe A et al. Genotyping increases the yield of angiotensin-converting enzyme in sarcoidosis—a systematic review. Dan Med J 2014;61:A4815. [PMID: 24814734] Heinie R et al. Diagnostic criteria for sarcoidosis. Autoimmun Rev 2014;13:383. [PMID: 24424172] Keir G et al. Assessing pulmonary disease and response to therapy: which test? Semin Respir Crit Care Med 2010;31:409. [PMID: 20665391]

	Antibody screen	Antidiuretic hormone

Test/Range/Collection	Physiologic Basis	Interpretation	Comments
Antibody screen, serum or plasma Red or lavender/pink $ Properly identified and labeled blood specimens are critical.	Detects antibodies to non-ABO red blood cell antigens in recipient's serum or plasma, using reagent red cells selected to possess antigens against which common antibodies can be produced. Further identification of the specificity of any antibody detected (using panels of red cells of known antigenicity) makes it possible to test donor blood for the absence of the corresponding antigen. Primary response to first antigen exposure requires 20–120 days; antibody is largely IgM with a small quantity of IgG. Secondary response requires 1–14 days; antibody is mostly IgG.	**Positive in:** Presence of alloantibody, autoantibodies.	In practice, a type and screen (ABO and Rh grouping and antibody screen) is adequate work-up for patients undergoing operative procedures unlikely to require transfusion. A negative antibody screen implies that a recipient can receive type-specific (ABO-Rh identical) blood with minimal risk. Some antibody activity (eg, anti-Jk^a, anti-E) may become so weak as to be undetectable but increase rapidly after secondary stimulation with the same antigen. *Technical Manual of the American Association of Blood Banks,* 18th ed. American Association of Blood Banks, 2014.
Antidiuretic hormone, plasma (ADH) If serum osmolality > 290 mosm/kg H$_2$O: 2–12 pg/mL If serum osmolality <290 mosm/kg H$_2$O: <2 pg/mL Lavender, pink $$$$ Draw in two chilled tubes and deliver to lab on ice. Specimen for serum osmolality must be drawn at same time.	Antidiuretic hormone, also known as arginine vasopressin (AVP), is a hormone secreted from the posterior pituitary that acts on the distal nephron to conserve water and regulate the tonicity of body fluids. Water deprivation provides both an osmotic and a volume stimulus for ADH release by increasing plasma osmolality and decreasing plasma volume. Water administration lowers plasma osmolality and expands blood volume, inhibiting the release of ADH by the osmoreceptor and the atrial volume receptor mechanisms.	**Increased in:** Nephrogenic diabetes insipidus, syndrome of inappropriate antidiuretic hormone (SIADH), brain tumor. Drugs: nicotine, morphine, chlorpropamide, clofibrate, cyclophosphamide. **Normal relative to plasma osmolality in:** Primary polydipsia. **Decreased in:** Central (neurogenic) diabetes insipidus, water intoxication. Drugs: ethanol, phenytoin.	Test can help to diagnose diabetes insipidus and psychogenic water intoxication. Test very rarely indicated in diagnosis of SIADH: measurement of serum and urine osmolality usually suffices. Patients with SIADH show decreased plasma sodium and decreased plasma osmolality, usually with high urine osmolality relative to plasma. These findings in a normovolemic patient with normal thyroid and adrenal function are sufficient to make the diagnosis of SIADH without measuring ADH itself. Devuyst O et al. Physiopathology and diagnosis of nephrogenic diabetes insipidus. Ann Endocrinol (Paris) 2012;73:128. [PMID: 22503803] Knepper MA et al. Molecular physiology of water balance. N Engl J Med 2015;372:1349. [PMID: 25830425] Peri A et al. Management of euvolemic hyponatremia attributed to SIADH in the hospital setting. Minerva Endocrinol 2014;39:33. [PMID: 24513602]

Antiglobulin test, direct		Antiglobulin test, indirect
Antiglobulin test, direct, red cells (direct Coombs, DAT) Negative Lavender/pink or red $ Blood anticoagulated with EDTA is used to prevent *in vitro* uptake of complement components. A red top tube may be used, if necessary. Direct antiglobulin test (DAT) is used to demonstrate *in vivo* coating of red cells with globulins, in particular IgG and C3d. DAT is performed with a polyspecific reagent that detects both IgG and C3d. If positive, tests with monospecific reagents (anti-IgG and anti-complement) should be performed to characterize the immune process involved.	**Positive in:** Autoimmune hemolytic anemia, hemolytic disease of the newborn, alloimmune reactions to recently transfused cells, and drug-induced hemolysis. Drugs may induce the formation of antibodies, either against the drug itself or against intrinsic red cell antigens. This may lead to a positive DAT, immune red cell destruction, or both. Some of the antibodies produced appear to be dependent on the presence of the drug (eg, penicillin, quinidine, ceftriaxone), whereas others are independent of the continued presence of the inciting drug (eg, methyldopa, levodopa, procainamide, cephalosporins, fludarabine).	A positive DAT implies *in vivo* red cell coating by immunoglobulins or complement. Such red cell coating may or may not be associated with immune hemolytic anemia. The DAT can detect a level of 100–500 molecules of IgG per red cell and 400–1100 molecules of C3d per red cell, depending on the reagent and technique used. Positive DATs without clinical manifestations of immune-mediated red cell destruction are reported in the range of 1 in 1000 up to 1 in 14,000 blood donors and 1–15% of hospital patients. A false-positive DAT is often seen in patients with hypergammaglobulinemia, eg, in some HIV-positive patients. *Technical Manual of the American Association of Blood Banks*, 18th ed. American Association of Blood Banks, 2014.
Antiglobulin test, indirect, serum or plasma (indirect Coombs) Negative Red or lavender, pink $ Indirect antiglobulin test is used to demonstrate the presence in the patient's serum/plasma of unexpected antibody to ABO and Rh-compatible reagent red blood cells. Patient serum or plasma is incubated *in vitro* with reagent red cells, which are then washed to remove unbound globulins. Agglutination that occurs when antihuman globulin (AHG, Coombs) reagent is added indicates that antibody has bound to a specific antigen present on the red cells.	**Positive in:** Presence of alloantibody or autoantibody. Drugs: methyldopa.	The technique is used in antibody detection and identification, and in the AHG crossmatch prior to transfusion (see Type and crossmatch). *Technical Manual of the American Association of Blood Banks*, 18th ed. American Association of Blood Banks, 2014.

(*Continued*)

	Test/Range/Collection	Physiologic Basis	Interpretation	Comments
Antithrombin	**Antithrombin (AT),** plasma 84–123% (enzymatic activity, qualitative) 80–130% (antigen, quantitative) Blue $$ Transport to lab on ice. Plasma must be separated and frozen in a polypropylene tube within 2 hrs.	Antithrombin is a serine protease inhibitor that protects against thrombus formation by inhibiting thrombin and other factors, including IXa, Xa, XIa. It accounts for 70–90% of the anticoagulant activity of human plasma. Its activity is enhanced up to 1000-fold by heparin. There are two types of assay: functional/enzymatic (activity) and immunologic (antigen). Since the immunologic assay cannot rule out functional AT deficiency, a functional assay should be ordered first. Functional assays test AT activity in inhibiting thrombin or factor Xa. Given an abnormal functional assay, the immunologic test indicates whether there is decreased production of AT (type I deficiency) or intact synthesis of a dysfunctional protein (type II deficiency).	**Decreased in:** Congenital and acquired AT deficiency (nephrotic syndrome, chronic liver disease), oral contraceptive use, chronic disseminated intravascular coagulation (DIC), acute venous thrombosis (consumption), L-asparaginase treatment (decreased synthesis) and heparin therapy (consumption).	Congenital or acquired AT deficiency results in a hypercoagulable state, venous thromboembolism, and heparin resistance. Congenital AT deficiency is present in 1:2000–1:3000 people and is autosomal codominant. Heterozygotes have AT levels 20–60% of normal. Evaluation of AT should be considered in patients with venous thrombosis, especially for thrombosis in unusual sites or associated with heparin resistance. Testing should be performed at least 2 months after the thrombotic event, at a time when the patient is not receiving anticoagulants. Cooper PC et al. The phenotypic and genetic assessment of antithrombin deficiency. Int J Lab Hematol 2011;33:227. [PMID: 21401902] Khor B et al. Laboratory tests for antithrombin deficiency. Am J Hematol 2010;85:947. [PMID: 21108326] MacCallum P et al. Diagnosis and management of heritable thrombophilias. BMJ 2014;349:g4387. [PMID: 25035247]
α₁-Antitrypsin	**α₁-Antitrypsin (AAT)** **(α₁-Antiprotease)** serum or plasma 110–270 mg/dL [1.1–2.7 g/L] SST, red, PPT (light green), lavender, pink $$	AAT is an α₁ globulin glycoprotein serine protease inhibitor, encoded by a gene that is located on the long arm of chromosome 14. The designation of PiMM is given to homozygosity for the normal gene alleles. AAT deficiency (inherited via autosomal co-dominant transmission) leads to excessive protease activity and panacinar emphysema in adults or liver disease in children (seen in PiZZ homozygosity and PiSZ compound heterozygosity genotypes). Cirrhosis of the liver and liver cancer in adults are also associated with the PI*ZZ genotype.	**Increased in:** Inflammation, infection, rheumatic disease, malignancy, and pregnancy as an acute-phase reactant. **Decreased in:** Congenital α₁-antitrypsin deficiency (blood AAT levels: deficient, <35% of the average normal functional level), nephrotic syndrome.	The diagnosis of AAT deficiency by measuring serum/plasma AAT level (eg, by nephelometry) can be followed by phenotyping (eg, by isoelectric focusing) or genotyping. Smoking is a much more common cause of chronic obstructive pulmonary disease in adults than is α₁-antitrypsin deficiency. Testing for α₁-antitrypsin deficiency should be done in young patients (<50 year-old with exercise limitation from emphysema), those with emphysema in absence of cigarette smoking, and in presence of familial clustering of emphysema and/or liver disease, basilar predominance of emphysema, or unexplained cirrhosis. Campos MA et al. α1 Antitrypsin deficiency: current best practice in testing and augmentation therapy. Ther Adv Respir Dis 2014;8:150. [PMID: 25013223] Stockley RA. Alpha1-antitrypsin review. Clin Chest Med 2014;35:39. [PMID: 24507836] Teckman JH et al. Advances in alpha-1-antitrypsin deficiency liver disease. Curr Gastroenterol Rep 2014;16:367. [PMID: 24338605]

	Arterial blood gases	Aspartate aminotransferase	B cell immunoglobulin gene rearrangement
Test/Specimen	**Arterial blood gases (ABG)**, whole blood Heparinized syringe $$$ Collect arterial blood in a heparinized syringe, and send to laboratory immediately.	**Aspartate aminotransferase**, serum or plasma (AST, SGOT, GOT) 0–35 IU/L [0–0.58 mckat/L] (laboratory-specific) SST, red, PPT (light green) $	**B-cell immunoglobulin gene rearrangement** Whole blood, bone marrow, frozen or paraffin-embedded tissue Lavender $$$$
Description	Blood gas measurements provide information about cardiopulmonary (oxygen and carbon dioxide exchange) and metabolic (acid-base) status. When integrated with the history and physical examination, the rapidly available arterial blood gas (ABG) analysis is useful in the care of the acutely ill or injured patient.	Intracellular enzyme involved in amino acid metabolism. It catalyzes the reversible transfer of an alpha-amino group between aspartate and glutamate. Present in large concentrations in liver, skeletal muscle, brain, red cells, kidneys and heart. Released into the bloodstream when tissue is damaged, especially in liver injury.	In general, the percentage of B lymphocytes with identical immunoglobulin (heavy chain and/or kappa light chain) gene rearrangements is very low; in malignancies, however, the clonal expansion of one population leads to a large number of cells with identical B-cell immunoglobulin gene rearrangements. B-cell clonality can be assessed by restriction fragment Southern blot, by hybridization, by polymerase chain reaction (PCR) or by DNA sequencing.
Interpretation	See Carbon Dioxide (p. 67), Oxygen (p. 168), and pH (p. 172).	**Increased in:** Acute viral hepatitis (ALT > AST), biliary tract obstruction (cholangitis, choledocholithiasis), alcoholic hepatitis and cirrhosis (AST > ALT), liver abscess, metastatic or primary liver cancer; right heart failure, ischemic or hypoxic injury to liver ("shock liver"), myocardial infarction, acute hemolysis, extensive muscle trauma. Drugs that cause cholestasis or hepatotoxicity. **Decreased in:** Pyridoxine (vitamin B_6) deficiency.	**Positive in:** B-cell neoplasms such as lymphoma/leukemia (monoclonal B-cell proliferation), plasma cell neoplasms.
Comments/References	In addition to the measurement of pH and partial pressures of oxygen and carbon dioxide, the bicarbonate concentration is calculated. Wagner PD. The physiological basis of pulmonary gas exchange: implications for clinical interpretation of arterial blood gases. Eur Respir J 2015;45:227. [PMID: 25323225]	Test is not indicated for diagnosis of myocardial infarction. AST/ALT ratio >1 suggests cirrhosis in patients with hepatitis C. Lee TH et al. Evaluation of elevated liver enzymes. Clin Liver Dis 2012;16:183. [PMID: 22541694] Woreta TA et al. Evaluation of abnormal liver tests. Med Clin North Am 2014;98:1. [PMID: 24266911]	The diagnostic sensitivity and specificity are heterogeneous and laboratory and method-specific. Results of the test must always be interpreted in the context of morphologic and other relevant data (eg, flow cytometry) and should not be used alone for a diagnosis of malignancy. The test is primarily for initial diagnosis, but may also be used to detect minimal residual disease based on unique DNA signatures present at the initial diagnosis. Fan H et al. Detection of clonal immunoglobulin heavy chain gene rearrangements by the polymerase chain reaction and capillary gel electrophoresis. Methods Mol Biol 2013;999:151. [PMID: 23666696] Kokovic I et al. Diagnostic value of immunoglobulin κ light chain gene rearrangement analysis in B-cell lymphomas. Int J Oncol 2015;46:953. [PMID: 25501347]

(Continued)

	BCR/ABL, t(9;22) translocation by RT-PCR	
Test/Range/Collection	**Physiologic Basis**	**Interpretation**	**Comments**
---	---	---	---
BCR-ABL, t(9;22) translocation by RT-PCR Negative Blood, bone marrow Lavender $$$$	Approximately 95% of cases of chronic myelogenous leukemia (CML) have the characteristic t(9;22)(q34;q11) that results in a *BCR-ABL* gene fusion on the derived chromosome 22, called the Philadelphia (Ph) chromosome. The remaining cases either have a cryptic translocation between 9q34 and 22q11 that cannot be identified by routine cytogenetic analysis, or have variant translocations involving a third or even a fourth chromosome besides 9 and 22. The *BCR-ABL* fusion transcript is found in all cases of CML, including those with a cryptic or variant translocation. A subset of acute lymphoblastic leukemia (ALL) and occasionally acute myelogenous leukemia (AML, mostly CML blast crisis) also have the Ph chromosome, and therefore are positive for *BCR-ABL*, t(9;22) translocation.	**Positive in:** All CML, a subset of acute lymphoblastic leukemia (ALL), and rare acute myeloid leukemia (eg, CML blast crisis).	This assay can also be used to distinguish between the major and minor transcripts. The major transcript, characterized by the p210 fusion gene product, is typically detected in CML. The minor transcript, characterized by the p190 fusion gene product, is typically detected in ALL. Detection limit of RT-PCR based assays is at least 1 in 100,000 cells. Small amounts of p190 transcript can be detected in most patients with CML, due to alternative splicing of the *BCR* gene. Both qualitative and quantitative RT-PCR assays for BCR-ABL/t(9;22) are used. The qualitative assay is typically used for the initial diagnosis. For treatment monitoring and follow-up, a quantitative assay should be used (every 3–6 months). Note that the quantitative assay may not distinguish between the major and minor *BCR-ABL* products, although separate quantitative assays for the major (p210) and minor (p190) fusion forms have become available. Quantitative RT-PCR assay that is standardized to the International Scale is recommended. Baccarani M et al. European LeukemiaNet recommendations for the management of chronic myeloid leukemia: 2013. Blood 2013;122:872. [PMID: 23803709] Press RD et al. BCR-ABL1 RT-qPCR for monitoring the molecular response to tyrosine kinase inhibitors in chronic myeloid leukemia. J Mol Diagn 2013;15:565. [PMID: 23810242] Zhen C et al. Molecular monitoring of chronic myeloid leukemia: international standardization of BCR-ABL1 quantitation. J Mol Diagn 2013;15:556. [PMID: 23876601]

BCR/ABL mutation analysis		
BCR-ABL mutation analysis (BCR-ABL genotyping) Blood, bone marrow Lavender $$$$	The analysis involves direct DNA sequencing of the PCR-amplified *BCR-ABL* products. The sequence is then compared with an ABL kinase domain (KD) reference sequence to identify single or multiple mutations. Mutation analysis is usually performed after patients experience TKI (tyrosine kinase inhibitor) treatment resistance, and the results may guide the selection of subsequent TKIs. Next-generation sequencing based mutation analysis is available.	**Positive in:** TKI (eg, imatinib)-resistant chronic myeloid leukemia; TKI (eg, imatinib)-resistant Ph-positive precursor B-lymphoblastic leukemia.	The first and second generations of *BCR-ABL* TKIs (imatinib, dasatinib, nilotinib) are generally effective in Philadelphia chromosome–positive (Ph-positive) leukemias (eg, chronic myeloid leukemia, CML). However, a small but significant fraction of patients may have an inferior response to a TKI, either failing to respond to primary therapy (primary resistance) or demonstrating progression (or relapse) after an initial response (secondary resistance). TKI resistance is mainly due to leukemic subclones with *BCR-ABL* mutation(s) in the ABL kinase domain that interfere with drug binding and activity. The *BCR-ABL* mutation analysis can assist physicians in evaluating resistance to TKI therapy and facilitate appropriate adjustments to treatment (eg, increasing dosage, or switching to another TKI or a non-TKI drug). Mutations at >17 different amino acid positions within the BCR-ABL kinase domain have been associated with clinical resistance to imatinib. Patients with the T315I mutation are also resistant to dasatinib and nilotinib, but not to ponatinib (a third-generation TKI). Alikian M et al. *BCR-ABL1* kinase domain mutations: methodology and clinical evaluation. Am J Hematol 2012;87:298. [PMID: 22231203] Drake JM et al. Clinical targeting of mutated and wild-type protein tyrosine kinases in cancer. Mol Cell Biol 2014;34:1722. [PMID: 24567371] Soverini S et al. Implications of *BCR-ABL1* kinase domain-mediated resistance in chronic myeloid leukemia. Leuk Res 2014;38:10. [PMID: 24131888]

(Continued)

	Beta-D-Glucan, serum	

Test/Range/Collection	Physiologic Basis	Interpretation	Comments
(1,3)-Beta-D-Glucan, serum <60 pg/mL (Fungitell); <20 pg/mL (Fungitec G); <11 pg/mL (Wako) (assay-dependent) Red Separate serum from cells within 2 hrs of collection, and refrigerate. $$$	(1,3)-Beta-D-Glucan (BDG) is a cell wall polysaccharide present in most pathogenic fungi. It is sloughed and released into the bloodstream of patients with invasive fungal infections (eg, aspergillosis or candidiasis). Monitoring serum for evidence of elevated and rising levels of BDG provides a convenient surrogate marker for invasive fungal disease. Test performance and diagnostic cutoff values differ among serum BDG assays, including the Fungitell assay, Fungitec G test, and Wako test.	**Positive in:** Invasive fungal infections caused by *Candida* species, *Acremonium*, *Aspergillus* species, *Coccidioides immitis*, *Fusarium* species, *Histoplasma capsulatum*, *Trichosporon* species, *Sporothrix schenskii*, *Saccharomyces cerevisiae*, and *Pneumocystis jirovecii*. **Negative in:** Invasive fungal infections caused by Zygomycetes (eg, *Absidia*, *Mucor and Rhizopus*).	The BDG test is indicated for presumptive diagnosis of invasive fungal (mold) infection. It should be used in conjunction with other diagnostic procedures. A negative test result does not rule out invasive fungal disease. Test may not detect the yeast phase of *Blastomyces dermatitidis* and certain fungal species such as genus *Cryptococcus*, which produce very little BDG. Patients with renal failure on hemodialysis utilizing cellulose membranes may have false positive results. Patients require 3–4 days for the return to baseline levels of BDG, after surgical exposure to BDG-containing sponges and gauze. The timing of sampling of surgical patients should take this into consideration. Beirão F et al. State of the art diagnostic of mold diseases: a practical guide for clinicians. Eur J Clin Microbiol Infect Dis 2013;32:3. [PMID: 22903167] Frange P et al. An update on pediatric invasive aspergillosis. Med Mal Infect 2015;45:189. [PMID: 26026226] Karageorgopoulos D et al. β-D-glucan assay for the diagnosis of invasive fungal infections: a meta-analysis. Clin Infect Dis 2011;52:750. [PMID 21367728] Schuetz AN. Invasive fungal infections: biomarkers and molecular approaches to diagnosis. Clin Lab Med 2013;33:505. [PMID: 23931836]

Beta-hCG		
Beta-hCG, quantitative, serum Males and nonpregnant females: undetectable or <5 mIU/mL [IU/L] SST, red $$	Human chorionic gonadotropin (hCG) is a glycoprotein made up of two subunits (α and β). The β-subunit is specific for hCG. hCG is produced by trophoblastic tissue, and its detection in serum or urine is the basis for pregnancy testing. Serum hCG can be detected as early as 24 hrs after implantation at a concentration of 5 mIU/mL. During normal pregnancy, serum levels double every 2–3 days and are 50–100 mIU/mL at the time of the first missed menstrual period. Peak levels are reached 60–80 days after the last menstrual period (LMP) (30,000–100,000 mIU/mL), and levels then decrease to a plateau of 5,000–10,000 mIU/mL at about 120 days after LMP and persist until delivery. Regular hCG produced by differentiated syncytiotrophoblast cells primarily functions to promote progesterone production and to maintain the myometrial and the placental vascular supply during the first trimester. Hyperglycosylated hCG (hCG-H) is produced by undifferentiated extravillous cytotrophoblast cells and maintains trophoblast invasion, eg, in implantation of pregnancy. Hyperglyco-sylated hCG and/or free β-subunit are also produced by a high proportion of malignant gestational trophoblastic diseases.	**Increased in:** Pregnancy (including ectopic pregnancy), hyperemesis gravidarum, tropho-blastic tumors (hydatidiform mole, choriocar-cinoma), some germ cell tumors (teratomas, seminoma), ectopic hCG production by other malignancies. **Decreasing over time:** Threatened abortion.	Routine pregnancy testing is done by rapid *qualitative* urine hCG test, or less commonly quantitative serum hCG test. Test is positive (>50 mIU/mL) in most pregnant women at the time of or shortly after the first missed menstrual period. Urine hCG tests are prone to false-negative results; if available, blood hCG test is preferred. *Quantitative* hCG test detects hCG levels as low as 1.0 mIU/mL. It is preferred for the evaluation of suspected ectopic pregnancy and threatened abortion. In both situations, hCG levels fail to demon-strate the normal early pregnancy increase. Test is also indicated for following the course of trophoblastic and germ cell tumors. Most commercially available hCG tests detect only regular hCG. In patients with malignancies that produce primarily hyperglycosyl-ated hCG (hCG-H), the test should be interpreted with caution. Kirk E et al. Diagnosing ectopic pregnancy and current concepts in the management of pregnancy of unknown location. Hum Reprod Update 2014;20:250. [PMID: 24101604] Montagnana M et al. Human chorionic gonadotropin in pregnancy diagnostics. Clin Chim Acta 2011;412:1515. [PMID: 21635878] Stenman UH et al. Determination of human chorionic gonadotro-pin. Best Pract Res Clin Endocrinol Metab 2013;27:783. [PMID: 24275190]

(Continued)

	Bilirubin	Blood urea nitrogen

Test/Range/Collection	Physiologic Basis	Interpretation	Comments
Bilirubin, serum or plasma 0.1–1.2 mg/dL [2–21 mcmol/L] Direct (conjugated to glucuronide) bilirubin: 0.1–0.4 mg/dL [<7 mcmol/L]; Indirect (unconjugated) bilirubin: 0.2–0.7 mg/dL [<12 mcmol/L] SST, PPT (light green) $$	Bilirubin is the orange-yellow pigment derived from the breakdown of hemoglobin (heme). The majority of bilirubin comes from senescent red cells. It is biotransformed in the liver and excreted in bile and urine. The conjugated form is water-soluble and reacts directly with diazo dyes in the absence of reaction accelerator, and is therefore called direct bilirubin. The unconjugated form is fat-soluble and reacts with diazo dyes only in the presence of accelerator; so it is called indirect. Some conjugated bilirubin is bound to serum albumin, so-called D (delta) bilirubin.	**Increased in:** Acute or chronic hepatitis, cirrhosis, biliary tract obstruction, toxic hepatitis, neonatal jaundice (neonatal hyperbilirubinemia), congenital liver enzyme abnormalities (Dubin-Johnson, Rotor, Gilbert, Crigler-Najjar syndromes), fasting, hemolytic disorders. Hepatotoxic drugs.	Assay of total bilirubin includes conjugated (direct) and unconjugated (indirect) bilirubin. The unconjugated (indirect) form is the difference between total bilirubin (with reaction accelerator) and the direct bilirubin fraction. Delta bilirubin is determined together with conjugated bilirubin. Delta bilirubin (half-life is about 17 days) accounts for relatively slow regression of jaundice. Only conjugated bilirubin appears in the urine, and it is indicative of cholestatic and parenchymal liver diseases. Hemolysis is associated with increased unconjugated bilirubin. Unbound (free) serum or plasma bilirubin level correlates better than total bilirubin with CNS bilirubin concentrations and bilirubin encephalopathy (kernicterus) in newborn jaundice. Muchowski KE. Evaluation and treatment of neonatal hyperbilirubinemia. Am Fam Physician 2014;89:873. [PMID: 25077393] Sticova E et al. New insights in bilirubin metabolism and their clinical implications. World J Gastroenterol 2013;19:6398. [PMID: 24151358] Woreta TA et al. Evaluation of abnormal liver tests. Med Clin North Am 2014;98:1. [PMID: 24266911]
Blood urea nitrogen, serum or plasma (BUN) 8–20 mg/dL [2.9–7.1 mmol/L] SST, PPT (light green) $	Urea is the end product of protein metabolism, which is excreted by the kidney. BUN is directly related to protein intake and nitrogen metabolism and inversely related to the rate of excretion of urea. Urea concentration in glomerular filtrate is the same as in plasma, but its tubular reabsorption is inversely related to the rate of urine formation. Thus, BUN is a less useful measure of glomerular filtration rate than the serum/plasma creatinine (Cr).	**Increased in:** Renal failure (acute or chronic), urinary tract obstruction, dehydration, shock, burns, HF, GI bleeding, nephrotoxic drugs (eg, gentamicin). **Decreased in:** Hepatic failure, nephrotic syndrome, cachexia (low-protein and high carbohydrate diets).	BUN is used to evaluate renal function. It is typically tested along with serum creatinine (Cr). BUN/Cr ratio (normal 10:1–20:1) is decreased in acute tubular necrosis, advanced liver disease, low protein intake, and following hemodialysis. BUN/Cr ratio is increased in dehydration, GI bleeding, and increased catabolism. Bellomo R et al. Acute kidney injury. Lancet 2012;380:756. [PMID: 22617274] Wang H et al. Urea. Subcell Biochem 2014;73:7. [PMID: 25298336]

B-type natriuretic peptide		
B-type natriuretic peptide (BNP), plasma Lavender, pink 0–100 pg/mL [0–347 pmol/L] $$ Point-of-care immunoassays also available.	BNP has biologic effects similar to those of atrial natriuretic peptide (ANP) and is stored mainly in the myocardium of the cardiac ventricles. Blood BNP levels are elevated in hypervolemic states such as heart failure (HF). BNP is useful for guiding and monitoring heart failure treatment and for predicting prognosis. BNP test serves to establish diagnosis and prognosis of HF, and to help guide HF management.	**Increased in:** HF (cutoff concentration: >100 pg/mL yields a sensitivity of 90%, specificity, 73%. BNP <100 pg/mL has a negative predictive value of 90%. BNP >400 pg/mL suggests HF with specificity exceeding 90%). BNP is also increased in a variety of other cardiac and noncardiac diseases including acute coronary syndrome, left ventricular dysfunction, valvular aortic stenosis, pulmonary embolism, and renal insufficiency.	BNP testing is not a substitute for careful cardiopulmonary evaluation and should not be the sole criterion for admission/discharge of a patient. Although normal levels indicate a low probability of HF, they do not exclude it or other serious cardiopulmonary disorders. Moderately increased levels are not specific for HF and can occur with a variety of cardiac and noncardiac diseases. BNP is not recommended for screening for left ventricular dysfunction or hypertrophy in the general population. It is also unnecessary to test BNP in patients with obvious HF (eg, NYHA class IV). Treatment of HF has been reported to decrease BNP levels in parallel with clinical improvement. Tests for N-terminal fragment of pro-BNP (NT-pro-BNP) are also available, and diagnostic performance is comparable to that of BNP. The normal reference intervals of pro-BNP are laboratory-dependent and vary with age and sex. Gaggin HK et al. Biomarkers and diagnostics in heart failure. Biochim Biophys Acta 2013;1832:2442. [PMID: 23313577] Oremus M et al. A systematic review of BNP and NT-proBNP in the management of heart failure: overview and methods. Heart Fail Rev 2014;19:413. [PMID: 24953975] Troughton R et al. Natriuretic peptide–guided heart failure management. Eur Heart J 2014;35:16. [PMID: 24216390]

(Continued)

	BRCA1 and BRCA2 genotyping		
Test/Range/Collection	Physiologic Basis	Interpretation	Comments
BRCA1 and BRCA2 genotyping, whole blood Negative for pathogenic mutations Lavender, pink, or yellow Keep specimen refrigerated during shipment. $$$$	Inactivating germline mutations in tumor suppressor genes BRCA1 and BRCA2 can lead to significantly increased lifetime risks for breast and ovarian cancer, causing a hereditary breast and ovarian cancer syndrome. Pathogenic mutations in BRCA1/2 account for up to 80% of breast and ovarian cancer in families with multiple cases of either disease. It is also associated with higher risk of other types of cancer, including fallopian tube, peritoneal, pancreatic, gastric, prostate, and male breast cancers. Test uses next-generation sequencing technology, Sanger sequencing technology, and PCR techniques.	**Positive in:** Autosomal dominant, pathogenic BRCA1/2 mutations, present in approximately 1 in 400 of the general population in the U.S. Prevalence of mutations varies among different ethnic groups — Ashkenazi Jews: BRCA1 8-10%, BRCA2 1%; Hispanics: BRCA1 3-4%; Caucasians (non-Ashkenazi Jews): BRCA1 2-3%, BRCA2 2%; African Americans: BRCA1 0.5%, BRCA2 2.5%; Asian Americans: BRCA1 0.5%.	Test is indicated for individuals with early onset of breast or ovarian cancer or a strong family history of breast and/or ovarian cancer. Test should not be used as a screening test for the general population. Test results can help choose cancer chemotherapy and novel targeted treatments (eg, poly [ADP-ribose] polymerase inhibitors), and can help determine the extent of surgery, if it is deemed indicated. Testing provides risk estimates for specific populations depending on test results. A true negative test indicates no increased risk for breast or ovarian cancer. A positive test warrants expert genetic counseling. Risk-reducing mastectomy and salpingo-oophorectomy can be effective in reducing occurrence of breast and ovarian cancers. Eccles DM et al. BRCA1 and BRCA2 genetic testing — pitfalls and recommendations for managing variants of uncertain clinical significance. Ann Oncol 2015;26:2057. PMID: 26153499] Kast K et al. Familial breast cancer — targeted therapy in secondary and tertiary prevention. Breast Care (Basel) 2015;10:27. [PMID: 25960722] Nelson HD et al. Risk Assessment, Genetic Counseling, and Genetic Testing for BRCA-Related Cancer: Systematic Review to Update the U.S. Preventive Services Task Force Recommendation [Internet]. Rockville (MD): Agency for Healthcare Research and Quality (US); 2013 Dec. [PMID: 24432435]

| Brucella antibodies, serum

Negative

SST, red

$ | Patients with acute brucellosis generally develop an agglutinating antibody titer of >1:160 within 3 weeks.
The titer may rise during the acute infection, with relapses, brucellergin skin testing, or use of certain vaccines (see Interpretation).
The agglutinin titer usually declines after 3 months or after successful therapy.
Low titers may persist for years.
Indirect enzyme-linked immunosorbent assays (ELISA) measuring IgM, IgG, and IgA antibodies have higher sensitivity and specificity than the agglutinating antibody test.
Routine use of PCR and RT-PCR assays for diagnosis of human brucellosis needs further clinical evaluation. | **Positive in:** *Brucella* infection (except *B. canis*) (97% within 3 weeks of illness); recent brucellergin skin test; infections with *Francisella tularensis, Yersinia enterocolitica,* salmonella, Rocky Mountain spotted fever; vaccinations for cholera and tularemia.
Negative in: *B. canis* infection. | This test detects antibodies against all of the *Brucella* species except *B. canis.* Test is not internationally standardized.
A fourfold or greater rise in titer in separate specimens drawn 1–4 weeks apart is indicative of recent exposure.
Since titers can remain high for a prolonged period despite successful therapy, they are not suitable for patient follow-up.
Specimens testing positive or equivocal for *Brucella* antibodies by ELISA should be confirmed by bacterial agglutination. Final diagnosis depends on isolation of organism by culture.
Al Dahouk S et al. New developments in the diagnostic procedures for zoonotic brucellosis in humans. Rev Sci Tech 2013;32:177. [PMID: 23837375]
Ulu-Kilic A et al. Clinical presentations and diagnosis of brucellosis. Recent Pat Antiinfect Drug Discov 2013;8:34. [PMID: 22873352] |

Brucella antibody

(Continued)

	C-peptide	
Test/Range/Collection	**Physiologic Basis**	**Interpretation**	**Comments**

Test/Range/Collection	Physiologic Basis	Interpretation	Comments
C-peptide, serum or plasma 0.8–4.0 ng/mL [mcg/L] (0.26–1.3 nmol/L) SST, PPT (light green), lavender $$$ Fasting sample preferred.	C-peptide is an inactive by-product of the cleavage of proinsulin to active insulin. It is produced in equal amounts to insulin and its presence indicates endogenous release of insulin. The half-life of C-peptide in the blood is about 30 min. C-peptide is largely excreted by the kidney.	**Increased in:** Renal failure, ingestion of oral hypoglycemic drugs, insulinomas, Beta-cell transplants. **Decreased in:** Factitious hypoglycemia due to insulin administration, pancreatectomy, type 1 diabetes mellitus (decreased or undetectable).	Test is most useful to detect factitious insulin injection (increased insulin, decreased C-peptide) or endogenous insulin production in diabetic patients receiving insulin (C-peptide present). A random C-peptide level has reasonable discriminatory power for determining type 1 vs type 2 diabetes. A molar ratio of insulin to C-peptide >1.0 in peripheral venous blood in a hypoglycemic patient is consistent with surreptitious or inadvertent insulin administration but not insulinoma. Measurement of insulin release using C-peptide can assist in classification and management of diabetes. Persistent and substantial insulin secretion suggests type 2 diabetes, whereas absence of C-peptide indicates the appropriateness of type 1 diabetes management strategies including insulin therapy. C-peptide levels of 2 nmol/L or greater suggest insulinoma. Besser RE. Determination of C-peptide in children: when is it useful? Pediatr Endocrinol Rev 2013;10:494. [PMID: 23957200] Jones AG et al. The clinical utility of C-peptide measurement in the care of patients with diabetes. Diabet Med 2013;30:803. [PMID: 23413806] Pietropaolo M. Persistent C-peptide: what does it mean? Curr Opin Endocrinol Diabetes Obes 2013;20:279. [PMID: 23743645]

C-reactive protein, high sensitivity

| **C-reactive protein, high sensitivity (hs-CRP)**, serum or plasma

<1.0 mg/L (lower 95th percentile)

SST, light green PPT

$ | CRP is an acute–phase reactant protein. Hepatic secretion is stimulated in response to inflammatory cytokines. Unlike other acute-phase proteins, CRP is not affected by hormones. CRP activates the complement system, binds to Fc receptors, and serves as an opsonin for some microorganisms.
Rapid, marked increases in CRP occur with inflammation, infection, trauma and tissue necrosis, malignancies, and autoimmune disorders.
CRP levels are also valuable in assessing vascular inflammation and cardiovascular risk stratification. CRP level has been shown to be an independent risk factor for atherosclerotic disease. Elevated CRP levels are associated with increased cardiovascular morbidity and mortality in patients with coronary artery disease. | **Increased in:** Inflammatory states, including arteriosclerotic disorders. | CRP is a very sensitive but nonspecific marker of inflammation. A variety of conditions other than arteriosclerosis may cause dramatic increases in CRP levels. CRP levels increase within 2 hrs of acute insult (eg, surgery, infection) and should peak and begin decreasing within 48 hrs if no other inflammatory event occurs. In patients with rheumatoid arthritis, persistently elevated CRP concentrations are present when the disease is active and usually fall to normal during periods of complete remission.
Patients with high hs-CRP concentrations are more likely to develop stroke, myocardial infarction, and severe peripheral vascular disease. hs-CRP results are used to assign risk as follows: <1.0 mg/L lowest tertile, lowest risk; 1.0–3.0 mg/L middle tertile, average risk; >3.0 mg/L highest tertile, highest risk.
Noncardiovascular cause should be considered if CRP values are >10 mg/L with repeat measurements.
Algarra M et al. Current analytical strategies for C-reactive protein quantification in blood. Clin Chim Acta 2013;415:1. [PMID: 22975530]
Dallmeier D et al. Strategies for vascular disease prevention: the role of lipids and related markers including apolipoproteins, LDL particle size, hs-CRP, Lp-PLA₂ and Lp(a). Best Pract Res Clin Endocrinol Metab 2014;28:281. [PMID: 24840259]
Rudolf J et al. Cholesterol, lipoproteins, high-sensitivity C-reactive protein, and other risk factors for atherosclerosis. Clin Lab Med 2014;34:113. [PMID: 24507791]. |

(Continued)

C1 esterase inhibitor (C1-INH)			
Test/Range/Collection	**Physiologic Basis**	**Interpretation**	**Comments**
C1 esterase inhibitor (C1 INH), serum 20–40 mg/dL (antigenic); >68% of normal (functional) (method-dependent) SST $$ Separate serum from cells ASAP or within 2 hrs of collection, and freeze if test cannot be performed within 2 hrs.	C1 esterase inhibitor (complement 1 inhibitor or C1 INH) is an acute-phase reactant protein and a broad-spectrum protease inhibitor. It controls the first stage of the classic complement pathway and also inhibits thrombin, plasmin, activated Hageman factor (factor XIIa) and kallikrein. C1 INH deficiency results in spontaneous activation of C1, leading to consumption of C2 and C4. Deficiency also causes release of bradykinin, leading to angioedema. Both antigenic and functional C1 INH assays are available. The antigen level is measured by immunoassay (eg, quantitative nephelometry). The functional assay measures the function of C1 INH, by its inhibition of the hydrolysis of a substrate ester by C1 esterase.	**Decreased in:** Hereditary angioedema (HAE), acquired angioedema (eg, related to B-cell lymphoma or autoimmune disorder).	C1 esterase inhibitor deficiency is an uncommon cause of angioedema. There are three subtypes of HAE. In type 1 (~85%), both antigenic and functional levels are low; in type 2 (~15%), antigenic level is normal but functional level is decreased; in type 3 (rare), the C1-INH levels are normal. Types 1 and 2 are caused by autosomal dominant mutations of the C1 INH gene. In some families, type 3 HAE has been linked to mutations in the Hageman factor (so-called FXII-HAE). Acquired angioedema has been attributed to massive consumption of C1 INH (presumably by tumor or lymphoma-related immune complexes) or to anti-C1 INH autoantibodies. When clinical suspicion exists, a serum C4 level screens for HAE. Low levels of C4 are present in all cases during an attack. C1 INH levels are indicated if the C4 level is low or there is a very high clinical suspicion of HAE in a patient with normal C4 during an asymptomatic phase between attacks. Recombinant human C1 INH (rhC1-INH) has been approved for the treatment of HAE. Altman KA et al. Hereditary angioedema: a brief review of new developments. Curr Med Res Opin 2014;30:923. [PMID: 24432781] Bork K et al. Overview of hereditary angioedema caused by C1-inhibitor deficiency: assessment and clinical management. Eur Ann Allergy Clin Immunol 2013;45:7. [PMID: 23678554] Cicardi M et al. Classification, diagnosis, and approach to treatment for angioedema: consensus report from the Hereditary Angioedema International Working Group. Allergy 2014;69:602. [PMID: 24673465]

	Calcitonin	Calcium, serum or plasma
Test / Specimen / Reference Range	Calcitonin, plasma or serum Males: <8 pg/mL [ng/L] Females: <6 pg/mL [ng/L] Green, SST $$$ Separate serum/plasma from cells ASAP or within 2 hrs and refrigerate or freeze	Calcium, serum or plasma (Ca^{2+}) 8.5–10.5 mg/dL [2.1–2.6 mmol/L] **Panic:** <6.5 or >13.5 mg/dL SST, PPT (light green) $ Prolonged venous stasis during collection causes false increase in serum calcium.
Physiologic Basis	Calcitonin is a 32-amino-acid polypeptide hormone secreted by the parafollicular C cells of the thyroid. It decreases osteoclastic bone resorption and lowers serum calcium levels.	Serum calcium is the sum of ionized calcium plus complexed calcium and calcium bound to proteins (mostly albumin). Level of ionized calcium is regulated by parathyroid hormone and vitamin D.
Interpretation	**Increased in:** Medullary thyroid carcinoma, Zollinger-Ellison syndrome, pernicious anemia, pregnancy (at term), newborns, carcinoma (breast, lung, pancreas), leukemia, myeloproliferative disorders, chronic renal failure.	**Increased in:** Hyperparathyroidism, malignancies secreting parathyroid hormone-related protein (PTHrP) (especially squamous cell carcinoma of lung and renal cell carcinoma), vitamin D excess, milk-alkali syndrome, multiple myeloma, Paget disease of bone with immobilization, sarcoidosis, other granulomatous disorders, familial hypocalciuria, vitamin A intoxication, thyrotoxicosis, Addison disease. Drugs: antacids (some), calcium salts, chronic diuretic use (eg, thiazides), lithium, others. **Decreased in:** Hypoparathyroidism (acquired or familial), vitamin D deficiency, renal insufficiency, pseudohypoparathyroidism, magnesium deficiency, hyperphosphatemia, massive transfusion, hypoalbuminemia. Drugs: phenytoin, colchicine.
Comments	Test is useful to diagnose and monitor medullary thyroid carcinoma, although stimulation tests may be necessary (using, eg, pentagastrin or calcium as the stimulant). Genetic testing (eg, *RET* mutation test) is now available for the diagnosis and management of multiple endocrine neoplasia type II, and for early disease detection in asymptomatic carriers and high-risk patients. (MEN II is the most common familial form of medullary thyroid carcinoma.) Griebeler ML et al. Medullary thyroid carcinoma. Endocr Pract 2013;19:703. [PMID: 23512389] Trimboli P et al. Medullary thyroid cancer diagnosis: an appraisal. Head Neck 2014;36:1216. [PMID: 23955938] Verburg FA et al. Calcium stimulated calcitonin measurement: a procedural proposal. Exp Clin Endocrinol Diabetes 2013;121:318. [PMID: 23430575]	Need to know serum albumin to interpret total calcium level. For every decrease in albumin by 1 mg/dL, calcium should be corrected upward by 0.8 mg/dL. In 10% of patients with malignancies, hypercalcemia is attributable to coexistent hyperparathyroidism, suggesting that serum PTH levels should be measured at initial presentation of all hypercalcemic patients (see Figure 9–15). Ahmad S et al. Hypercalcemic crisis: a clinical review. Am J Med 2015;128:239. [PMID: 25447624] Eastell R et al. Diagnosis of asymptomatic primary hyperparathyroidism: proceedings of the Fourth International Workshop. J Clin Endocrinol Metab 2014;99:3570. [PMID: 25162666] Michels TC et al. Parathyroid disorders. Am Fam Physician 2013;88:249. [PMID: 23944728]

(Continued)

Test/Range/Collection	Physiologic Basis	Interpretation	Comments
Calcium, ionized, serum or whole blood	Calcium circulates in three forms: as free Ca^{2+} (50–55%), protein-bound to albumin and globulins (40–45%), and as calcium-ligand complexes (5–10%) (with citrate, bicarbonate, lactate, phosphate, and sulfate). Protein binding is highly pH-dependent, and acidosis results in an increased free calcium fraction.	**Increased in:** ↓ Blood pH. **Decreased in:** ↑ Blood pH, citrate, EDTA.	Ionized calcium measurements are not needed except in special circumstances, eg, massive blood transfusion, transfusion of whole blood in neonates, liver transplantation, neonatal hypocalcemia, cardiac bypass surgery, critical illness, and possibly monitoring of patients with secondary hyperparathyroidism from renal failure. Validity of test depends on sample integrity.
4.4–5.4 mg/dL (at pH 7.4) [1.1–1.3 mmol/L]	Ionized Ca^{2+} is the form that is physiologically active. Ionized calcium is a more accurate reflection of physiologic status than total calcium in patients with altered serum proteins (renal failure, nephrotic syndrome, multiple myeloma, etc), altered concentrations of calcium-binding ligands, and acid-base disturbances. Measurement of ionized calcium is by ion-selective electrodes.		Ionized calcium normalized to pH 7.4 should be interpreted with caution and along with patient's acid/base status. See diagnostic algorithms for hypercalcemia and hypocalcemia (Figures 9–15 and 9–17).
Whole blood specimen must be collected anaerobically and anticoagulated with standardized amounts of heparin. Tourniquet application must be brief. Specimen should be analyzed promptly.			French S et al. Calcium abnormalities in hospitalized patients. South Med J 2012;105:231. [PMID: 22475676]
SST, green (for whole blood)	Ionized calcium levels vary inversely with pH, about 0.2 mg/dL per 0.1 pH unit change.		Kelly A et al. Hypocalcemia in the critically ill patient. J Intensive Care Med 2013;28:166. [PMID: 21841146]
$			

Calcium, ionized

Calcium, urine, 24-hour		
Calcium, urine (U_{Ca}), 24 hour 20–300 mg/24 hr [2.5–7.5 mmol/24 hr or 2.3–3.3 mmol/12 hr] (for persons with average calcium intake, ie, 600–800 mg/day) Urine bottle containing hydrochloric acid $$$ Collect 24-hour urine or 12-hour overnight urine. Refrigerate during collection.	Calcium is one of the most common elements in the body. It is excreted in urine. Ordinarily, there is moderate urinary calcium excretion, the amount depending on dietary calcium, parathyroid hormone (PTH) level, and protein intake. Renal calculi occur much more often in those with hyperparathyroidism than in other hypercalcemic states.	**Increased in:** Hyperparathyroidism, osteolytic bone metastases, myeloma, osteoporosis, vitamin D intoxication, distal renal tubular acidosis (RTA), idiopathic hypercalciuria, milk-alkali syndrome, thyrotoxicosis, Paget disease, Fanconi syndrome, hepatolenticular degeneration, schistosomiasis, sarcoidosis, malignancy (breast, bladder), osteitis deformans, immobilization. Drugs: acetazolamide, calcium salts, cholestyramine, corticosteroids, dihydrotachysterol, initial diuretic use (eg, furosemide), others. **Decreased in:** Hypoparathyroidism, pseudo-hypoparathyroidism, rickets, osteomalacia, nephrotic syndrome, acute glomerulo-nephritis, osteoblastic bone metastases, hypothyroidism, celiac disease (gluten enteropathy), steatorrhea, familial hypocalciuric hypercalcemia, other causes of hypocalcemia. Drugs: aspirin, bicarbonate, chronic diuretic use (eg, thiazides, chlorthalidone), estrogens, indomethacin, lithium, neomycin, oral contraceptives.	Approximately one third of patients with hyperparathyroidism have normal urine calcium excretion. The extent of calcium excretion can be expressed as a urine calcium (U_{Ca})/urine creatinine (U_{Cr}) ratio. Normally, $$\frac{U_{Ca}\,(mg/dL)}{U_{Cr}\,(mg/dL)} < 0.14$$ or $$\frac{U_{Ca}\,(mmol/L)}{U_{Cr}\,(mmol/L)} < 0.40$$ Hypercalciuria is defined as a ratio of >0.22 or >0.57, respectively. Test is useful in the evaluation of renal stones but is not usually needed for the diagnosis of hyperparathyroidism, which can be made using serum calcium (see above) and PTH measurements (see Figure 10–8). It may be useful in hypercalcemic patients to rule out familial hypocalciuric hypercalcemia in which patients have urine calcium/creatinine ratio <0.01 and urine calcium <200 mg/day. This autosomal dominant condition usually does not require treatment. Interpret a random urine calcium/creatinine ratio with caution. For hypercalciuria detection, a 24-hr urine calcium is preferred. Christensen SE et al. Familial hypocalciuric hypercalcaemia: a review. Curr Opin Endocrinol Diabetes Obes 2011;18:359. [PMID: 21986511] Jones AN et al. Fasting and postprandial spot urine calcium-to-creatinine ratios do not detect hypercalciuria. Osteoporos Int 2012;23:553. [PMID: 21347742] Pak CY et al. Defining hypercalciuria in nephrolithiasis. Kidney Int 2011;80:777. [PMID: 21775970]

(Continued)

Test/Range/Collection	Physiologic Basis	Interpretation	Comments
Calreticulin mutation analysis (*CALR* mutation), whole blood Lavender, yellow $$$$	Calreticulin is a multifunctional calcium-binding protein localized in the endoplasmic reticulum. Somatic frame-shift mutation (insertions or deletions) in exon 9 of the *CALR* gene is present in the majority of *JAK2/MPL* unmutated cases of essential thrombocythemia (ET) and primary myelofibrosis (PMF). *CALR* mutation is therefore an important diagnostic marker in ET and PMF. Its pathogenic role in ET/PMF remains to be elucidated.	**Positive in:** Myeloproliferative neoplasma, ie, in ~25% of cases of essential thrombocythemia (ET) and ~35% of cases of primary myelofibrosis (PMF); ~10% of patients with refractory anemia with ring sideroblasts and marked thrombocytosis (RARS-T).	*JAK2* V617F mutation is the most frequent genetic mutation in ET and PMF, present in 60–65% of cases. *MPL* gene mutation is seen in an additional 3–5% of ET and PMF cases. Among *JAK2/MPL*-unmutated ET/PMF cases, 70–88% have *CALR* mutation. *CALR* mutation and *JAK2/MPL* mutation are mutually exclusive in ET/PMF. *CALR* mutation has not been found in polycythemia vera patients. The most common *CALR* mutation types (85%) are 52 bp deletion (type 1) and 5 bp insertion (type 2) in exon 9 of the gene. While a positive result helps to establish the diagnosis of myeloproliferative neoplasm (ET and PMF), a negative result does not rule it out. Compared with *JAK2* mutation, *CALR* mutations are associated with lower Hgb level, lower leukocyte count, higher platelet count, and probably better survival in ET/PMF patients. Klampfl T et al. Somatic mutations of calreticulin in myeloproliferative neoplasms. N Engl J Med 2013;369:2379. [PMID: 24325356] Nangalia J et al. Somatic *CALR* mutations in myeloproliferative neoplasms with nonmutated *JAK2*. N Engl J Med 2013;369:2391. [PMID: 24325359] Tefferi A et al. An overview on *CALR* and *CSF3R* mutations and a proposal for revision of WHO diagnostic criteria for myeloproliferative neoplasms. Leukemia 2014;28:1407. [PMID: 24441292]
Carbon dioxide, partial pressure (PCO₂), whole blood Arterial: 32–48 mm Hg (4.26–6.38 kPa) Heparinized syringe $$$ Specimen must be collected in heparinized syringe and immediately transported on ice to lab without exposure to air.	The partial pressure of carbon dioxide in arterial blood (PCO_2) provides important information with regard to adequacy of ventilation-perfusion, and acid–base status.	**Increased in:** Respiratory acidosis: decreased alveolar ventilation (eg, COPD, respiratory depressants), ventilation-perfusion imbalance, neuromuscular diseases (eg, myasthenia gravis). **Decreased in:** Respiratory alkalosis: hyperventilation (eg, anxiety), sepsis, liver disease, fever, early salicylate poisoning, and excessive artificial ventilation.	See laboratory characteristics of acid–base disturbances (Figure 9–1, Table 8–1). Wagner PD. The physiological basis of pulmonary gas exchange: implications for clinical interpretation of arterial blood gases. Eur Respir J 2015;45:227. [PMID: 25323225] West JB. Causes of and compensations for hypoxemia and hypercapnia. Compr Physiol 2011;1:1541. [PMID: 23733653]

Calreticulin (*CALR*) mutation analysis | **Carbon dioxide, partial pressure**

(Continued)

	Carbon dioxide (total bicarbonate)	Carboxyhemoglobin (COHb)
Test/Specimen	**Carbon dioxide (total bicarbonate),** serum or plasma 22–28 meq/L [mmol/L] **Panic:** <15 or >40 meq/L [mmol/L] SST, PPT (light green) $	**Carboxyhemoglobin (COHb),** whole blood (COHb, %) <2% [non-smokers] <9% [smokers] Blood gas syringe or green $$ Specimen should be collected before treatment with oxygen is started. Do not remove stopper or cap. Refrigerate within 30 min after collection, if needed.
Physiologic Basis	Bicarbonate–carbonic acid buffer is one of the most important buffer systems in maintaining normal body fluid pH. Total carbon dioxide (CO_2) is measured as the sum of bicarbonate (HCO_3^-) concentration and dissolved CO_2 (carbonic acid concentration plus dissolved free CO_2). Total CO_2 measurements use either electrode-based or enzymatic methods. Because HCO_3^- makes up 90–95% of the total CO_2 content, total CO_2 is a useful surrogate for HCO_3^- concentration.	Carbon monoxide (CO) is an odorless and nonirritating gas formed by hydrocarbon combustion. CO binds to hemoglobin with much greater affinity (~240 times) than oxygen, forming carboxyhemoglobin (COHb) and resulting in impaired oxygen transport/delivery and utilization. CO can also precipitate an inflammatory cascade that results in CNS lipid peroxidation and delayed neurologic sequelae.
Interpretation	**Increased in:** Primary metabolic alkalosis, compensated respiratory acidosis, volume contraction, mineralocorticoid excess, congenital chloridorrhea. Drugs: diuretics (eg, thiazide, furosemide). **Decreased in:** Metabolic acidosis, compensated respiratory alkalosis. Fanconi syndrome, volume overload. Drugs: acetazolamide, outdated tetracycline.	**Increased in:** Carbon monoxide poisoning, exposure to automobile exhaust, smoke from fires, coal gas, and defective furnaces. Cigarette smokers can have up to 9% carboxyhemoglobin, while nonsmokers have <2%.
Comments	Total CO_2 determination is indicated for all seriously ill patients on admission. Simultaneous measurement of HCO_3^-, pH, and PCO_2 is required to fully characterize a patient's acid–base status. See Acid–base disturbance (Table 8–1; Figure 9–1). Brown D et al. Molecular mechanisms of acid-base sensing by the kidney. J Am Soc Nephrol 2012;23:774. [PMID: 22362904] Curthoys NP et al. Proximal tubule function and response to acidosis. Clin J Am Soc Nephrol 2014;9:1627. [PMID: 23908456] Wagner PD. The physiological basis of pulmonary gas exchange: implications for clinical interpretation of arterial blood gases. Eur Respir J 2015;45:227. [PMID: 25323225]	Laboratory CO-oximetry is widely available for rapid evaluation of CO poisoning. Toxic effects (headache, dizziness, nausea, confusion, and/or unconsciousness) occur if the COHb level is >10–15%. Levels >40% may be fatal if not treated immediately with oxygen. PO_2 is usually normal in CO poisoning. Guzman JA. Carbon monoxide poisoning. Crit Care Clin 2012;28:537. [PMID: 22998990] Hampson NB et al. Practice recommendations in the diagnosis, management, and prevention of carbon monoxide poisoning. Am J Respir Crit Care Med 2012;186:1095. [PMID: 23087025]

Test/Range/Collection	Physiologic Basis	Interpretation	Comments
Carcinoembryonic antigen (CEA)			
Carcinoembryonic antigen, serum (CEA) <2.5 ng/mL [mcg/L] SST $$ Separate serum from cells ASAP or within 2 hr of collection	CEA is an oncofetal antigen, a glycoprotein associated with certain malignancies, particularly epithelial tumors (eg, colorectal cancer, pancreatic cancer, etc).	**Increased in:** Colorectal cancer (72%), lung cancer (76%), pancreatic cancer (91%), stomach cancer (61%), cigarette smokers, benign acute (50%) and chronic (90%) liver disease, benign GI disease (peptic ulcer, pancreatitis, colitis). Elevations >20 ng/mL are generally associated with malignancy. For breast cancer recurrence (using 5 ng/mL cutoff), sensitivity is 44.4% and specificity, 95.5%.	**Screening:** Test is not sensitive or specific enough to be useful in cancer screening. CEA levels should be used in conjunction with clinical evaluation and other diagnostic procedures. **Monitoring after surgery:** Test is used to detect recurrence of colorectal cancer after surgery (elevated CEA levels suggest recurrence 3–6 months before other clinical indicators), although such monitoring has not yet been shown to improve survival rates. If monitoring is done, the same assay method must be used consistently to eliminate any method-dependent variability. CEA levels in pancreatic cyst fluid may help manage mucinous cystic neoplasm, although the accuracy and the cut-off level vary among laboratories. Bhutani MS et al. Pancreatic cyst fluid analysis—a review. J Gastrointestin Liver Dis 2011;20:175. [PMID: 21725515] Fahy BN. Follow-up after curative resection of colorectal cancer. Ann Surg Oncol 2014;21:738. [PMID: 24271157] Grunnet M et al. Carcinoembryonic antigen (CEA) as tumor marker in lung cancer. Lung Cancer 2012;76:138. [PMID: 22153832]
CD4 cell count			
CD4 cell count, absolute, whole blood CD4: 359–1725 cells/mcL (29–61%) Lavender, yellow $$$ For an absolute CD4 count, order T-cell subsets and a CBC with differential.	Lymphocyte identification depends on specific cell surface CD (clusters of differentiation) antigens, which can be detected by flow cytometry analysis using monoclonal antibodies. The CD4 cells (helper T cells) express both CD3 (a pan–T-cell marker) and CD4. The CD8 cells (suppressor T cells) express both CD3 and CD8. CD4 cell levels are used to categorize HIV-related clinical conditions by CDC's classification system for HIV infection. The measurement of CD4 cell levels has been used to establish decision points for initiating prophylaxis for various opportunistic infections and for monitoring the efficacy of antiretroviral therapy.	**Increased in:** Rheumatoid arthritis, type 1 diabetes mellitus, SLE without renal disease, primary biliary cirrhosis, atopic dermatitis, Sézary syndrome, psoriasis, chronic autoimmune hepatitis. **Decreased in:** AIDS/HIV infection, SLE with renal disease, acute cytomegalovirus (CMV) infection, burns, graft-versus-host disease, sunburn, myelodysplastic syndromes, acute lymphoblastic leukemia in remission, recovery from bone marrow transplantation, herpes infection, infectious mononucleosis, measles, ataxia-telangiectasia, vigorous exercise.	During HIV infection, when the absolute CD4 count drops below 200 cells/mcL, therapeutic prophylaxis against *Pneumocystis jirovecii* pneumonia (PCP) and other opportunistic infections may be initiated. When the absolute CD4 count drops below 100 cells/mcL, prophylaxis against *Mycobacterium avium* complex is recommended. For patients who are doing well on therapy (virologically suppressed, CD4 count >300/mcL), monitoring the CD4 cell count more than once a year is unnecessary. For longitudinal studies involving serial monitoring, specimen collections should be performed at the same time of day. Anglemyer A et al. Early initiation of antiretroviral therapy in HIV-infected adults and adolescents: a systematic review. AIDS 2014;28:S105. [PMID: 24849469] Ford N et al. The future role of CD4 cell count for monitoring antiretroviral therapy. Lancet Infect Dis 2015;15:241. [PMID: 25467647] Gale HB et al. Is frequent CD4+ T-lymphocyte count monitoring necessary for persons with counts ≥300 cells/μL and HIV-1 suppression? Clin Infect Dis 2013;56:1340. [PMID: 23315315]

	Positive in:	
Celiac disease (gluten enteropathy) serologic testing, serum Negative SST, red $$$$ Patient on gluten-containing diet. Separate serum from cells ASAP or within 2 hrs of collection, then refrigerate or freeze.	**Positive in:** Celiac disease (gluten enteropathy) (anti-tTG sensitivity, 90%; specificity ~95%).	Celiac disease (gluten-sensitive enteropathy) is associated with a variety of autoantibodies, including IgA anti-tissue transglutaminase (tTG) antibodies. Although the IgA isotype of these antibodies usually predominates in celiac disease (gluten enteropathy), individuals may also produce IgG isotypes, particularly those who are IgA deficient. The most sensitive and specific serologic test is the tTG antibody test. For patients with IgA deficiency, serum IgG anti-tTG, should be tested.	Useful for evaluating patients suspected of having celiac disease (gluten enteropathy), including patients with compatible symptoms, those with atypical symptoms, and those at increased risk (family history and/or positivity for HLA DQ2 and/or DQ8 alleles). Those with positive laboratory results should then be referred for small intestinal (duodenum) biopsy to confirm the diagnosis. Celiac disease (gluten enteropathy) is caused by a combination of genetic (HLA DQ2 and/or DQ8 alleles) and environmental (gluten ingestion) factors. Genotyping for HLA-DQ2/DQ8 may be useful in ruling out celiac disease (gluten enteropathy) in certain clinical situations (eg, equivocal duodenal biopsy finding in a seronegative patient). Lebwohl B et al. Diagnosis of celiac disease. Gastrointest Endosc Clin N Am 2012;22:661. [PMID: 23083985] Tonutti E et al. Diagnosis and classification of celiac disease and gluten sensitivity. Autoimmun Rev 2014;13:472. [PMID: 24440147]
Centromere antibodies, serum (ACA) Negative SST $$ Separate serum from cells ASAP or within 2 hrs of collection, refrigerate or freeze.	**Positive in:** CREST syndrome (calcinosis, Raynaud phenomenon, esophageal dysmotility, sclerodactyly, and telangiectasia) (80–90%), diffuse scleroderma (5–10%), Raynaud disease (20–30%).	Centromere antibodies (ACA) are antibodies to nuclear proteins, specifically CENP-A, -B, and -C. The CENP-B is the primary autoantigen and is recognized by all sera that contain ACA. Presence of ACA predicts a favorable prognosis for systemic sclerosis. Both immunofluorescent antibody testing (IFA)- and enzyme-linked immunosorbent assay (ELISA)-based assays are available for ACA detection.	ACA correlate with limited skin involvement and high risk of vascular complications, eg, pulmonary hypertension. In patients with connective tissue disease, the predictive value of a positive ACA test is >95% for scleroderma or related disease (CREST syndrome, Raynaud disease). Nevertheless, diagnosis of CREST syndrome is made clinically. The presence of detectable ACA may antedate the development of clinical CREST syndrome by several years. In addition to ACA, tests for autoantibodies targeting topoisomerase-I and RNA polymerase also help diagnose and subclassify systemic sclerosis. ACA is also present in a small percentage of patients with primary biliary cirrhosis, rheumatoid arthritis and systemic lupus erythematosus. (See also Autoantibodies, Table 8–7.) Saketkoo LA et al. The primary care physician in the early diagnosis of systemic sclerosis: the cornerstone of recognition and hope. Am J Med Sci 2014;347:54. [PMID: 24366221] Tyndall A et al. The differential diagnosis of systemic sclerosis. Curr Opin Rheumatol 2013;25:692. [PMID: 24061074] Villalta D et al. Diagnostic accuracy and predictive value of extended autoantibody profile in systemic sclerosis. Autoimmun Rev 2012;12:114. [PMID: 22776784]

(Continued)

	Ceruloplasmin, serum or plasma

Test/Range/Collection	Physiologic Basis	Interpretation	Comments
Ceruloplasmin, serum or plasma 20–50 mg/dL [200–500 mg/L] (age-dependent) SST, PPT (light green) (fasting specimen is preferred) $$	Ceruloplasmin, a 120,000–160,000 MW α_2-glycoprotein with oxidase activity synthesized by the liver, is the main (95%) copper-carrying protein in human serum. Any failure during its synthesis whereby copper cannot be incorporated into ceruloplasmin results in secretion of an apoceruloplasmin. The apo form has a short half-life and is rapidly metabolized, leading to reduced serum level of ceruloplasmin. ATP7B (an ATPase required for hepatic copper transport) is deficient in Wilson disease, leading to progressive copper accumulation in the liver and/or brain with organ damage.	**Increased in:** Acute and chronic inflammation, pregnancy. Drugs: oral contraceptives, phenytoin. **Decreased in:** Wilson disease (hepatolenticular degeneration) (95%), CNS disease other than Wilson (15%), liver disease other than Wilson (23%), malabsorption (enteropathy), malnutrition, primary biliary cirrhosis, nephrotic syndrome, severe copper deficiency, Menkes disease (X-linked inherited copper deficiency), hereditary aceruloplasminemia.	Serum ceruloplasmin level and slit-lamp examination for Kayser-Fleischer rings are initial tests recommended for suspected cases of Wilson disease. Slit-lamp exam is only 50–60% sensitive in patients without neurologic symptoms. Initial tests may also include serum copper (total and free). Equivocal cases may need 24-hour urinary copper excretion and/or liver copper measurement. Direct genetic testing for *ATP7B* mutations is increasingly available to confirm the clinical diagnosis of Wilson disease. Serum/plasma ceruloplasmin alone is not reliable for diagnosis of Wilson disease in asymptomatic patients. There is as yet no effective biomarker or method suitable for newborn screening for the disease. Bandmann O et al. Wilson's disease and other neurological copper disorders. Lancet Neurol 2015;14:103. [PMID: 25496901] Hahn SH. Population screening for Wilson's disease. Ann N Y Acad Sci 2014;1315:64. [PMID: 24731025] Lutsenko S. Modifying factors and phenotypic diversity in Wilson's disease. Ann NY Acad Sci 2014;1315:56. [PMID: 24702697]

		Chloride
Chloride, serum or plasma (Cl⁻) 98–107 meq/L [mmol/L] SST, PPT (light green) $	Chloride, the principal inorganic anion of extracellular fluid, is important in maintaining proper body water distribution, osmotic pressure, and normal acid–base balance. If chloride is lost (as HCl or NH₄Cl), alkalosis ensues; if chloride is ingested or retained, acidosis ensues. Chloride level is partially regulated by the kidney.	**Increased in:** Renal failure, nephrotic syndrome, renal tubular acidosis, dehydration, overtreatment with saline, hyperparathyroidism, diabetes insipidus, metabolic acidosis from diarrhea (loss of HCO₃⁻), respiratory alkalosis, hyperadrenocorticism. Drugs: acetazolamide (hyperchloremic acidosis), androgens, hydrochlorothiazide, salicylates (intoxication). **Decreased in:** Vomiting, diarrhea, gastrointestinal suction, renal failure combined with salt deprivation, over-treatment with diuretics, chronic respiratory acidosis, diabetic ketoacidosis, excessive sweating, SIADH, salt-losing nephropathy, acute intermittent porphyria, water intoxication, expansion of extracellular fluid volume, adrenal insufficiency, hyperaldosteronism, metabolic alkalosis. Drugs: chronic laxative or bicarbonate ingestion, corticosteroids, diuretics.	Test is helpful in assessing normal and increased anion gap metabolic acidosis. It is somewhat helpful in distinguishing hypercalcemia due to primary hyperparathyroidism (high serum chloride) from that due to malignancy (normal serum chloride). When assessing serum/plasma electrolytes, abnormal chloride levels alone usually signify an underlying metabolic disorder. Sweat chloride test is often used to help diagnose cystic fibrosis. Berend K et al. Chloride: the queen of electrolytes? Eur J Intern Med 2012;23:203. [PMID: 22385875] Wall SM et al. Cortical distal nephron Cl(−) transport in volume homeostasis and blood pressure regulation. Am J Physiol Renal Physiol 2013;305:F427. [PMID: 23637202]

(Continued)

Cholesterol, Serum or Plasma

Test/Range/Collection	Physiologic Basis	Interpretation	Comments
Cholesterol, serum or plasma Desirable: <200 mg/dL [<5.2 mmol/L], adults Borderline: 200–239 mg/dL [5.2–6.1 mmol/L], adults High risk: >240 mg/dL [>6.2 mmol/L], adults (age-dependent) SST, light green PPT $ Fasting specimen is required for LDL-C determination. HDL-C and total cholesterol can be measured with nonfasting specimen.	Cholesterol level is determined by lipid metabolism, which is in turn influenced by heredity, diet, and liver, kidney, thyroid, and other endocrine organ functions. Screening for total cholesterol (TC) may be done with nonfasting specimens, but a complete lipoprotein profile or LDL cholesterol (LDL-C) determination must be performed on fasting specimens. TC, triglyceride (TG), and high-density lipoprotein cholesterol (HDL-C) are directly measured. Although methods have become available for direct LDL-C measurement, in practice, LDL-C is often indirectly determined by use of the Friedewald equation: $[LDL-C] = [TC] - [HDL-C] - [TG/5]$ Note that this calculation is not valid for specimens having TG >400 mg/dL [>4.52 mmol/L], for patients with type III hyperlipoproteinemia or chylomicronemia, or nonfasting specimens.	**Increased in:** Primary disorders: polygenic hypercholesterolemia, familial hypercholesterolemia (deficiency of LDL receptors), familial combined hyperlipidemia, familial dysbetalipoproteinemia. Secondary disorders: hypothyroidism, uncontrolled diabetes mellitus, nephrotic syndrome, biliary obstruction, anorexia nervosa, hepatocellular carcinoma, Cushing syndrome, acute intermittent porphyria. Drugs: corticosteroids. **Decreased in:** Severe liver disease (acute hepatitis, cirrhosis, malignancy), hyperthyroidism, severe acute or chronic illness, malnutrition, malabsorption (eg, HIV), extensive burns, familial (Gaucher disease, Tangier disease), abetalipoproteinemia, intestinal lymphangiectasia.	Coronary heart disease (CHD) risk depends on the LDL cholesterol and non-HDL cholesterol levels. The HDL-C is inversely associated with risk of CHD and remains a key component of predicting cardiovascular risk. Treatment decisions should be based on CHD risk. The risk reduction is proportional primarily to the reduction in LDL cholesterol achieved with treatment. Treatment decisions and therapeutic goals are traditionally based on LDL-C concentrations: the recommended LDL-C intervention goals are <100 mg/dL for high-risk patients (eg, patients with CHD), <130 mg/dL for moderate-risk patients (≥2 risk factors), and <160 mg/dL for low-risk patients (no or 1 risk factor). New guideline recommends cholesterol-lowering treatment using evidence-based fixed-dose statin therapy without specific LDL-C target levels. A 2015 risk assessment tool for estimating a patient's 10-year risk of suffering a myocardial infarction, incorporating both total and HDL cholesterol levels, is available at: http://cvdrisk.nhlbi.nih.gov/ Goldstein JL et al. A century of cholesterol and coronaries: from plaques to genes to statins. Cell 2015;161:161. [PMID: 25815993] Martin SS et al. Clinician–patient risk discussion for atherosclerotic cardiovascular disease prevention: importance to implementation of the 2013 ACC/AHA Guidelines. J Am Coll Cardiol 2015;65:1361. [PMID: 25835448] Rader DJ et al. HDL and cardiovascular disease. Lancet 2014;384:618. [PMID: 25131981] Smith SC Jr et al. 2013 ACC/AHA guideline recommends fixed-dose strategies instead of targeted goals to lower blood cholesterol. J Am Coll Cardiol 2014;64:601. [PMID: 25104531]

Clostridium difficile toxins		
Clostridium difficile toxins, stool Negative Urine or stool container for collection of diarrheal (unformed) stool $$$ Must be tested within 12 hrs of collection because toxin (B) is labile.	*Clostridium difficile*, a motile, gram-positive rod, is the major agent of nosocomial, antibiotic-associated diarrhea, which is toxigenic in origin (see Antibiotic-associated colitis, Chapter 5). There are two toxins (A and B) produced by *C. difficile*; toxin A is an enterotoxin and toxin B is a cytotoxin. Cytotoxicity assay performed in cell culture is used to detect the cytopathic effect of the toxins, whose identity is confirmed by neutralization with specific antitoxins. The assay sensitivity and specificity are 95% and 90%, respectively. However, the assay is expensive and requires 24–48 hrs before results become available. Toxin A (more weakly cytopathic in cell culture) is enterotoxic and produces enteric disease. Toxin B (more easily detected in standard cell culture assays) fails to produce intestinal disease.	**Positive in:** Antibiotic-associated diarrhea (15–25%), antibiotic-associated colitis (50–75%), and pseudomembranous colitis (90–100%). About 3% of healthy adults and 10–20% of hospitalized patients have *C. difficile* in their colonic flora. There is also a high carrier rate of *C. difficile* and its toxin in healthy neonates.	Diagnostic testing for *C. difficile* infection should be performed only in symptomatic patients. Rapid enzyme immunoassay (EIA) (2–4 hour) tests for toxin A or toxins A and B have been used as an alternative to the cytotoxicity assay but are less sensitive and thus suboptimal. New guidelines recommend a two-step testing process, which includes an initial screening of stool samples with a rapid immunoassay for glutamate dehydrogenase (GDH), a common enzyme produced by *C. difficile*. A negative GDH assay effectively rules out infection, while a positive assay requires confirmation with a more specific assay, ie, the cell cytotoxicity assay or toxigenic culture, or a nucleic acid amplification test (NAAT). Rapid PCR-based NAAT assays that amplify the genes responsible for *C. difficile* toxins are highly sensitive and specific, and are used by many laboratories for patient management but their place among the various diagnostic options remains to be defined. Repeat testing during the same episode of diarrhea is of limited value and should be discouraged. Direct visualization with histopathologic examination of pseudomembranes on lower gastrointestinal endoscopy only detects 50–55% of *C. difficile* cases. Bagdasarian N et al. Diagnosis and treatment of *Clostridium difficile* in adults: a systematic review. JAMA 2015;313:398. [PMID: 25626036] Barbut F et al. New molecular methods for the diagnosis of *Clostridium difficile* infections. Drugs Today (Barc) 2012;48:673. [PMID: 23110263] Tenover FC et al. Laboratory diagnosis of *Clostridium difficile* infection: can molecular amplification methods move us out of uncertainty? J Mol Diagn 2011;13:573. [PMID: 21854871]

(Continued)

Test/Range/Collection	Physiologic Basis	Interpretation	Comments
Coccidioides antibodies, serum or CSF Negative SST or red (serum); glass or plastic (CSF) $$	Screens for presence of antibodies to *Coccidioides immitis*. Some centers use the mycelial-phase antigen, coccidioidin, to detect antibody. IgM antibodies appear early in disease in 75% of patients, begin to decrease after week 3, and are rarely seen after 5 months. They may persist in disseminated cases, usually in immunocompromised patients. IgG antibodies appear later in the course of the disease. Meningeal disease may have negative serum IgG and require CSF IgG antibody titers.	**Positive in:** Infection by coccidioides (90%). **Negative in:** Coccidioidin skin testing, many patients with chronic cavitary coccidioides; 5% of meningeal coccidioides negative by CSF complement fixation (CF) test.	Diagnosis of coccidiodomycosis is based on serologic testing, culture and tissue biopsy. Precipitin (immunodiffusion) and complement fixation (CF) tests detect 90% of primary symptomatic cases. Precipitin test (for IgM and IgG antibodies) is most effective in detecting early primary infection or an exacerbation of existing disease. Test is diagnostic but not prognostic. CF test (for IgG antibody) becomes positive later than precipitin test, and titers can be used to assess severity of infection. Titers rise as the disease progresses and decline as the patient improves. ELISA-based test is also available; data suggest good test performance characteristics. In coccidiodomycosis, routine CSF testing is not recommended. Malo I et al. Update on the diagnosis of pulmonary coccidioidomycosis. Ann Am Thorac Soc 2014;11:243. [PMID: 24575994] Thompson G et al. Routine CSF analysis in coccidiodomycosis is not required. PLoS One 2013;8:e64249. [PMID: 23717579]
Cold agglutinins, serum <1:32 titer Red, SST $$ Specimen should be kept in warm water (at 37°C) before separation of serum from cells.	Cold agglutinins are IgM (rarely IgG or IgA) autoantibodies that are capable of agglutinating red blood cells (RBCs) at temperatures below 35°C (strongly at 4°C, weakly at 24°C, and weakly or not at all at 37°C). Cold agglutinins can be monoclonal or polyclonal, and have been associated with various diseases, particularly infections, neoplasms, and collagen vascular diseases. Cold agglutinins are not necessarily pathologic, and may be detected in asymptomatic individuals during routine blood typing and crossmatching. If the agglutination is not reversible after incubation at 37°C, then the reaction is not due to cold agglutinins.	**Present in:** Chronic cold agglutinin disease or lymphoproliferative disorders (eg, Waldenström macroglobulinemia, chronic lymphocytic leukemia), autoimmune hemolytic anemia, myeloma, collagen-vascular diseases, *Mycoplasma pneumoniae* pneumonia, infectious mononucleosis, mumps orchitis, cytomegalovirus, listeriosis (ie, *Listeria monocytogenes*), legionella, tropical diseases (eg, trypanosomiasis, malaria).	Cold agglutinins are seen in a spectrum of conditions, ranging from "benign" cold agglutinin disease to malignant lymphoma. Primary chronic cold agglutinin disease is a clonal lymphoproliferative disorder, affecting 10–15% of patients with autoimmune hemolytic anemia. Cold agglutinins regularly occur during the course of two infections, *Mycoplasma pneumonia* pneumonia and infectious mononucleosis. Patients develop anti-I or anti-i antibodies, respectively, which are usually of the IgM class and react with adult human RBCs at temperatures below 35°C, resulting in agglutination. In *Mycoplasma* pneumonia, titers of anti-I rise late in the first week or during the second week, are maximal at 3–4 weeks after onset, and then disappear rapidly. A rise in cold agglutinin antibody titer is suggestive of recent mycoplasma infection. Berentsen S et al. Diagnosis and treatment of cold agglutinin-mediated autoimmune hemolytic anemia. Blood Rev 2012;26:107. [PMID: 22330255] Swiecicki PL et al. Cold agglutinin disease. Blood 2013;122:1114. [PMID: 23757733]

Complement C3			
Complement C3, serum 64–200 mg/dL [640–2000 mg/L] (age-dependent) SST $$ Separate serum from cells ASAP or within 2 hrs of collection.	**Increased in:** Many inflammatory conditions as an acute-phase reactant, active phase of rheumatic diseases (eg, rheumatoid arthritis, SLE), acute viral hepatitis, myocardial infarction, cancer, diabetes mellitus, pregnancy, sarcoidosis, amyloidosis, thyroiditis. **Decreased by:** Decreased synthesis (protein malnutrition, congenital deficiency, severe liver disease), increased catabolism (immune complex disease, membranoproliferative glomerulonephritis [75%], SLE, Sjögren syndrome, rheumatoid arthritis, DIC, paroxysmal nocturnal hemoglobinuria, autoimmune hemolytic anemia, gram-negative bacteremia or sepsis), increased loss (burns, gastroenteropathies).	C3 is the central component in complement activation. The classic and alternative complement pathways converge at the C3 step in the complement cascade (see Figure 10-3). Low levels indicate activation by one or both pathways. Most diseases with immune complexes show decreased C3 levels. Deficiency of C3 is associated with recurrent infections. Test is usually performed as an immunoassay (by radial immunodiffusion or nephelometry).	Complement C3 levels may be useful in following the activity of immune complex diseases. The best test to detect inherited deficiencies is CH50 (complement activity assay). Complement-mediated membranoproliferative glomerulonephritis could benefit from targeted anti-complement therapy (eg, eculizumab). Lupu F et al. Crosstalk between the coagulation and complement systems in sepsis. Thromb Res 2014;13:S28. [PMID: 24759136] Popat RJ et al. Complement and glomerular diseases. Nephron Clin Pract 2014;128:238. [PMID: 25412932] Tichaczek-Goska D. Deficiencies and excessive human complement system activation in disorders of multifarious etiology. Adv Clin Exp Med 2012;21:105. [PMID: 23214307]
Complement C4			
Complement C4, serum or plasma 15–45 mg/dL [150–450 mg/dL] (age-dependent) SST, lavender, green $$ Separate serum from cells ASAP or within 2 hrs of collection.	**Increased in:** Various malignancies (not clinically useful). **Decreased by:** Decreased synthesis (congenital deficiency), increased catabolism (SLE, rheumatoid arthritis, proliferative glomerulonephritis, hereditary angioedema [HAE]), and increased loss (burns, protein-losing enteropathies).	C4 is a component of the classic complement pathway. Depressed levels usually indicate classic pathway activation. Deficiency of C4 or another early component of the classical pathway (C1q, C2) is often associated with autoimmune diseases (eg, SLE-like), whereas deficiency of properdin, C3 or a terminal pathway component (C5 to C9) leads to recurrent bacterial infections. Test is usually performed as an immunoassay and not a functional assay.	C4 is often ordered together with C3 for monitoring activity of rheumatologic diseases. Normal C4 levels with decrease in C3 may be seen in complement-mediated atypical hemolytic uremic syndrome (aHUS). Low C4 level accompanies acute attacks of HAE, and C4 is used as a first-line test for the disease. C1 esterase inhibitor (C1-INH) levels are generally not indicated for the evaluation of HAE unless C4 level is low. Congenital C4 deficiency occurs with an SLE-like syndrome. Elkon KB et al. Complement, interferon and lupus. Curr Opin Immunol 2012;24:665. [PMID: 22999705] Grumach AS et al. Are complement deficiencies really rare? Overview on prevalence, clinical importance and modern diagnostic approach. Mol Immunol 2014;61:110. [PMID: 25037634] Mayilyan KR. Complement genetics, deficiencies, and disease associations. Protein Cell 2012;3:487. [PMID: 22773339]

(Continued)

Test/Range/Collection	Physiologic Basis	Interpretation	Comments
Complement, total, serum (also known as **CH50**) 30–75 U/mL (laboratory-specific) Red $$$	Traditionally, the test uses sheep red blood cells coated with antibodies. Addition of serum complement causes lysis of the sensitized red cells. The amount of hemolysis is evaluated quantitatively. Test measures the integrity and activity of the classical pathway components (C1-C9), and does not depend on the alternative pathway components (Figure 10-3). For precise titrations of hemolytic complement, the dilution of serum that lyses 50% of the indicator red cells is determined as the CH50. An automated method using antibody-coated liposomes (in lieu of red cells) with entrapped indicator enzyme (eg, G6PD) has been developed. Serum complement causes lysis of liposomes and the released enzyme activity is then measured. The assay correlates with the CH50 assay, has lower variability and is easier to perform.	**Decreased with:** >50–80% deficiency of classic pathway complement components (congenital or acquired deficiencies). **Normal in:** Deficiencies of the alternative pathway complement components.	This is a functional assay of biologic activity of the classical complement pathway. Sensitivity to decreased levels of complement components depends on exactly how the test is performed. It is used to monitor disease activity in patients with SLE and glomerulonephritis, and to detect congenital and acquired severe deficiency in the classic complement pathway. Liszewski KM et al. Complement regulators in human disease: lessons from modern genetics. J Intern Med 2015;277:294. [PMID: 25495259] Mastellos DC et al. Complement in paroxysmal nocturnal hemoglobinuria: exploiting our current knowledge to improve the treatment landscape. Expert Rev Hematol 2014;7:583. [PMID: 25213458] Sarma JV et al. The complement system. Cell Tissue Res 2011;343:227. [PMID: 20838815]

Complete blood cell count		
Complete blood cell count (CBC), blood Refer to individual test for reference range Lavender $$	The CBC consists of a panel of tests that examines whole blood and includes the following: total white blood cell count (WBC, $\times 10^3$/mcL) and white blood cell differential (%) (p. 220), red blood cell count (RBC, $\times 10^6$/mcL) (p. 188), hemoglobin concentration (Hb, g/L) (p. 116), hematocrit (Hct, %) (p. 112), platelet count (Plt, 10^3/mcL) (p. 175), red cell indices including mean corpuscular volume (MCV, fL) (p. 156), mean corpuscular hemoglobin (MCH) (p. 155), mean corpuscular hemoglobin concentration (MCHC, g/L) (p. 156), and red cell distribution width (RDW, %). Several new quantitative CBC parameters are being introduced, including nucleated red blood cells (nRBCs), immature granulocytes (IGs), immature reticulocyte fraction (IRF), immature platelet fraction (IPF), red cell fragments (schistocytes) as well as new parameters for detection of functional iron deficiency (eg, reticulocyte hemoglobin content, CHr). Automated laboratory hematology analyzers are widely available. The basic principles used for the cell counting and white cell differential are instrument-dependent.	Refer to individual test for detailed information.	The CBC provides important information about the types and numbers of cells in the blood, especially red cells, white cells, and platelets. It helps in evaluating symptoms (eg, weakness, fatigue, fever or bruising), diagnosing conditions or diseases (eg, anemia, infection, leukemia, lymphoma, and many other disorders), and determining the stages of a particular disease (eg, chronic myeloid leukemia). Hct, MCH, and MCHC are typically calculated from RBC, Hb, and MCV. If significantly abnormal CBC values are obtained, a peripheral blood smear should be prepared and examined (eg, red cell morphology, WBC differential, platelet count estimation, identification of immature and malignant cells). Most new parameters are specific for certain analyzers, and results from different manufacturers may not be comparable. Ford J. Red blood cell morphology. Int J Lab Hematol 2013;35:351. [PMID: 23480230] Gulati G et al. Purpose and criteria for blood smear scan, blood smear examination, and blood smear review. Ann Lab Med 2013;33:1. [PMID: 23301216] Leach M. Interpretation of the full blood count in systemic disease—a guide for the physician. J R Coll Physicians Edinb 2014;44:36. [PMID: 24995446] Lecompte TP et al. Novel parameters in blood cell counters. Clin Lab Med 2015;35:209. [PMID: 25676381]

(Continued)

Test/Range/Collection	Physiologic Basis	Interpretation	Comments
Cortisol, serum or plasma	Cortisol, serum or plasma		
Cortisol, plasma or serum 8:00 AM: 5–20 mcg/dL [140–550 nmol/L] (time-dependent) 8 hrs post 1 mg dexamethasone given at midnight: 0–5 mcg/dL; 30–60 min post 25 units Cosyntropin [intravenously]: >20 mcg/dL SST, PPT (light green) $$	Release of corticotropin-releasing factor (CRF) from the hypothalamus stimulates release of ACTH from the pituitary, which in turn stimulates release of cortisol from the adrenal. Cortisol provides negative feedback to this system. Test measures both free cortisol and cortisol bound to cortisol-binding globulin (CBG). Morning levels are higher than evening levels (eg, 5–20 mcg/dL at 8 AM vs. 0–9 mcg/dL at 8 PM).	**Increased in:** Cushing syndrome, acute illness, surgery, trauma, septic shock, depression, anxiety, alcoholism, starvation, chronic renal failure, increased CBG (congenital, pregnancy, estrogen therapy). **Decreased in:** Addison disease; decreased CBG (congenital, liver disease, nephrotic syndrome).	Cortisol levels are used to evaluate Cushing syndrome and adrenal insufficiency. Cortisol levels are useful only in the context of standardized suppression or stimulation tests. See Cosyntropin stimulation test and Dexamethasone suppression tests for details. Low-dose dexamethasone suppression, late-night salivary cortisol, and 24-hr urinary free cortisol are regarded as screening tests of choice for Cushing syndrome (Figure 9-8). Circadian fluctuations in cortisol levels limit usefulness of single measurements. Analysis of diurnal variation of cortisol is not useful diagnostically. Brandão Neto RA et al. Diagnosis and classification of Addison's disease (autoimmune adrenalitis). Autoimmun Rev 2014;13(4–5):408. [PMID: 24424183] Deutschbein T et al. Screening for Cushing's syndrome: new immunoassays require adequate normative data. Horm Metab Res 2013;45:118. [PMID: 23417245] Turpeinen U et al. Determination of cortisol in serum, saliva and urine. Best Pract Res Clin Endocrinol Metab 2013;27:795. [PMID: 24275191]
Cortisol (urinary free)	Cortisol (urinary free)		
Cortisol (urinary free), urine 10–110 mcg/24 hr [30–300 nmol/d] Urine bottle containing boric acid. $$$ Collect 24-hour urine. Refrigerate during collection.	Urinary free cortisol measurement is useful in the initial evaluation of suspected Cushing syndrome (see Cushing syndrome algorithm, Figure 9–8).	**Increased in:** Cushing syndrome, acute illness, stress. **Not increased in:** Obesity.	24-hour urinary free cortisol is one of the initial diagnostic tests of choice for Cushing syndrome, although the sensitivity and specificity are less than ideal. Not useful for the definitive diagnosis of adrenal insufficiency. Baseline urinary free cortisol excretion <5 mcg/24 hr may be consistent with adrenal insufficiency. A shorter (12-hour) overnight collection and measurement of the ratio of urine-free cortisol to urine creatinine appears to perform nearly as well as a 24-hour collection for urine-free cortisol. Urinary free cortisol to creatinine ratio can also be obtained from a random urine collection. Alexandraki KI et al. Is urinary free cortisol of value in the diagnosis of Cushing's syndrome? Curr Opin Endocrinol Diabetes Obes 2011;18:259. [PMID: 21681089] Deutschbein T et al. Screening for Cushing's syndrome: new immunoassays require adequate normative data. Horm Metab Res 2013;45:118. [PMID: 23417245]

Cosyntropin/cortrosyn stimulation test		
Cosyntropin (Cortrosyn) stimulation test, serum or plasma SST, light green PPT, or lavender $$$ First draw a cortisol level. Then administer cosyntropin (250 mcg IV or IM). Draw another cortisol level in 30 to 60 minutes.	Cosyntropin (also known as Cortrosyn, a synthetic peptide analogue of ACTH) stimulates the adrenal to release cortisol. A normal response is a doubling of basal levels or a significant increase to a level above 20 mcg/dL (>552 nmol/L). A poor cortisol response to cosyntropin indicates adrenal insufficiency (see Adrenocortical insufficiency algorithm, Figure 9–3).	**Decreased in:** Acute adrenal insufficiency (adrenal crisis), chronic adrenal insufficiency (Addison disease), pituitary insufficiency, AIDS.	ACTH stimulation test itself does not distinguish primary from secondary (pituitary) chronic adrenal insufficiency, because in secondary adrenal insufficiency the atrophic adrenal may be unresponsive to cosyntropin. Test may not reliably detect pituitary insufficiency. Metyrapone test may be useful to assess the pituitary–adrenal axis. Serum/plasma baseline ACTH is markedly elevated if patient has primary adrenal disease, whereas ACTH is decreased in secondary (pituitary) adrenal insufficiency. AIDS patients with adrenal insufficiency may have normal ACTH stimulation tests. Charmandari E et al. Adrenal insufficiency. Lancet 2014;383:2152. [PMID: 24503135] Husebye ES et al. Consensus statement on the diagnosis, treatment and follow-up of patients with primary adrenal insufficiency. J Intern Med 2014;275:104. [PMID: 24330030] Raff H et al. Physiological basis for the etiology, diagnosis, and treatment of adrenal disorders: Cushing's syndrome, adrenal insufficiency, and congenital adrenal hyperplasia. Compr Physiol 2014;4:739. [PMID: 24715566]

(Continued)

	Creatine kinase, total

Test/Range/Collection	Physiologic Basis	Interpretation	Comments
Creatine kinase, total, serum or plasma (CK) 20–200 IU/L (age- and method-dependent) SST, PPT $	Creatine kinase is an enzyme which catalyses the interconversion of creatine and phospho-creatine (PCr). Skeletal muscle, myocardium, and brain are rich in the enzyme. CK is released when there is tissue damage (eg. myocardial infarction [MI], myopathy).	**Increased in:** MI, myocarditis, muscle trauma, rhabdomyolysis, muscular dystrophy, polymyositis, severe muscular exertion, malignant hyperthermia, hypothyroidism, cerebral infarction, surgery, Reye syndrome, tetanus, generalized convulsions, alcoholism, DC countershock. Drugs: clofibrate, HMG-CoA reductase inhibitors (statins).	CK is as sensitive a test as aldolase for muscle damage (eg. myositis), so aldolase is not needed for this condition. CK values may be increased up to 50-fold in active polymyositis and other inflammatory myopathies. A urine myoglobin may also be ordered for these conditions. During an MI, serum CK level rises rapidly (within 3–5 hrs); elevation persists for 2–3 days post-MI. Total CK is not specific enough for use in diagnosis of MI, but a normal total CK has a high negative predictive value. A more specific test is needed for diagnosis of MI or acute coronary syndrome (eg, cardiac troponin I, which has largely replaced CK-MB). Amato AA et al. Overview of the muscular dystrophies. Handb Clin Neurol 2011;101:1. [PMID: 21496621] Milisenda JC et al. The diagnosis and classification of polymyositis. J Autoimmun 2014;48:118. [PMID: 24461380] van der Kooi AJ et al. Idiopathic inflammatory myopathies. Handb Clin Neurol 2014;119:495. [PMID: 24365315]

Creatine kinase, MB		
Creatine kinase, MB, (CK-MB) <16 IU/L <5% of total CK or <5 mcg/L mass units (laboratory-specific) SST, PPT, green $$	CK consists of three isoenzymes, made up of 2 subunits, M and B. The fraction with the greatest electrophoretic mobility is CK1 (BB), CK2 (MB) is intermediate, and CK3 (MM) moves slowest toward the anode. Skeletal muscle is characterized by isoenzyme MM and brain by isoenzyme BB. Myocardium has MB isoenzyme. Assay techniques include isoenzyme separation by electrophoresis or by immunoassay using antibody specific for MB fraction (mass units).	**Increased in:** Myocardial infarction (MI), cardiac trauma or intervention procedure, certain muscular dystrophies, and polymyositis. Slight persistent elevation reported in patients with chronic heart failure and chronic renal failure.	CK-MB is a relatively specific test for MI. It appears in serum approximately 4 hrs after infarction, peaks at 12−24 hrs, and declines over 48−72 hrs. CK-MB mass concentration is a sensitive marker of MI within 4−12 hrs after infarction. Because cardiac troponins (cTnI and cTnT) are tissue-specific and are now the markers of choice for the diagnosis of acute MI, high sensitivity cardiac troponin I (cTnI) test has replaced the conventional CK-MB assay. Measurement of CK-MB remains useful in evaluating patients who are already cTnI positive (eg, due to chronic heart or renal failure) and have recurrent chest pain. Periprocedual (eg, emergency or elective percutaneous coronary intervention) CK-MB is considered a better prognostic indicator of myocardial injury and risk of procedural morbidity and mortality than cTnI. Estimation of CK-MM and CK-BB is not clinically useful. Use total CK. Gollop ND et al. Is periprocedural CK-MB a better indicator of prognosis after emergency and elective percutaneous coronary intervention compared with post-procedural cardiac troponins? Interact Cardiovasc Thorac Surg 2013;17:867. [PMID: 23842761] Sluss PM. Methodologies for measurement of cardiac markers. Clin Lab Med 2014;34:167. [PMID: 24507795] Tehrani DM et al. Third universal definition of myocardial infarction: update, caveats, differential diagnoses. Cleve Clin J Med 2013;80:777. [PMID: 24307162]

(Continued)

Test/Range/Collection	Physiologic Basis	Interpretation	Comments
Creatinine, serum or plasma (Cr) 0.6–1.2 mg/dL [50–100 mcmol/L] SST, PPT $	Endogenous creatinine is excreted by filtration through the glomerulus and by tubular secretion. Creatinine clearance is an acceptable clinical measure of glomerular filtration rate (GFR), although it sometimes overestimates GFR (eg, in cirrhosis). For each 50% reduction in GFR, serum creatinine approximately doubles.	**Increased in:** Acute or chronic renal failure, urinary tract obstruction, nephrotoxic drugs, hypothyroidism. **Decreased in:** Reduced muscle mass, cachexia, aging.	Serum or plasma creatinine should not be used as a stand-alone source for assessing renal function. Estimated GFR (eGFRcr) should also be reported. In the alkaline picrate method, substances other than Cr (eg, acetoacetate, acetone, β-hydroxybutyrate, α-ketoglutarate, pyruvate, glucose) may give falsely high results. Therefore, patients with diabetic ketoacidosis may have spuriously elevated Cr. Increased bilirubin may spuriously decrease Cr. Chronic renal insufficiency may be underrecognized, as the Cr-based GFR estimating equations tend to overestimate kidney function. Age, male sex, and black race are predictors of kidney disease. Early diagnosis is important and should be pursued in at-risk populations. Serum/plasma creatinine levels may not reflect decreased renal function because creatinine production rate is decreased with reduced lean body mass. Increased intravascular volume and increased volume of distribution associated with anasarca may also mask decreased renal function by reducing serum creatinine levels. The use of changes in Cr as a surrogate of GFR has limited value in critically ill patients. See Glomerular filtration rate, estimated (eGFR) (p. 105). Levey AS et al. GFR estimation: from physiology to public health. Am J Kidney Dis 2014;63:820. [PMID: 24485147] Macedo E et al. Measuring renal function in critically ill patients: tools and strategies for assessing glomerular filtration rate. Curr Opin Crit Care 2013;19:560. [PMID: 24240821]

Creatinine, serum or plasma

(Continued)

	Creatinine clearance			Cryoglobulins, qualitative, serum

Creatinine clearance (Cl_Cr)

Adults: 90–130 mL/min/ 1.73 m² BSA

$$

Collect carefully timed 24-hour urine and simultaneous serum/plasma creatinine sample. Record patient's weight and height.

Widely used test of glomerular filtration rate. Theoretically reliable, but often compromised by incomplete urine collection. Creatinine clearance is calculated from measurement of urine creatinine (U_{Cr} [mg/dL]), plasma/serum creatinine (P_{Cr} [mg/dL]), and urine flow rate (V [mL/min]) according to the formula:

$$Cl_{Cr}(mL/min) = \frac{U_{Cr} \times V}{P_{Cr}}$$

where

$$V(mL/min) = \frac{24\text{-hour urine volume}(mL)}{1440(min/24h)}$$

Creatinine clearance is often "corrected" for body surface area (BSA [m²]) according to the formula:

$$Cl_{Cr}(corrected) = Cl_{Cr}(uncorrected) \times \frac{1.73}{BSA}$$

Increased in: High cardiac output, exercise, acromegaly, diabetes mellitus (early stage), infections, hypothyroidism.

Decreased in: Acute or chronic renal failure, decreased renal blood flow (shock, hemorrhage, dehydration, HF). Drugs: nephrotoxic drugs.

Serum or plasma Cr may, in practice, be a more reliable indicator of renal function than 24-hour Cl_Cr unless urine collection is carefully monitored. An 8-hour collection provides results similar to those obtained with a 24-hour collection.

Cl_Cr will overestimate glomerular filtration rate to the extent that Cr is secreted by the renal tubules (eg, in cirrhosis).

Cl_Cr can be estimated from the serum/plasma creatinine using the following formula:

$$\frac{Cl_{Cr}}{(mL/min)} = \frac{(140-Age) \times Wt(kg)}{72 - P_{Cr}}$$

Serial decline in Cl_Cr is the most reliable indicator of progressive renal dysfunction.

Also see GFR, estimated (eGFR) (p. 105).

Levey AS et al. Glomerular filtration rate and albuminuria for detection and staging of acute and chronic kidney disease in adults: a systematic review. JAMA 2015;313:837. [PMID: 25710660]

Levey AS et al. GFR estimation: from physiology to public health. Am J Kidney Dis 2014;63(5):820. [PMID: 24485147]

Macedo E et al. Measuring renal function in critically ill patients: tools and strategies for assessing glomerular filtration rate. Curr Opin Crit Care 2013;19:560. [PMID: 24240821]

Cryoglobulins, qualitative, serum

Negative at 72 hrs

Red

$

Fasting specimen required, and blood sample must be drawn in a pre-warmed vacutainer tube, kept at 37°C and immediately transported to the laboratory.

Cryoglobulins are immunoglobulins (IgG, IgM, IgA, or light chains) that precipitate on exposure to the cold. The serum sample is stored at 4°C and examined for the presence or absence of precipitation over a period of 3 days.

Type I cryoglobulins (25%) are monoclonal immunoglobulins, most commonly IgM, occasionally IgA, and rarely IgA or Bence Jones protein.

Type II (25%) are mixed cryoglobulins with a monoclonal component (usually IgM) that complexes with polyclonal IgG in the cryoprecipitate.

Type III (50%) are mixed polyclonal cryoglobulins (IgG and IgM).

Positive in: Immunoproliferative disorders (multiple myeloma, Waldenström macroglobulinemia, chronic lymphocytic leukemia, B-cell lymphoma), collagen vascular disease (SLE, polyarteritis nodosa, rheumatoid arthritis, Sjögren syndrome), hemolytic anemia, infections (eg, HCV, HIV), glomerulonephritis, chronic liver disease. The term "essential mixed cryoglobulinemia" (a vasculitic syndrome) is used to refer to patients with no primary disease other than Sjögren syndrome; other cases are classified as secondary mixed cryoglobulinemia.

All types of cryoglobulins may cause cold-induced symptoms, including Raynaud phenomenon, vascular purpura, and urticaria.

Patients with type I cryoglobulinemia usually suffer from underlying disease (eg, multiple myeloma).

Patients with type I and III cryoglobulinemia often have immune complex disease, with vascular purpura, bleeding tendencies, arthritis, and nephritis.

Typing of cryoglobulins by electrophoresis is not necessary for diagnosis or clinical management.

About 50% of essential mixed cryoglobulinemia patients have evidence of hepatitis C infection.

Motyckova G et al. Laboratory testing for cryoglobulins. Am J Hematol 2011;86:500. [PMID: 21594887]

Retamozo S et al. Cryoglobulinemic disease. Oncology (Williston Park) 2013;27:1098. [PMID: 24575538]

Takada S et al. Cryoglobulinemia (review). Mol Med Rep. 2012;6:3. [PMID: 22484457]

	Cryptococcal antigen, serum and CSF		
Test/Range/Collection	**Physiologic Basis**	**Interpretation**	**Comments**
Cryptococcal antigen, serum or CSF Negative Red or SST (serum), or glass or plastic tube (CSF) $$	Most infections with *Cryptococcus neoformans* occur in the lungs. However, fungal meningitis and encephalitis can occur as a secondary infection in AIDS patients and other individuals at risk. The capsular polysaccharide of *Cryptococcus neoformans* potentiates opportunistic infections by the yeast. The cryptococcal antigen test used is a latex agglutination or enzyme immunoassay test. A titer is usually performed on positive specimens.	**Positive in:** Cryptococcal infection (eg, Cryptococcal meningitis).	False-positive and false-negative results have been reported. False positives due to rheumatoid factor can be reduced by pretreatment of serum using pronase before testing. Sensitivity and specificity of serum cryptococcal antigen titer for cryptococcal meningitis are 91% and 83%, respectively. Cryptococcal antigen testing performed on CSF specimens needs to be confirmed by culture. Antibody test for Cryptococcus is also available for serum and CSF specimens. Molecular techniques are under clinical evaluation. Ninety-six percent of cryptococcal infections occur in HIV/AIDS patients. Arvanitis M et al. Molecular and nonmolecular diagnostic methods for invasive fungal infections. Clin Microbiol Rev 2014;27:490. [PMID: 24982319] Kaplan JE et al. Cryptococcal antigen screening and early antifungal treatment to prevent cryptococcal meningitis: a review of the literature. J Acquir Immune Defic Syndr 2015;68:S331. [PMID: 25768872] Schelenz S et al. British Society for Medical Mycology best practice recommendations for the diagnosis of serious fungal diseases. Lancet Infect Dis 2015;15:461. [PMID: 25771341]

Test / Range / Specimen	Increased in	Comments	Notes
C-telopeptide, beta-cross-linked (CTX-beta), serum Adult male: 60–850 pg/mL Adult female: premenopausal 60–650 pg/mL; postmenopausal 104–1010 pg/mL (age and laboratory-specific). SST, red $$$$ Fasting specimen is preferred. For patients on supplement biotin (>5 mg/day), specimen should not be collected until >8 hr after the last dose.	**Increased in:** Osteoporosis, osteopenia, osteomalacia, rickets, Paget disease, hyperparathyroidism, and hyperthyroidism.	During bone resorption, osteoclasts secrete a mixture of proteases that degrade the type I collagen fibrils into fragments including C-terminal telopeptide (CTX). One of the fragments is beta-CTX, which is released into blood and is considered a specific marker for increased bone resorption.	Test aids in the diagnosis of medical conditions associated with increased bone turnover, but cannot replace bone mineral density to diagnose osteoporosis. Test may be useful for monitoring antiresorptive treatment in postmenopausal women treated for osteoporosis and individuals diagnosed with osteopenia. Reduced renal function may lead to reduced urinary excretion of beta-CTX and consequent increase in the serum beta-CTX concentration. For treatment monitoring, blood specimen should be collected at a designated time of day to minimize circadian variation. Serum CTX is preferred to the urine NTX test as a marker for bone turnover, (see N-telopeptide, cross-linked, p. 163 and serum PINP test (procollagen type 1 intact N-terminal propeptide), p. 179). Biver E. Use of bone turnover markers in clinical practice. Curr Opin Endocrinol Diabetes Obes 2012;19:468. [PMID: 23128576] Chubb SA. Measurement of C-terminal telopeptide of type I collagen (CTX) in serum. Clin Biochem 2012;45:928. [PMID: 22504058] Lee J et al. Current recommendations for laboratory testing and use of bone turnover markers in management of osteoporosis. Ann Lab Med 2012;32:105. [PMID: 22389876]
Cyclic citrullinated protein antibody (anti-CCP), serum Negative SST, red $$$$	**Increased in:** RA (sensitivity 70–80%, specificity 93–98%), deforming erosive arthritis in SLE (sensitivity 30–70%, specificity 80–97%)	Post-translational deamination of arginine residues by peptidyl arginine deaminase (citrullination) during inflammation results in production of antigenic epitope. IgG antibodies to citrullinated proteins (particularly filaggrin) are frequently elevated in rheumatoid arthritis (RA) and are also elevated in erosive arthritis in patients with systemic lupus erythematosus (SLE).	Specificity of anti-CCP for RA is higher than that of rheumatoid factor (RF). CCP antibodies may be present in the preclinical phase of RA, are associated with future RA development, and may predict radiographic joint destruction. Patients with weak positive results should be monitored and testing repeated. Anti-CCP antibodies are also very specific markers for erosive arthritis in SLE. Budhram A et al. Anti-cyclic citrullinated peptide antibody as a marker of erosive arthritis in patients with systemic lupus erythematosus: a systematic review and meta-analysis. Lupus 2014;23:1156. [PMID: 24900382] Farid SSh et al. Anti-citrullinated protein antibodies and their clinical utility in rheumatoid arthritis. Int J Rheum Dis 2013;16:379. [PMID: 23992255] Kourilovitch M et al. Diagnosis and classification of rheumatoid arthritis. J Autoimmun 2014;48-49:26. [PMID: 24568777]

(Continued)

Test/Range/Collection	Physiologic Basis	Interpretation	Comments
Cystatin C, serum or plasma 0.5–1.3 mg/L (age and method-dependent) eGFR >60 mL/min/BSA Red, SST, PPT $$$	Cystatin C (CyC) is a 13 kDa cysteine proteinase inhibitor, which is produced by all nucleated cells in the body. It is produced at a constant rate and freely filtered by the kidneys. Unlike creatinine, CyC is completely reabsorbed and metabolized by proximal renal tubules. Its blood level is less influenced by age, race, sex, body mass, diet or drugs than is creatinine. CyC may be used as an alternative to creatinine for assessing renal function. It is considered a superior marker, especially when creatinine use is clinically inappropriate, for example, in patients with cirrhosis or morbid obesity, are malnourished, or have decreased muscle mass.	**Increased in:** Chronic kidney disease, renal dysfunction/failure.	CyC based eGFR (eGFRcys) has been proposed as a superior alternative to eGFRcr, especially where there is decreased muscle mass, eGFRcys should be calculated using the 2012 CKD-EPI equation. See also glomerular filtration rate, estimated (eGFR, p. 105). Elevated serum or plasma CyC level is independently associated with cardiovascular risk and all-cause mortality in elderly people. Limitations on widespread use of CyC as a routine test of kidney function include incomplete understanding of non–GFR factors affecting serum or plasma CyC level, incomplete assay standardization, and significantly higher costs. Levey AS et al. Glomerular filtration rate and albuminuria for detection and staging of acute and chronic kidney disease in adults: a systematic review. JAMA 2015;313:837. [PMID: 25710660] Shlipak MG et al. Update on cystatin C: incorporation into clinical practice. Am J Kidney Dis 2013;62:595. [PMID: 23701892]
Cytomegalovirus antibodies, IgG and IgM, serum (CMV serology) Negative SST $$$	Detects the presence of antibodies to CMV, either IgG or IgM. CMV infection is usually acquired during childhood or early adulthood. By age 20–40 years, 40–90% of the population has CMV antibodies. Antibodies play an important role in protection against CMV infection and disease (including mother-to-fetus transmission), but the level of protection is incomplete.	**Increased in:** Previous or active CMV infection. False-positive CMV IgM tests occur when rheumatoid factor or infectious mononucleosis is present.	Serial specimens exhibiting a greater than fourfold titer rise suggest a recent infection. Active CMV infection can be documented by viral isolation. Viremia is commonly confirmed by either an antigenemia assay or a quantitative nucleic acid test (ie, viral load in plasma or whole blood). Serology test is useful for screening of potential organ donors and recipients. Detection of CMV IgM antibody in the serum of a newborn usually indicates congenital infection. Detection of CMV IgG antibody is not diagnostic, because maternal CMV IgG antibody passed via the placenta can persist in newborn's serum for 6 months. CMV seronegative blood and leukocyte-reduced blood are used to prevent transfusion-acquired CMV infection. Kotton CN. CMV: Prevention, diagnosis and therapy. Am J Transplant 2013;13:S24. [PMID: 23347212] Revello MG et al. Role of human cytomegalovirus (HCMV)-specific antibody in HCMV-infected pregnant women. Early Hum Dev 2014;90:S32. [PMID: 24709453] Schleiss MR. Cytomegalovirus in the neonate: immune correlates of infection and protection. Clin Dev Immunol 2013;2013:501801. [PMID: 24023565]

Cytomegalovirus antibodies (IgG and IgM), serum

D-dimer		
D-dimer, plasma	D-dimer is one of the terminal fibrin degrada-tion products. The presence of D-dimers indicates that a fibrin clot was formed and subsequently degraded by plasmin. Essentially, D-dimer is elevated whenever the coagulation system has been activated, followed by fibrinolysis.	**Increased in:** Deep vein thrombosis (DVT), venous thromboembolism (VTE), pulmonary embolism (PE), disseminated intravascular coagulation (DIC), arterial thromboembolism, pregnancy (especially postpartum period), malignancy, surgery, thrombolytic therapy.	D-dimer assay is a sensitive test for DIC, DVT and VTE or PE. The D-dimer can be measured by a variety of methods, for example, semiquantitative latex agglutination and quantitative high sensitivity immunoassay (eg, ELISA). The D-dimer test may help to exclude DVT/PE in patients with low or intermediate clinical probability. A D-dimer level below the cutoff of 400 ng/mL [or (age×10) ng/mL in patients 50 years or older] essentially rules out PE/VTE, but a positive test does not confirm the diagnosis, and further testing (eg, ultrasound, CT angiography) is recommended. See Figure 9–29 for its use in pulmo-nary embolism evaluation.
<400 ng/mL			
Blue			D-dimer is often markedly elevated in DIC.
$$			Righini M et al. Age-adjusted D-dimer cutoff levels to rule out pulmo-nary embolism: the ADJUST-PE study. JAMA 2014;311:1117. [PMID: 24643601]
			Rodger MA et al. Clinical decision rules and D-Dimer in venous throm-boembolism: current controversies and future research priorities. Thromb Res 2014;134:763. [PMID: 25129416]
			Wells P et al. The diagnosis and treatment of venous thromboembolism. Hematology Am Soc Hematol Educ Program 2013;2013:457. [PMID: 24319219]

(Continued)

Dehydroepiandrosterone sulfate (DHEA-S)

Test/Range/Collection	Physiologic Basis	Interpretation	Comments
Dehydroepiandrosterone sulfate (DHEA-S), serum or plasma Male: 40–500 mcg/dL Female: 20–320 mcg/dL (age and sex dependent) SST, PPT, green, lavender/pink $$$$	DHEA is a 19-carbon endogenous steroid hormone secreted by the adrenal glands. It is converted to DHEA-S in the adrenals, liver, and small intestine. DHEA-S is albumin-bound in the circulation, and there is no diurnal variation in DHEA-S levels. Levels of DHEA-S are about 300× higher than DHEA and more stable. It serves as the precursor of androgens and estrogens.	**Increased in:** Adrenal hyperplasia, adrenal cancer, congenital adrenal hyperplasia, polycystic ovary syndrome (PCOS). **Decreased in:** Adrenal insufficiency, hypo-pituitarism, rheumatoid arthritis (females), insulin, corticosteroids.	DHEA-S serves as an indicator of adrenal androgen production. Its measurement is typically used along with other steroid and peptide hormones to evaluate adrenal function, to help diagnose adrenal cortex tumors and PCOS (in females). For evaluating central adrenal insufficiency, baseline levels of both serum/plasma cortisol and DHEA-S should be obtained. Orally ingested DHEA is converted to DHEA-S when passing through intestines and liver. People taking DHEA supplements have elevated blood levels of DHEA-S. Use by athletes is prohibited by the World Anti-doping Agency. Al-Aridi R et al. Biochemical diagnosis of adrenal insufficiency: the added value of dehydroepiandrosterone sulfate measurements. Endocr Pract 2011;17:261. [PMID: 21134877] Goodarzi MO et al. DHEA, DHEAS and PCOS. J Steroid Biochem Mol Biol 2015;145:213. [PMID: 25008465] Rachoń D. Differential diagnosis of hyperandrogenism in women with polycystic ovary syndrome. Exp Clin Endocrinol Diabetes 2012;120:205. [PMID: 22421986]

Dexamethasone suppression test (low dose, overnight)		
Dexamethasone suppression test (low dose, overnight), serum or plasma 8:00 AM serum cortisol level: <5 mcg/dL [<140 nmol/L] SST, PPT, green $$ Give 1 mg dexamethasone at 11:00 PM. At 8:00 AM, draw serum/plasma cortisol level.	For diagnosis of Cushing syndrome, the 1 mg overnight dexamethasone suppression test is most commonly performed. In normal patients, dexamethasone suppresses the 8:00 AM serum cortisol level below 5 mcg/dL. Patients with Cushing syndrome have 8:00 AM levels >10 mcg/dL (>276 nmol/L).	**Positive in:** Cushing syndrome (sensitivity is high in severe cases but less so in mild ones; specificity is only 70–90% in patients with chronic illness in hospitalized patients).	The test serves as a good screening test for Cushing syndrome. If this test is abnormal, use high-dose dexamethasone suppression test (see p. 90) to determine etiology. (See also Cushing syndrome algorithm, Figure 9–8.) For subclinical Cushing syndrome evaluation, a lower cut-off of 3.0 mcg/dL has been recommended but this produces more false-positive results. Patients taking phenytoin may fail to suppress because of enhanced dexamethasone metabolism. Depressed patients may also fail to suppress morning cortisol level. Other initial screening tests for Cushing syndrome include determinations of late-night salivary cortisol and 24-hr urine free cortisol. The 2 day, 2 mg dexamethasone suppression test is an alternative test, which appears to be more accurate in patients with alcoholism, diabetes mellitus or psychiatric disorders. Carroll TB et al. The diagnosis of Cushing's syndrome. Rev Endocr Metab Disord 2010;11:147. [PMID: 20821267] Raff H et al. Physiological basis for the etiology, diagnosis, and treatment of adrenal disorders: Cushing's syndrome, adrenal insufficiency, and congenital adrenal hyperplasia. Compr Physiol 2014;4:739. [PMID: 24715566] Starker LF et al. Subclinical Cushing syndrome: a review. Surg Clin North Am 2014;94:657. [PMID: 24857582]

(Continued)

Test/Range/Collection	Physiologic Basis	Interpretation	Comments
Dexamethasone suppression test (high-dose, overnight), serum or plasma 8:00 AM serum cortisol level: <5 mcg/dL [<140 nmol/L] SST, PPT, green $$ Give 8 mg dexamethasone dose at 11:00 PM. At 8:00 AM, draw cortisol level.	Suppression of plasma cortisol levels to <50% of baseline with dexamethasone indicates Cushing disease (pituitary-dependent ACTH hypersecretion, usually from a pituitary adenoma) and differentiates this from adrenal and ectopic causes of Cushing syndrome (see Cushing syndrome algorithm, Figure 9–8).	**Positive in:** Cushing disease (88–92% sensitivity; specificity 57–100%).	High-dose dexamethasone suppression test is indicated only after a positive low-dose dexamethasone suppression test (see p. 89). Sensitivity and specificity depend on sampling time and diagnostic criteria. Bilateral sampling of the inferior petrosal sinuses for ACTH after administration of corticotropin-releasing hormone has been used to identify the site of a pituitary adenoma before surgery. Carroll TB et al. The diagnosis of Cushing's syndrome. Rev Endocr Metab Disord 2010;11:147. [PMID: 20821267] Raff H et al. Physiological basis for the etiology, diagnosis, and treatment of adrenal disorders: Cushing's syndrome, adrenal insufficiency, and congenital adrenal hyperplasia. Compr Physiol 2014;4:739. [PMID: 24715566]
Double-stranded-DNA antibody (ds-DNA Ab), serum Negative (ELISA) or <1:10 titer (IFA) SST $$	IgG or IgM antibodies directed against host double-stranded DNA. Anti-dsDNA Ab are considered the serological hallmark of systemic lupus erythematosus (SLE). Test is not standardized across laboratories.	**Increased in:** Systemic lupus erythematosus (SLE; 60–70% sensitivity, 95% specificity, based on >1:10 titer). **Not increased in:** Drug-induced lupus.	Double-stranded DNA antibodies can be screened by a qualitative enzyme-linked immunosorbent assay (ELISA) assay, and, if positive, semi-quantitative immunofluorescent antibody testing (IFA) is then performed. High titers are seen only in SLE. Titers of ds-DNA antibody correlate moderately well with occurrence of glomerulonephritis (lupus nephritis) and renal disease activity. Autoantibodies against histones, Sm and nucleosomes may be detected and are also considered biomarkers for SLE. (See also Autoantibodies, Table 8–7.) Pisetsky DS. Standardization of anti-DNA antibody assays. Immunol Res 2013;56:420. [PMID: 23579774] Rekvig OP. Anti-dsDNA antibodies as a classification criterion and a diagnostic marker for systemic lupus erythematosus: critical remarks. Clin Exp Immunol 2015;179:5. [PMID: 24533624] Yu C et al. Diagnostic criteria for systemic lupus erythematosus: a critical review. J Autoimmun 2014;48:10. [PMID: 24461385]

		Positive/Increased in	Comments
Drug abuse screen, urine (urine toxicology drug screen, urine drug screen) Negative $	Testing for drugs of abuse (illicit) and drugs for pain treatment (prescribed) usually involves testing a single urine specimen for a number of drugs, eg, cocaine, opiates, barbiturates, amphetamines, benzodiazepines, cannabinoids, methadone, oxycodone, phencyclidine (PCP), tricyclic antidepressants. Screening tests are often immunoassays, which may not be specific for the tested drug. A positive test may warrant further confirmatory test by gas chromatography-mass spectrometry (GC/MS), the most widely accepted method of drug confirmation. Interpretation of results must take into account that urine concentrations can vary extensively with fluid intake and other biological variables. Adulteration of a urine specimen may also cause erroneous results.	**Positive in:** Chronic and casual drug users (sensitivity and specificity are assay-dependent), consumption of poppy seed containing foods.	It is important to know which drugs are included in the drug abuse screen and to understand that the test is qualitative and not quantitative. A single urine drug test detects only fairly recent drug use, and does not differentiate casual use from chronic drug use. The latter requires sequential drug testing and clinical evaluation. Urine drug testing does not determine the degree of impairment, the dose and frequency of drug taken, or the exact time of drug use. In a pain management setting, a negative result could be due to rapid metabolism/clearance of the drug, not taking drug as prescribed, diversion or stockpiling of prescribed drugs, or urine sample substitution. Poppy seeds contain small amounts of morphine and codeine and can produce a positive opiate result. Magnani B et al. Urine drug testing for pain management. Clin Lab Med 2012;32:379. [PMID: 22939297] Tenore PL. Advanced urine toxicology testing. J Addict Dis 2010;29:436. [PMID: 20924879]
Epstein-Barr virus antibodies, serum (EBV Ab) Negative SST $$	Antiviral capsid antibodies (anti-VCA) (IgM) appear early and last up to 3 months; anti-VCA IgG antibodies peak at 2–4 weeks after onset of clinical symptoms, decline slightly and then persist for life. Early antigen antibodies (anti-EA) are next to develop, are most often positive at 1 month after presentation, typically last for 2–3 months, and may last up to 6 months in low titers. Anti-EA may also be found in some patients with Hodgkin disease, chronic lymphocytic leukemia, and some other malignancies. Anti-EB nuclear antigen (anti-EBNA) antibody begins to appear in a minority of patients 2–4 months after onset of symptoms but is uniformly present by 6 months. It persists for the rest of a person's life.	**Positive/Increased in:** EB virus infection, infectious mononucleosis. Antibodies to the diffuse (D) form of antigen (detected in the cytoplasm and nucleus of infected cells) are greatly elevated in nasopharyngeal carcinoma. Antibodies to the restricted (R) form of antigen (detected only in the cytoplasm of infected cells) are greatly elevated in Burkitt lymphoma.	EBV antibodies are not usually needed to diagnose infectious mononucleosis, which is often a clinical diagnosis. Testing is most useful in diagnosing infectious mononucleosis in patients who have the clinical and hematologic criteria for the disease but who fail to develop heterophile agglutinins (10%) (see Heterophile antibody, p.126). The interpretation of EBV antibody tests requires familiarity with these tests and access to patient's clinical information. EBV antibodies cannot be used to diagnose "chronic" mononucleosis. Chronic fatigue syndrome is not caused by EBV. The best indicator of primary infection is a positive anti-VCA IgM (check for false positives caused by rheumatoid factor). The presence of anti-VCA IgG and anti-EBNA suggests past infection. EBV viral load could serve as a useful tool for the early diagnosis of infectious mononucleosis in cases with inconclusive serological results. Lennon P et al. Infectious mononucleosis. BMJ 2015; 350:h1825. [PMID: 25891165] Ruf S et al. Determining EBV load: current best practice and future requirements. Expert Rev Clin Immunol 2013;9:139. [PMID: 23390945]

(Continued)

Test/Range/Collection	Physiologic Basis	Interpretation	Comments
Erythrocyte sedimentation rate, whole blood (ESR) Males: <10 mm/h Females: <15 mm/h (laboratory-specific) Lavender; black $ Test must be run within 8 hrs after sample collection.	In plasma, erythrocytes (red blood cells [RBCs]) usually settle slowly. However, if they aggregate for any reason (usually because of plasma proteins called acute-phase reactants, eg, fibrinogen), they settle rapidly. Sedimentation of RBCs occurs because their density is greater than plasma. ESR measures the distance in millimeters that erythrocytes fall during 1 hour.	**Increased in:** Infections (osteomyelitis, pelvic inflammatory disease [75%]), inflammatory disease (giant cell arteritis [temporal arteritis], polymyalgia rheumatica, rheumatic fever), malignant neoplasms, paraproteinemias, anemia, pregnancy, chronic renal failure, inflammatory bowel disease (ulcerative colitis, regional ileitis). For endocarditis, sensitivity is approximately 93%. **Decreased in:** Polycythemia, sickle cell anemia, spherocytosis, anisocytosis, poikilocytosis, hypofibrinogenemia, hypogammaglobulinemia, heart failure, microcytosis, certain drugs (eg, high-dose corticosteroids).	There is often good correlation between ESR and C-reactive protein (CRP), but discordance between ESR and CRP has been noted in certain inflammatory disorders. Test is typically indicated for diagnosis and monitoring of temporal arteritis, systemic vasculitis and polymyalgia rheumatica. The test is not sensitive or specific for other conditions, although an extremely elevated ESR (eg, >100 mm/h) is useful in developing a rheumatic disease differential diagnosis. The ESR is higher in women, blacks, and older persons. A low value is of no diagnostic significance. The ESR should not be used to screen asymptomatic persons for disease because of its low sensitivity and specificity. Menes SB et al. A meta-analysis of the utility of C-reactive protein, erythrocyte sedimentation rate, fecal calprotectin, and fecal lactoferrin to exclude inflammatory bowel disease in adults with IBS. Am J Gastroenterol 2015;110:444. [PMID: 25732419] Weyand CM et al. Clinical practice. Giant-cell arteritis and polymyalgia rheumatica. N Engl J Med 2014;371:50. [PMID: 24988557]
Erythropoietin, serum or plasma (EPO) 5–30 mIU/mL [5–30 IU/L] [hematocrit-dependent] SST, PPT $$$	Erythropoietin (EPO) is a glycoprotein hormone produced in the kidney (peritubular capillary endothelial cells) that induces RBC production by stimulating proliferation, differentiation, and maturation of erythroid precursors. Hypoxia is the usual stimulus for production of EPO. EPO has also been shown to have an important cytoprotective function in the neuronal and cardiovascular systems.	**Increased in:** Anemias associated with bone marrow hyporesponsiveness (aplastic anemia, iron deficiency anemia), hemolytic anemia, secondary polycythemia (high-altitude hypoxia, COPD, pulmonary fibrosis), EPO-producing tumors (cerebellar hemangioblastomas, pheochromocytomas, renal tumors), kidney transplant rejection, pregnancy, polycystic kidney disease, treatment with recombinant human EPO. **Decreased in:** Anemia of chronic disease, renal failure, inflammatory states, primary polycythemia (polycythemia vera) (39%), congenital polycythemia (EPOR mutation), HIV infection with AZT treatment.	EPO levels are useful in differentiating primary from secondary polycythemia and in detecting recurrence of EPO-producing tumors. See diagnostic evaluation of polycythemia (Figure 9–26). Because virtually all patients with severe anemia due to chronic renal failure respond to EPO therapy, pre-therapy EPO levels are not necessary. EPO levels <500 IU/L predict response to recombinant human EPO treatment of symptomatic anemia in patients with myelodysplastic syndrome or myelofibrosis. Patients receiving recombinant human EPO as chronic therapy should have iron studies performed routinely. Koulnis M et al. Erythropoiesis: from molecular pathways to system properties. Adv Exp Med Biol 2014;844:37. [PMID: 25480636] Kremyanskaya M et al. Why does my patient have erythrocytosis? Hematol Oncol Clin North Am 2012;26:267. [PMID: 22463827] Tefferi A et al. Polycythemia vera and essential thrombocythemia: 2015 update on diagnosis, risk-stratification and management. Am J Hematol 2015;90:162. [PMID: 25611051]

Estradiol		
Estradiol (E2), serum or plasma Adult males: 10–40 pg/mL Adult females: Premenopausal: 30–400 pg/mL* Postmenopausal: 2–20 pg/mL (Adult males: 37–147 pmol/L). (Adult females: Premenopausal: 110–1480 pmol/L* Postmenopausal: 7–73 pmol/L) *E2 levels vary widely through the menstrual cycle. SST, red, lavender, PPT (light green) $$$$	In women, estradiol (E2) is produced primarily by the granulosa cells of the ovaries by aromatization of androstenedione to estrone (E1), followed by conversion of estrone to estradiol by 17β-hydroxysteroid dehydrogenase. Smaller amounts of estradiol and estrone are also produced by the adrenal cortex and some peripheral tissues (eg, fat cells), and by the testes (in men). E2 is the predominant sex hormone in premenopausal women. It is responsible for the development of secondary sex characteristics (eg, breast development). E1 is the primary estrogen in men and postmenopausal women, at much lower levels. E2 levels in premenopausal women fluctuate during the menstrual cycle. They are low at menstruation (<50 pg/mL), rise with follicular development (peak 200–400 pg/mL), drop briefly at ovulation, rise again during the luteal phase, and then drop to menstrual levels. During pregnancy, estrogen levels, including estradiol, rise steadily toward term. Estriol (E3) is produced by the placenta during pregnancy.	**Increased in:** Feminization, gynecomastia, precocious puberty, estrogen-producing tumors, hepatic cirrhosis, hyperthyroidism. **Decreased in:** Primary and secondary hypogonadism (ovarian failure).	E2 measurement is of value, together with gonadotropins, in evaluating menstrual and fertility problems in adult females. It is also useful in the evaluation of feminization (including gynecomastia) and estrogen-producing tumors in males. E2 test is used in therapeutic monitoring of human menopausal gonadotropin therapy, estrogen replacement therapy, and antiestrogen therapy (eg, aromatase inhibitor therapy). It is also used for monitoring ovarian hyperstimulation during *in vitro* fertilization treatment. Amato MC et al. Low estradiol-to-testosterone ratio is associated with oligo-anovulatory cycles and atherogenic lipidic pattern in women with polycystic ovary syndrome. Gynecol Endocrinol 2011;27:579. [PMID: 20608809] Prossnitz ER et al. Estrogen biology: new insights into GPER function and clinical opportunities. Mol Cell Endocrinol 2014;389:71. [PMID: 24530924] Rosner W et al. Challenges to the measurement of estradiol: an Endocrine Society position statement. J Clin Endocrinol Metab 2013;98:1376. [PMID: 23463657]

(Continued)

Test/Range/Collection	Physiologic Basis	Interpretation	Comments
Ethanol, serum or plasma (EtOH) Undetectable (unit: mg/dL or mmol/L) SST, red, lavender, PPT $$ Do not use alcohol swab. Do not remove stopper.	Test measures serum level of ethyl alcohol (ethanol). Ethanol is metabolized by alcohol dehydrogenase and the cytochrome P450 drug metabolizing enzyme. Toxic concentrations may cause inebriation, CNS depression, respiratory depression, mental and motor impairment and liver damage. In children, ethanol ingestion may cause hypoglycemia.	**Present in:** Ethanol ingestion.	Whole blood alcohol concentrations are about 15% lower than serum concentrations. Each 100 mg/dL of ethanol contributes about 22 mosm/kg to serum osmolality (see Table 8–14). Legal intoxication in many states is defined as >80 mg/dL (>17 mmol/L). For law enforcement determination of impaired driving, a breath alcohol test is now most commonly used. Chan LN et al. Pharmacokinetic and pharmacodynamic drug interactions with ethanol (alcohol). Clin Pharmacokinet 2014;53:1115. [PMID: 25267448] Donovan JE. The burden of alcohol use: focus on children and preadolescents. Alcohol Res 2013;35:186. [PMID: 24881327] Szabo G et al. Converging actions of alcohol on liver and brain immune signaling. Int Rev Neurobiol 2014;118:359. [PMID: 25175869]
Factor assays (coagulation factors II, V, VII, VIII, IX, X, XI, and XII) Blood Blue 50–150% $$$ Deliver immediately to laboratory on ice. Stable for 2 hrs. Freeze if assay is delayed > 2 hrs.	The partial thromboplastin time (PTT) and prothrombin time (PT) are the bases for factor assays. Factors VIII, IX, XI, and XII are PTT-based. Factors II, V, VII, and X are PT-based. The factor assay is based on the ability of patient plasma to correct the PTT or PT of specific factor-deficient plasma (<1% activity for the factor being measured). Quantitative results are obtained by comparing with a standard curve made from dilutions of normal reference plasma. Historically, a pool of normal plasma was used in factor assays and was assumed to have a factor activity of 100% (100 IU/dL, 1.0 IU/mL). This has now been replaced by commercial plasma standards and the activity levels of the various coagulation factors in the reference plasma are provided by the manufacturer. Multiple dilutions are often performed to rule out inhibitor interference (ie, non-parallelism).	**Increased in:** Acute- phase reactant response (elevated factor VIII). **Decreased in:** Hereditary factor deficiency (eg, hemophilia A, B); acquired factor deficiency secondary to acquired factor-specific inhibitor (eg, factor VIII inhibitor), liver disease (except factor VIII) and DIC (consumptive coagulopathy); vitamin K deficiency or warfarin therapy (II, VII, IX, and X), etc. Severe factor II deficiency may occur in rare patients with lupus anticoagulant. Acquired factor X deficiency may occur in patients with amyloidosis. Patients with von Willebrand disease may have low factor VIII levels (eg, type 3 vWD).	Factor assays are commonly undertaken when there is prolongation of the PTT and/or PT suggesting a deficiency of one or more clotting factors. Occasionally, factor VIII assay may be ordered as part of a hypercoagulability work-up. Although factor assays are typically PTT- or PT-based, chromogenic and immunogenic factor assays are also available for some factors including factors X and VIII. Heparin and direct thrombin inhibitors (eg, argatroban) can act as factor inhibitors and interfere with specific factor assays. Factor assay result needs to be interpreted with caution if non-parallelism is present (eg, lupus anticoagulant, factor-specific inhibitor). Chromogenic assay is more reliable in this setting. Astermark J. FVIII inhibitors: pathogenesis and avoidance. Blood 2015;125:2045. [PMID: 25712994] James P et al. Rare bleeding disorders—bleeding assessment tools, laboratory aspects and phenotype and therapy of FXI deficiency. Haemophilia 2014;20:571. [PMID: 24762279] Tiede A et al. Laboratory diagnosis of acquired hemophilia A: limitations, consequences, and challenges. Semin Thromb Hemost 2014;40:803. [PMID: 25299927] Wool GD et al. Pathology consultation on anticoagulation monitoring: factor X-related assays. Am J Clin Pathol 2013;140:623. [PMID: 24124140]

Factor II (prothrombin) mutation		
Factor II (prothrombin) G20210A mutation Blood Lavender $$$$	The factor II (prothrombin) 20210A mutation is a common genetic risk factor for thrombosis and is associated with elevated prothrombin levels. Higher concentrations of prothrombin lead to increased rates of thrombin generation, resulting in excessive growth of fibrin clots. It is an autosomal dominant disorder, with heterozygosity being at a 3- to 11-fold greater risk for thrombosis. Although homozygosity is rare, inheritance of two G20210A mutations would further increase the risk for developing thrombosis. The estimated frequency of factor II G20210A in white populations is between 1% and 6%. Prothrombin 20210A mutation is often ordered along with factor V Leiden (resistance to activated protein C) analysis to help diagnose the cause of recurrent venous thrombosis and/ or thromboembolism (VTE).	**Positive in:** Hypercoagulability secondary to factor II (prothrombin) G20210A mutation (sensitivity and specificity approach 100%).	Most carriers never experience a deep vein thrombosis (DVT) or pulmonary embolism (PE). Test result does not affect acute management and rarely affects the long term management of VTE. Testing should not be routinely ordered for patients with DVT or PE without determination of how and why the test result would alter management. Prothrombin mutation is associated with abdominal vein thrombosis, especially portal vein thrombosis. Polymerase chain reaction (PCR) is the most commonly used method for the detection of factor II G20210A mutation. Johnson NV et al. Advances in laboratory testing for thrombophilia. Am J Hematol 2012;87:S108. [PMID: 22473489] Leebeek FW et al. Prothrombotic disorders in abdominal vein thrombosis. Neth J Med 2012;70:400. [PMID: 23123534] MacCallum P et al. Diagnosis and management of heritable thrombophilias. BMJ 2014;349:g4387. [PMID: 25035247]

(Continued)

	Factor V Leiden mutation	
Test/Range/Collection	Physiologic Basis	Interpretation	Comments
Factor V Leiden Mutation Blood Lavender $$$$	The Leiden mutation is a single nucleotide base mutation (G1691A) in the factor V gene, leading to an amino acid substitution (Arg-506Glu) at one of the sites where coagulation factor V is cleaved by activated protein C (APC). This mutation results in a substantially reduced anticoagulant response to APC, because factor Va Leiden is inactivated about 10 times more slowly than normal factor Va. The frequency of factor V Leiden in white populations is between 2–15%. Factor V mutations may be present in up to half of the cases of unexplained venous thrombosis and are seen in more than 90% of patients with APC resistance.	**Positive in:** Hypercoagulability secondary to factor V Leiden mutation (sensitivity and specificity approach 100%).	The factor V Leiden mutation is the most common inherited risk factor for thrombosis and accounts for > 90% of cases with APC resistance. The presence of the mutation is only a risk factor for thrombosis, not an absolute marker for disease. Homozygotes have a 50- to 100-fold increase in risk of thrombosis (relative to the general population), and heterozygotes have a 7-fold increase in risk. Besides deep vein thrombosis (DVT), factor V Leiden is also associated with abdominal vein thrombosis, especially Budd Chiari syndrome, which requires immediate and long-term anticoagulation treatment. Most carriers never experience a DVT or pulmonary embolism (PE). Test result does not affect acute management and rarely affects the long-term management of venous thromboembolism. Testing should not be routinely ordered for patients with DVT or PE without determination of how and why the test result would alter management. Polymerase chain reaction (PCR) is the most commonly used method for the detection of the Leiden mutation of factor V. Franchini M. Utility of testing for factor V Leiden. Blood Transfus 2012;10:257. [PMID: 22889815] Leebeek FW et al. Prothrombotic disorders in abdominal vein thrombosis. Neth J Med 2012;70:400. [PMID: 23123534] MacCallum P et al. Diagnosis and management of heritable thrombophilias. BMJ 2014;349:g4387. [PMID: 25035247] Middeldorp S. Is thrombophilia testing useful? Hematology Am Soc Hematol Educ Program 2011;2011:150. [PMID: 22160027]

	Factor VIII assay	Fecal fat, quantification
Test / Specimen / Cost	**Factor VIII assay,** plasma 50–150% of normal (varies with age) Blue $$ Deliver immediately to laboratory on ice. Stable for 2 hrs. Freeze if assay is delayed for > 2 hrs. $$	**Fecal fat,** stool Random: < 60 droplets of fat/high power field 72-hour: < 7 g/day $$$ Qualitative: Random stool sample is adequate. Quantitative: Dietary fat should be about 100 g/day for 5 days before and during stool collection. Then all stools should be collected for 72 hrs and refrigerated.
Physiologic Basis	Test measures activity of factor VIII (antihemophilic factor), a key factor of the intrinsic pathway of the coagulation cascade (Figure 10–2). Factor VIII is produced by vascular endothelial cells and is the only coagulation factor that is not produced by hepatocytes. Factor VIII is carried by von Willebrand factor in the circulation. Clotting-based assay is commonly used. For patients with lupus anticoagulant, factor activity may be falsely low due to nonparallelism.	In healthy people, most dietary fat is completely absorbed in the small intestine. Normal small intestinal lining, bile acids, and pancreatic enzymes are required for normal fat absorption.
Interpretation	**Increased in:** Inflammatory states (acute-phase reactant), last trimester of pregnancy, oral contraceptives. **Decreased in:** Hemophilia A, von Willebrand disease (types 1, 3, 2N), DIC, acquired factor VIII inhibitor (acquired hemophilia).	**Increased in:** Malabsorption from small bowel disease (regional enteritis, celiac disease (gluten enteropathy), tropical sprue), pancreatic insufficiency, diarrhea with or without fat malabsorption.
Comments	Normal hemostasis requires at least 25% of factor VIII activity. Symptomatic hemophiliacs usually have levels ≤5%. Disease levels are defined as severe (< 1%), moderate (1–5%), and mild (> 5%). Factor VIII assays are used to guide replacement therapy in patients with hemophilia. Factor deficiency can be distinguished from factor inhibitor by an inhibitor screen and by nonparallelism on coagulation factor assays. Astermark J. FVIII inhibitors: pathogenesis and avoidance. Blood 2015;125:2045. [PMID: 25712994] Coppola A et al. Current and evolving features in the clinical management of haemophilia. Blood Transfus 2014;12:S554. [PMID: 24922295] Tuddenham E. In search of the source of factor VIII. Blood; 2014;123:3691. [PMID: 24926070]	72-hr fecal fat quantification is considered the gold standard for the diagnosis of pancreatic exocrine insufficiency. However, the test is cumbersome and unpleasant for patient and testing personnel. Test not routinely available. A random, qualitative fecal fat (so-called Sudan stain) is useful only if positive. Furthermore, it does not correlate well with quantitative measurements. Sudan stain appears to detect triglycerides and lipolytic by-products, whereas 72-hour fecal fat measures fatty acids from a variety of sources, including phospholipids, cholesteryl esters, and triglycerides. The quantitative method can be used to measure the degree of fat malabsorption initially and then after a therapeutic intervention. A normal quantitative stool fat reliably rules out pancreatic insufficiency and most forms of generalized small intestine disease. Besides fecal fat quantification, fecal pancreatic elastase 1 (see p. 168) can be used to evaluate pancreatic insufficiency with excellent sensitivity. The ^{13}C-mixed triglycerides breath test has also been introduced and adopted by many laboratories. Domínguez-Muñoz JE. Pancreatic exocrine insufficiency: diagnosis and treatment. J Gastroenterol Hepatol. 2011;26:S12. [PMID: 21323992] Lindkvist B. Diagnosis and treatment of pancreatic exocrine insufficiency. World J Gastroenterol 2013;19:7258. [PMID: 24259956]

(Continued)

	Fecal occult blood tests		
Test/Range/Collection	Physiologic Basis	Interpretation	Comments
Fecal occult blood tests (FOBT), stool Negative $ Dietary (meat, fish, turnips, horseradish) and medication (aspirin, nonsteroidal anti-inflammatory drugs) restrictions are often recommended to reduce false positive results, but available evidence does not suggest large effect on positivity rates in non-rehydrated testing. To avoid false-negatives, patients should avoid taking vitamin C. Patient collects two specimens from three consecutive bowel movements.	Traditionally, tests detect blood in the stool using gum guaiac as an indicator reagent (gFOBT). In gFOBT, gum guaiac is impregnated in a test paper that is smeared with stool using an applicator. Hydrogen peroxide is used as a developer solution. The resultant phenolic oxidation of guaiac in the presence of blood in the stool yields a blue color. The fecal immunochemical test (FIT) for hemoglobin is a better test for colorectal cancer screening.	**Positive in:** Upper GI disease (peptic ulcer, gastritis, variceal bleeding, esophageal and gastric cancer), lower GI disease (diverticulosis, colonic polyps, colorectal cancer, inflammatory bowel disease, vascular ectasias, hemorrhoids).	Although fecal occult blood testing is an accepted screening test for colorectal cancer, the sensitivity and specificity of an individual test are low. The usefulness of fecal occult blood testing after digital rectal examination is low. The quantitative fecal immunochemical test (FIT) is superior to gFOBT because there are no dietary and drug restrictions and it is more amenable to standardization and quality control. It is specific for hemoglobin, and clinically more sensitive for cancers and advanced adenomas. FIT screening has largely replaced gFOBT for noninvasive screening for colorectal cancer. Stool DNA tests have also gained approval for screening average risk adults ≥50 years for colorectal cancer, Imperiale TF et al. Multitarget stool DNA testing for colorectal cancer screening. N Engl J Med 2014;370:1287. [PMID: 24645800] Lee JK et al. Accuracy of fecal immunochemical tests for colorectal cancer: systematic review and meta-analysis. Ann Intern Med 2014;160:171. [PMID: 24658694] Young GP et al. Advances in fecal occult blood tests: the FIT revolution. Dig Dis Sci 2015;60:609. [PMID: 25492500]

Ferritin		
Ferritin, serum or plasma Males: 30–500 ng/mL [mcg/L] Females: 12–300 ng/mL [mcg/L] SST, PPT, lavender/pink, green (age-dependent) $$	Ferritin is the body's major iron storage protein. The serum ferritin level correlates with total body iron stores. The test is used to detect iron deficiency, to monitor response to iron therapy, and, in iron overload states, to monitor iron removal therapy. It is also used to predict homozygosity for hemochromatosis in relatives of affected patients. In the absence of liver disease and infection/inflammation, it is a more sensitive test for iron deficiency than serum iron and iron-binding capacity (transferrin saturation).	**Increased in:** Iron overload (hemochromatosis, hemosiderosis), acute or chronic liver disease, alcoholism, various malignancies (eg, leukemia, Hodgkin disease), chronic inflammatory disorders (eg, rheumatoid arthritis, adult Still disease), hemophagocytic lymphohistiocytosis, thalassemia minor, hyperthyroidism, HIV infection, non-insulin–dependent diabetes mellitus, blood transfusion, and postpartum state. **Decreased in:** Iron deficiency (60–75%).	Serum ferritin is clinically useful in distinguishing between iron deficiency anemia (serum ferritin levels diminished) and anemia of chronic disease or thalassemia (levels usually normal or elevated). Test of choice for diagnosis of iron deficiency anemia. **Ferritin (ng/mL)** — **Likelihood Ratio (LR) for Iron Deficiency** > 100 — 0.08 45–100 — 0.54 35–45 — 1.83 25–35 — 2.54 15–25 — 8.83 ≤ 15 — 52.00 Liver disease and conditions with acute-phase reactant response increase serum ferritin levels and may mask the diagnosis of iron deficiency. Serum soluble transferrin receptor (sTfR) measurement is helpful in determining iron deficiency status. Serum ferritin < 1000 ng/mL may predict absence of cirrhosis in hemochromatosis. Beck KL et al. Dietary determinants of and possible solutions to iron deficiency for young women living in industrialized countries: a review. Nutrients 2014;6:3747. [PMID: 25244367] Janka GE et al. Hemophagocytic lymphohistiocytosis: pathogenesis and treatment. Hematology Am Soc Hematol Educ Program 2013;2013:605. [PMID: 24319239] Kanwar P et al. Diagnosis and treatment of hereditary hemochromatosis: an update. Expert Rev Gastroenterol Hepatol 2013;7:517. [PMID: 23985001] Nemeth E et al. anemia of inflammation. Hematol Oncol Clin North Am 2014;28:671. [PMID: 25064707]

(*Continued*)

	α-Fetoprotein (AFP)		
Test/Range/Collection	Physiologic Basis	Interpretation	Comments
α-Fetoprotein, serum (AFP) 0–9 ng/mL [mcg/L] (age-dependent) SST, red $$ Avoid hemolysis.	α-fetoprotein (AFP) is a glycoprotein produced both early in fetal life and by some tumors. Serum AFP is a useful tumor marker.	**Increased in:** Hepatocellular carcinoma (72%), massive hepatic necrosis (74%), viral hepatitis (34%), chronic active hepatitis (29%), cirrhosis (11%), regional enteritis (5%), benign gynecologic diseases (22%), testicular carcinoma (embryonal) (70%), teratocarcinoma (64%), teratoma (37%), ovarian carcinoma (57%), endometrial cancer (50%), cervical cancer (53%), pancreatic cancer (23%), gastric cancer (18%), and colon cancer (5%). **Negative in:** Seminoma.	The test is not sensitive or specific enough to be used as a general screening test for hepatocellular carcinoma (HCC). However, screening may be justified in populations at very high risk for hepatocellular cancer. Combined testing of AFP with des-gamma-carboxyprothrombin and *Lens culinaris* agglutinin–reactive fraction of AFP (AFP-L3) increases the sensitivity of HCC diagnosis. In hepatocellular cancer or germ cell tumors associated with elevated AFP, the test may be helpful in monitoring recurrence after therapy. AFP is also used to screen pregnant women at 15–20 weeks gestation for possible fetal neural tube defects. AFP level in maternal serum or amniotic fluid is compared with levels expected at a given gestational age. Toyoda H et al. Tumor markers for hepatocellular carcinoma: simple and significant predictors of outcome in patients with HCC. Liver Cancer 2015;4:126. [PMID: 26020034] Wilson RD et al. Prenatal screening, diagnosis, and pregnancy management of fetal neural tube defects. J Obstet Gynaecol Can 2014;36:927. [PMID: 25375307] Wong RJ et al. Elevated alpha-fetoprotein: differential diagnosis—hepatocellular carcinoma and other disorders. Clin Liver Dis 2015;19:309. [PMID: 25921665]

(Continued)

Fibrinogen (functional)		Fluorescent treponemal antibody-absorbed

Fibrinogen (functional), plasma

150–400 mg/dL

[1.5–4.0 g/L]

Panic: < 75 mg/dL

Blue

$$

Fibrinogen is synthesized in the liver and has a half-life of about 4 days.

Thrombin cleaves fibrinogen to form insoluble fibrin monomers, which polymerize to form a clot.

Increased in: Inflammatory states (acute-phase reactant), use of oral contraceptives, pregnancy, postmenopausal women, smoking, and exercise.

Decreased in: Acquired deficiency: liver disease, consumptive coagulopathies such as DIC, and thrombolytic therapy; hereditary deficiency, resulting in an abnormal (dysfibrinogenemia), reduced (hypofibrinogenemia), or absent (afibrinogenemia) fibrinogen.

Fibrinogen assay is typically performed in the investigation of unexplained bleeding, prolonged PT or PTT, or as part of a DIC panel.

An elevated fibrinogen level has also been used as a predictor of arterial thrombotic events.

Fibrinogen is generally measured by a clotting-based functional (activity) assay. The Clauss assay, based on a high concentration of thrombin added to diluted patient plasma, is the most commonly used method. Direct thrombin inhibitor therapy may interfere with the assay.

Diagnosis of dysfibrinogenemia depends upon the discrepancy between antigen (measured by enzyme-linked immunosorbent assay, ELISA) and activity levels.

Hereditary afibrinogenemia is associated with mild-to-severe bleeding, whereas hypofibrinogenemia is most often asymptomatic. Dysfibrinogenemia is commonly associated with bleeding, thrombophilia, or both; however, most individuals are asymptomatic.

de Moerloose P et al. Congenital fibrinogen disorders: an update. Semin Thromb Hemost 2013;39:585. [PMID: 23852822]

Feinstein DI. Disseminated intravascular coagulation in patients with solid tumors. Oncology (Williston Park) 2015;29:96. [PMID: 25683828]

Peyvandi F et al. Rare bleeding disorders. Haemophilia 2012;18:S148. [PMID: 22726099]

Fluorescent Treponema pallidum antibody-absorbed (FTA-ABS), serum

Nonreactive

SST

$$

A syphilis test. Detects specific antibodies against *Treponema pallidum*.

Patient's serum is first diluted with nonpathogenic treponemal antigens (to bind nonspecific antibodies). The absorbed serum is placed on a slide that contains fixed *T. pallidum*. Fluorescein-labeled antihuman gamma globulin is then added to bind to and visualize (under a fluorescence microscope) the patient's antibody on treponemes.

Reactive in: Syphilis: primary (95%), secondary (100%), late (96%), late latent (100%); also rarely positive in collagen vascular diseases in the presence of antinuclear antibody.

Historically, this test was used to confirm a reactive nontreponemal screening serologic test for syphilis such as RPR or VDRL. A new syphilis testing algorithm using treponemal tests for screening and nontreponemal serologic tests for confirmation has been proposed (see also Table 8–21 and Syphilis testing, p. 200).

Once positive, the FTA-ABS may remain positive for life. However, one study found that at 36 months after treatment, 24% of patients had nonreactive FTA-ABS tests.

Seña AC et al. Novel *Treponema pallidum* serologic tests: a paradigm shift in syphilis screening for the 21st century. Clin Infect Dis 2010;51:700. [PMID: 20687840]

Tucker JD et al. Accelerating worldwide syphilis screening through rapid testing: a systematic review. Lancet Infect Dis 2010;10:381. [PMID: 20510278]

	Folic acid (Folate)		
Test/Range/Collection	**Physiologic Basis**	**Interpretation**	**Comments**
Folic acid (Folate), whole blood (RBC), serum or plasma 165–760 ng/mL (370–1720 nmol/L) (RBC); 4–20 ng/mL (9–45 nmol/L) (serum or plasma) Lavender, SST, PPT $$	Folate is a vitamin necessary for methyl group transfer in thymidine formation, and hence DNA synthesis. Deficiency can result in megaloblastic anemia. The naturally occurring folate polyglutamates are hydrolyzed to monoglutamate forms before absorption by the small intestine. In the liver, folate monoglutamates are converted to N^5-methyltetrahydrofolate (MeTHF), which is excreted in bile. This methylated form of folate is reabsorbed from the gut but not taken up by the liver and therefore becomes the major circulating form of folate. Red cell folate has been considered more important because it reflects tissue folate level; however, it is also more cumbersome and not always routinely available. Evidence from the literature indicates that serum/plasma folate measurements provide equivalent information when determining whether folate deficiency is present.	**Decreased in:** Tissue folate deficiency (from dietary folate deficiency), vitamin B_{12} deficiency (50–60%, since cellular uptake of folate depends on vitamin B_{12}).	A low red cell folate level may indicate either folate or vitamin B_{12} deficiency. A therapeutic trial of folate (and not red cell or serum folate testing) is indicated when the clinical and dietary history is strongly suggestive of folate deficiency and the peripheral smear shows hypersegmented neutrophils. However, the possibility of vitamin B_{12} deficiency must always be considered in the setting of megaloblastic anemia, since folate therapy treats the hematologic, but not the neurologic, sequelae of vitamin B_{12} deficiency. Folate deficiency has become a rare event in developed countries, and folate measurement is only indicated in unexplained macrocytosis and inborn errors of metabolism. Routine folate test is not recommended. Lassi ZS et al. Folic acid supplementation during pregnancy for maternal health and pregnancy outcomes. Cochrane Database Syst Rev 2013;3:CD006896. [PMID: 23543547] Gilfix BM. Utility of measuring serum or red blood cell folate in the era of folate fortification of flour. Clin Biochem 2014;47:533. [PMID: 24488651] Reynolds EH. The neurology of folic acid deficiency. Handb Clin Neurol 2014;120:927. [PMID: 24365361]

	Follicle-stimulating hormone	
Follicle-stimulating hormone (FSH), serum or plasma Males: 1–10 mIU/mL Females: (mIU/mL) Follicular 4–13 Luteal 2–13 Midcycle 5–22 Postmenopausal 20–138 (laboratory-specific) SST, PPT, green $$	FSH is stimulated by the hypothalamic hormone GnRH and is then secreted from the anterior pituitary in a pulsatile fashion. Levels rise during the preovulatory phase of the menstrual cycle and then decline. FSH is necessary for normal pubertal development and fertility in males and females.	**Increased in:** Primary or premature ovarian failure (eg, autoimmune oophoritis, Turner syndrome), ovarian or testicular agenesis, castration, gonadotoxic cancer treatment, postmenopause, Klinefelter syndrome, drugs. **Decreased in:** Hypothalamic disorders, pituitary disorders, pregnancy, anorexia nervosa. Drugs: corticosteroids, oral contraceptives.	Test indicated in the work-up of amenorrhea in women (see Amenorrhea algorithm, Figure 9–4) and delayed puberty, impotence, or infertility in men. Impotence work-up should begin with serum testosterone measurement. Basal FSH levels in premenopausal women depend on age, smoking history, and menstrual cycle length and regularity. Because of its variability, FSH is an unreliable guide to menopausal status during the transition into menopause. For ovarian reserve assessment, antimüllerian hormone is more informative than baseline FSH testing. Check JH. Premature ovarian insufficiency—fertility challenge. Minerva Ginecol 2014;66:133. [PMID: 24848073] Klein DA et al. Amenorrhea: an approach to diagnosis and management. Am Fam Physician 2013;87:781. [PMID: 23939500] Toner JP et al. Why we may abandon basal follicle-stimulating hormone testing: a sea change in determining ovarian reserve using antimüllerian hormone. Fertil Steril 2013;99:1825. [PMID: 23548941]

(Continued)

Test/Range/Collection	Physiologic Basis	Interpretation	Comments
Fructosamine, serum or plasma 0.16–0.27 mmol/L SST, lavender, green $	Glycation of plasma protein produces fructosamine, a less expensive marker of glycemic control than HbA$_{1c}$. The test is particularly useful if rapid monitoring of glycemic control is required (eg, during pregnancy) or if red cell life span is altered (eg, hemolysis, hemoglobin variants, blood loss, kidney diseases). Its level reflects glycemia over the previous 2–3 weeks. Tests are not standardized and there are no established clinical cutoff points.	**Increased in:** Diabetes mellitus, gestational diabetes.	Fructosamine correlates well with fasting plasma glucose ($r = 0.74$) but cannot be used to predict precisely the HbA$_{1c}$. Although various equations have been developed to convert fructosamine to an "HbA1$_c$ equivalent," it is not recommended as a substitute for HbA$_{1c}$ except in specific clinical situations where HbA1$_c$ testing is known to be problematic or short-term changes in glycemia are of clinical importance. In clinical studies where fasting glucose or HbA1$_c$ measurements are not available but where serum or plasma specimens were collected, fructosamine may be useful to identify individuals with undiagnosed hyperglycemia. Parrinello CM et al. Beyond HbA1$_c$ and glucose: the role of nontraditional glycemic markers in diabetes diagnosis, prognosis, and management. Curr Diab Rep 2014;14:548. [PMID: 25249070] Virally M et al. Methods for the screening and diagnosis of gestational diabetes mellitus between 24 and 28 weeks of pregnancy. Diabetes Metab. 2010;36:549. [PMID: 21163420]
Gamma-glutamyl transpeptidase (GGT), serum or plasma 9–85 U/L [0.15–1.42 mckat/L] (laboratory-specific) SST, PPT, green $	GGT is an enzyme present in liver, kidney, and pancreas. It is induced by alcohol intake and is an extremely sensitive indicator of liver disease, particularly alcoholic liver disease.	**Increased in:** Liver disease: acute viral or toxic hepatitis, chronic or subacute hepatitis, alcoholic hepatitis, cirrhosis, biliary tract obstruction (intrahepatic or extrahepatic), primary or metastatic liver neoplasm, and mononucleosis. Drugs (by enzyme induction): phenytoin, carbamazepine, barbiturates, alcohol.	GGT is useful in follow-up of alcoholics undergoing treatment because the test is sensitive to modest alcohol intake. GGT is elevated in 90% of patients with liver disease. Elevated GGT activity has prognostic significance. GGT is used to confirm hepatic origin of elevated serum alkaline phosphatase. Carobene A et al. A systematic review of data on biological variation for alanine aminotransferase, aspartate aminotransferase and γ-glutamyl transferase. Clin Chem Lab Med 2013;51:1997. [PMID: 24072574] Kunutsor SK et al. Liver enzymes and risk of all-cause mortality in general populations: a systematic review and meta-analysis. Int J Epidemiol 2014;43:187. [PMID: 24585856]

Test / Range / Specimen		Interpretation	Comments
	Gastrin		
Gastrin, serum <100 pg/mL [ng/L] (assay-dependent) SST $$ Overnight fasting required.	Gastrin is secreted from G cells in the stomach antrum and stimulates acid secretion from the gastric parietal cells. It is also considered a biomarker of cancer risk. Values fluctuate throughout the day but are lowest in the early morning.	**Increased in:** Gastrinoma (Zollinger-Ellison syndrome) (80–93% sensitivity), antral G cell hyperplasia, hypochlorhydria, achlorhydria, chronic atrophic gastritis, pernicious anemia. Drugs: antacids, cimetidine and other H_2 blockers; omeprazole and other proton pump inhibitors. **Decreased in:** Antrectomy with vagotomy.	Tests are performed primarily for the diagnosis of gastrin-producing tumors (gastrinomas). Gastrin circulates as several bioactive peptides, and the peptide pattern in gastrinoma patients often deviates from normal. Gastrin is the first-line test for determining whether a patient with active ulcer disease has a gastrinoma. Gastric acid analysis is not indicated. Before interpreting an elevated level, be sure that the patient is not taking antacids, H_2 blockers, or proton pump inhibitors. Both fasting and post-secretin infusion levels may be required for diagnosis. Epelboym I et al. Zollinger-Ellison syndrome: classical considerations and current controversies. Oncologist 2014;19:44. [PMID: 24319020] Ito T et al. Zollinger-Ellison syndrome: recent advances and controversies. Curr Opin Gastroenterol 2013;29:650. [PMID: 24100728] Rehfeld JF et al. Pitfalls in diagnostic gastrin measurements. Clin Chem 2012;58:831. [PMID: 22419747]
	Glomerular filtration rate, estimated (eGFR)		
Glomerular filtration rate, estimated (eGFR) (see Creatinine and cystatin C, serum or plasma) > 60 mL/min/1.73 m²	The National Kidney Disease Education Program (NKDEP) recommends the use of the estimation of GFR from serum creatinine in adults (> 18 years) with chronic kidney disease (CKD) and those at risk for CKD (diabetes mellitus, hypertension, and family history of kidney failure). Estimated GFR (eGFR) provides a clinically more useful measure of kidney function than creatinine alone. GFR calculators recommended by MDRD (Modification of Diet in Renal Disease) and CKD-EPI (CKD Epidemiology Collaboration) are available at the NKDEP website: http://nkdep.nih.gov/lab-evaluation/gfr-calculators.shtml.	**Decreased in:** CKD, kidney failure.	CKD is defined as either kidney damage or GFR < 60 mL/min/1.73 m² for at least 3 months. Kidney damage is defined as pathologic abnormalities or markers of damage, including abnormalities in blood or urine tests (eg, albuminuria) or imaging studies. Kidney failure is defined as GFR <15 mL/min. Cystatin C (CyC)-based eGFR (eGFRcys) has been proposed as a superior alternative, especially for conditions (eg, decreased muscle mass, kidney transplant, cirrhosis) where the creatinine-based eGFR (eGFRcr) is less reliable Harman G et al. Accuracy of cystatin C-based estimates of glomerular filtration rate in kidney transplant recipients: a systematic review. Nephrol Dial Transplant 2013;28:741. [PMID: 23275574] Levey AS et al. Glomerular filtration rate and albuminuria for detection and staging of acute and chronic kidney disease in adults: a systematic review. JAMA 2015;313:837. [PMID: 25710660] Shlipak MG et al. Update on cystatin C: incorporation into clinical practice. Am J Kidney Dis 2013;62:595. [PMID: 23701892]

(Continued)

	Glucagon

Test/Range/Collection	Physiologic Basis	Interpretation	Comments
Glucagon, plasma 20–100 pg/mL [20–100 ng/L] (age and laboratory-specific) Lavender $$$$ Fasting specimen collected in pre-chilled lavender tube is required. After drawing specimen, chill tube in wet ice for 10 minutes before centrifugation.	Glucagon is a peptide hormone secreted by the pancreatic alpha islet cells. Glucagon secretion is stimulated by low levels of blood glucose. It stimulates the production of glucose in the liver by glycogenolysis. Excessive glucagon secretion can lead to hyperglycemia. Glucagon-secreting tumors are associated with necrolytic migratory erythema, diabetes mellitus, thrombosis, and neuropsychiatric features.	**Increased in:** Glucagonoma and other glucagon-secreting tumors, familial hyperglucagonemia. **Decreased in:** Diabetes mellitus (type 1) with pronounced hypoglycemic features, chronic pancreatitis, post-pancreatectomy.	Useful as a tumor marker for diagnosis and follow-up of glucagon-secreting tumors. Results obtained with different glucagon assays can differ substantially. Different glucagon assays may exhibit variable cross-reactivity with different isoforms of glucagon, not all of which are biologically active. Serial measurements should, therefore, always be performed using the same assay. Kanakis G et al. Biochemical markers for gastroenteropancreatic neuroendocrine tumours (GEP-NETs). Best Pract Res Clin Gastroenterol 2012;26:791. [PMID: 23582919] Lund A et al. Glucagon and type 2 diabetes: the return of the alpha cell. Curr Diab Rep 2014;14:555. [PMID: 25344790] Sandoval DA et al. Physiology of proglucagon peptides: role of glucagon and GLP-1 in health and disease. Physiol Rev 2015;95:513. [PMID: 25834231]

Glucose			
Glucose, serum or plasma 60–110 mg/dL [3.3–6.1 mmol/L] ***Panic:*** < 40 or > 500 mg/dL SST, PPT, gray $ Overnight fasting usually required.	Normally, the glucose concentration in extracellular fluid is closely regulated so that a source of energy is readily available to tissues and so that no glucose is excreted in the urine.	**Increased in:** Diabetes mellitus, Cushing syndrome (10–15%), chronic pancreatitis (30%). Drugs: corticosteroids, phenytoin, estrogen, thiazides. **Decreased in:** Pancreatic islet cell disease with increased insulin, insulinoma, adrenocortical insufficiency, hypopituitarism, diffuse liver disease, malignancy (adrenocortical, stomach, fibrosarcoma), infant of a diabetic mother, enzyme deficiency diseases (eg, galactosemia). Drugs: insulin, ethanol, propranolol; sulfonylureas, tolbutamide, and other oral hypoglycemic agents.	Diagnosis of diabetes mellitus requires a fasting plasma glucose of > 126 mg/dL (7.0 mmol/L) on more than one occasion, a casual plasma glucose level ≥200 mg/dL (11.1 mmol/L) or HbA$_{1c}$ ≥ 6.5% along with symptoms of diabetes. Patients with fasting blood glucose levels 110 mg/dL (6.1 mmol/L) to 126 mg/dL (7.0 mmol/L) are considered to have impaired fasting glucose. Hypoglycemia is defined as a glucose of < 50 mg/dL in men and < 40 mg/dL in women. While random serum glucose levels correlate with home glucose monitoring results (weekly mean capillary glucose values), there is wide fluctuation within individuals. Thus, glycosylated hemoglobin levels are favored to monitor glycemic control. The American Diabetes Association recommends that adults age 45 years or older should be evaluated for diabetes by measuring fasting glucose levels at 3-year intervals. Long-term outcome studies are needed to provide evidence for this recommendation. Campos C. Chronic hyperglycemia and glucose toxicity: pathology and clinical sequelae. Postgrad Med 2012;124:90. [PMID: 23322142] Laiteerapong N et al. Screening for prediabetes and type 2 diabetes mellitus. JAMA 2016;315:697. [PMID: 26881373] Thomas CC et al. Update on diabetes classification. Med Clin North Am. 2015;99:1. [PMID: 25456640]

(Continued)

Glucose tolerance test

Test/Range/Collection	Physiologic Basis	Interpretation	Comments
Glucose tolerance test (oral), serum or plasma Fasting: < 100 mg/dL 1-hour: < 180 mg/dL 2-hour: < 140 mg/dL [Fasting: < 5.6 mmol/L 1-hour: < 10.0 mmol/L 2-hour: < 7.7 mmol/L] SST, PPT (light green), gray $$ Subjects should receive a 150- to 200-g per day carbohydrate diet for at least 3 days before the test. A 75-g glucose dose is dissolved in 300 mL of water for adults (1.75 g/kg for children) and given after an overnight fast. Serial determinations of plasma or serum venous blood glucoses are obtained at baseline, 1 hour, and 2 hours.	Oral glucose tolerance test (OGTT) determines the ability of a patient to respond appropriately to a glucose load. It is one of the three screening tests (fasting blood glucose, HbA$_{1c}$ and OGTT) for type 2 diabetes in adults.	**Increased glucose rise (decreased glucose tolerance) in:** Diabetes mellitus, impaired glucose tolerance, gestational diabetes, severe liver disease, hyperthyroidism, stress (infection), increased absorption of glucose from GI tract (hyperthyroidism, gastrectomy, gastroenterostomy, vagotomy, excess glucose intake), Cushing syndrome, pheochromocytoma. Drugs: diuretics, oral contraceptives, glucocorticoids, nicotinic acid, phenytoin. **Decreased glucose rise (flat glucose curve) in:** Intestinal disease (celiac disease [gluten enteropathy], Whipple disease), adrenal insufficiency (Addison disease, hypopituitarism), pancreatic islet cell tumors or hyperplasia.	Test is not generally required for diagnosis of type 2 diabetes mellitus. In screening for gestational diabetes, the glucose tolerance test is performed between 24 and 28 weeks of gestation. There are 2 strategies used in the United States. In the 2-step approach, a 50-g OGTT is performed in a nonfasting state. If the screening threshold is met or exceeded, patients receive the 100-g OGTT after a fasting glucose level is obtained. Glucose levels are evaluated after 1, 2, and 3 hours. A diagnosis is made when 2 or more glucose values fall at or above the specified glucose thresholds. Alternatively, in the 1-step approach, a 75-g glucose load is administered after fasting and blood glucose levels are evaluated after 1 and 2 hours. Gestational diabetes is diagnosed if 1 glucose value falls at or above the specified glucose threshold. Laiteerapong N et al. Screening for prediabetes and type 2 diabetes mellitus. JAMA 2016;315:697. [PMID: 26881373] Macaulay S et al. Gestational diabetes mellitus in Africa: a systematic review. PLoS One 2014;9:e97871. [PMID: 24892280] McIntyre HD et al. Counterpoint: establishing consensus in the diagnosis of GDM following the HAPO study. Curr Diab Rep 2014;14:497. [PMID: 24777652] Waugh NR et al. Screening for type 2 diabetes: a short report for the National Screening Committee. Health Technol Assess 2013;17:1. [PMID: 23972041]

G6PD (Glucose-6-phosphate dehydrogenase)		
Glucose-6-phosphate dehydrogenase, whole blood (G6PD) 5–15 units/g Hb Yellow, green, lavender or pink $$	G6PD is an enzyme in the hexose monophosphate shunt that is essential in generating NADPH and reduced glutathione, which protect hemoglobin from oxidative denaturation. Numerous G6PD isoenzymes have been identified. Inherited G6PD deficiency causes neonatal hyperbilirubinemia and chronic hemolytic anemia; exposure to oxidative stressors such as certain drugs, foods or infections, can elicit significant acute hemolysis. The wild-type is G6PD-B. Most African Americans have G6PD-A(+) isoenzyme. 10–15% have G6PD-A(–), which has moderately decreased enzyme activity. It is transmitted in an X-linked recessive manner. Some Mediterranean and Middle Eastern people have the G6PD-B(–) variant (known as G6PD^{Med}), which has markedly decreased enzyme activity. Uncommon variants that are associated with severely decreased enzyme activity include G6PD^{Canton} and G6PD^{Iowa}.	**Increased in:** Young erythrocytes (reticulocytosis). **Decreased in:** G6PD deficiency (enzyme activity level is dependent on the type of G6PD variant).	In deficient patients, hemolytic anemia can be triggered by oxidant agents: antimalarial drugs (eg, chloroquine, primaquine), methylene blue, naphthalene, nalidixic acid, nitrofurantoin, isoniazid, dapsone, phenacetin, rasburicase, vitamin C (high dose), sulfasalazine and other "sulfa" drugs. Patients from high risk groups (eg, African American and people from the Mediterranean region) should be screened for G6PD deficiency before taking an oxidant drug. Hemolytic episodes can also occur in deficient patients who eat fava beans (favism) or bitter melon/gourd, with diabetic ketoacidosis, and in infections. G6PD deficiency may be the cause of hemolytic disease of newborns in Asians and Mediterraneans. Besides laboratory evidence of hemolysis (eg, increase in LDH and bilirubin), "bite cells" may be seen on routine blood smear, and "Heinz bodies" inside red cells on a specially stained blood smear. G6PD activity levels may be measured as normal during an acute episode, because mostly nonhemolyzed young and less deficienct red cells are assessed. If deficiency is still suspected, assay should be repeated in 2–3 months when cells of all ages are present. Patients who have recently received blood transfusions may have falsely normal enzyme activity level. G6PD mutation analysis is available but is only indicated for patients with established enzyme deficiency, ie, to determine the exact G6PD mutant variant. Luzzatto L et al. G6PD deficiency: a classic example of pharmacogenetics with on-going clinical implications. Br J Haematol 2014;164:469. [PMID: 24372186] Watchko JF et al. Should we screen newborns for glucose-6-phosphate dehydrogenase deficiency in the United States? J Perinatol 2013;33:499. [PMID: 23429543]

(Continued)

	Growth hormone	
Test/Range/Collection	**Physiologic Basis**	**Interpretation**	**Comments**
---	---	---	---
Growth hormone, serum or plasma (GH) 0–5 ng/mL [mcg/L] (age-dependent) SST, PPT, green $$$ Patient must be fasting and at complete rest for 30 minutes before blood sample collection.	Human GH is secreted by the anterior pituitary. It stimulates hepatic IGF-1 (insulin-like growth factor 1), mobilizes fatty acids, and stimulates collagen and protein synthesis. GH levels are subject to wide fluctuations during the day and, because it is secreted in surges, a single, one-time test is of limited diagnostic value.	**Increased in:** Acromegaly (90% have GH levels > 10 ng/mL), McCune-Albright syndrome with acromegaly, Laron dwarfism (defective GH receptor), starvation. Drugs: dopamine, levodopa. **Decreased in:** Pituitary dwarfism, hypopituitarism, congenital or acquired GH deficiency.	Elevated levels of human GH indicate the possibility of acromegaly, but must be confirmed with stimulation and suppression testing. IGF-1 test is preferred for acromegaly screen. If IGF level is high (or equivocal), then GH should be measured after oral glucose administration. Inadequate suppression of GH levels to < 2 ng/mL 2 hrs after 75 or 100 g oral glucose confirms the diagnosis of acromegaly. Random determinations of GH are rarely useful in the diagnosis of acromegaly. For the diagnosis of hypopituitarism or GH deficiency in children, an insulin-induced hypoglycemia test has been used. Failure to increase GH levels to > 5 ng/mL in children or >4 ng/mL in adults after insulin (0.1 unit/kg) is consistent with GH deficiency. Arginine and/or GH-releasing hormone stimulation tests have also been used. Alatzoglou KS et al. Isolated growth hormone deficiency (GHD) in childhood and adolescence: recent advances. Endocr Rev 2014;35:376. [PMID: 24450934] Andersen M. Management of endocrine disease: GH excess: diagnosis and medical therapy. Eur J Endocrinol 2013;170:R31. [PMID: 24144967] Hawkes CP et al. Measuring growth hormone and insulin-like growth factor-I in infants: what is normal? Pediatr Endocrinol Rev 2013;11:126. [PMID: 24575549]

Test/Specimen	Physiologic Basis	Interpretation	Comments
Haptoglobin, serum or plasma 46–316 mg/dL [0.5–3.2 g/L] (method-dependent) SST, PPT, green, lavender $$ Fasting specimen preferred.	Haptoglobin is a glycoprotein primarily produced in the liver that binds free hemoglobin. Its scavenging function counteracts the potentially harmful oxidative and nitric oxide–scavenging effects associated with free hemoglobin released from lysed red blood cells *in vivo*.	**Increased in:** Acute and chronic infection (acute-phase reactant), malignancy, biliary obstruction, ulcerative colitis, myocardial infarction, and diabetes mellitus. **Decreased in:** Newborns and children, post-transfusion, intravascular hemolysis, autoimmune hemolytic anemia, liver disease (10%), hemodilution. May be decreased following uneventful transfusion (10%) for unknown reasons.	Haptoglobin levels become depleted in the presence of large amounts of free hemoglobin, and so decreased haptoglobin is a marker of hemolysis. However, it is of uncertain clinical predictive value due to its low specificity and because of occasional normal individuals who have very low levels. Test result needs to be correlated with clinical and other laboratory findings. High normal levels probably rule out significant intravascular hemolysis. Low haptoglobin levels can aid in early recognition of the HELLP syndrome (**h**emolytic anemia, **e**levated **l**iver enzymes, and **l**ow **p**latelet count) in pregnant women. Alayash AI. Haptoglobin: old protein with new functions. Clin Chim Acta 2011;412:493. [PMID: 21159311] Schaer DJ et al. Haptoglobin, hemopexin, and related defense pathways-basic science, clinical perspectives, and drug development. Front Physiol 2014;5:415. [PMID: 25389409] Shih AW et al. Haptoglobin testing in hemolysis: measurement and interpretation. Am J Hematol 2014;89:443. [PMID: 24809098]
***Helicobacter pylori* antibody**, serum or plasma Negative SST, lavender/pink, green $$	*Helicobacter pylori* is a gram-negative spiral bacterium that is found on gastric mucosa. It induces acute and chronic inflammation in the gastric mucosa and a positive serologic antibody response. Serologic testing for *H. pylori* antibody (IgG, IgM and IgA) is by semi-quantitative enzyme-linked immunosorbent assay (ELISA).	**Increased (positive) in:** Histologic (chronic or chronic active) gastritis due to *H. pylori* infection (with or without peptic ulcer disease). Sensitivity 98%, specificity 48%. Asymptomatic adults: 15–50%.	The prevalence of *H. pylori*-positive serologic tests in asymptomatic adults is approximately 35% overall but is > 50% in patients over age 60. Fewer than one in six adults with *H. pylori* antibody develop peptic ulcer disease. Treatment of asymptomatic adults with positive serology is not currently recommended. After successful eradication, serologic titers fall over a 3- to 6-month period but remain positive in up to 50% of patients at 1 year. The noninvasive fecal antigen immunoassay and the urea breath test have excellent sensitivity and specificity (> 95%) for active infection. Bacterial culture from gastric biopsy is the gold standard. Lopes AI et al. *Helicobacter pylori* infection-recent developments in diagnosis. World J Gastroenterol 2014;20:9299. [PMID: 25071324] Mégraud F et al. Diagnosis of *Helicobacter pylori* infection. Helicobacter 2014;19(Suppl 1):6. [PMID: 25167939]

(Continued)

	Hematocrit		
Test/Range/Collection	Physiologic Basis	Interpretation	Comments
Hematocrit, whole blood (Hct) Males: 39–49% Females: 35–45% (age-dependent) Lavender 5	The Hct represents the percentage of whole blood volume composed of erythrocytes. Laboratory instruments calculate Hct from the erythrocyte count (RBC) and the mean corpuscular volume (MCV) by the formula: Hct = (RBC × MCV)/10 Manual spun hematocrit (microhematocrit) is 1.5–3% higher than that from an automated hematology instrument and is less reliable.	**Increased in:** Hemoconcentration (as in dehydration, burns, vomiting), polycythemia (erythrocytosis), extreme physical exercise. **Decreased in:** Macrocytic anemia (liver disease, hypothyroidism, vitamin B_{12} deficiency, folate deficiency, myelodysplasia, HIV infection, alcoholism), normocytic anemia (early iron deficiency, anemia of chronic disease, hemolytic anemia, acute hemorrhage, bone marrow infiltrates of leukemia, lymphoma, myeloma or metastatic tumor), and microcytic anemia (iron deficiency, thalassemia, sideroblastic anemia). Hemodilution.	Conversion from hemoglobin (Hb) to hematocrit is roughly Hb × 3 = Hct. This does not apply if there is a significant hypochromic red cell population present. The Hct reported by clinical laboratories is not a spun Hct. The spun Hct may be spuriously high if the centrifuge is not calibrated, if the specimen is not spun to constant volume, or if there is "trapped plasma." Spun Hct is rarely needed. In determining transfusion need, the clinical picture must be considered in addition to the Hct and hemoglobin concentration (g/dL). Hct is used to monitor the effects of therapy for polycythemia vera with a goal of keeping the Hct < 45%. Point-of-care instruments may not measure Hct accurately in all patients. In hemodialysis patients, erythropoiesis-stimulating agents have been used to maintain an Hct of 33–36% (hemoglobin of 11–12 g/dL) to reduce blood transfusions and improve quality of life, but recent data led to an FDA black box warning regarding a risk of myocardial infarction, stroke, and death associated with the use of these agents at higher than recommended doses. Barbui T et al. Rethinking the diagnostic criteria of polycythemia vera. Leukemia 2014;28:1191. [PMID: 24352199] Leach M. Interpretation of the full blood count in systemic disease—a guide for the physician. J R Coll Physicians Edinb 2014;44:36. [PMID: 24995446] Sireci AN. Hematology testing in urgent care and resource-poor settings: an overview of point of care and satellite testing. Clin Lab Med 2015;35:197. [PMID: 25676380]

	Hemoglobin A1c, blood			Hemoglobin A$_2$

Hemoglobin A$_{1c}$ (Glycohemoglobin, HbA$_{1c}$), blood

4.0–5.6%
[20–38 mmol/mol] (method-dependent)

Lavender, pink

$$

During the life span of each RBC, glucose combines with hemoglobin to produce stable glycated hemoglobin.

The level of glycated hemoglobin is related to the mean plasma glucose level during the previous 1–3 months. The HbA$_{1c}$ level can be used to estimate the average blood glucose levels (eAG), ie, eAG (mg/dL) = (28.7 x %HbA1c) – 46.7.

There are three glycated A hemoglobins: HbA$_{1a}$, HbA$_{1b}$, and HbA$_{1c}$. Some assays quantitate HbA$_{1c}$, some quantitate total HbA$_1$, and some quantitate all glycated hemoglobins, not just A.

Hemoglobin variants may interfere with HbA$_{1c}$ determinations.

Increased in: Diabetes mellitus, splenectomy. Falsely high results can occur depending on the method used and may be due to presence of hemoglobin F or uremia.

Decreased in: Any condition that shortens red cell life span (hemolytic anemias, congenital spherocytosis, acute or chronic blood loss, sickle cell disease, hemoglobinopathies).

HbA$_{1c}$ is useful for monitoring glycemic control and for quantifying the risk of diabetic complications. There is a clear relationship between glycemic control as reflected by HbA$_{1c}$ and the progression of microvascular complications in both type I and type II diabetes. Intervention to lower blood glucose in clinical trials led to a reduction in the microvascular complications of diabetes.

HbA$_{1c}$ values of 5.7–6.4% indicate an increased risk for developing diabetes. An HbA$_{1c}$ value of 6.5% or higher is considered a diagnostic criterion for diabetes mellitus.

Laiteerapong N et al. Screening for prediabetes and type 2 diabetes mellitus. JAMA 2016;315:697. [PMID: 26881373]

Garber AJ. Treat-to-target trials: uses, interpretation and review of concepts. Diabetes Obes Metab 2014;16:193. [PMID: 23668598]

Nathan DM et al. Translating the A$_{1c}$ assay into estimated average glucose values. Diabetes Care 2008;31:1473. [PMID: 18540046]

Rhea JM et al. Pathology consultation on HbA(1c) methods and interferences. Am J Clin Pathol 2014;141:5. [PMID: 24343732]

Weykamp C. HbA$_{1c}$: a review of analytical and clinical aspects. Ann Lab Med 2013;33:393. [PMID: 24205486]

Hemoglobin A$_2$, whole blood (HbA$_2$)

1.5–3.5% of total hemoglobin (Hb)

Lavender

$$

HbA$_2$ is a minor component of normal adult hemoglobin (<3.5% of total Hb).

Increased in: β-Thalassemia minor (HbA$_2$ levels 4–9% of total Hb, HbF 1–5%), β-thalassemia major (HbA$_2$ levels normal or increased, HbF 80–100%).

Decreased in: Untreated iron deficiency, hemoglobin H disease, hemoglobin Lepore major (rare).

Patients with the combination of iron deficiency and β-thalassemia may have a normal HbA$_2$ level.

Test is useful in the diagnosis of β-thalassemia minor (in absence of iron deficiency, which decreases HbA$_2$ and can mask the diagnosis). Quantitated by column chromatographic or automated HPLC techniques.

Normal HbA$_2$ levels are seen in δ-thalassemia or very mild β-thalassemias.

See thalassemia syndromes (Table 8–22).

Amid A et al. Screening for thalassemia carriers in populations with a high rate of iron deficiency: revisiting the applicability of the Mentzer Index and the effect of iron deficiency on HbA$_2$ levels. Hemoglobin 2015;39:141. [PMID: 25806419]

Mosca A et al. Analytical goals for the determination of HbA$_2$. Clin Chem Lab Med 2013;51:937. [PMID: 23027585]

(Continued)

Hemoglobin electrophoresis and evaluation

Test/Range/Collection	Physiologic Basis	Interpretation	Comments
Hemoglobin (Hb) electrophoresis and evaluation, whole blood HbA: > 95% HbA$_2$: 1.5–3.5% HbF: < 2% (age-dependent) Lavender, blue, or green $$	Hemoglobin electrophoresis is used as a screening test to detect and differentiate variant and abnormal hemoglobins. Alkaline and/or citrate agar electrophoresis is the commonly used method. Separation of hemoglobins is based on different rates of migration of charged hemoglobin molecules in an electric field. HPLC and capillary zone electrophoresis are useful alternative methods for hemoglobin analysis, and are being increasingly used for diagnosis of hemoglobinopathy. Molecular tests are also used to confirm hemoglobinopathy (eg, β-thalassemia).	Presence of HbS with HbA > HbS: sickle cell trait (HbAS) or sickle α-thalassemia; HbS and F, no HbA: sickle cell anemia (HbSS), sickle β^0-thalassemia, or sickle-HPFH (hereditary persistence of fetal hemoglobin); HbS > HbA and F: sickle β$^+$-thalassemia. Presence of HbC: HbA > HbC: HbC trait (HbAC); HbC and F, no HbA: HbC disease (HbCC), HbC-β^0-thalassemia, or HbC-HPFH; HbC > HbA: HbC β$^+$-thalassemia. Presence of HbS and HbC: HbSC disease. Presence of HbH: HbH disease. Increased HbA$_2$: β-thalassemia minor. Increased HbF: Hereditary persistence of fetal hemoglobin, sickle cell anemia, β-thalassemia major, HbC disease, HbE disease.	Evaluation of a suspected hemoglobinopathy should include electrophoresis of a hemolysate to detect abnormal hemoglobins, quantitation of hemoglobins A$_2$ and F by column chromatography, and solubility test if HbS is detected. Interpretation of Hb electrophoresis results should be put in the clinical context, including the family history, serum iron studies, red cell morphology, hemoglobin, hematocrit, and red cell indices (eg, RBC and MCV). Molecular testing aids in genetic counseling of patients with thalassemia and combined hemoglobinopathies. Next-generation sequencing based hemoglobin gene evaluation is being developed. Bain BJ. Haemoglobinopathy diagnosis: algorithms, lessons and pitfalls. Blood Rev 2011;25:205. [PMID: 21596464] Piel FB et al. The α-thalassemias. N Engl J Med 2014;371:1908. [PMID: 25390741] Traeger-Synodinos J et al. Advances in technologies for screening and diagnosis of hemoglobinopathies. Biomark Med 2014;8:119. [PMID: 24325233]

Hemoglobin, fetal		
Hemoglobin, fetal, whole blood (HbF) Adult: < 2% (varies with age) Lavender, blue, or green $$	Fetal hemoglobin constitutes about 75% of total hemoglobin at birth and declines to 50% at 6 weeks, 5% at 6 months, and < 1.5% by 1 year. Within the first year, adult hemoglobin (HbA) becomes the predominant hemoglobin. Fetal to adult hemoglobin switching (HbF-to-HbA switch) is regulated by nuclear factors (eg, BCL11A).	**Increased in:** Hereditary disorders: eg, β-thalassemia major (20–100% of total Hb is HbF), β-thalassemia minor (2–5% HbF), HbF β⁰-thalassemia (10–80% HbF), sickle cell anemia (5–20% HbF), hereditary persistence of fetal hemoglobin (10–40% HbF). Acquired disorders (< 10% HbF): aplastic anemia, megaloblastic anemia, paroxysmal nocturnal hemoglobinuria (PNH), leukemia (eg, juvenile myelomonocytic leukemia). **Decreased in:** Hemolytic anemia of the newborn.	Semiquantitative acid elution test (Kleihauer-Betke test) provides an estimate of fetal hemoglobin only and varies widely between laboratories. It is useful in distinguishing hereditary persistence of fetal hemoglobin (all RBCs show an increase in fetal hemoglobin) from β-thalassemia major (only a portion of RBCs are affected). Enzyme-linked antiglobulin test and flow cytometry are also used to detect fetal red cells in the Rh(−) maternal circulation in suspected cases of Rh sensitization and to determine the amount of RhoGAM to administer (1 vial/15 mL fetal RBC). Prenatal diagnosis of hemoglobinopathies may be made from quantitative hemoglobin levels using HPLC or molecular diagnostic techniques. Bain BJ. Haemoglobinopathy diagnosis: algorithms, lessons and pitfalls. Blood Rev 2011;25:205. [PMID: 21596464] Perrine SP et al. Targeted fetal hemoglobin induction for treatment of beta hemoglobinopathies. Hematol Oncol Clin North Am 2014;28:233. [PMID: 24589264] Sankaran VG. Targeted therapeutic strategies for fetal hemoglobin induction. Hematology Am Soc Hematol Educ Program 2011. 2011;459. [PMID: 22160074]

(Continued)

	Hemoglobin, total		
Test/Range/Collection	Physiologic Basis	Interpretation	Comments
Hemoglobin, total, whole blood (Hb) Males: 13.6–17.5 g/dL Females: 12.0–15.5 g/dL (age-dependent) [Males: 136–175 g/L Females: 120–155 g/L] **Panic:** ≤ 7 g/dL Lavender S	Hemoglobin is the major protein of erythrocytes that transports oxygen from the lungs to peripheral tissues. It is commonly measured by spectrophotometry on automated instruments after lysis of red cells and conversion of all hemoglobin to cyanmethemoglobin (hemoglobinocyanide method).	**Increased in:** Hemoconcentration (as in dehydration, burns, vomiting), polycythemia (erythrocytosis), extreme physical exercise. **Decreased in:** Macrocytic anemia (liver disease, hypothyroidism, vitamin B_{12} deficiency, folate deficiency, myelodysplasia, HIV infection, alcoholism), normocytic anemia (early iron deficiency, anemia of chronic disease, hemolytic anemia, acute hemorrhage, bone marrow infiltrates of leukemia, lymphoma, myeloma or metastatic tumor), and microcytic anemia (iron deficiency, thalassemia, sideroblastic anemia). Hemodilution.	The cyanmethemoglobin technique is the method of choice for hemoglobin determination and is selected by the International Committee for Standardization in Hematology. The method measures all hemoglobin derivatives except sulfhemoglobin by hemolyzing the specimen and adding a reducing agent. As such, this method does not distinguish between intracellular versus extracellular hemoglobin (hemolysis). Hypertriglyceridemia and very high white blood cell counts can cause false elevations of Hb. Murphy WG. The sex difference in haemoglobin levels in adults—mechanisms, causes, and consequences. Blood Rev 2014;28:41. [PMID: 24491804] Sankaran VG et al. Anemia: progress in molecular mechanisms and therapies. Nat Med 2015;21:221. [PMID: 25742458] Sireci AN. Hematology testing in urgent care and resource-poor settings: an overview of point of care and satellite testing. Clin Lab Med 2015;35:197. [PMID: 25676380]

Heparin anti-Xa assay, chromogenic		
Heparin anti-Xa assay, chromogenic, plasma Undetectable (< 0.05 U/mL) Blue $$ Separate plasma from cells within 1 hr, and as needed freeze plasma for storage and shipment.	The anti-Xa assay is a chromogenic assay that measures heparin level indirectly. Factor Xa is used as assay reagent. Heparin in patient's plasma binds with antithrombin and inhibits excess Xa. The quantity of residual Xa is then measured using a chromogenic substrate, and the released colored compound is measured spectrophotometrically. The quantity of residual Xa is inversely proportional to the amount of heparin present in plasma. The chromogenic anti-Xa assay can be calibrated specifically for unfractionated heparin (UFH), low molecular weight heparin (LMWH), or fondaparinux.	**Therapeutic ranges:** Unfractionated heparin (IV): 0.30–0.70 U/mL. Low molecular weight heparin (LMWH, SQ): 0.50–1.10 U/mL (twice-daily dose) or 1.1–2.0 U/mL (once-daily dose). Fondaparinux (SQ): 0.6–1.5 U/mL (adults) or 0.5–1.0 U/mL (children). Note that the therapeutic ranges are laboratory- and method-specific.	The test can precisely determine the level of heparin in patient's plasma, and is used to monitor therapy with heparins. PTT is the most commonly used test for monitoring unfractionated heparin (UFH) therapy. For patients with documented lupus anticoagulant or deficiency in a contact system factor (eg, factor XII), PTT monitoring is problematic and therefore heparin level by anti-Xa assay should be used. In addition, patients with "heparin resistance" (ie, patient requires >35,000 U/day to achieve a therapeutic PTT) should also be monitored with anti-Xa assay. Some institutions have switched from PTT to anti-Xa assays for monitoring all patients receiving UFH. Low molecular weight heparin (LMWH) and fondaparinux are administered subcutaneously, and generally do not prolong the PTT. The anti-Xa assay has to be used if monitoring is required (eg, in obesity with >100 kg body weight, cachexia, renal insufficiency, neonates, and pregnancy). Blood sample is typically collected 4 hrs and 3 hrs after subcutaneous injection of LMWH and fondaparinux, respectively. Routine monitoring of LMWH therapy with anti-Xa measurements in obese patients remains controversial. Di Nisio M et al. Prevention of venous thromboembolism in hospitalized acutely ill medical patients: focus on the clinical utility of (low-dose) fondaparinux. Drug Des Devel Ther 2013;7:973. [PMID: 24068866] Egan G et al. Measuring anti-factor Xa activity to monitor low-molecular-weight heparin in obesity: a critical review. Can J Hosp Pharm 2015;68:33. [PMID: 25762818] Wool GD et al. Pathology consultation on anticoagulation monitoring: factor X-related assays. Am J Clin Pathol 2013;140:623. [PMID: 24124140]

(Continued)

	Heparin-induced thrombocytopenia (HIT) antibodies		
Test/Range/Collection	Physiologic Basis	Interpretation	Comments
Heparin-induced thrombocytopenia (HIT) antibodies, serum Negative Red, SST $$ Separate serum from cells ASAP or within 2 hrs of collection. Freeze and ship on dry ice.	Heparin-induced thrombocytopenia (HIT) is an adverse reaction and prothrombotic complication of heparin therapy that is strongly associated with venous and arterial thrombosis, which requires urgent detection and treatment with a nonheparin anticoagulant. The HIT antibodies are directed at heparin and platelet factor 4 (PF4) and may appear on exposure to heparin. The formed immune complexes propagate platelet activation, leading to release of more PF4 and thrombosis. However, only a minority of patients who form HIT antibodies actually develop thrombocytopenia and/or thrombosis (clinical HIT). An enzyme-linked immunosorbent assay (ELISA) method is typically used for the detection of heparin-associated PF4 antibodies.	**Positive in:** Heparin-induced thrombocytopenia, type II.	There are two types of HIT. Type I HIT is generally considered a benign condition and is not antibody-mediated. In type II HIT, which typically occurs between days 5–10 of heparin therapy, thrombocytopenia is usually more severe and is antibody-mediated. Patients with type II HIT are at risk for developing arterial or venous thrombosis if heparin therapy is continued. The ELISA-based antigenic assay is very sensitive and is designed to detect antibody binding to PF4/heparin (usually IgG). However, the test is relatively nonspecific because it may also detect nonpathogenic IgA and IgM antibodies. Results should be used in conjunction with clinical findings, platelet counts, and other laboratory results. If available, ELISA assay that exclusively detects anti-PF4/heparin IgG antibodies (the pathogenic antibodies) should be used. Positive ELISA results are typically reflexed to functional assays, such as serotonin release assay, heparin-induced platelet aggregation study, and flow cytometry analysis. Functional assays are more specific, but are technically demanding and usually done in reference laboratories. Besides ELISA, a few rapid assays for HIT antibodies (results available within 10–30 min) have become available, such as the PF4/heparin particle gel immunoassay and lateral flow immunoassay. Their limitations are moderate specificity and variable test performance. Bakchoul T et al. Current insights into the laboratory diagnosis of HIT. Int J Lab Hematol 2014;36:296. [PMID: 24750676] Grouzi E. Update on argatroban for the prophylaxis and treatment of heparin-induced thrombocytopenia type II. J Blood Med 2014;5:131. [PMID: 25152637] McKenzie SE. Advances in the pathophysiology and treatment of heparin-induced thrombocytopenia. Curr Opin Hematol 2014;21:380. [PMID: 24992313]

(Continued)

	Hepatitis A virus antibody		
Hepatitis A virus antibody, serum or plasma (Anti-HAV) Negative SST, PPT, lavender or pink $$	Hepatitis A is caused by a nonenveloped 27-nm RNA virus of the enterovirus-picornavirus group and is usually acquired by the fecal–oral route. IgM antibody is detectable within 1 week after symptoms develop and persists for 6 months. IgG antibody appears 4 weeks later than IgM and persists for years (see Figure 10–5 for time course of serologic changes). Hepatitis A appears only as an acute infection and does not become chronic. IgG antibody is positive after successful hepatitis A vaccination.	**Positive in:** Acute hepatitis A (IgM), convalescence from hepatitis A (IgG), after hepatitis A vaccination (IgG).	The most commonly used test for hepatitis A antibody is an immunoassay that detects total IgG and IgM antibodies. This test can be used to establish immune status. To diagnose acute hepatitis A virus infection, order hepatitis A IgM antibody. IgG antibody positivity is found in 40–50% of adults in the United States and Europe (higher rates in developing nations). Testing for anti-HAV (IgG) may reduce cost of HAV vaccination programs. Those who are at risk of HAV infection and negative for anti-HAV antibody need to be vaccinated. Hepatitis A vaccine is also recommended for postexposure prophylaxis, although immunoglobulin G is an acceptable alternative. Matheny SC et al. Hepatitis A. Am Fam Physician 2012;86:1027. [PMID: 23198670] Vaughan G et al. Hepatitis A virus: host interactions, molecular epidemiology and evolution. Infect Genet Evol 2014;21:227. [PMID: 24200587]
	Hepatitis B surface antigen		
Hepatitis B virus surface antigen, serum or plasma (HBsAg) Negative SST, PPT (light green), blue $$	In hepatitis B virus infection, surface antigen is detectable 2–5 weeks before onset of symptoms, rises in titer, and peaks at about the time of onset of clinical illness. Generally, it persists for 1–5 months, declining in titer and disappearing with resolution of clinical symptoms (see Figure 10–6 for time course of serologic changes).	**Present In:** Acute hepatitis B, chronic hepatitis B (persistence of HBsAg for > 6 months, positive HBcAb [total]), asymptomatic HBV carriers. May be undetectable in acute hepatitis B infection. If clinical suspicion is high, HBcAb (IgM) test is then indicated.	First-line test for the diagnosis of acute or chronic hepatitis B. If positive, HBV DNA testing is often performed to provide further information on the disease status. HBsAg quantification has been considered useful for monitoring natural history and treatment outcomes. Chen CH et al. Serum hepatitis B surface antigen levels predict treatment response to nucleos(t)ide analogues. World J Gastroenterol 2014;20:7686. [PMID: 24976706] Chou R et al. Screening for hepatitis B virus infection in adolescents and adults: a systematic review to update the U.S. Preventive Services Task Force recommendation. Ann Intern Med 2014;161:31. [PMID: 24861032] Martinot-Peignoux M et al. HBsAg quantification: useful for monitoring natural history and treatment outcome. Liver Int. 2014;34:597. [PMID: 24373085]

Test/Range/Collection	Physiologic Basis	Interpretation	Comments
Hepatitis B virus surface antibody (HBsAb, anti-HBs), serum or plasma Negative SST, lavender (light green), blue $$	Hepatitis B virus (HBV) is a DNA virus. This test detects antibodies to HBV surface antigen, which confer immunity to hepatitis B virus infection.	**Present in:** Hepatitis B immunity due to HBV infection or prior hepatitis B vaccination. **Absent in:** Hepatitis B carrier state, nonexposure to HBV.	Test indicates immune status for HBV. It is not useful for the evaluation of acute or chronic hepatitis. Antibodies against hepatitis B surface antigen (HBsAb) wane over time after vaccination for HBV. Booster dose vaccination should be administered as needed. (See Figure 10–6 for time course of serologic changes.) Schönberger K et al. Determinants of long-term protection after hepatitis B vaccination in infancy: a meta-analysis. Pediatr Infect Dis J 2013;32:307. [PMID: 23249904] You CR et al. Update on hepatitis B virus infection. World J Gastroenterol 2014;20:13293. [PMID: 25309066]
Hepatitis B virus core antibody, total, (HBcAb, anti-HBc), serum or plasma Negative SST, PPT (light green), blue $$	HBcAb (IgG and IgM) become positive (as IgM) about 2 months after exposure to hepatitis B virus. Its persistent positivity may reflect chronic hepatitis (IgM) or recovery (IgG). HBcAb IgG persists for a lifetime after HBV exposure, with or without development of HBsAb. (See Figure 10–6 for time course of serologic changes.)	**Positive in:** Hepatitis B (acute and chronic), hepatitis B carriers, prior hepatitis B (immune) when IgG is present in low titer with or without HBsAb. **Negative:** After hepatitis B vaccination.	HBcAb (total) is useful in evaluation of acute or chronic hepatitis only if HBsAg is negative. An HBcAb (IgM) test is then indicated only if the HBcAb (total) is positive. HBcAb (IgM) may be the only serologic indication of acute HBV infection and occult HBV infection. HBcAb positive, HBsAg negative patients may reactivate their hepatitis B if given chemotherapy (eg, rituximab), and prophylaxis with anti-HBV therapy should be given. You CR et al. Update on hepatitis B virus infection. World J Gastroenterol 2014;20:13293. [PMID: 25309066]

Hepatitis B e antigen	
Hepatitis B e antigen/ antibody (HBeAg/Ab), serum or plasma Negative SST, PPT (light green) $$	HBeAg is a soluble protein secreted by HBV, related to HBcAg, indicating viral replication and infectivity. Two distinct serologic types of hepatitis B have been described, one with a positive HBeAg, and the other with a negative HBeAg and a positive anti-HBe antibody. HBeAg negative variants have been identified, which harbor mutations in the precore stop codon or the basal core promoter, reducing or abrogating HBeAg production. These variants are associated with active chronic hepatitis and less favorable clinical course.
Increased (positive) in: HBV (acute, chronic) hepatitis.	All patients positive for HBeAg are considered infectious. During the natural course of hepatitis B infection, loss of HBeAg and accumulation of HBeAb (seroconversion) are associated with decreased infectivity. After the HBeAg seroconversion, patients may become "inactive HBsAg carriers." However, over time precore and/or basal core promoter mutant variants may emerge and be selected for, leading to so-called HBeAg-negative chronic hepatitis B with high levels of viral replication and active hepatitis. Therefore, seroconversion status (HBeAg negative, HBeAb positive) may not correlate with disease activity, and HBV viral load test should be performed to help monitor and manage patients with chronic hepatitis B infection. Alexopoulou A et al. HBeAg negative variants and their role in the natural history of chronic hepatitis B virus infection. World J Gastroenterol 2014;20:7644. [PMID: 24976702] You CR et al. Update on hepatitis B virus infection. World J Gastroenterol 2014;20:13293. [PMID: 25309066]

(Continued)

	Hepatitis B virus DNA, quantitative		
Test/Range/Collection	**Physiologic Basis**	**Interpretation**	**Comments**
Hepatitis B virus DNA, quantitative (HBV-DNA by PCR), plasma or serum Quantification range 1.3–8.2 log IU/mL (20–170,000,000 IU/mL) (laboratory-specific) 1 IU/mL is approximately 5 copies/mL Lavender, pink, SST $$$$	The presence of HBV-DNA in serum or plasma confirms active hepatitis B infection and implies infectivity of blood. Current use of the assay is primarily for assessing responses of hepatitis B to therapy, such as entecavir, tenofovir, or peginterferon. HBV-DNA is also used before and after liver transplantation to detect low-level viral replication, and for patients infected by mutant strains of HBV that do not make the surface or e antigen. In patients with chronic hepatitis B, HBV DNA levels in blood correlate with the risk of cirrhosis and hepatocellular carcinoma, and thus have prognostic value. HBV-DNA can be detected using very sensitive techniques (eg, quantitative real-time PCR) even in patients thought to have recovered from HBV infection who are positive for anti-HBs and anti-HBc.	**Positive in:** Acute hepatitis B, chronic hepatitis B, silent HBV carriers, occult HBV infection.	HBV-DNA levels are useful in determining the status of chronic HBV infection by differentiating between active and inactive disease states, and in monitoring patient's response to anti-HBV therapy. It is essential in evaluating patients infected with HBeAg negative mutant variants because HBV-DNA is the only reliable marker of active HBV replication. Viral load fluctuates over time in most patients and may vary by as much as 10^2–10^4 in serial measurements. The World Health Organization has recognized an international standard, a genotype A subtype adw2 isolate, for HBV-DNA quantification. Assays are commonly reported in International Units (IU) based on comparison with the standard. However, correlation between copies/mL and IU is variable. Marcellin P et al. Long-term therapy for chronic hepatitis B: hepatitis B virus DNA suppression leading to cirrhosis reversal. J Gastroenterol Hepatol 2013;28:912. [PMID: 23573915] Pazienza V et al. Advance in molecular diagnostic tools for hepatitis B virus detection. Clin Chem Lab Med 2013;51:1707. [PMID: 23612658] You CR et al. Update on hepatitis B virus infection. World J Gastroenterol 2014;20:13293. [PMID: 25309066]

Hepatitis C virus antibody			
Hepatitis C virus antibody, serum or plasma (HCV Ab, anti-HCV) Negative SST, PPT (light green) $$	Detects antibody to hepatitis C virus, which is a single-stranded RNA virus of the Flaviviridae family. The screening test (enzyme immunoassay [EIA] or chemiluminescent immunoassay [CIA]) detects antibodies to proteins encoded by putative structural (HC34) and nonstructural (HC31, C100-3) regions of the HCV genome. The presence of these antibodies indicates that the patient has been infected with HCV, may harbor infectious HCV, and may be capable of transmitting HCV. A recombinant immunoblot assay (RIBA), equivalent to Western blot, is available as a confirmatory test. HCV RNA tests are preferred for confirming active infection if the screening test is positive. See Figure 10–7 for hepatitis C serologic changes.	**Increased in:** Acute hepatitis C (only 20–50%; seroconversion may take 3 months or more), posttransfusion chronic hepatitis (70–90%), blood donors (0.5–1%), non–blood-donating general public (2–3%), hemophiliacs (75%), intravenous drug users (40–80%), hemodialysis patients (1–30%), male homosexuals (4%).	Sensitivity of screening assays for HCV infection is 86%, specificity 99.5%. Anti-HCV positivity documents previous exposure, not necessarily active infection. HCV-RNA or HCV core antigen assay could serve to confirm active infection. Samples that are weakly positive (signal-to-cutoff ratio < 3.8 for EIA assay or < 8 for CIA assay) require reflex HCV-RNA or RIBA testing. Samples that are negative on screening test usually require no further testing. However, HCV-RNA is generally obtained if there is high clinical suspicion of HCV despite a negative anti-HCV, especially in immunocompromised persons or in the setting of acute hepatitis. During an acute infection, anti-HCV and the RIBA often do not become positive; seroconversion may take 3 months or more. HCV RNA test is preferred if clinically indicated, because viral RNAs become detectable within 2–3 weeks after exposure. Kamili S et al. Laboratory diagnostics for hepatitis C virus infection. Clin Infect Dis 2012;55:S43. [PMID: 22715213] Marwaha N et al. Current testing strategies for hepatitis C virus infection in blood donors and the way forward. World J Gastroenterol 2014;20:2948. [PMID: 24659885] Saludes V et al. Tools for the diagnosis of hepatitis C virus infection and hepatic fibrosis staging. World J Gastroenterol 2014;20:3431. [PMID: 24707126]

(Continued)

Test/Range/Collection	Physiologic Basis	Interpretation	Comments
Hepatitis C virus genotyping			
Hepatitis C virus genotyping PPT (light green), SST, or lavender $$$$ Separate serum or plasma from cells within 2 hrs of collection.	HCV genotyping is a tool used to optimize anti-viral treatment regimens. HCV RNA is assayed using reverse transcriptase polymerase chain reaction (RT-PCR) to amplify a specific portion of the 5' untranslated region of the hepatitis C virus. The amplified nucleic acid is sequenced bidirectionally. Another technique is the HCV line probe assay that uses genotype-specific probes to detect sequence variations in the 5' untranslated region and the core region of the viral genome. The test may be unsuccessful if the HCV RNA viral load is less than 1,000 HCV RNA copies per mL.	**Positive in:** Hepatitis C. Isolates of hepatitis C virus are grouped into six major genotypes. These genotypes are sub-typed according to sequence characteristics and are designated as 1a, 1b, 2a, 2b, 3a, 3b, 4, 5a, and 6a.	Six major genotypes of HCV have been discovered around the world. Genotypes 1, 2, and 3 are the most common types in North America and Europe. The HCV genotype should be assessed before the start of treatment because it determines the treatment length and drug dose and also offers prognostic information on treatment outcomes as certain genotypes respond more favorably to treatment (measured by rate of sustained virological response, defined as the absence of HCV-RNA 24 weeks after completion of treatment). HCV genotype 1 (60–75% of HCV infections in the U.S.) is traditionally more difficult to cure than genotypes 2 or 3. However, with the introduction of direct-acting antivirals (eg, sofosbuvir), the majority of HCV infected patients, including those infected with genotypes 4, 5 and 6, have the potential for achieving sustained virological response. Treatment selection varies by genotype and other patient factors. AASLD/IDSA HCV Guidance Panel. Hepatitis C Guidance: AASLD-IDSA recommendations for testing, managing, and treating adults infected with hepatitis C virus. Hepatology 2015;62:932. [PMID: 26111063] Chevaliez S. Virological tools to diagnose and monitor hepatitis C virus infection. Clin Microbiol Infect 2011;17:116. [PMID: 21054664] Irshad M et al. An insight into the diagnosis and pathogenesis of hepatitis C virus infection. World J Gastroenterol 2013;19:7896. [PMID: 24307784] Kohli A et al. Treatment of hepatitis C: a systematic review. JAMA 2014;312:631. [PMID: 25117132] Lawitz EJ et al. Response-guided therapy in patients with genotype 1 hepatitis C virus: current status and future prospects. J Gastroenterol Hepatol 2014;29:1574. [PMID: 24852401] Wyles DL et al. Importance of HCV genotype 1 subtypes for drug resis-tance and response to therapy. J Viral Hepat 2014;21:229. [PMID: 24597691]

(Continued)

Hepatitis C virus RNA (HCV-RNA), quantitative	Hepatitis Delta antibody

Hepatitis C virus RNA (HCV RNA), quantitative (HCV viral load)

Negative (detection limit: 12 IU/mL, assay-specific)

PPT (light green), SST, or lavender.

$$$

Analysis should be done within 2 hrs. Otherwise, separate serum or plasma and freeze at −20°C within 2 hrs for testing at a later time.

Detection of HCV RNA is used to confirm active infection and to monitor antiviral treatment. Widely used methods include reverse-transcriptase PCR (RT-PCR) and branched DNA (b-DNA) transcription-mediated amplification (TMA).

For each viral load assay, a linear range exists that encompasses the upper and lower limits of quantification (ULOQ and LLOQ, respectively). HCV RNA that is detectable but below the LLOQ value by PCR is reported as "<LLOQ, detected". A result of "<LLOQ, not detected" or "target not detected" indicates that no PCR amplification can be achieved in a sample.

Positive in: Hepatitis C infection (active).

RNA is very susceptible to degradation; thus, improper specimen handling can cause false-negative results. Assays are generally reported in IU/mL, with standardization using WHO reference material.

A less than 2 log (or 100-fold) decrease in viral load after 12 weeks of treatment indicates lack of response to therapy.

For treatment monitoring, sustained virological response is defined as undetectable HCV-RNA (aviremia) 24 weeks after completion of antiviral treatment.

Cobb B et al. HCV RNA viral load assessments in the era of direct-acting antivirals. Am J Gastroenterol 2013;108:471. [PMID: 23552304] Irshad M et al. An insight into the diagnosis and pathogenesis of hepatitis C virus infection. World J Gastroenterol 2013;19:7896. [PMID: 24307784]

Hepatitis Delta virus antibody (anti-HDV), serum or plasma

Negative

SST, red, PPT (light green), lavender

$$

This antibody is a marker for acute or persisting infection with the delta agent, a defective RNA virus that can infect only HBsAg-positive patients. HDV requires HBsAg for complete replication and transmission. Eight HDV genotypes (1 to 8) have been identified.

HBV plus hepatitis D virus (HDV) infection may be more severe than HBV infection alone. Antibody to HDV ordinarily persists for about 6 months after acute infection. Further persistence indicates carrier status.

Positive in: Hepatitis D coinfection or superinfection with HBV.

Test only indicated in HBsAg-positive patients. Chronic HDV hepatitis occurs in 80–90% of HBsAg carriers who are superinfected with delta virus.

The test detects total antibodies (IgG and IgM) to the delta agent. If anti-HDV is positive, HDV RNA testing can help determine ongoing active infection (RNA positive) versus past infection (RNA negative). Alvarado-Mora MV et al. An update on HDV: virology, pathogenesis and treatment. Antivir Ther 2013;18:541. [PMID: 23792471] Olivero A et al. Hepatitis delta virus diagnosis. Semin Liver Dis 2012;32:220. [PMID: 22932970]

Test/Range/Collection	Physiologic Basis	Interpretation	Comments
Hepatitis E virus antibody (anti-HEV), serum or plasma Negative Red, SST, lavender $$$	Hepatitis E virus (HEV) is a small single-stranded RNA virus that causes hepatitis. The virus has a single serotype but 4 genotypes; genotypes 1 and 2 infect only humans, whereas genotypes 3 and 4 primarily infect other mammals, particularly pigs, but occasionally cause human disease as well. The virus is acquired through the fecal-oral route, usually through contaminated water supplies. HEV can also be transmitted by blood transfusion. Perinatal transmission from infected mother to infant has also been reported. HEV generally causes a self-limited acute infection. Chronic hepatitis does not develop after acute infection, except in transplant or immunocompromised patients (eg, HIV).	**Positive in:** Acute hepatitis E (IgM), convalescence from hepatitis E (IgG).	Both anti-HEV IgM and anti-HEV IgG ELISA assays are available. False positive or negative result may occur. Detection of HEV RNA by RT-PCR in blood or stool is the confirmatory test for acute hepatitis E and has been used for both epidemiologic and diagnostic purposes. Blood donation screening with microarrays has been proposed. Aggarwal R. Diagnosis of hepatitis E. Nat Rev Gastroenterol Hepatol 2013;10:24. [PMID: 23026902] Arends JE et al. Hepatitis E: an emerging infection in high income countries. J Clin Virol 2014;59:81. [PMID: 24388207]
Heterophile antibody, serum (Monospot, Paul-Bunnell test) Negative SST, red $	Infectious mononucleosis (IM) is an acute, usually self-limited saliva-transmitted infectious disease due to the Epstein-Barr virus (EBV). The virus preferentially infects B cells and causes immune responses including the activation of T cells. Heterophile (Paul-Bunnell) antibodies (IgM) appear in 60% of mononucleosis patients within 1–2 weeks and in 80–90% within the first month. They are not specific for EBV but are only rarely found in other disorders. The monospot test, a form of the heterophile antibody test, is a rapid test for infectious mononucleosis due to EBV. The test relies on the agglutination of horse RBCs by heterophile antibodies in patient's serum. Titers are substantially diminished by 3 months after primary infection and are not detectable by 6 months.	**Positive in:** Infectious mononucleosis (90–95%). **Negative in:** Heterophile-negative mononucleosis: CMV, heterophile-negative EBV, toxoplasmosis, hepatitis viruses, HIV-1 seroconversion, listeriosis, tularemia, brucellosis, cat-scratch disease, Lyme disease, syphilis, rickettsial infections, medications (phenytoin, sulfasalazine, dapsone), collagen vascular diseases (especially systemic lupus erythematosus), subacute infective endocarditis.	The test is used as an aid in the diagnosis of infectious mononucleosis. Its three classic laboratory features are a lymphocytosis, a significant number (>10–20%) of atypical lymphocytes (reactive T cells) on peripheral blood smear, and a positive heterophile antibody test. If heterophile test is negative in the setting of hematologic and clinical evidence of a mononucleosis-like illness, a repeat test in 1–2 weeks may be positive. EBV serology (anti-VCA, anti-EBNA, anti-EA) may also be indicated, especially in children and teenage patients who may have negative heterophile tests. PCR-based EBV tests (qualitative and/or quantitative) can help diagnose early mononucleosis in cases with inconclusive serological results. Hatton OL et al. The interplay between Epstein-Barr virus and B lymphocytes: implications for infection, immunity, and disease. Immunol Res 2014;58:268. [PMID: 24619311] Vouloumanou EK et al. Current diagnosis and management of infectious mononucleosis. Curr Opin Hematol 2012;19:14. [PMID: 22123662]

Histoplasma capsulatum antigen		
Histoplasma capsulatum antigen, urine, serum, CSF (HPA) Negative SST (serum) $$ Deliver urine, CSF in a clean plastic or glass container tube. Urine is the best specimen for the test.	Histoplasmosis is the most common systemic fungal infection and typically starts as a pulmonary infection with influenza-like symptoms. This may heal, progress, or lie dormant with reinfection occurring at a later time. Heat-stable *H. capsulatum* polysaccharide is detected by antigen enzyme immunoassay (EIA) using alkaline phosphatase or horseradish peroxidase-conjugated antibodies.	**Increased in:** Disseminated histoplasmosis (90–97% in urine, 50–78% in blood, and approximately 42% in CSF), localized disease (16% in urine), blastomycosis (urine and serum), coccidioidomycosis (CSF).	Histoplasmosis is usually seen in the Mississippi and Ohio River valleys but may appear elsewhere. Detection of *Histoplasma* antigenemia or antigenuria is recommended for the diagnosis of disseminated histoplasmosis and may be useful in the early acute stage of pulmonary histoplasmosis before the appearance of antibodies. The test can also be used to monitor therapy or to follow relapse in immunocompromised patients. Quantitative EIA for *H. capsulatum* var *capsulatum* polysaccharide antigen in urine is a useful test in diagnosis of disseminated histoplasmosis and in assessing efficacy of treatment or in detecting relapse, especially in AIDS patients and when serologic tests for antibodies may be negative. It is not useful for ruling out localized pulmonary histoplasmosis. In bronchoalveolar lavage fluid, HPA has 70% sensitivity for the diagnosis of pulmonary histoplasmosis. The EIA test should be used in conjunction with other diagnostic procedures (eg, *Histoplasma* antibodies, microbiological culture, tissue biopsy, imaging study) to help diagnose histoplasmosis. Couturier MR et al. Urine antigen tests for the diagnosis of respiratory infections: legionellosis, histoplasmosis, pneumococcal pneumonia. Clin Lab Med 2014;34:219. [PMID: 24856525] McKinsey DS et al. Pulmonary histoplasmosis. Semin Respir Crit Care Med 2011;32:735. [PMID: 22167401]

(Continued)

Test/Range/Collection	Physiologic Basis	Interpretation	Comments
Histoplasma capsulatum antibodies by immunodiffusion			
Histoplasma capsulatum **antibodies by immunodiffusion,** serum Negative SST (acute and convalescent samples, collected 2–3 weeks apart) $$	This test screens for *Histoplasma* antibodies by detecting precipitins to specific antigens ("H" and "M" bands) by immunodiffusion. The "M" band often appears first and may occur without the "H" band. "M" precipitin is present in approximately 70% of acute and chronic histoplasmosis cases. Only 10% of patients have both "M" and "H" precipitins. Positive "H" band indicates active infection, but is rarely found alone; "M" band indicates acute or chronic infection or prior skin testing. Presence of both is highly suggestive of active histoplasmosis.	**Positive in:** Previous, chronic, or acute histoplasma infection, recent histoplasmin skin testing. Cross-reactions at low levels in patients with blastomycosis and coccidioidomycosis.	Test is useful as a screening test or as an adjunct to complement fixation test (see below) in diagnosis of systemic histoplasmosis. McKinsey DS et al. Pulmonary histoplasmosis. Semin Respir Crit Care Med 2011;32:735. [PMID: 22167401]
Histoplasma capsulatum antibodies by CF			
Histoplasma capsulatum **antibodies by complement fixation (CF)** serum, CSF < 1:4 titer SST $$ Submit paired sera—one specimen collected within 1 week after onset of illness and another 2 weeks later.	The standard method for the diagnosis of histoplasmosis remains culture isolation and identification of the organism. However, culture often requires 2–4 weeks. Antibody detection offers a more rapid alternative and is valuable in the diagnosis of acute, chronic, disseminated, and meningeal histoplasmosis. Antibodies in primary pulmonary infections are generally found within 4 weeks after exposure and frequently are present at the time symptoms appear. Two types of CF test are available based on mycelial antigen and yeast phase antigen. The yeast phase test is considerably more sensitive. Latex agglutination (LA) and enzyme-linked immunosorbent assay (ELISA) tests are also available but are less reliable.	**Increased in:** Previous, chronic, or acute histoplasma infection (75–80%), recent histoplasmin skin testing (20%), other fungal disease, leishmaniasis. Cross-reactions in patients with blastomycosis and coccidioidomycosis.	Elevated CF titers > 1:16 are suggestive of infection. Titers > 1:32 or rising titers are usually indicative of active infection. Histoplasmin skin test is not recommended for diagnosis because it interferes with subsequent serologic tests. The CF test is usually positive in CSF from patients with chronic meningitis. About 3.5–12% of clinically normal persons have positive titers, usually less than 1:16. McKinsey DS et al. Pulmonary histoplasmosis. Semin Respir Crit Care Med 2011;32:735. [PMID: 22167401]

HIV antibody		
HIV screening, serum or plasma Negative SST, PPT, lavender, green $$	Originally, the human immunodeficiency virus (HIV) screening tests detected antibodies against both HIV-1 and HIV-2. HIV-1 is found worldwide and is the etiologic agent of most HIV infections in the U.S. HIV-2 is less common than HIV-1 and is found mostly in West Africa. The HIV antibody test is considered positive only when confirmed by a Western blot analysis. The currently used 4th-generation screening test uses combined antibody and p24 antigen immunoassay to identify HIV-1 and HIV-2 infections. If the results are positive, follow-up immunoassay is performed to differentiate between HIV-1 and HIV-2, to help guide the choice of combination antiretroviral therapy. The 4th-generation testing can screen for and confirm HIV infection in a few hrs, and has been recommended as the initial screening testing for HIV infection.	**Positive in:** HIV infection	The U.S. Preventive Services Task Force recommends routine HIV screening for all persons 15 to 65 years of age (including all pregnant women), unless a patient refuses. Those younger than 15 and older than 65 with risk factors should also be screened. HIV antibodies become detectable 3–4 weeks after viral infection. The 4th-generation test can become positive in 2 weeks. Qualitative and quantitative HIV-1 nucleic acid PCR tests are positive 10–12 days from initial HIV infection; however, these tests are not typically used for screening purposes. An over-the-counter in-home rapid HIV test is also available. However, test sensitivity is only about 92% when the test is self-administered. Positive results require confirmation with a 4th-generation test or Western blot analysis. Ibitoye M et al. Home testing past, present and future: lessons learned and implications for HIV home test. AIDS Behav 2014;18:933. [PMID: 24281697] Peters PJ et al. Screening Yield of HIV Antigen/Antibody Combination and Pooled HIV RNA Testing for Acute HIV Infection in a High-Prevalence Population. JAMA 2016;315:682. [PMID: 26881371] Sherin K et al. What is new in HIV infection? Am Fam Physician 2014;89:265. [PMID: 24695446] Taylor D et al. Probability of a false-negative HIV antibody test result during the window period: a tool for pre- and post-test counselling. Int J STD AIDS 2015;26:215. [PMID: 25033879]

(*Continued*)

	HIV RNA, quantitative		HIV resistance testing
Test/Range/Collection	**Physiologic Basis**	**Interpretation**	**Comments**
HIV RNA, quantitative (viral load), plasma < 40 [copies per mL] (assay-specific) Lavender, PPT (light green) $$$$	Monitoring HIV-1 RNA level (viral load) in plasma of infected patients is used to assess disease progression and patient response to combination antiretroviral therapy. Commonly used assays are either based on RT-PCR target amplification (eg, Roche Amplicor HIV Monitor and Abbott m2000) or branched-chain DNA (bDNA) signal amplification (eg, Versant HIV-1 RNA 3.0 Assay bDNA). For each viral load assay, a linear range exists that encompasses the upper and lower limits of quantification (ULOQ and LLOQ, respectively). HIV RNA that is detectable but below the LLOQ value by PCR is reported as "<LLOQ, detected." A result of "<LLOQ, not detected" or "target not detected" indicates that no PCR amplification can be achieved in a sample.	The real-time PCR based assays (eg, Abbott m2000, Roche Amplicor) have a broad dynamic range from 40–75 copies per mL to 1×10^7 copies per mL. The bDNA-based assay (Versant HIV-1 RNA) has a measurement range of 75–500,000 copies per mL.	The clinical significance of changes in HIV-1 viral load has not been fully established; however, a threefold change (0.5 log) in copies/mL may be significant. Caution should be taken in the interpretation of any single viral load determination. Dried blood spots have been used instead of plasma for viral load monitoring in remote settings. Bonner K et al. Viral load monitoring as a tool to reinforce adherence: a systematic review. J Acquir Immune Defic Syndr 2013;64:74. [PMID: 23774877] Smit PW et al. Systematic review of the use of dried blood spots for monitoring HIV viral load and for early infant diagnosis. PLoS One 2014;9:e86461. [PMID: 24603442] Stephan C et al. Impact of baseline HIV-1 RNA levels on initial highly active antiretroviral therapy outcome: a meta-analysis of 12,370 patients in 21 clinical trials. HIV Med 2013;14:284. [PMID: 23171153]
HIV resistance testing Lavender, PPT (light green) $$$$	Testing for resistance to antiretroviral agents is considered to be standard of care and is widely used in the management of HIV-infected persons. It is an important tool in optimizing the efficacy of combination antiretroviral therapy. The identification of resistance allows selection of antiviral agents with maximum therapeutic benefit and minimum toxic side effects. Both phenotypic and genotypic resistance tests are available. The resistance tests require a viral load of > 1000 copies per mL.	**Positive in:** HIV-1 infection with drug resistance.	Phenotypic resistance tests evaluate the ability of the virus to proliferate in the presence of various drugs and thus give direct information on how well the drugs inhibit the virus. Genotypic resistance assays detect specific mutations in the viral genome that are associated with resistance to various antiretroviral agents. Combined phenotypic/genotypic assays are also available. Clotet B et al. Interpretation of resistance data from randomized trials of first-line antiretroviral treatment. AIDS Rev 2012;14:247. [PMID: 23258299] Dunn DT et al. Genotypic resistance testing in routine clinical care. Curr Opin HIV AIDS 2011;6:251. [PMID: 21646877] Kumarasamy N et al. Beyond first-line HIV treatment regimens: the current state of antiretroviral regimens, viral load monitoring, and resistance testing in resource-limited settings. Curr Opin HIV AIDS 2013;8:586. [PMID: 24100872] Stadeli KM et al. Rates of emergence of HIV drug resistance in resource-limited settings: a systematic review. Antivir Ther 2013;18:115. [PMID: 23052978]

(Continued)

	HLA typing	HLA-B27 typing
HLA (human leukocyte antigen) typing (HLA typing) Yellow, lavender or green (30–50 mL) $$$$ Keep whole blood samples at room temperature, and do not spin tubes.	The human leukocyte antigen (HLA) class I and class II system consists of six closely linked loci (HLA-A, B, C, DR, DQ and DP) located on the short arm of chromosome 6. The previous standard technique for HLA typing was the complement-dependent cytotoxicity test (serotyping). This is a complement-mediated serologic assay in which antiserum containing specific anti-HLA antibodies is added to peripheral blood lymphocytes. Cell death indicates that the lymphocytes carried the specific targeted antigen. The three HLA-A, –B, and –C are determined in this manner. The HLA-D locus is determined by mixed lymphocyte culture. DNA sequencing based methods for HLA typing (genotyping) have largely replaced traditional HLA serotyping. Both intermediate and high resolution genotyping techniques are routinely used. **Useful in:** Evaluation of transplant candidates and potential donors, paternity and forensic testing, and evaluation of HLA-associated diseases or adverse drug reactions.	HLA typing is usually performed for matching transplantation candidates and potential donors, in blood product matching (eg, platelets), and in paternity testing. It is also helpful in diagnosis of certain HLA-associated diseases (eg, B27 for ankylosing spondylitis) and prevention of adverse drug reactions associated with particular HLA antigens (eg, B*5701 for abacavir sensitivity). The most important HLA alleles responsible for the immune response to a transplanted organ are HLA-A, B and DR. HLA alleles of less importance in transplant immunology are HLA-C and DQ. Next-generation sequencing techniques allow faster, more accurate and more cost-effective HLA typing. Erlich H. HLA DNA typing: past, present, and future. Tissue Antigens 2012;80:1. [PMID: 22651253] Latham K et al. An overview of HLA typing for hematopoietic stem cell transplantation. Methods Mol Biol 2014;1109:73. [PMID: 24473779]
HLA-B27 typing, whole blood Per report Lavender, pink, yellow $$$	The human leukocyte antigen B27 (HLA-B27) allele is found in approximately 8% of the U.S. white population. It occurs less frequently in the African American population. Although serotyping is available, PCR-based HLA-B27 genotyping testing is routinely used. **Present in:** Spondyloarthritis (88% of Caucasian patients with ankylosing spondylitis); reactive arthritis (formerly Reiter syndrome) (80%) following infection with enteric organisms such as *Yersinia, Shigella* or *Salmonella*); anterior uveitis; psoriatic arthritis; and inflammatory bowel disease.	2–8% of individuals with HLA-B27 develop ankylosing spondylitis (low penetrance). The best diagnostic tests for ankylosing spondylitis are lumbosacral spine and sacroiliac joint films and not HLA-B27 typing. HLA-B27 testing is not usually clinically indicated. Chatzikyriakidou A et al. What is the role of HLA-B27 in spondyloarthropathies? Autoimmun Rev 2011;10:464. [PMID: 21296192] Reveille JD et al. The epidemiology of back pain, axial spondyloarthritis and HLA-B27 in the United States. Am J Med Sci 2013;345:431. [PMID: 23841117]

	HLA-B51 typing	
Test/Range/Collection	**Physiologic Basis**	**Interpretation**	**Comments**

Test/Range/Collection	Physiologic Basis	Interpretation	Comments
HLA-B51 typing, whole blood Per report Lavender, pink, yellow $$$	Risk of developing Behçet disease is increased in the presence of certain human leukocyte antigens, particularly HLA-B51/B5. Presence of an HLA-B51/B5 allele may also be associated with more severe disease. Both serotyping and genotyping tests are available.	**Increased in:** Behçet disease (50–80%).	Behçet disease is a rare systemic inflammatory disorder characterized by chronic vasculitis of arteries and veins of all sizes, and manifested as recurrent oral and genital ulcers, ocular and skin involvement, and other multisystem problems. The exact contribution of HLA-B51 in the pathogenesis of Behçet disease has not been elucidated, but the associated neutrophil hyperfunction may play a role. Kaya TI. Genetics of Behçet's disease. Patholog Res Int 2012;2012:912589. [PMID: 22013548] Maldini C et al. Relationships of HLA-B51 or B5 genotype with Behçet's disease clinical characteristics: systematic review and meta-analyses of observational studies. Rheumatology (Oxford) 2012;51:887. [PMID: 22240504] Mat MC et al. Behçet's disease as a systemic disease. Clin Dermatol 2014;32:435. [PMID: 24767193]

Homocysteine

Homocysteine, plasma or serum Males: 4–12 mcmol/L Females: 4–10 mcmol/L (method and age-dependent) SST, green (Fasting specimen is required; plasma or serum must be separated from cells within 1 hour of collection.) $$	Homocysteine is a naturally occurring, sulfur-containing amino acid produced during catabolism of methionine, an essential amino acid. It is metabolized by two major pathways: remethylation and transsulfuration. Several vitamins function as cofactors and substrates in these pathways, including folic acid, vitamin B_{12} and vitamin B_6. Deficiencies in one or more of these vitamins can lead to acquired hyperhomocysteinemia. Inherited homocystinuria is a rare autosomal recessive disorder that usually results from defective activity of cystathione β-synthase.	**Increased in:** Homocystinuria due to defects in cystathionine β-synthase, methionine synthase or intracellular cobalamin metabolism, *MTHFR C677T* mutation, deficiency of folic acid or B vitamins (eg, B_{12}, B_6), cigarette smoking, chronic alcohol ingestion, renal failure, systemic lupus erythematosus, hypothyroidism, diabetes mellitus, certain medications (eg, methotrexate, nicotinic acid, theophylline, L-dopa), and advanced age. **Decreased in:** Down syndrome, hyperthyroidism.	Hyperhomocysteinemia is typically defined as a total homocysteine level above the 95th percentile of a control population, which in most studies is approximately 15 mcmol/L. Hyperhomocysteinemia may be classified as moderate (16–30), intermediate (31–100), and severe (> 100 mcmol/L). Clinical and epidemiologic studies have demonstrated that hyperhomocysteinemia is an independent risk factor for atherosclerosis and coronary heart disease and for arterial and venous thromboembolism. Nevertheless, due to the lack of definitive evidence for clinical treatment outcome benefits from reducing homocysteine levels, routine screening for hyperhomocysteinemia is not recommended. For patients with elevated homocysteine concentration, it is important to check their vitamin status. A causal relationship between high homocysteine level and risk of developing dementia has not been established. Andras A et al. Homocysteine lowering interventions for peripheral arterial disease and bypass grafts. Cochrane Database Syst Rev 2013;7:CD003285. [PMID: 23881650] Cacciapuoti F. Lowering homocysteine levels with folic acid and B-vitamins do not reduce early atherosclerosis, but could interfere with cognitive decline and Alzheimer's disease. J Thromb Thrombolysis 2013;36:258. [PMID: 23224755]

(Continued)

Test/Range/Collection	Physiologic Basis	Interpretation	Comments
5-Hydroxyindoleacetic acid, urine (5-HIAA) 0–8 mg/24 hr [0–40 mcmol/d] $$ Collect 24-hr or random urine, and refrigerate. Patients should abstain from medications that may affect metabolism of serotonin and avoid foods that are rich in serotonin (eg, avocados, bananas, pineapple, eggplant) for at least 72 hrs before and during urine collection.	Serotonin (5-hydroxytryptamine) is a neurotransmitter that is metabolized by monoamine oxidase (MAO) to 5-HIAA and then excreted into the urine. Intestinal carcinoid tumors along with neuroendocrine tumors can produce excess amounts of serotonin and 5-HIAA, especially in individuals with carcinoid syndrome. Biochemical diagnosis of gastrointestinal carcinoids is established by demonstrating elevation of urinary 5-HIAA or plasma serotonin or chromogranin A.	**Increased in:** Metastatic carcinoid tumor (foregut, midgut, and bronchial). Nontropical sprue (slight increase). Diet: Bananas, walnuts, avocado, eggplant, pineapple, plums. Drugs: reserpine. **Negative in:** Rectal carcinoids (usually), renal insufficiency. Drugs: MAO inhibitors, phenothiazines. Test is often falsely positive if pretest probability is low. Using 5-HIAA/Cr ratio may improve performance, especially if the urine collection is random or other than 24-hr.	Urinary 5-HIAA excretion is used as a biochemical tumor marker for clinical diagnosis, to monitor treatment effects, and as a prognostic predictor. A very high concentration of urinary 5-HIAA is an indicator that a gastrointestinal carcinoid tumor is malignant. Because most carcinoid tumors drain into the portal vein and serotonin is rapidly cleared by the liver, the carcinoid syndrome (flushing, bronchial constriction, diarrhea, hypotension, and cardiac valvular lesions) associated with secretion of serotonin and other vasoactive substances is a late manifestation of carcinoid tumors, appearing only after hepatic metastasis has occurred. Bolanowski M et al. Neuroendocrine neoplasms of the small intestine and the appendix—management guidelines. Endokrynol Pol 2013;64:480. [PMID: 24431119] Kunz PL et al. Consensus guidelines for the management and treatment of neuroendocrine tumors. Pancreas 2013;42:557. [PMID: 23591432] Strosberg J. Neuroendocrine tumours of the small intestine. Best Pract Res Clin Gastroenterol 2012;26:755. [PMID: 23582917]
IgG index, serum and CSF 0.29–0.69 ratio SST or red (serum), glass or plastic tube (CSF) $$$ Collect serum and CSF simultaneously.	This test compares CSF IgG and albumin levels with serum levels. The formula used for CSF IgG index calculation is: (CSF IgG/CSF albumin)/(serum IgG/serum albumin). The CSF index is an indicator of the relative amount of CSF IgG compared to serum. An increased ratio reflects synthesis of IgG within the central nervous system. The index is independent of the activity of the demyelinating process.	**Increased in:** Multiple sclerosis (~80%), neurosyphilis, acute inflammatory polyradiculoneuropathy, subacute sclerosing panencephalitis, other inflammatory and infectious CNS diseases.	Test is reasonably sensitive but not specific for multiple sclerosis. There is no predictable correlation between the IgG index values and the oligoclonal IgG band number in patients with multiple sclerosis. The use of CSF IgG index plus oligoclonal banding has been reported to increase the sensitivity to over 90% (see Oligoclonal bands, p. 164). Deangelis TM et al. Diagnosis of multiple sclerosis. Handb Clin Neurol 2014;122:317. [PMID: 24507524] Fitzner B et al. Molecular biomarkers in cerebrospinal fluid of multiple sclerosis patients. Autoimmun Rev 2015;14:903. [PMID: 26071103]

Test/Range/Collection	Physiologic Basis/Interpretation	Comments
IgG subclasses (immunoglobulin G subclasses) (1,2,3,4) Subclass 1: 240–1120 mg/dL; subclass 2: 125–550 mg/dL; subclass 3: 20–135 mg/dL; subclass 4: 7–90 mg/dL Age-dependent $$$$ SST, green Separate serum or plasma from cells ASAP or within 2 hrs of collection, and refrigerate.	IgG proteins consist of 4 subclasses (IgG1, IgG2, IgG3 and IgG4), which differ in the structure of the gamma heavy chain. Test is used for evaluating patients with possible humoral immunodeficiency or combined immunodeficiency (cellular and humoral), with or without hypogammaglobulinemia. It is also used for evaluating potential IgG4-related diseases (IgG4-RD), characterized by chronic fibrotic inflammation with unique pathological features.	**Decrease in all subclasses:** Common variable immunodeficiency, combined immunodeficiency, ataxia telangiectasia, other primary and acquired immunodeficiency disorders. **Decrease in IgG2:** Recurrent sinopulmonary infection with or without concomitant IgA deficiency. **Increase in IgG4:** IgG4-related disease.	The test is not a first-order test for patients suspected of having an immunodeficiency disease. Levels of total IgG, IgA and IgM levels, along with other first-order tests for immunodeficiency, should be performed first. Isolated deficiencies of IgG3 or IgG4 occur rarely, and the clinical significance of these findings is not clear. Elevated levels of IgG4 supports the diagnosis of an IgG4-related disease (e.g., type 1 autoimmune pancreatitis). Albin S et al. An update on the use of immunoglobulin for the treatment of immunodeficiency disorders. Immunotherapy 2014;6:1113. [PMID: 25428649] Beyer G et al. IgG4-related disease: a new kid on the block or an old aquaintance? United European Gastroenterol J 2014;2:165. [PMID: 25360299] Driessen G et al. Educational paper: primary antibody deficiencies. Eur J Pediatr 2011;170:693. [PMID: 21544519]

(Continued)

Test/Range/Collection	Physiologic Basis	Interpretation	Comments
Immunofixation electrophoresis (IFE), serum or urine Negative SST (serum) $$$	IFE is used to identify specific immunoglobulin (Ig) classes. Proteins are separated electrophoretically on several tracks on a gel. Antisera specific to individual classes of molecules are added to each track. If specific classes of heavy or light chain are present, insoluble complexes form with the antisera, which can then be stained and detected.	**Positive in:** Presence of identifiable monoclonal protein: plasma cell neoplasms (myeloma, Waldenström macroglobulinemia, heavy chain disease, primary amyloidosis, monoclonal gammopathy of undetermined significance, plasmacytoma), certain B-cell lymphomas and leukemias. The most common M-protein seen in myeloma is the IgG type, followed by IgA and light chain only.	IFE is indicated to define an overt or suspicious Ig spike seen on serum protein electrophoresis (SPEP) or urine protein electrophoresis (UPEP), to differentiate a polyclonal from a monoclonal increase (eg, M-protein in serum, Bence Jones protein in urine), and to identify the specific type of a monoclonal increase. The IFE detection limit for M-protein is approximately 25 mg/dL. Immuno-subtraction capillary zone electrophoresis (CZE immunotyping) is an equivalent test to IFE, and is increasingly used in clinical laboratories. Serum free light chain analysis and heavy/light chain analysis (Hevylite) are also used in the diagnosis and monitoring of plasma cell neoplasms. Jenner E. Serum free light chains in clinical laboratory diagnostics. Clin Chim Acta 2014;427:15. [PMID: 23999048] Protein Testing in Patients with Multiple Myeloma: A Review of Clinical Effectiveness and Guidelines [Internet]. Ottawa (ON): Canadian Agency for Drugs and Technologies in Health; 2015 Jan. [PMID: 25632494] Rajkumar SV et al. International Myeloma Working Group updated criteria for the diagnosis of multiple myeloma. Lancet Oncol 2014;15:e538. [PMID: 25439696]

Immunofixation electrophoresis

(Continued)

Test / Specimen	Physiologic Basis	Interpretation	Comments
Immunoglobulins, serum (Ig) IgA: 0.78–3.67 g/L IgG: 5.83–17.6 g/L IgM: 0.52–3.35 g/L SST $$$	IgG makes up about 85% of total serum immunoglobulins and predominates late in immune responses. It is the only immunoglobulin to cross the placenta. IgM antibody predominates early in immune responses. Secretory IgA plays an important role in host defense mechanisms by blocking transport of microbes across mucosal surfaces.	↑ **IgG:** Polyclonal: Autoimmune diseases (eg, SLE, rheumatoid arthritis), sarcoidosis, chronic liver diseases, some parasitic diseases, chronic or recurrent infections. Monoclonal: Multiple myeloma (IgG type), lymphomas, or other malignancies. ↑ **IgM:** Polyclonal: Isolated infections such as viral hepatitis, infectious mononucleosis, early response to bacterial or parasitic infection. Monoclonal: Waldenström macroglobulinemia, lymphoma. ↑ **IgA:** Polyclonal: Chronic liver disease, chronic infections (especially of the GI and respiratory tracts). Monoclonal: Multiple myeloma (IgA). ↓ **IgG:** Immunosuppressive therapy, genetic (severe combined immunodeficiency disease [SCID], Wiskott Aldrich syndrome, common variable immunodeficiency). ↓ **IgM:** Immunosuppressive therapy. ↓ **IgA:** Inherited IgA deficiency (ataxia telangiectasia, combined immunodeficiency disorders).	Quantitative immunoglobulin levels are indicated in the evaluation of immunodeficiency. In X-linked agammaglobulinemia (also known as Bruton agammaglobulinemia), immunoglobulins of all classes are nearly undetectable, and there is a complete lack of circulating B cells. IgG deficiency is associated with recurrent and occasionally severe pyogenic infections. Protein electrophoresis (PEP, serum and/or urine), IFE and serum free light chain analysis help detect and characterize monoclonal immunoglobulin (paraprotein in serum, Bence Jones protein in urine). The most common form of multiple myeloma is the IgG type, followed by IgA type. Myeloma of IgM, IgD, or IgE type is rare. Quantitation of the serum paraprotein is used for treatment monitoring and patient follow-up. Caers J et al. Diagnosis and follow-up of monoclonal gammopathies of undetermined significance; information for referring physicians. Ann Med 2013;45:413. [PMID: 23767978] Cunningham-Rundles C. The many faces of common variable immunodeficiency. Hematology Am Soc Hematol Educ Program 2012;2012:301. [PMID: 23233596] Oza A et al. Waldenström macroglobulinemia: prognosis and management. Blood Cancer J 2015;5:e394. [PMID: 25815903]
Inhibitor screen (1:1 mix), plasma Negative Blue $$ Fill tube completely.	Test is useful for evaluating a prolonged PTT and/or PT. (Presence of heparin should first be excluded.) Patient's plasma is mixed with pooled normal plasma (1:1 mix) and PTT and/or PT are performed. If the patient has a factor deficiency, the post-mixing PTT/PT will be normal (correction). If an inhibitor is present, the post-mixing PTT/PT will remain prolonged (no correction) immediately and/or after incubation (at 37°C for 1 or 2 hours).	**Positive in:** Presence of inhibitor: Antiphospholipid antibodies (lupus anticoagulant, LAC), factor-specific antibodies, or both. **Negative in:** Factor deficiencies. See evaluation of isolated prolongation of PTT (Figure 9–28).	Lupus anticoagulant is a nonspecific inhibitor, which prolongs PTT on inhibitor screen (1:1 mix study) both immediately and after 1–2 hours' incubation. 1-hour to 2-hour incubation period is often needed to detect factor-specific antibodies with low *in vitro* affinities (eg, post-mixing PTT is normal immediately, but is prolonged after incubation). Dependent on the result of the 1:1 mix study, follow-up testing is often performed, ie, dilute Russell's viper venom time (DRVVT) if lupus anticoagulant is suspected or factor assays if factor deficiency is considered. Ortel TL. Antiphospholipid syndrome: laboratory testing and diagnostic strategies. Am J Hematol 2012;87:S75. [PMID: 22473619] Sakurai Y et al. Acquired hemophilia A: a frequently overlooked autoimmune hemorrhagic disorder. J Immunol Res 2014;2014:320674. [PMID: 24741588]

	Insulin antibody		
Test/Range/Collection	Physiologic Basis	Interpretation	Comments
Insulin antibody, serum Negative SST, red $$$	This assay quantitatively measures human serum autoantibodies to endogenous insulin or antibodies to exogenous insulin. In type 1 diabetes mellitus, the four islet autoantibodies are directed against insulin, glutamic acid decarboxylase (GAD), tyrosine phosphatase-like insulinoma antigen (IA-2), and zinc transporter 8 (ZnT8). Autoantibodies directed against insulin, GAD, IA-2, and ZnT8 usually precede the clinical onset of disease. Insulin antibodies develop in nearly all diabetics treated with insulin of animal origin. Most such antibodies are IgG and generally do not cause clinical problems. Occasionally, high-affinity antibodies can bind to exogenous insulin and cause insulin resistance.	**Present in:** Insulin therapy, type 1 diabetes mellitus before treatment (~55%), factitious hypoglycemia (surreptitious injection of insulin).	Insulin antibodies interfere with most assays for total insulin and C-peptide. Free insulin and free C-peptide can be measured instead in patients with insulin antibodies. Insulin antibody test is not sensitive or specific for the detection of surreptitious insulin use; use C-peptide level instead. If anti-insulin antibody or another islet antibody is present in a child with diabetes who is not insulin-treated, the diagnosis of type 1 diabetes is confirmed. In non-diabetics, the presence of insulin antibody can help to predict future development of type 1 diabetes, when used in conjunction with family history, HLA typing and other islet autoantibodies. The detection of anti-insulin antibody in insulin-treated patients is of no diagnostic utility. Anti-insulin antibody only roughly correlates with insulin requirements in patients with diabetes. Kawasaki E. Type 1 diabetes and autoimmunity. Clin Pediatr Endocrinol 2014;23:99. [PMID: 25374439] Pipi E et al. Distinct clinical and laboratory characteristics of latent autoimmune diabetes in adults in relation to type 1 and type 2 diabetes mellitus. World J Diabetes 2014;5:505. [PMID: 25126396] Simmons K et al. Lessons from type 1 diabetes for understanding natural history and prevention of autoimmune disease. Rheum Dis Clin North Am 2014;40:797. [PMID: 25437293]

Insulin, immunoreactive			
Insulin, immunoreactive, serum or plasma 3–25 mcU/mL SST, PPT, lavender $$ Fasting sample required. Measure glucose concurrently.	Insulin is a peptide hormone produced by the beta cells in the pancreatic islets. It regulates the uptake and utilization of glucose. Test measures blood levels of insulin, either endogenous or exogenous. The test has cross-reactivity with recombinant human insulin, as well as certain insulin analogues. Insulin antibody may interfere with the assay, causing inaccurate results.	**Increased in:** Insulin-resistant states (eg, obesity, type 2 diabetes mellitus, uremia, glucocorticoids, acromegaly), liver disease, surreptitious use of insulin or oral hypoglycemic agents, insulinoma (pancreatic islet cell tumor). **Decreased in:** Type 1 diabetes mellitus, hypopituitarism.	Measurement of serum insulin level has little clinical value except in the diagnosis of fasting hypoglycemia caused by insulinoma. An insulin-to-glucose ratio > 0.3 is presumptive evidence of insulinoma. Levels of proinsulin and C-peptide are also increased. C-peptide should be used as well as serum insulin to distinguish insulinoma from surreptitious insulin use, since C-peptide will be absent with exogenous insulin use. Insulin levels decline in patients with type 1 diabetes, but are either normal or elevated in the early stage of type 2 diabetes. In patients with confirmed insulin antibody, free insulin level should be obtained instead. Antonakis PT et al. Pancreatic insulinomas: laparoscopic management. World J Gastrointest Endosc 2015;7:1197. [PMID: 26566426] Lambadiari V et al. Insulin action in muscle and adipose tissue in type 2 diabetes: the significance of blood flow. World J Diabetes 2015;6:626. [PMID: 25987960] Martens P et al. Approach to the patient with spontaneous hypoglycemia. Eur J Intern Med 2014;25:415. [PMID: 24641805]

(Continued)

Test/Range/Collection	Physiologic Basis	Interpretation	Comments
Insulin-like growth factor-1, serum (IGF-1, previously known as somatomedin C) 123–463 ng/mL (age- and sex-specific reference interval must be used) SST, red $$$$	Insulin-like growth factor-1 is a growth hormone (GH)-dependent plasma peptide produced by the liver. It mediates the growth-promoting effect of GH. It has an anabolic, insulin-like action on fat and muscle and stimulates collagen and protein synthesis. Its level is relatively constant throughout the day. Its concentration is regulated by genetic factors, nutrient intake, GH, and other hormones such as T4, cortisol, and sex steroids. Blood IGF is the cornerstone and often the stand-alone test in the diagnosis and follow-up of patients with acromegaly.	**Increased in:** Acromegaly (level correlates with disease activity better than GH level). **Decreased in:** Pituitary dwarfism, hypopituitarism, Laron dwarfism (end-organ resistance to GH), fasting for 5–6 days, poor nutrition, hypothyroidism, cirrhosis. Values may be normal in GH-deficient patients with hyperprolactinemia or craniopharyngioma.	IGF-1 is a sensitive test for acromegaly. An elevated IGF level and non-suppression of GH after oral glucose load to a nadir < 0.4 ng/mL are considered diagnostic of acromegaly. Normal IGF-1 levels rule out active acromegaly. In acromegaly, IGF-1 levels are useful for assessing the relative degree of GH excess, because changes in IGF-1 correlate with changes in symptoms and soft tissue growth. IGF-1 is also very useful in monitoring the symptomatic response to therapy. IGF-1 can be decreased in adult GH deficiency, but it is not a sensitive diagnostic test. Measurement of IGF-1 can help to assess nutritional status, and to adjust GH dose during treatment of GH deficiency. Kannan S et al. Diagnosis of acromegaly: state of the art. Expert Opin Med Diagn 2013;7:443. [PMID: 23971897] Livingstone C. Insulin-like growth factor-1 (IGF-1) and clinical nutrition. Clin Sci (Lond) 2013;125:265. [PMID: 23721057] Pawlikowska-Haddal A et al. How useful are serum IGF-1 measurements for managing GH replacement therapy in adults and children? Pituitary 2012;15:126. [PMID: 21909971]

Insulin-like growth factor-1

(Continued)

Test/Specimen	Description	Interpretation	Comments
Intrinsic factor blocking antibody (IFBA), serum Negative SST, red $$$$	Vitamin B_{12} (cobalamin) deficiency can lead to megaloblastic anemia and neurologic deficits. The most common cause of B_{12} deficiency in developed countries is pernicious anemia (PA). Pernicious anemia is an autoimmune disorder that results in diminished or absent gastric acid, pepsin, and intrinsic factor (IF) production. Most PA patients have autoanti-bodies against gastric parietal cells or IF, with the latter being very specific but present in only 50–60% of cases. Parietal cell antibodies are more sensitive but less specific. Measurement of serum B_{12}, either preceded or followed by serum methylmalonic acid (MMA) test, is the first step in diagnosing pernicious anemia (PA). If these tests support B_{12} deficiency, then intrinsic factor blocking antibody (IFBA) testing may be indicated to confirm PA as the etiology.	**Positive in:** Pernicious anemia (sensitivity 50–60%, specificity >95%).	A positive IFBA test supports very strongly a diagnosis of PA. However, since the diagnostic sensitivity of IFBA testing for PA is only 50–60%, an indeterminate or negative IFBA test does not exclude the diagnosis of PA. In these patients, either PA or another etiology, such as malnutrition, may still be present. Measurement of serum gastrin levels will help in these cases. In patients with PA, fasting serum gastrin is elevated (>200 pg/mL) as a compensatory response to the achlorhydria that is present in this condition. Do not order IFBA testing in patients who received a vitamin B_{12} injection within the previous 2 weeks because high levels of vitamin B_{12} can interfere with the assay. Bizzaro N et al. Diagnosis and classification of pernicious anemia. Autoimmun Rev 2014;13:565. [PMID: 24424200] Osborne D et al. Autoimmune mechanisms in pernicious anaemia & thyroid disease. Autoimmun Rev 2015;14:763. [PMID: 25936607] Shipton MJ et al. Vitamin B_{12} deficiency—a 21st century perspective. Clin Med (Lond) 2015;15:145. [PMID: 25824066]
Iodine, 24-hr urine 90–1000 mcg/24 hr [0.7–7.9 mcmol/24 hr] Requires refrigerated aliquot of >10 mL of well-mixed 24-hour urine collection. Do not freeze. $$$$	Iodine is a trace mineral essential for the production of thyroid hormones. Symptoms and signs of iodine deficiency include thyroid goiter, mental retardation, and stunted growth in children. 90% of ingested iodine is excreted in urine. The measurement of urinary iodine excretion serves as an index and estimate of dietary iodine intake.	**Increased in:** Excess iodine intake, iodine-containing drug therapy or contrast media exposure. **Decreased in:** Deficiency in dietary iodine.	Test is used to detect iodine deficiency. Plant foods are poor sources of iodine so vegetarians are at risk for iodine deficiency, especially if they avoid iodine enriched salt. Useful for monitoring iodine excretion rate as an index of daily iodine replacement therapy, and for correlating total body iodine load with ^{131}I-uptake studies in assessing thyroid function. Values >1000 mcg/24 hr may indicate dietary excess, but more frequently suggest recent drug or contrast media exposure. Iodine excess has been linked to the development of autoimmune thyroiditis. Guideline: Fortification of Food-Grade Salt with Iodine for the Prevention and Control of Iodine Deficiency Disorders. Geneva: 2014 WHO Guide-lines Approved by the Guidelines Review Committee. [PMID: 25473709] Rohner F et al. Biomarkers of nutrition for development—iodine review. J Nutr 2014;144:1322S. [PMID: 24966410]

Test/Range/Collection	Physiologic Basis	Interpretation	Comments
Iron (Fe), serum or plasma 50–175 mcg/dL [9–31 mcmol/L] SST, PPT $ Hemolyzed sample unacceptable.	Plasma iron concentration is determined by absorption from the intestine; storage in the intestine, liver, spleen, bone marrow; rate of breakdown or loss of hemoglobin; and rate of synthesis of new hemoglobin. The key regulator of iron homeostasis is hepcidin. Hepcidin excess or deficiency contributes to the dysregulation of iron homeostasis in hereditary and acquired iron disorders.	**Increased in:** Hemosiderosis (eg, multiple transfusions, excess iron administration), acute Fe poisoning (children), hemolytic anemia, pernicious anemia, aplastic or hypoplastic anemia, viral hepatitis, lead poisoning, thalassemia, hemochromatosis. Drugs: estrogens, ethanol, oral contraceptives. **Decreased in:** Iron deficiency, nephrotic syndrome, chronic renal failure, anemia of inflammation, iron–refractory iron deficiency anemia (IRIDA), many infections, active hematopoiesis, remission of pernicious anemia, hypothyroidism, malignancy (carcinoma), Waldenström macroglobulinemia, postoperative state, kwashiorkor.	Absence of stainable iron on bone marrow aspirate differentiates iron deficiency from other causes of microcytic anemia (eg, thalassemia, sideroblastic anemia, some chronic disease anemias); the procedure is invasive and expensive. Serum iron, iron–binding capacity, transferrin saturation, serum ferritin or soluble transferrin receptor may obviate the need for bone marrow examination. Serum iron, transferrin saturation and ferritin are useful in screening family members for hereditary hemochromatosis. Recent transfusion confounds the test results. Kaitha S et al. Iron deficiency anemia in inflammatory bowel disease. World J Gastrointest Pathophysiol 2015;6:62. [PMID: 26301120] Nemeth E et al. Anemia of inflammation. Hematol Oncol Clin North Am 2014;28:671. [PMID: 25064707] Ruchala P et al. The pathophysiology and pharmacology of hepcidin. Trends Pharmacol Sci 2014;35:155. [PMID: 24552640]
Iron-binding capacity, total, serum (TIBC) 250–460 mcg/dL [45–82 mcmol/L] SST $$	Iron is transported in plasma complexed to transferrin, which is synthesized in the liver. Total iron-binding capacity is calculated from transferrin levels measured immunologically. Each molecule of transferrin has two iron-binding sites; so its iron-binding capacity is 1.47 mg/g. Normally, transferrin carries an amount of iron representing about 16–60% of its capacity to bind iron (eg, % saturation of iron-binding capacity is 16–60%).	**Increased in:** Iron deficiency anemia, late pregnancy, infancy, acute hepatitis. Drugs: oral contraceptives. **Decreased in:** Hypoproteinemic states (eg, nephrotic syndrome, starvation, malnutrition, cancer), hemochromatosis, thalassemia, hyperthyroidism, chronic infections, chronic inflammatory disorders, chronic liver disease, other chronic disease.	Serum iron, TIBC, and % saturation are used for the diagnosis of iron deficiency, but serum ferritin is a more sensitive test for assessing iron status. TIBC correlates with serum transferrin, but the relationship is not linear over a wide range of transferrin values and is disrupted in diseases affecting transferrin-binding capacity or other iron-binding proteins. Increased % transferrin saturation with iron is seen in iron overload (iron poisoning, hemolytic anemia, sideroblastic anemia, thalassemia, hemochromatosis, pyridoxine deficiency, aplastic anemia, RBC transfusions). Decreased % transferrin saturation with iron is seen in iron deficiency (usually saturation <16%). Transferrin levels can also be used to assess nutritional status. Recent transfusion confounds the test results. Burke RM et al. Identification, prevention and treatment of iron deficiency during the first 1000 days. Nutrients 2014;6:4093. [PMID: 25310252] Crownover BK et al. Hereditary hemochromatosis. Am Fam Physician 2013;87:183. [PMID: 23418762] Steinbicker AU et al. Out of balance–systemic iron homeostasis in iron-related disorders. Nutrients 2013;5:3034. [PMID: 23917168]

Islet cell antibodies		
Islet cell antibodies (ICAs), IgG, serum Negative SST $$$$	Islet cell antibodies (ICAs) are associated with type 1 diabetes or insulin–dependent diabetes mellitus (IDDM). ICAs attack pancreatic islet cells, leading to insulin deficiency. ICAs are present in the serum of patients during the prediabetic phase and predict development of type 1 disease. ICAs are detected on thin frozen sections of human pancreas by indirect immunofluorescence assay (IFA), which measures a variety of autoantibodies and is semi-quantitative. ICAs include antibodies directed against several islet cell autoantigens, including insulin, glutamic acid decarboxylase (GAD), insulinoma-associated protein 2 (IA2), and efflux zinc transporter 8 (ZnT8). Immunoassays are available for evaluating specific insulin, GAD, IA2 and ZnT8 autoantibodies, which are more reliable markers for the prediabetic state. Insulin is the only B cell-specific autoantigen.	**Increased in:** Type 1 diabetes mellitus; individuals at risk for developing type 1 diabetes mellitus.	Useful in assessing risk and predicting onset of type 1 diabetes. Measurements of insulin, GAD Ab, IA2, and ZnT8 antibodies are useful adjuncts to measuring ICAs. Predictive value for the development of type I diabetes in first-degree relatives of patients with type 1 diabetes increases to 90–100% when the ICAs are strongly and persistently positive, ICAs are present in combination with insulin or GAD antibodies, or when 2 or more of insulin, GAD, IA2, and ZnT8 autoantibodies are present. Although not required for diagnosis, an assay for ICAs can be useful in aiding the differential diagnosis of type 1 (eg, latent autoimmune diabetes) versus type 2 diabetes. ICAs are present in 85% of newly diagnosed type 1 diabetic patients, but are rarely detected in type 2 diabetic patients. Pipi E et al. Distinct clinical and laboratory characteristics of latent autoimmune diabetes in adults in relation to type 1 and type 2 diabetes mellitus. World J Diabetes 2014;5(4):505. [PMID: 25126396] Simmons K et al. Lessons from type 1 diabetes for understanding natural history and prevention of autoimmune disease. Rheum Dis Clin North Am 2014;40:797. [PMID: 25437293] Tooley JE et al. Biomarkers in type 1 diabetes: application to the clinical trial setting. Curr Opin Endocrinol Diabetes Obes 2014;21:287. [PMID: 24937037]

(Continued)

Test/Range/Collection	Physiologic Basis	Interpretation	Comments
JAK2 (V617F) mutation, blood or bone marrow Lavender $$$$	*JAK2* stands for the Janus Kinase 2. Detection of the *JAK2* V617F mutation provides a qualitative marker for the non-chronic myelogenous leukemia subgroup of myeloproliferative neoplasms, including polycythemia vera (PV), essential thrombocythemia (ET), and primary myelofibrosis (PMF). The V617F mutation, a valine-to-phenylalanine substitution at codon 617, leads to constitutive tyrosine phosphorylation activity, which is believed to confer independence and/or hypersensitivity of myeloid progenitors to cytokines (eg, erythropoietin).	**Positive in:** PV (~90%), ET (~65%), PMF (~55%).	A positive result identifying a *JAK2* V617F mutation supports a diagnosis of PV, ET, or PMF. It is particularly useful for establishing a diagnosis of PV in patients with marked erythrocytosis (eg, hemoglobin > 18.5 g/dL in males or > 16.5 g/dL in females) because up to 90% patients with PV carry the mutation. A negative result does not rule out the possibility of diagnosis of PV, ET, or PMF. Reflex testing for *JAK2* exon 12/13 mutations is indicated for possible PV, and *CALR* and *MPL* mutation analysis is indicated for possible ET and PMF. The absence of *JAK2* V617F and exon 12/13 mutations makes the diagnosis of PV unlikely, whereas 35–45% of patients with ET and PMF are negative for *Jak2* V617F mutation. See diagnostic evaluation for polycythemia and thrombocytosis (Figures 9–26 and 9–33). Silvennoinen O et al. Molecular insights into regulation of *JAK2* in myeloproliferative neoplasms. Blood 2015;125:3388. [PMID: 25824690] Skoda RC et al. Pathogenesis of myeloproliferative neoplasms. Exp Hematol 2015;43:599. [PMID: 26209551] Tefferi A et al. Essential thrombocythemia and polycythemia vera: focus on clinical practice. Mayo Clin Proc 2015;90:1283. [PMID: 26355403]

JAK2 (V617F) mutation

Kappa and lambda free light chains with ratio			
Kappa and lambda free light chains with ratio, quantitative, serum Free kappa (κ): 0.57–2.63 mg/dL Free lambda (λ): 0.33–1.94 mg/dL Free kappa/lambda ratio: 0.26–1.65 [Free kappa: 5.7–26.3 × 10³ g/L] [Free lambda: 3.3–19.4 × 10³ g/L] SST, red $	Plasma cells produce 1 of the 5 heavy chains (A, M, G, D, E) together with kappa (κ) or lambda (λ) molecules. There is an excess free light chain (FLC) production over heavy chain synthesis. Serum kappa FLCs are normally monomeric, while lambda FLCs tend to be dimeric, joined by disulphide bonds. The half-lives of serum FLCs are short (kappa 2–4 hours; lambda 3–6 hours). The serum Ig FLC nephelometric immunoassay measures levels of free kappa and lambda light chains. Serum levels of FLC are dependent on the balance between production by plasma cells and renal clearance. When there is increased polyclonal Ig production and/or renal impairment, both kappa and lambda FLC concentrations can increase up to 30–40 fold. However, the κ/λ ratio remains unchanged. In contrast, plasma cell dyscrasias produce an excess of only one of the light-chain types (monoclonal), often with suppression of the alternate light chain, so κ/λ ratios become highly abnormal, either increased or decreased.	**Increased, with abnormal κ/λ ratio:** Multiple myeloma including intact Ig producing myeloma, light-chain-only myeloma and "nonsecretory" myeloma, primary amyloidosis (light-chain amyloidosis, AL), plasmacytoma, and high-risk monoclonal gammopathy of undetermined significance (MGUS), non-Hodgkin B-cell lymphoma (eg, chronic lymphocytic leukemia) or small lymphocyte lymphoma. **Increased, with normal κ/λ ratio:** Infection, renal impairment that is unrelated to plasma cell disorder.	Serum FLC assays are used to help detect, diagnose, monitor and prognosticate plasma cell disorders. The serum FLC assay, in combination with serum protein electrophoresis (SPEP) and immunofixation, yields high sensitivity in disease screening and has eliminated the need for 24-hr urine studies for diagnosis of plasma cell dyscrasias. Serum Hevylite assays have also become available and will further improve the diagnostic accuracy of monoclonal gammopathies. Involved/uninvolved serum FLC ratio ≥100 has been accepted as a defining criterion for multiple myeloma. The baseline FLC levels are of prognostic value in all plasma cell dyscrasias. Because of short half-lives, FLC concentrations allow more rapid assessment of the effects of treatment than do those of intact monoclonal Ig (eg, the half-life of IgG is 21 days, and of IgA, 5 days). FLC molecules at high levels are frequently nephrotoxic. The FLC measurements thus can guide patient management. Jenner E. Serum free light chains in clinical laboratory diagnostics. Clin Chim Acta 2014;427:15. [PMID: 23990048] Landgren O et al. Biologic frontiers in multiple myeloma: from biomarker identification to clinical practice. Clin Cancer Res 2014;20:804. [PMID: 24270684] Rajkumar SV et al. International Myeloma Working Group updated criteria for the diagnosis of multiple myeloma. Lancet Oncol 2014;15:e538. [PMID: 25439696]

(Continued)

Test/Range/Collection	Physiologic Basis	Interpretation	Comments
Lactate dehydrogenase (LDH), serum or plasma 88–230 U/L [1.46–3.82 mckat/L] (laboratory-specific) SST, PPT ≤ Hemolyzed specimens are unacceptable.	LDH is an enzyme that catalyzes the interconversion of lactate and pyruvate in the presence of NAD/NADH. It is widely distributed in body cells and fluids. Because LDH is highly concentrated in RBCs, spuriously elevated serum levels occur if RBCs are hemolyzed during specimen collection.	**Increased in:** Tissue necrosis, especially in acute injury of cardiac muscle, RBCs, kidney, skeletal muscle, liver, lung, and skin. Commonly elevated in various carcinomas, in *Pneumocystis jiroveci* pneumonia (78–94%), and in non-Hodgkin lymphomas. Marked elevations occur in hemolytic anemias, megaloblastic anemia (vitamin B$_{12}$ and/or folate deficiency), polycythemia vera, thrombotic thrombocytopenic purpura, hepatitis, cirrhosis, obstructive jaundice, renal disease, musculoskeletal disease, and heart failure. Drugs causing hepatotoxicity (eg, acetaminophen) or hemolysis. **Decreased in:** Drugs: clofibrate, fluoride (low dose).	LDH is an important prognostic marker for various non-Hodgkin lymphomas. It also correlates with disease transformation in patients with low-grade lymphomas. Serum LDH is a useful prognostic biomarker in metastatic melanoma and is incorporated in its TNM classification. However, like other biomarkers (eg, serum S100B protein, osteopontin), the positive predictive value of LDH is limited by its false-positive rate. LDH is not a useful liver function test, and it is not specific enough for the diagnosis of hemolytic or megaloblastic anemias. In diagnosis of myocardial infarction, serum LDH has been replaced by cardiac-specific troponin I levels. LDH isoenzymes are not clinically useful. Freedman A. Follicular lymphoma: 2014 update on diagnosis and management. Am J Hematol 2014;89:429. [PMID: 24687887] Jain P et al. Richter's transformation in chronic lymphocytic leukemia. Oncology (Williston Park) 2012;26:1146. [PMID: 23413591] Karagiannis P et al. Evaluating biomarkers in melanoma. Front Oncol 2015;4:383. [PMID: 25667918]

Lactate dehydrogenase

Lactate			
Lactate, venous blood 0.5–2.0 meq/L [mmol/L] 4.5–18 mg/dL Gray $$ Collect on ice in gray-top tube containing fluoride to inhibit *in vitro* glycolysis and lactic acid production, and process within 15 minutes.	Severe tissue hypoperfusion and hypoxia lead to anaerobic glucose metabolism with production of lactic acid (type A lactic acidosis). In other disorders (with increased production or decreased clearance of lactate), lactic acidosis (type B) occurs with no clinical evidence of inadequate tissue oxygen delivery. Lactate is a useful laboratory marker for monitoring tissue perfusion status in critically ill patients, particularly those with sepsis and septic shock.	**Increased in:** Lactic acidosis, ethanol intoxication, sepsis, shock (septic, cardiogenic, hypovolemic, obstructive), liver disease, diabetic ketoacidosis, seizure, trauma, excessive exercise, hypoxia, HIV infection and treatment, regional hypoperfusion (bowel ischemia), prolonged use of a tourniquet (spurious elevation), MELAS (mitochondrial myopathy, encephalopathy, lactic acidosis, and stroke-like episodes), type I glycogen storage disease, fructose 1,6-diphosphatase deficiency (rare), pyruvate dehydrogenase deficiency, thiamine deficiency, non-Hodgkin and Burkitt lymphoma (rare). Drugs: phenformin, metformin (debated), epinephrine, isoniazid toxicity, nucleoside reverse-transcriptase inhibitors, propofol, theophylline.	Lactic acidosis should be suspected when there is a markedly increased anion gap (> 18 meq/L) in the absence of other causes (eg, renal failure, ketosis, ethanol, methanol, or salicylate). Lactic acidosis is characterized by lactate levels > 5 mmol/L and serum pH < 7.35. However, hypoalbuminemia may mask the anion gap and concomitant alkalosis may raise the pH. Blood lactate levels may indicate whether perfusion is being restored by therapy. High levels (≥ 4 mmol/L) of serum lactate are associated with increased risk of death independent of organ failure and shock. Patients with sepsis and elevated lactate levels have higher rates of in-hospital and 30-day mortality. Andersen LW et al. Etiology and therapeutic approach to elevated lactate levels. Mayo Clin Proc 2013;88:1127. [PMID: 24079682] Inzucchi SE et al. Metformin in patients with type 2 diabetes and kidney disease: a systematic review. JAMA 2014;312:2668. [PMID: 25536258] Reddy AJ et al. Lactic acidosis: clinical implications and management strategies. Cleve Clin J Med 2015;82:615. [PMID: 26366959]

(Continued)

Lead

Test/Range/Collection	Physiologic Basis	Interpretation	Comments
Lead, whole blood (Pb) Child (<6 yr): <10 mcg/dL Child (>6 yr): <25 mcg/dL [Child (<6 yr): <0.48 mcmol/L Child (>6 yr): <1.21 mcmol/L] Adult: <40 mcg/dL [Adult: <1.93 mcmol/L] Industrial workers' limit: <50 mcg/dL [Industrial workers' limit: <2.42 mcmol/L] Navy $$ Use trace metal-free navy blue top tube with heparin.	Lead salts are absorbed through ingestion, inhalation, or the skin. About 5–10% of ingested lead is found in blood, and 95% of this is in erythrocytes; 80–90% is taken up by bone, where it is relatively inactive. Lead poisons enzymes by binding to protein disulfide groups, leading to cell death. It also causes oxidative stress and damage to cells. Lead levels fluctuate. Several specimens may be needed to rule out lead poisoning. There is substantial individual variability in vulnerability to lead.	**Increased in:** Lead poisoning, including abnormal ingestion (especially lead-containing paint, water from lead plumbing, moonshine whiskey), occupational exposures (metal smelters, miners, welders, storage battery workers, auto manufacturers, ship builders, paint manufacturers, printing workers, pottery workers, gasoline refinery workers, demolition and tank cleaning workers), retained bullets.	Cognition may be impaired by modest elevations of blood lead concentrations. Neurologic impairment may be detectable in children with lead levels of 15 mcg/dL and in adults at 30 mcg/dL; full-blown symptoms appear at > 60 mcg/dL. Most chronic lead poisoning leads to a moderate anemia with basophilic stippling of erythrocytes on peripheral blood smear. Acute poisoning is rare and associated with abdominal pain and constipation. Recent studies have demonstrated that harmful effects can occur in children with blood lead levels less than the current limit of 10 mcg/dL, and a new cutoff value of 5 mcg/dL has been recommended. Blood lead levels are more reflective of acute exposure, whereas bone lead levels better reflect cumulative exposure over time. Jaishankar M et al. Toxicity, mechanism and health effects of some heavy metals. Interdiscip Toxicol 2014;7:60. [PMID: 26109881] Mason LH et al. Pb neurotoxicity: neuropsychological effects of lead toxicity. Biomed Res Int 2014;2014:840547. [PMID: 24516855] Zhai Q et al. Dietary strategies for the treatment of cadmium and lead toxicity. Nutrients 2015;7:552. [PMID: 25594439]

Legionella antibody		
Legionella antibody, serum <1:32 titer SST $$$ Submit paired sera, one collected within 2 weeks of illness and another 2–3 weeks later.	*Legionella pneumophila* is a weakly staining gram-negative bacillus that causes Pontiac fever (acute influenza-like illness) and legionnaires disease (a pneumonia that may progress to a severe multisystem illness). It does not grow on routine bacteriologic culture media. There are at least 6 serogroups of *L. pneumophila* and at least 22 species of *Legionella*. Indirect immunofluorescent assays for *L. pneumophila* serogroup 1 (IgM and/or IgG) and serogroups 1–6 (IgM and/or IgG) are both available.	**Increased in:** *Legionella* infection (80% of patients with pneumonia have a fourfold rise in titer); cross-reactions with other infectious agents (*Yersinia pestis* [plague], *Francisella tularensis* [tularemia], *Bacteroides fragilis, Mycoplasma pneumoniae, Leptospira interrogans*, campylobacter serotypes).	The test provides only a retrospective laboratory diagnosis because it generally takes more than 3 weeks to mount a detectable antibody response. More than a fourfold rise in titer to > 1:128 in specimens gathered more than 3 weeks apart indicates recent infection. A single titer of > 1:256 is considered diagnostic. About 50–60% of cases of legionellosis may have a positive direct fluorescent antibody test. Culture can have a sensitivity of 50%. All three methods may increase sensitivity to 90%. This test is species-specific. Polyvalent antiserum is needed to test for all serogroups and species. Urine *Legionella* antigen testing, in adjunct to cultures, may provide a rapid turnaround for results. The urine antigen test is very specific, but the sensitivity ranges from 70% to 90% because it detects primarily serogroup 1 infections. Abdel-Nour M et al. Biofilms: the stronghold of *Legionella pneumophila*. Int J Mol Sci 2013;14:21660. [PMID: 24185913] Isaac DT et al. Master manipulators: an update on *Legionella pneumophila* Icm/Dot translocated substrates and their host targets. Future Microbiol 2014;9:343. [PMID: 24762308] van Duin D. Diagnostic challenges and opportunities in older adults with infectious diseases. Clin Infect Dis 2012;54:973. [PMID: 22186775]

(Continued)

Leukemia/lymphoma phenotyping by flow cytometry			
Test/Range/Collection	Physiologic Basis	Interpretation	Comments
Leukemia/lymphoma phenotyping by flow cytometry Blood, bone marrow aspirates, fine-needle aspirates, fresh tissue biopsies, body fluids. Lavender or yellow (blood, bone marrow), green (bone marrow) Specimen should be delivered within 24 hours. $$$$	Immunophenotyping by multiparameter flow cytometry is an integral part of the diagnosis and classification systems for leukemias and malignant lymphomas. The majority of immunophenotyping markers are the cluster of differentiation antigens, or CD antigens. Other commonly used markers include glycophorin A, HLA-DR, immunoglobulin (Ig) light chains, MPO (myeloperoxidase), TdT (terminal deoxynucleotidyl transferase), and ZAP-70 (zeta-chain associated protein kinase 70). Detection of certain cellular antigens also has prognostic (eg, ZAP-70) and therapeutic (eg, CD20, CD33, CD52) significance.	**Abnormal phenotype profile present in:** Acute myeloid leukemias, acute lymphoblastic leukemias, B- and T-cell non-Hodgkin lymphomas, plasma cell myeloma. **Markers expressed mainly in hematopoietic precursors:** HLA-DR, TdT, CD34; **B cells:** CD19, CD20, CD22, CD24, CD10, CD79, Ig heavy chains (γ, α, μ, δ), and light chains (κ, λ); **T cells:** CD3, CD7, CD5, CD2, CD4, CD8; **myeloid cells:** MPO, CD13, CD33, CD11, CD117. **Markers that suggest megakaryocytic differentiation:** CD41, CD42, CD61; **erythroid differentiation:** glycophorin, hemoglobin A; **monocytic differentiation:** CD14, CD15, CD64, CD68; **NK cells:** CD16, CD56; **hairy cell leukemia:** CD103 on clonal B cells; **plasma cells:** CD38 and cytoplasmic light chain restriction; **paroxysmal nocturnal hemoglobinuria cells:** absence of CD55, CD59 and fluorescent aerolysin.	Each leukemia/lymphoma has a unique diagnostic immunopheno-type (Table 8–13). An interpretative report should be generated for each specimen analyzed. Multicolor analysis may be performed, allowing for an accurate definition of the surface and cytoplasmic antigen profile of specific cells. Two simultaneous hematologic malignancies may be detected within the same tissue site. Morphologic features remain the cornerstone of the evaluation of leukemia/lymphoma, but ancillary studies including immunophe-notyping, cytogenetics, and/or molecular genetic testing are needed in most, if not all, cases. Multiparametric and high-sensitivity flow cytometric analysis is needed to detect minimal residual disease (eg, acute lymphoblastic leukemia, multiple myeloma). Gaipa G et al. Detection of minimal residual disease in pediatric acute lymphoblastic leukemia. Cytometry B Clin Cytom 2013;84:359. [PMID: 23757107] Paiva B et al. New criteria for response assessment: role of minimal residual disease in multiple myeloma. Blood 2015;125:3059. [PMID: 25883846] Preis M et al. Laboratory tests for paroxysmal nocturnal hemoglobin-uria. Am J Hematol 2014;89:339. [PMID: 24127129] Woo J et al. Recent advancements of flow cytometry: new applications in hematology and oncology. Expert Rev Mol Diagn 2014;14:67. [PMID: 24308362]

(Continued)

	Lipase	Lipoprotein(a)
Lipase, serum or plasma 0–160 U/L [0–2.66 mckat/L] (laboratory-specific) SST, PPT $$	Lipases are responsible for hydrolysis of glycerol esters of long-chain fatty acids to produce fatty acids and glycerol. Lipases are produced in the liver, intestine, tongue, stomach, and many other cells. Assays are highly dependent on the substrate used.	**Increased in:** Acute, recurrent, or chronic pancreatitis, pancreatic pseudocyst, pancreatic malignancy, pancreatic trauma, peritonitis, biliary disease, hepatic disease, diabetes mellitus (especially diabetic ketoacidosis), intestinal disease, gastric malignancy or perforation, cystic fibrosis, inflammatory bowel disease (Crohn disease and ulcerative colitis).	Serum lipase may be a more reliable test than serum amylase for the initial diagnosis of acute pancreatitis, because of its increased sensitivity in acute alcoholic pancreatitis and because lipase remains elevated longer than amylase. Most current guidelines indicate that lipase should be preferred over total and pancreatic amylase. Cut-offs of 2–4 times the upper limit of the reference interval are recommended. The specificity of lipase and amylase in acute pancreatitis is similar, although both are poor. Simultaneous measurement of serum amylase and lipase does not improve diagnostic accuracy. Measurement of serum lipase does not help in determining the severity or cause of acute pancreatitis, and daily measurements are of no value in assessing the patient's clinical progress or ultimate prognosis. Test sensitivity is not very good for chronic pancreatitis or pancreatic cancer. For chronic pancreatic insufficiency, fecal pancreatic elastase (p. 168) has excellent sensitivity. Lippi G et al. Laboratory diagnosis of acute pancreatitis: in search of the Holy Grail. Crit Rev Clin Lab Sci 2012;49:18. [PMID: 22339380] Mahajan A et al. Utility of serum pancreatic enzyme levels in diagnosing blunt trauma to the pancreas: a prospective study with systematic review. Injury 2014;45:1384. [PMID: 24702828]
Lipoprotein(a) [Lp(a)], serum or plasma ≤ 30 mg/dL SST, red, PPT, green, lavender Overnight fasting; separate serum or plasma from cells ASAP or within 2 hours of collection. $$	Lipoprotein(a) [Lp(a)] is an LDL-like molecule consisting of an apolipoprotein B-100 particle attached to apoprotein (a) via a disulfide bridge. Lp(a) is both proatherogenic and prothrombotic. Elevated Lp(a) level is a risk factor for cardiovascular diseases, and is an independent predictor of coronary artery disease and myocardial infarction. Lp(a) is also a risk factor for venous thrombosis, ischemic stroke and aortic valve stenosis.	**Increased in** ~15% of general population. Lp(a) levels > 30 mg/dL are associated with a 2–3 fold increased risk of cardiovascular events independent of other risk factors.	Test is not recommended as a screening test in the healthy population, largely because there is a lack of very effective medications to lower Lp(a). Levels of Lp(a) are related to genetic factors, and are largely unaffected by diet, exercise and lipid-lowering medications. Lp(a)-lowering therapy might be beneficial in patients with high Lp(a) levels, especially for patients with additional risk factors for coronary artery disease. Lp(a) levels vary significantly among different ethnic groups. African Americans, for example, have much higher levels than Caucasians, independent of isoform variations. Kostner KM et al. When should we measure lipoprotein(a)? Eur Heart J 2013;34:3268. [PMID: 23735860] Malaguarnera M et al. Lipoprotein(a) in cardiovascular diseases. Biomed Res Int 2013;2013:650989. [PMID: 23484137]

Test/Range/Collection	Physiologic Basis	Interpretation	Comments
Lipoprotein-associated phospholipase A$_2$ (Lp-PLA$_2$), serum or plasma < 235 ng/mL (age- and sex-dependent) SST, red, green, lavender Separate serum or plasma from cells ASAP or within 2 hours of collection, and refrigerate. \$\$	Lp-PLA$_2$ is an inflammatory protein lipase produced mostly by monocytes and macrophages in the vascular intima. It facilitates hydrolysis of phospholipids in the arterial wall and generation of pro-atherogenic metabolites. Due to its pro-inflammatory and pro-oxidative effects, Lp-PLA$_2$ plays an important role in the pathogenesis of atherosclerosis. In the bloodstream, it mostly binds to LDL (> 80%), and also to other lipoproteins (eg, to HDL, ~10%).	**Increased in:** Atherosclerosis (eg, coronary artery disease, carotid stenosis and associated ischemic stroke)	Elevated levels of Lp-PLA$_2$ have been associated with higher plaque burden and increased cardiovascular risk. Individuals with elevated levels of Lp-PLA$_2$ are at increased risk of cardiovascular events, including myocardial infarction and ischemic stroke. The use of Lp-PLA$_2$ is helpful in patients at moderate cardiovascular risk (> 2 risk factors) and in those at high-risk, in whom assessment of Lp-PLA$_2$ activity levels can guide the lipid-lowering treatment. Darapladib is an Lp-PLA$_2$ inhibitor that has shown beneficial effects in patients with atherosclerosis. Test is not recommended for cardiovascular disease risk assessment in asymptomatic adults. Jensen MK et al. Novel metabolic biomarkers of cardiovascular disease. Nat Rev Endocrinol 2014;10:659. [PMID: 25178732] Maiolino G et al. Lipoprotein-associated phospholipase A$_2$ prognostic role in atherosclerotic complications. World J Cardiol 2015;7:609. [PMID: 26516415]

Lipoprotein associated phospholipase A$_2$ (Lp-PLA$_2$)

Luteinizing hormone

Luteinizing hormone, serum or plasma (LH) Males: 1–10 mIU/mL Females: (mIU/mL) Follicular 1–18 Luteal 0.4–20 Midcycle peak 24–105 Postmenopausal 15–62 (laboratory-specific) SST, PPT, green $$	LH is stimulated by the hypothalamic hormone gonadotropin-releasing hormone (GnRH). It is secreted from the anterior pituitary and acts on the gonads. LH is the principal regulator of steroid biosynthesis in the ovary and testis, and is essential for fertility in men and women. LH, along with FSH (follicle-stimulating hormone), acts on the FSH-stimulated follicle and is eventually responsible for luteinization and ovulation. The LH/chorinic gonadotropin receptor (LHCGR) belongs to the G protein-coupled receptor superfamily.	**Increased in:** Primary hypogonadism, polycystic ovary syndrome, postmenopause, endometriosis, after depot leuprolide injection; immunoassay result may be falsely elevated in pregnancy. **Decreased in:** Pituitary or hypothalamic failure, anorexia nervosa, bulimia, advanced prostate cancer, severe stress, malnutrition, Kallman syndrome (gonadotropin deficiency associated with anosmia). Drugs: digoxin, oral contraceptives, phenothiazines.	In male hypogonadism, serum LH and FSH levels can distinguish between primary (hypergonadotropic) and secondary (hypogonadotropic) hypogonadism. Hypogonadism associated with aging (andropause) may present a mixed picture, with low testosterone levels and low to low-normal gonadotropin levels. Repeated measurement may be required to diagnose gonadotropin deficiencies. Elevated serum LH levels are a common feature in polycystic ovary syndrome, but measurement of total testosterone is the test of choice to diagnose polycystic ovary syndrome. The use of a single LH measurement should be discouraged due to its intrinsic variability. LH measurements can help differentiate normogonadotropic amenorrhoea and hypothalamic amenorrhoea. Andersen CY et al. Human steroidogenesis: implications for controlled ovarian stimulation with exogenous gonadotropins. Reprod Biol Endocrinol 2014;12:128. [PMID: 25543693] Conway G et al. The polycystic ovary syndrome: a position statement from the European Society of Endocrinology. Eur J Endocrinol 2014;171:1. [PMID: 24849517] Klein DA et al. Amenorrhea: an approach to diagnosis and management. Am Fam Physician 2013;87:781. [PMID: 23939500] Sansone A et al. Endocrine evaluation of erectile dysfunction. Endocrine 2014;46:423. [PMID: 24705931]

(Continued)

Lyme disease antibody

Test/Range/Collection	Physiologic Basis	Interpretation	Comments
Lyme disease antibodies, total, serum ELISA: negative (<1:8 titer) Western blot: nonreactive SST $$	Test detects the presence of antibody to *Borrelia burgdorferi*, the etiologic agent in Lyme disease, an inflammatory disorder transmitted by the ticks *Ixodes dammini, I pacificus,* and *I scapularis* in the northeastern and midwestern, western, and southeastern United States, respectively. Culture of *B burgdorferi* requires special medium that is not routinely available. The number of organisms present in blood and CSF is very low. As a result, the sensitivity of cultures is only about 10%. Even polymerase chain reaction–based testing does not substantially increase the rate of bacterial detection. The diagnosis thus relies on testing for host antibodies to *B burgdorferi* infection. Test detects IgM antibody, which develops within 3–6 weeks after the onset of rash, and IgG antibody, which develops within 6–8 weeks after the onset of disease and which may persist for months.	**Positive in:** Lyme disease (~30 days after infection), asymptomatic individuals living in endemic areas, immunization with recombinant outer-surface protein A (OspA) Lyme disease vaccine, tick-borne relapsing fever (*Borrelia hermsii*). **Negative in:** First 30 days of *Borrelia* infection or after early antibiotic therapy.	Test is not recommended for patients who do not have symptoms typical of Lyme disease. Test is less sensitive in patients with only an acute rash (ie, ~50% sensitivity). Because culture or direct visualization of the organism is difficult, serologic diagnosis (by enzyme immunoassay, EIA) is indicated. Two-step serologic testing has been recommended using an EIA, followed by separate IgM and IgG Western blot test. Positive or equivocal serologic testing (IgM and IgG) by sensitive EIA on specimens < 30 days after appearance of skin rash needs to be confirmed by Western blot tests (IgM and IgG), which use strict criteria and therefore provide specificity. Only IgG Western blot is needed in the chronic stage (> 30 days after disease onset). Both steps can be done using the same blood sample. Results are considered positive only if the EIA and the Western blots are both positive. The two-step assay has low sensitivity in early infection, but is highly sensitive and specific after 6–8 weeks of untreated infection. Bockenstedt LK et al. Review: unraveling Lyme disease. Arthritis Rheumatol 2014;66:2313. [PMID: 24965960] Halperin JJ. Chronic Lyme disease: misconceptions and challenges for patient management. Infect Drug Resist 2015;8:119. [PMID: 26028977] Oliveira CR et al. Update on persistent symptoms associated with Lyme disease. Curr Opin Pediatr 2015;27:100. [PMID: 25490690]

(Continued)

	Magnesium		Mean corpuscular hemoglobin
Magnesium, serum or plasma (Mg²⁺) 1.8–3.0 mg/dL [0.75–1.25 mmol/L] **Panic:** < 0.5 or > 4.5 mg/dL [<0.2 or > 1.85 mmol/L] Red, green $	Magnesium is primarily an intracellular cation (second most abundant, 60% found in bone); it is a necessary cofactor in numerous enzyme systems, particularly ATPases. By regulating enzymes controlling intracellular calcium, Mg²⁺ affects smooth muscle vasoconstriction, important to the underlying pathophysiology of several critical illnesses. In extracellular fluid, it influences neuromuscular response and irritability. Magnesium concentration is determined by intestinal absorption, renal excretion, and exchange with bone and intracellular fluid.	**Increased in:** Dehydration, tissue trauma, renal failure, hypoadrenocorticism, hypothyroidism. Drugs: aspirin (prolonged use), lithium, magnesium salts, laxatives, enemas, progesterone, triamterene. **Decreased in:** Chronic diarrhea, enteric fistula, starvation, chronic alcoholism, total parenteral nutrition with inadequate replacement, hypoparathyroidism (especially post-parathyroid surgery), acute pancreatitis, chronic glomerulonephritis, hyperaldosteronism, diabetic ketoacidosis, heart failure, critical illness, Gitelman syndrome (familial hypokalemia– hypomagnesemia– hypocalciuria), hereditary isolated magnesium wasting, induced hypothermia. Drugs: albuterol, amphotericin B, calcium salts, platinum derivates (cisplatin, carboplatinum), citrates (blood transfusion), cyclosporine, rapamycin, diuretics (furosemide, thiazide), proton pump inhibitors (omeprazole, pantoprazole, etc), ethacrynic acid.	Magnesium deficiency correlates with higher mortality and poorer clinical outcome in the ICU and is directly implicated in hypokalemia, hypocalcemia, tetany, and dysrhythmia. Hypomagnesemia is relatively common, and is associated with tetany, weakness, disorientation, and somnolence. A magnesium deficit may exist with little or no apparent change in serum level. Prolonged hypomagnesemia can cause refractory hypokalemia as well as functional hypoparathyroidism. There is a progressive reduction in serum magnesium level during normal pregnancy (related to hemodilution). Due to the kidney's ability to increase excretion to nearly 100% after the renal magnesium threshold is exceeded, clinically significant hypermagnesemia is rare. Ayuk J et al. Contemporary view of the clinical relevance of magnesium homeostasis. Ann Clin Biochem 2014;51(Pt 2):179. [PMID: 24402002] DeBaaij JH et al. Magnesium in man: implications for health and disease. Physiol Rev 2015;95:1. [PMID: 25540137]
Mean corpuscular hemoglobin, blood (MCH) 27–33 pg Lavender $	MCH indicates the amount of hemoglobin per RBC in absolute units. MCH is calculated from measured values of hemoglobin (Hb) (g/dL) and RBC ($\times 10^{12}$/L) by the formula: $MCH = (Hb/RBC) \times 10$	**Increased in:** Macrocytosis, hemochromatosis. **Decreased in:** Microcytosis (iron deficiency, thalassemia), hypochromia (lead poisoning, sideroblastic anemia, anemia of chronic disease).	Low MCH can mean hypochromia or microcytosis or both. High MCH is evidence of macrocytosis. Brugnara C et al. Red cell indices in classification and treatment of anemias: from M.M. Wintrobe's original 1934 classification to the third millennium. Curr Opin Hematol 2013; 20:222. [PMID: 23449069] Bryan LJ et al. Why is my patient anemic? Hematol Oncol Clin North Am 2012;26:205. [PMID: 22463824]

Test/Range/Collection	Physiologic Basis	Interpretation	Comments
Mean corpuscular hemoglobin concentration, blood (MCHC) 31–36 g/dL [310–360 g/L] Lavender $	MCHC is the average hemoglobin concentration in RBCs. It is calculated from hemoglobin concentration of whole blood (Hb, g/dL) and hematocrit (MCV × RBC): $$MCHC = \dfrac{Hb}{MCV \times RBC}$$	**Increased in:** Marked spherocytosis (hereditary spherocytosis or immune hemolysis). Spuriously increased in autoagglutination (eg, cold agglutinins), lipemia, cellular dehydration syndromes, hereditary xerocytosis. **Decreased in:** Hypochromic anemia (iron deficiency, thalassemia, lead poisoning), sideroblastic anemia, anemia of chronic disease. Spuriously decreased with markedly high white blood cell count.	For a given patient, the MCHC is fairly constant, and therefore delta check of MCHC is a useful parameter to ensure accuracy of red cell indices. The MCHC value may be misleading in the presence of a dimorphic population of RBCs. Brugnara C et al. Red cell indices in classification and treatment of anemias: from M.M. Wintrobe's original 1934 classification to the third millennium. Curr Opin Hematol 2013;20:222. [PMID: 23449069] Bryan LJ et al. Why is my patient anemic? Hematol Oncol Clin North Am 2012;26:205. [PMID: 22463824]
Mean corpuscular volume, blood (MCV) 80–100 fL Lavender $	MCV is the average volume of the red cells, and it is measured by an automated hematology instrument based on electrical impedance or forward light scatter.	**Increased in:** Liver disease (alcoholic and non-alcoholic), alcohol abuse, HIV/AIDS, hemochromatosis, megaloblastic anemia (folate, vitamin B_{12} deficiencies), myelodysplastic syndrome, marked reticulocytosis (acute bleeding or hemorrhage), chemotherapy, post splenectomy, hypothyroidism, newborns. Spurious increase in autoagglutination, high white blood cell count. Drugs: methotrexate, phenytoin, zidovudine. **Decreased in:** Iron deficiency, polycythemia vera on phlebotomy therapy, thalassemia, sideroblastic anemia, lead poisoning, hereditary spherocytosis, and some anemias of chronic disease.	MCV can be normal in combined iron and folate deficiency. In patients with two red cell populations (macrocytic and microcytic), MCV may be normal. MCV is an insensitive test in the evaluation of anemia. It is not uncommon for patients with evolving iron deficiency anemia or pernicious anemia to have a normal MCV. A low MCV can be used as an indication of iron depletion in frequent blood donors and a guide to phlebotomy therapy for hemochromatosis. See anemias (Figure 9–5; Tables 8–2, 8–3). Briani C et al. Cobalamin deficiency: clinical picture and radiological findings. Nutrients 2013;5:4521. [PMID: 24248213] Brugnara C et al. Red cell indices in classification and treatment of anemias: from M.M. Wintrobe's original 1934 classification to the third millennium. Curr Opin Hematol 2013; 20:222. [PMID: 23449069] Bryan LJ et al. Why is my patient anemic? Hematol Oncol Clin North Am 2012;26:205. [PMID: 22463824] Schoorl M et al. Application of innovative hemocytometric parameters and algorithms for improvement of microcytic anemia discrimination. Hematol Rep 2015;7:5843. [PMID: 26331001]

Metanephrines, free (unconjugated), plasma		
Metanephrines, free (unconjugated), plasma Metanephrine, free: < 0.50 nmol/L Normetanephrine, free: < 0.9 nmol/L Lavender, green $$$ Collect specimen after at least 30 min rest. Place specimen tube on ice, centrifuge within 1 hour, separate plasma and freeze immediately.	Catecholamines (norepinephrine and epinephrine), secreted in excess by pheochromocytomas, are metabolized within tumor cells by the enzyme catechol-O-methyltransferase to metanephrines (normetanephrine and metanephrine), and these can be detected in plasma. Measurement of plasma concentrations of free (unconjugated) metanephrines offers several advantages for the detection of pheochromocytoma: independence of short-term changes noted in catecholamine secretion in response to change of posture, exercise, or intraoperative stress; good correlation with tumor mass; and only minor interference from drugs. In diagnosis of pheochromocytoma, determination of plasma free metanephrines is often more reliable and efficient than other biochemical tests.	**Increased in:** Pheochromocytoma (sensitivity 99%; specificity 89–94%).	The plasma free metanephrines test has been recommended as one of the first-line biochemical tests for the diagnosis of pheochromocytoma. (See Pheochromocytoma algorithm, Figure 9–25.) Sensitivity of plasma free metanephrines (99%) is higher than that of urinary fractionated metanephrines (97%), plasma catecholamines (84%), and urinary vanillylmandelic acid (64%). Specificity of plasma free metanephrines is 89–94% compared with urinary vanillylmandelic acid (95%), urinary total metanephrines (93%), urinary catecholamines (88%), plasma catecholamines (81%), and urinary fractionated metanephrines (69%). Free metanephrines levels are superior to deconjugated metanephrines levels for diagnosis of pheochromocytoma, especially in patients with concomitant renal failure. Plasma catecholamines are often spuriously increased when drawn in the hospital setting. Eisenhofer G et al. Laboratory evaluation of pheochromocytoma and paraganglioma. Clin Chem 2014;60:1486. [PMID: 25332315] Pamporaki C et al. Plasma-free vs. deconjugated metanephrines for diagnosis of phaeochromocytoma. Clin Endocrinol (Oxf) 2013;79:476. [PMID: 23461656] van Berkel A et al. Diagnosis of endocrine disease: biochemical diagnosis of phaeochromocytoma and paraganglioma. Eur J Endocrinol 2014;170:R109. [PMID: 24347425]

(Continued)

	Metanephrines, fractionated, urine		Methanol
Test/Range/Collection	**Physiologic Basis**	**Interpretation**	**Comments**
Metanephrines, fractionated, urine Metanephrine: 60–200 mcg/24 hr Normetanephrine: 120–510 mcg/24 hr Urine container containing boric acid or acetic acid $$$ Collect 24-hour urine.	Catecholamines (norepinephrine and epinephrine), secreted in excess by pheochromocytomas, are metabolized by the enzyme catechol-*O*-methyltransferase to metanephrines (normetanephrine and metanephrine), and these are excreted in the urine.	**Increased in:** Pheochromocytoma (98% sensitivity, 93% specificity), neuroblastoma, ganglioneuroma, significant physical stress. Drugs: Monoamine oxidase inhibitors, tricyclic antidepressants, levodopa.	Urinary fractionated metanephrines is often one of the first-line biochemical tests for the diagnostic evaluation of pheochromocytoma. (See Pheochromocytoma algorithm, Figure 9–25). Because < 0.1% of persons with hypertension have a pheochromocytoma, routine screening of all such people would yield a positive predictive value of < 10%. Avoid overutilization of tests. Do not order urine vanillylmandelic acid, urine catecholamines, and plasma metanephrines and catecholamines at the same time. Eisenhofer G et al. Laboratory evaluation of pheochromocytoma and paraganglioma. Clin Chem 2014;60:1486. [PMID: 25332315] Van Berkel A et al. Diagnosis of endocrine disease: biochemical diagnosis of phaeochromocytoma and paraganglioma. Eur J Endocrinol 2014;170:R109. [PMID: 24347425]
Methanol, whole blood Negative Green or lavender $$	Methanol is extensively metabolized by alcohol dehydrogenase to formaldehyde and by aldehyde dehydrogenase to formic acid, the major toxic metabolite. Serum methanol levels > 20 mg/dL are toxic and levels > 40 mg/dL are life-threatening.	**Increased in:** Methanol intoxication.	Methanol intoxication is associated with metabolic acidosis and an osmol gap (see Table 8–14). Methanol is commonly ingested in its pure form or in cleaning or copier solutions. Acute ingestion causes an optic neuritis that may result in blindness. Methanol poisoning can be fatal. Fomepizole, a competitive alcohol dehydrogenase inhibitor, can be used to treat methanol poisoning and can obviate the need for extracorporeal hemodialysis. Quantitative measurement of the serum methanol level using gas chromatography is expensive, time-consuming, and not always available. Because methanol is osmotically active and measurement of serum osmolality is easily performed, the osmolal gap is often used as a screening test. See Table 8–14. Kruse JA. Methanol and ethylene glycol intoxication. Crit Care Clin 2012;28:661. [PMID: 22998995] Roberts DM et al. Recommendations for the role of extracorporeal treatments in the management of acute methanol poisoning: a systematic review and consensus statement. Crit Care Med 2015;43:461. [PMID: 25493973]

(Continued)

		Methemoglobin	MTHFR mutation

Methemoglobin, whole blood (MetHb)

<0.15 g/dL [<23.25 mmol/L] or <1.5% of total Hb

Blood gas syringe (heparinized) (Lavender or green for total hemoglobin only)

$$

Don't remove the stopper or cap, analyze promptly.

Methemoglobin has its heme iron in the oxidized ferric state and thus cannot combine with and transport oxygen. Methemoglobin can be assayed spectrophotometrically by measuring the decrease in absorbance at 630–635 nm due to the conversion of methemoglobin to cyanmethemoglobin with cyanide. CO-oximetry is the gold standard and is useful for rapid quantitation of methemoglobin.

Increased in: Hereditary methemoglobinemia: structural hemoglobin variants (hemoglobin M) (rare), NADH-MetHb reductase (cytochrome b_5 reductase) deficiency. Acquired methemoglobinemia: Oxidant drugs such as sulfonamides, dapsone, sulfasalazine, silver sulfadiazine, primaquine, isoniazid, drug abuse (volatile nitrites, cocaine), nitroglycerin, nitrates, aniline dyes, phenacetin, hydralazine, topical anesthetics (eg, benzocaine, prilocaine), ifosfamide chemotherapy, chloramine toxicity during hemodialysis, infants with diarrhea or urinary tract infections (due to oxidant stress).

Levels of 1.5 g/dL (about 10% of total Hb) result in visible cyanosis. The diagnosis can be suspected by the characteristic chocolate brown color of a freshly obtained blood sample. Patients with levels of about 35% have headache, weakness, and breathlessness (tachycardia, tachypnea). Levels > 70% are usually fatal.

Administration of methylene blue facilitates the reduction of MetHb to Hb in the enzyme deficiency state and ameliorates the cyanosis but it has no effect in reducing Hb M variants or in relieving the cyanosis that they cause.

Ashurst J et al. Methemoglobinemia: a systematic review of the pathophysiology, detection, and treatment. Del Med J 2011;83:203. [PMID: 21954509]

Skold A et al. Methemoglobinemia: pathogenesis, diagnosis, and management. South Med J 2011;104:757. [PMID: 22024786]

Methylenetetrahydrofolate reductase (*MTHFR*) mutation

Blood

Lavender

$$$$

5,10-Methylenetetrahydrofolate reductase (MTHFR) plays a key role in folate metabolism. MTHFR enzyme deficiency leads to hyperhomocysteinemia. Increased plasma homocysteine is a risk factor for arteriosclerotic vascular disease and thrombosis. Two mutations in the human *MTHFR* gene, C667T and A1298C, result in moderate impairment of MTHFR activity (30–60% of normal). In addition, these mutations have been associated with an increased risk for various cancers, likely due to genomic DNA hypomethylation. *MTHFR* mutation test is ordered along with other inherited clotting risk testing, such as factor V Leiden and prothrombin 20210 mutation tests.

Positive in: Individuals with *MTHFR* C677T and/or A1298C mutations (sensitivity and specificity approach 100%).

The *MTHFR* mutation assay is indicated for patients with early-onset arteriosclerotic vascular disease or thrombosis, particularly those with hyperhomocysteinemia or significant family histories. See recommended testing for venous thrombosis (Figure 9–34). Both C677T and A1298C mutations should be examined when assessing genetic risk factors for hyperhomocysteinemia. Only those who are homozygous for C677T mutation or compound heterozygous for the C677T/A1298C mutations have significantly elevated plasma homocysteine levels. Double homozygotes have not been reported.

The association of thrombophilia (venous thromboembolism) in pregnancy with mutations in *MTHFR* is still controversial. The assay is typically polymerase chain reaction (PCR) based. Battinelli EM et al. The role of thrombophilia in pregnancy. Thrombosis 2013;2013:516420. [PMID: 24455235]

Rai V. Methylenetetrahydrofolate reductase A1298C polymorphism and breast cancer risk: a meta-analysis of 33 studies. Ann Med Health Sci 2014;4:841. [PMID: 25506474]

Trimmer EE. Methylenetetrahydrofolate reductase: biochemical characterization and medical significance. Curr Pharm Des 2013;19:2574. [PMID: 23116396]

	Methylmalonic acid	
Test/Range/Collection	**Physiologic Basis**	**Interpretation**	**Comments**
---	---	---	---
Methylmalonic acid (MMA), serum or plasma 0–0.4 mcmol/L (0–4.7 mcg/dL) SST, red, lavender, green $$	Elevation of serum methylmalonic acid (MMA) in cobalamin (B_{12}) deficiency results from impaired conversion of methylmalonyl-CoA to succinyl-CoA, a pathway involving methylmalonyl-CoA mutase as its enzyme and adenosylcobalamin as its coenzyme. Serum MMA is used to indirectly evaluate vitamin B_{12} status, mainly for confirming B_{12} deficiency in patients with low serum B_{12} levels. It is also a diagnostic marker for congenital methylmalonic acidemia, characterized by neonatal or infantile metabolic ketoacidosis, failure to thrive, and developmental delay.	**Increased in:** Vitamin B_{12} (cobalamin) deficiency (95%), pernicious anemia, renal insufficiency, pregnancy, elderly (5–15%).	If serum or plasma vitamin B_{12} level is 300 pg/mL or greater, B_{12} deficiency is unlikely and test for MMA is generally not indicated. Explanation of high frequency (5–15%) of increased serum MMA in the elderly with low or normal serum vitamin B_{12} levels is unclear. Benefits of B_{12} supplementation in this situation are unclear. Normal MMA levels can exclude vitamin B_{12} deficiency in the presence of unexplained low B_{12} levels found in lymphoid disorders. Test is usually normal in HIV patients who may have low serum vitamin B_{12} levels without actual vitamin B_{12} deficiency; these patients usually have low vitamin B_{12}–binding protein. For individuals with mildly elevated MMA levels (0.40–2.00 mcmol/L), vitamin B_{12} treatment normalizes MMA level but has no significant effect on hemoglobin, MCV, or anemic, neurologic, or gastroenterologic symptoms, at least in the short term. Urine MMA (reference interval: 0–3.6 mmol/mol creatinine) test is also available for evaluating B_{12} status as well as for monitoring patients with methylmalonic aciduria. Baumgartner MR et al. Proposed guidelines for the diagnosis and management of methylmalonic and propionic acidemia. Orphanet J Rare Dis 2014;9:130. [PMID: 25205257] Oberley MJ et al. Laboratory testing for cobalamin deficiency in megaloblastic anemia. Am J Hematol 2013;88:522. [PMID: 23423840] Wong CW. Vitamin B_{12} deficiency in the elderly: is it worth screening? Hong Kong Med J 2015;21:155. [PMID: 25756278]

β₂-Microglobulin		
β₂-Microglobulin, serum or plasma (β₂M) < 0.2 mg/dL [< 2.0 mg/L] SST, green, lavender $$$	β₂-Microglobulin is a low-molecular-weight protein that is the light chain of the class I MHC antigens. It is present on the surface of all nucleated cells and in all body fluids. It is almost totally reabsorbed and catabolized by the proximal renal tubules. It is increased in many conditions that are accompanied by high cell turnover and/or immune activation.	**Increased in:** Inflammatory conditions (eg, inflammatory bowel disease), infections (eg, HIV, CMV), graft rejection, autoimmune disorders, lymphoid malignancies (eg, lymphoplasmacytic lymphoma/Waldenström macroglobulinemia), multiple myeloma, chronic renal failure, myeloproliferative and myelodysplastic disorders.	Because of its accumulation with renal dysfunction and its ability to become glycosylated, form fibrils, and deposit in tissues, β₂M is a cause of long-term dialysis-associated amyloidosis. Of tests used to predict progression to AIDS in HIV-infected patients, CD4 cell number has the most predictive power, followed closely by β₂M. Serum β₂M levels are elevated in many hematological and lymphoid malignancies. An association has been found between serum β₂M levels and tumor burden in some disorders, particularly multiple myeloma, making it a valuable prognostic marker in these conditions. It has been incorporated into the international prognostic scoring systems for multiple myeloma and certain lymphomas. Bataille R et al. Multiple myeloma international staging system: "staging" or simply "aging" system? Clin Lymphoma Myeloma Leuk 2013;13:635. [PMID: 24035714] Gertz MA. Waldenström macroglobulinemia: 2013 update on diagnosis, risk stratification, and management. Am J Hematol 2013;88:703. [PMID: 23784973] Stoppini M et al. Systemic amyloidosis: lessons from β₂-microglobulin. J Biol Chem 2015;290:9951. [PMID: 25750126] Yoo C et al. Serum beta₂-microglobulin in malignant lymphomas: an old but powerful prognostic factor. Blood Res 2014;49:148. [PMID: 25325033]

(Continued)

Test/Range/Collection	Physiologic Basis	Interpretation	Comments
		Mitochondrial antibodies	
Mitochondrial antibodies (AMA), serum Negative (<1.0 U) SST $$	Originally demonstrated using immunofluorescence approaches, antimitochondrial antibodies can now be detected using commercially available enzyme-linked immunosorbent assays (ELISAs). Although ELISAs are more practical, they are slightly less sensitive than immunofluorescence techniques. In AMA-negative patients with a high suspicion of primary biliary cirrhosis (PBC), antimitochondrial autoantibodies can be sought using recombinant autoantigens. AMA positivity constitutes one of three major diagnostic criteria for PBC.	**Increased in:** Primary biliary cirrhosis (PBC) (85–95%), chronic active hepatitis (25–28%), occasionally in CREST syndrome and other autoimmune diseases; lower titers in viral hepatitis, infectious mononucleosis, neoplasms, cryptogenic cirrhosis (25–30%).	Primarily used to distinguish PBC (antibodies present) from extrahepatic biliary obstruction (antibodies absent). The antigens recognized by AMA have been designated M1–M9. AMA from patients with PBC recognize the M2 antigen complex, which includes enzymes of the 2-pyruvate dehydrogenase (PDH-E2) and 2-oxoglutarate dehydrogenase found on the inner mitochondrial membrane. AMA are both sensitive and specific for diagnosis and prediction of PBC and are usually present at high titer. But the titer or levels of AMA do not indicate PBC activity or progression. AMA subtype profiles do not predict prognosis in patients with PBC. Nakamura M. Clinical significance of autoantibodies in primary biliary cirrhosis. Semin Liver Dis 2014;34:334. [PMID: 25057956] Webb GJ et al. The immunogenetics of primary biliary cirrhosis: a comprehensive review. J Autoimmun 2015;64:42. [PMID: 26250073]
		Neutrophil cytoplasmic antibodies	
Neutrophil cytoplasmic antibodies, serum (ANCA) Negative SST, red $$$	Measurement of autoantibodies in serum against cytoplasmic constituents of neutrophils. (See also Autoantibodies, Table 8–7.) Dual testing by standard indirect immunofluorescence for serum cytoplasmic ANCA (cANCA) and perinuclear ANCA (pANCA) with reflex testing of myeloperoxidase (MPO) and proteinase 3 (PR3) antibodies is often recommended. In some laboratories, ANCA testing is performed with MPO and PR3 antibodies as a single panel. ANCA is commonly associated with small vessel vasculitis.	**Positive in:** Granulomatosis with polyangiitis (formerly Wegener granulomatosis), systemic vasculitis, pauci-immune crescentic glomerulonephritis, paraneoplastic vasculitis, Churg-Strauss angiitis, microscopic polyangiitis, drug-induced vasculitis, ulcerative colitis.	Only the antibodies against MPO and PR3 have clinical utilitiy. ANCA testing has a good positive predictive value only when the pre-test probability is high because the prevalence of primary vasculitis is very low. In the patient with systemic vasculitis, elevated ANCA levels imply active disease. Longitudinal measurement of ANCA is useful in monitoring disease activity since the titers fall after 3–4 months of treatment. Persistently elevated ANCA despite treatment predicts a higher chance of relapse. However, ANCA levels can be persistently elevated and should be used in conjunction with other clinical indices in treatment decisions. For ANCA-associated vasculitis, ANCA sensitivity, specificity, positive predictive value, and negative predictive value vary with method and population studied. Aggarwal A. Role of autoantibody testing. Best Pract Res Clin Rheumatol 2014;28:907. [PMID: 26096093] Kallenberg CG. Pathogenesis and treatment of ANCA-associated vasculitides. Clin Exp Rheumatol 2015;33(4 Suppl 92):S1. [PMID: 26457917] Silva de Souza AW. Autoantibodies in systemic vasculitis. Front Immunol 2015;6:184. [PMID: 25954277]

N-telopeptide, cross-linked			Nuclear antibody		

N-telopeptide, cross-linked (NTx), urine

Adults: 20–100 units

7–17 years old: 20–700 units

(NTx Units = nmol Bone Collagen Equivalents/mmol creatinine or nM BCE/mM creatinine)

(age-specific and laboratory-specific)

24-hour urine. Collect without preservative.

$$$$

Approximately 90% of the organic matrix of bone is type I collagen that is cross-linked at the N- and C-terminal ends of the molecule. Cross-linked N-terminal fragment of type I collagen (NTx) is a specific marker of increased bone resorption. The intra-individual coefficient of variation of urine NTx measurements is approximately 30%. Part of this variation is due to diurnal fluctuations, and a 24-hour collection is thus preferred.

Increased in: Osteoporosis, osteomalacia, rickets, Paget disease, hyperparathyroidism, hyperthyroidism, fractures, childhood growth, multiple myeloma, and cancer with bone metastasis.

Test may be useful for monitoring of antiresorptive treatment in patients with osteopenia, osteoporosis, Paget disease, or other disorders. Not useful during childhood growth and during fracture healing. Biologic variability of urine levels of NTx may limit its clinical usefulness. Serum C-terminal telopeptide (CTx) and procollagen type I N-terminal pro-peptide (PINP) are preferred over urine NTx for monitoring osteoporosis treatment. Serum CTx is considered the reference bone resorption marker. Urinary NTx may help detection and management of bone metastasis. Also see C-telopeptide, beta-cross-linked (p. 85) and PINP (p. 179).

Bandeira F et al. Bone markers and osteoporosis therapy. Arq Bras Endocrinol Metabol 2014;58:504. [PMID: 25166041]

Chiu L et al. Use of urinary markers in cancer setting: a literature review. J Bone Oncol 2015;4:18. [PMID: 26579485]

Lee J et al. Current recommendations for laboratory testing and use of bone turnover markers in management of osteoporosis. Ann Lab Med 2012;32:105. [PMID: 22389876]

Nuclear antibody, serum (anti-nuclear antibody, ANA)

<1:20

SST

$$

Heterogeneous antibodies to nuclear antigens (DNA and RNA, centromere, histone, and nonhistone proteins, nuclear membrane, nucleoli). Nuclear antibody is measured in serum by layering the patient's serum over human epithelial cells and detecting the antibody with fluorescein conjugated polyvalent antihuman immunoglobulin. Solid-phase assays such as enzyme-linked immunosorbent assay (ELISA) and laser bead assays are also available for ANA detection, but have lower sensitivity for systemic lupus erythematosus (SLE) compared with the gold standard immunofluorescence assay.

Elevated in: Patients over age 65 (35–75%, usually in low titers), SLE (98%), drug-induced lupus (100%), Sjögren syndrome (70–80%), rheumatoid arthritis (30–50%), scleroderma (50–80%), mixed connective tissue disease (100%), Felty syndrome, mononucleosis, hepatic or biliary cirrhosis, hepatitis, lymphocytic leukemia, myasthenia gravis, dermatomyositis, polymyositis (10–25%), chronic renal failure.

The ANA test is one of the most widely used autoantibody tests. If ANA is positive, the sub-specificities are identified using different assays. A negative ANA test does not completely rule out SLE, but alternative diagnoses should be considered. The pattern of ANA staining may give some clues to diagnoses. Test reports should mention the staining pattern (eg, homogeneous, speckled, centromere, nucleolar, etc), the titer (highest dilution at which the test is positive) and substrate used (eg, HEp2 cells). The rim (peripheral) pattern is highly specific (for SLE). Not useful as a screening test. Should be used only when there is clinical suspicion of SLE or other connective tissue disease.

Aggarwal A. Role of autoantibody testing. Best Pract Res Clin Rheumatol 2014;28:907. [PMID: 26096093]

Chan EK et al. Report of the first international consensus on standardized nomenclature of antinuclear antibody HEp-2 cell patterns 2014–2015. Front Immunol 2015;6:412. [PMID: 26347739]

(Continued)

Oligoclonal bands

Test/Range/Collection	Physiologic Basis	Interpretation	Comments
Oligoclonal bands, serum and CSF Negative SST or red (serum), glass or plastic tube (CSF) $$ Collect serum and CSF simultaneously.	Electrophoretic examination of IgG found in CSF may show oligoclonal bands not found in serum. It is considered positive for CSF oligoclonal bands if there are two or more bands in the CSF that are not present in the serum. This suggests local production in CSF of limited species of IgG. The pathogenesis of oligoclonal bands in multiple sclerosis is still obscure.	**Positive in:** Multiple sclerosis, CNS syphilis, subacute sclerosing panencephalitis, progressive multifocal leukoencephalopathy, Guillain-Barré syndrome, other CNS inflammatory diseases.	Test is indicated when multiple sclerosis is suspected clinically. CSF oligoclonal bands are not specific for multiple sclerosis, and only ~10% of patients with multiple sclerosis have oligoclonal bands detected. Nevertheless, the test is commonly used along with other clinical and laboratory tools to help diagnose the disease. Identical serum and CSF oligoclonal bands ("mirror pattern"), or no oligoclonal bands, suggest systemic immune activation. IgG index (see p. 134) is a more reliable test analytically, but neither test is specific for multiple sclerosis. There is no predictable correlation between the IgG index and the oligoclonal band number in the CSF of multiple sclerosis patients. Quantification of oligoclonal bands in CSF is an insensitive prognostic indicator and should not be used to influence treatment decisions. Disanto G et al. The evidence for a role of B cells in multiple sclerosis. Neurology 2012;78:823. [PMID: 22411958] Raphael I et al. Body fluid biomarkers in multiple sclerosis: how far we have come and how they could affect the clinic now and in the future. Expert Rev Clin Immunol 2015;11:69. [PMID: 25523168]

Osmolality, serum		
Osmolality, serum or plasma (Osm) 285–293 mosm/kg H₂O [mmol/kg H₂O] **Panic:** < 240 or > 320 mosm/kg H₂O SST, PPT $$	Test measures the osmotic pressure of serum by the freezing point depression method. Plasma and urine osmolality are more useful indicators of degree of hydration than BUN, hematocrit, or serum proteins. Serum osmolality can be estimated by the following formula: $$Osm = 2(Na^+) + \frac{BUN}{2.8} + \frac{Glucose}{18}$$ where Na⁺ is in meq/L and BUN and glucose are in mg/dL.	**Increased in:** Diabetic ketoacidosis, nonketotic hyperosmolar hyperglycemic coma, hypernatremia secondary to dehydration (diarrhea, severe burns, vomiting, fever, hyperventilation, inadequate water intake, central or nephrogenic diabetes insipidus, or osmotic diuresis), hypernatremia with normal hydration (hypothalamic disorders, defective osmostat), hypernatremia with overhydration (iatrogenic or accidental excessive NaCl or NaHCO₃ intake), alcohol or other toxic ingestion (see Comments), hypercalcemia; tube feedings. Drugs: corticosteroids, mannitol, glycerin. **Decreased in:** Pregnancy (third trimester), hyponatremia with hypovolemia (adrenal insufficiency, renal losses, diarrhea, vomiting, severe burns, peritonitis, pancreatitis), hyponatremia with normovolemia (SIADH), hyponatremia with hypervolemia (CHF, cirrhosis, nephrotic syndrome, postoperative state). Drugs: chlorthalidone, cyclophosphamide, thiazides.	If the difference between calculated and measured serum osmolality is greater than 10 mosm/kg H₂O, suspect the presence of a low-molecular-weight toxin (ethanol, methanol, isopropyl alcohol, ethylene glycol, acetone, ethyl ether, paraldehyde, or mannitol), ethanol being the most common. (See Table 8–14 for further explanation.) Every 100 mg/dL of ethanol increases serum osmolality by 22 mosm/kg H₂O (ethanol/4.6). Whereas the osmolal gap may overestimate the blood alcohol level, a normal serum osmolality excludes ethanol intoxication. Measurement of serum osmolality is an important first step in the laboratory evaluation of the hyponatremic patient. The simultaneous measurement of plasma ADH (vasopressin) and plasma osmolality in a dehydration test is the most powerful diagnostic tool in the differential diagnosis of polyuria/polydipsia. Cheuvront SN et al. Physiologic basis for understanding quantitative dehydration assessment. Am J Clin Nutr 2013;97:455. [PMID: 23343973] Nagler EV et al. Diagnosis and treatment of hyponatremia: a systemic review of clinical practice guidelines and consensus statements. BMC Med 2014;12:1. [PMID: 25539784] Pasquel FJ et al. Hyperosmolar hyperglycemic state: a historic review of the clinical presentation, diagnosis, and treatment. Diabetes Care 2014;37:3124. [PMID: 25342831]

(Continued)

Test/Range/Collection	Physiologic Basis	Interpretation	Comments
Osmolality, urine (Urine Osm) Random: 100–900 mosm/kg H_2O [mmol/kg H_2O] Urine container $$	Test measures renal tubular concentrating ability. Urine osmolality and specific gravity usually change in parallel with each other. When large molecules such as glucose and protein are present, however, the results diverge. Specific gravity is increased more, due to the weight of the molecules, whereas urine osmolality is increased less, reflecting the number of molecules.	**Increased in:** Hypovolemia, syndrome of inappropriate ADH secretion (SIADH). Drugs: anesthetic agents (during surgery), carbamazepine, chlorpropamide, cyclophosphamide, metolazone, vincristine. **Decreased in:** Diabetes insipidus, primary polydipsia, exercise, starvation. Drugs: acetohexamide, demeclocycline, glyburide, lithium, tolazamide.	In the hypoosmolar state (serum osmolality < 280 mosm/kg), urine osmolality is used to determine whether water excretion is normal or impaired. A urine osmolality value of < 100 mosm/kg indicates complete and appropriate suppression of antidiuretic hormone secretion. With average fluid intake, normal random urine osmolality is 100–900 mosm/kg H_2O. After 12-hour fluid restriction, normal random urine osmolality is > 850 mosm/kg H_2O. Capatina C et al. Diabetes insipidus after traumatic brain injury. J Clin Med 2015;4:1448. [PMID: 26239685] Oh JY et al. Syndrome of inappropriate antidiuretic hormone secretion and cerebral/renal salt wasting syndrome: similarities and differences. Front Pediatr 2015;2:146. [PMID: 25657991] Pasquel FJ et al. Hyperosmolar hyperglycemic state: a historic review of the clinical presentation, diagnosis, and treatment. Diabetes Care 2014;37:3124. [PMID: 25342831]

Osteocalcin

Osteocalcin, serum or plasma

Adults: 10–50 ng/mL

7–17-years-old:
25–300 ng/mL

(age-specific)

SST, red, lavender, pink or green

$$$$

Osteocalcin is a noncollagen protein of 49 amino acids in bone matrix, produced by osteoblasts. Its production is dependent on vitamin K and is stimulated by 1,25-dihydroxy vitamin D. It regulates hydroxyapatite size and shape, as well as glucose metabolism. Osteocalcin level has also been correlated with bone formation and osteoblast number, thus it is used as a marker of bone osteoblastic activity. Osteocalcin is released into the circulation from the matrix during bone resorption and is considered a marker of bone turnover, rather than a specific marker of bone formation. Osteocalcin levels are increased in metabolic bone diseases with increased bone or osteoid formation.

Both intact osteocalcin (amino acids 1–49) and the large N-terminal/midregion (N-MID) fragment (amino acids 1–43) are present in blood. Intact osteocalcin is unstable due to protease cleavage between amino acids 43 and 44. The N-MID-fragment, resulting from cleavage, is more stable. The test detects both the stable N-MID-fragment and intact osteocalcin.

Increased in: Osteoporosis, osteomalacia, rickets, Paget disease, hyperparathyroidism, renal osteodystrophy, thyrotoxicosis, fractures, acromegaly, and cancer with bone metastasis.
Decreased in: Hypoparathyroidism, hypothyroidism, and growth hormone deficiency.

Test may be useful for monitoring and assessing effectiveness of anti-resorptive therapy in patients treated for osteopenia, osteoporosis, Paget disease, or other disorders in which osteocalcin levels are elevated.
Test can also be used as an adjunct in the diagnosis of conditions associated with increased bone turnover, including Paget disease, cancer accompanied by bone metastases, primary hyperparathyroidism, and renal osteodystrophy.
Osteocalcin is cleared by the kidneys. In patients with renal failure, the osteocalcin levels can be elevated as a result of impaired clearance and renal osteodystrophy.
Further studies are needed to define the role of osteocalcin in the regulation of glucose metabolism and its clinical relevance.
Bandeira F et al. Bone markers and osteoporosis therapy. Arq Bras Endocrinol Metabol 2014;58:504. [PMID: 25166041]
Klein GL. Insulin and bone: recent developments. World J Diabetes 2014;5:14. [PMID: 24567798]
Lee J et al. Current recommendations for laboratory testing and use of bone turnover markers in management of osteoporosis. Ann Lab Med 2012;32:105. [PMID: 22389876]

(Continued)

Test/Range/Collection	Physiologic Basis	Interpretation	Comments
Oxygen, partial pressure (PO₂), whole blood 83–108 mm Hg [11.04–14.36 kPa] Heparinized syringe $$$ Collect arterial blood in a heparinized syringe. Send to laboratory immediately on ice.	Test measures the partial pressure of oxygen (oxygen tension) in arterial blood. Partial pressure of oxygen is critical because it determines (along with hemoglobin and blood supply) tissue oxygen supply.	**Increased in:** Oxygen therapy. **Decreased in:** Ventilation/perfusion mismatching (asthma, COPD, atelectasis, pulmonary embolism, pneumonia, interstitial lung disease, airway obstruction by foreign body, shock); alveolar hypoventilation (kyphoscoliosis, neuromuscular disease, head injury, stroke); right-to-left shunt (congenital heart disease). Drugs: barbiturates, opioids.	% Saturation of hemoglobin (Hb) (SO₂) is the percent of total Hb that is combined with O₂. SO₂ is dependent on the oxygen partial pressure. % Saturation on blood gas reports is calculated, not measured. It is calculated from PO₂ and pH using reference oxyhemoglobin dissociation curves for normal adult hemoglobin (lacking methemoglobin, carboxyhemoglobin, etc). At PO₂ < 60 mm Hg, the oxygen saturation (and content) cannot be reliably estimated from the PO₂. Therefore, oximetry should be used to determine % saturation directly. Damiani E et al. Arterial hypoxia and mortality in critically ill patients: a systemic review and meta-analysis. Crit Care 2014;18:711. [PMID: 25532567] Nitzan M et al. Pulse oximetry: fundamentals and technology update. Med Devices (Auckl) 2014;7:231. [PMID: 25031547] Wagner PD. The physiological basis of pulmonary gas exchange: implications for clinical interpretation of arterial blood gases. Eur Respir J 2015;45:227. [PMID: 25323225]
Pancreatic elastase, fecal >200 mcg/g $$$ Collect >1 g of random formed stool in clean, leak proof plastic container. Freeze immediately.	Fecal pancreatic elastase-1 (FE-1) is a protease synthesized by pancreatic acinar cells. It is highly stable during passage through the gastrointestinal tract, and its concentration can be measured in feces. The ELISA-based quantitative assay is a sensitive, specific, and noninvasive test for exocrine pancreatic insufficiency, superior to chymotrypsin. Sensitivity is 100% for severe, 77–100% for moderate, and 0–60% for mild pancreatic insufficiency, respectively. Specificity is 93% except for patients with small intestinal disease, eg, Crohn disease and gluten-sensitive enteropathy.	**Decreased in:** Exocrine pancreatic insufficiency (mild–moderate 100–200 mcg/g; severe <100 mcg/g).	Fecal elastase-1 (FE-1) is a marker of pancreatic exocrine secretion. There is a direct correlation between pancreatic elastase-1 levels in pancreatic fluid and stool. It is a superior marker to fecal chymotrypsin and 72-hour fecal fat analysis (see p. 97). Due to the limited availability of 72-hour fecal fat quantification, FE-1 based diagnostic criteria have been proposed for assessing the probability of pancreatic exocrine insufficiency, ie, FE-1 <15, high probability; FE-1 >200, low probability. Lindkvist B. Diagnosis and treatment of pancreatic exocrine insufficiency. World J Gastroenterol 2013;19:7258. [PMID: 24259956] Morera-Ocon FJ et al. Considerations on pancreatic exocrine function after pancreaticoduodenectomy. World J Gastrointest Oncol 2014;6:325. [PMID: 25232457]

Parathyroid hormone			
Parathyroid hormone, serum or plasma (PTH) "Intact" PTH: 11–54 pg/mL [1.2–5.7 pmol/L] (laboratory-specific) SST, lavender, green $$$$ Fasting sample preferred; simultaneous measurement of serum calcium and phosphorus is also required.	PTH is secreted from the parathyroid glands. It mobilizes calcium from bone, increases distal renal tubular reabsorption of calcium, decreases proximal renal tubular reabsorption of phosphorus, and stimulates 1,25-hydroxy vitamin D synthesis from 25-dihydroxy vitamin D by renal 1α-hydroxylase. The "intact" PTH molecule (84 amino acids) has a circulating half-life of about 5 minutes. Carboxyl terminal and mid-molecule fragments make up 90% of circulating PTH. They are biologically inactive, cleared by the kidney, and have half-lives of about 1–2 hours. The amino terminal fragment is biologically active and has a half-life of 1–2 minutes. Measurement of PTH by immunoassay depends on the specificity of the antibodies used. Intact PTH assays using two antibodies ("sandwich" immunoassay) are the standard assays. The second- and third-generation intact PTH assays are less prone to interference from large PTH fragments (eg, amino acids 7–84), and the enhanced assays measure only the biologically intact PTH molecule (amino acids 1–84).	**Increased in:** Primary hyperparathyroidism, secondary hyperparathyroidism due to renal disease, vitamin D deficiency. Drugs: lithium, furosemide, propofol, phosphates. **Decreased in:** Hypoparathyroidism, sarcoidosis, hyperthyroidism, hypomagnesemia, malignancy with hypercalcemia, nonparathyroid hypercalcemia.	Test is useful for the diagnosis and differential diagnosis of hypercalcemia, hyperparathyroidism (primary, secondary, tertiary) and hypoparathyroidism, and for monitoring patients with end-stage renal failure for possible renal osteodystrophy. PTH results must always be evaluated in light of concurrent serum calcium levels. PTH tests differ in sensitivity and specificity from assay to assay and from laboratory to laboratory. Carboxyl terminal antibody measures intact, carboxyl terminal and midmolecule fragments. It is 85% sensitive and 95% specific for primary hyperparathyroidism. Amino terminal antibody measures intact and amino terminal fragments. It is about 75% sensitive for hyperparathyroidism. Intact PTH assays are preferred because they detect PTH suppression in nonparathyroid hypercalcemia. Intact PTH is a better indicator of hyperparathyroidism in renal failure. Sensitivity of immunometric assays is 85–90% for primary hyperparathyroidism. Intraoperative quick PTH monitoring in patients undergoing parathyroidectomy can be used to confirm cure and predict long-term operative success in most cases. A low intraoperative PTH level during thyroid surgery is a predictor of postoperative hypocalcemia resulting from parathyroid gland ischemia. See diagnostic algorithms for hypercalcemia and hypocalcemia (Figures 9–15 and 9–17). Cusano NE et al. Use of parathyroid hormone in hypoparathyroidism. J Endocrinol Invest 2013;36:1121. [PMID: 24445125] Michels TC et al Parathyroid disorders. Am Fam Physician 2013;88:249. [PMID: 23944728] Moorthi RN et al. Recent advances in the noninvasive diagnosis of renal osteodystrophy. Kidney Int 2013;84:886. [PMID: 23802194]

(Continued)

Test/Range/Collection	Physiologic Basis	Interpretation	Comments
Parathyroid hormone-related protein (PTHrP), plasma Assay-specific (pmol/L or undetectable) Lavender Tube containing anticoagulant and protease inhibitors; specimen drawn without a tourniquet. $$	Parathyroid hormone-related protein (PTHrP) is a 139- to 173-amino acid protein with amino terminal homology to PTH. The homology explains the ability of PTHrP to bind to the PTH receptor and have PTH-like effects on bone and kidney. PTHrP induces increased plasma calcium, decreased plasma phosphorus, and increased urinary cAMP. PTHrP is found in keratinocytes, fibroblasts, placenta, brain, pituitary gland, adrenal gland, stomach, liver, testicular Leydig cells, and mammary glands. Its physiologic role in these diverse sites is unknown. PTHrP is secreted by solid malignant tumors (lung, breast, kidney; other squamous tumors) and produces humoral hypercalcemia of malignancy. PTHrP can act as an oncoprotein to regulate the growth and proliferation of many common malignancies and is a marker of cancers that metastasize to bone. PTHrP analysis is by immunoradiometric assay (IRMA). Assay of choice is amino terminal-specific IRMA. Two-site IRMA assays require sample collection in protease inhibitors because serum proteases destroy immunoreactivity.	**Increased in:** Humoral hypercalcemia of malignancy (80% of solid tumors).	Assays directed at the amino terminal portion of PTHrP are not influenced by renal failure. Increases in PTHrP concentrations are readily detectable with most current assays in the majority of patients with humoral hypercalcemia of malignancy. About 20% of patients with malignancy and hypercalcemia have low PTHrP levels because their hypercalcemia is caused by local osteolytic processes. Soki FN et al. The multifaceted actions of PTHrP in skeletal metastasis. Future Oncol 2012;8:803. [PMID: 22830401] Wysolmerski JJ. Parathyroid hormone-related protein: an update. J Clin Endocrinol Metab 2012; 97:2947. [PMID: 22745236]

Partial thromboplastin time

| Partial thromboplastin time, activated, plasma (aPTT)

25–35 seconds
(laboratory-specific)

Panic: ≥60 seconds
(off heparin)

Blue

$$

Do not contaminate specimen with heparin. | The aPTT is a clot-based test in which phospholipid reagent, an activator substance, and calcium are added to the patient's plasma, and the time for a fibrin clot to form is measured.

PTT evaluates the intrinsic and common coagulation pathways and adequacy of all coagulation factors except XIII and VII.

PTT is usually abnormal if any factor level drops below 25–40% of normal, depending on the PTT reagent used.

PTT is commonly used to monitor unfractionated heparin therapy. | **Increased in:** Deficiency of any individual coagulation factor except Factors XIII and VII, presence of nonspecific inhibitor (eg, lupus anticoagulant), specific factor inhibitor, von Willebrand disease (PTT may also be normal in its mild form), hemophilia A and B, DIC. Drugs: heparin, direct thrombin inhibitor (eg, hirudin, argatroban), warfarin. See evaluation of isolated prolongation of PTT (Figure 9–28) and bleeding disorders (Figure 9–7, Table 8–8).

Decreased in: Hypercoagulable states (eg, increased factor VIII levels). | PTT cannot be used to monitor very high doses of heparin (eg, cardiac bypass surgery) because the clotting time is beyond the analytical measurement range of PTT.

For patients with documented lupus anticoagulant, PTT cannot be used to monitor heparin therapy. Chromogenic anti-Xa assay is used instead.

Patients receiving low molecular weight heparin usually have normal PTT values.

PTT may be normal in patients with the mild form of von Willebrand disease and chronic DIC.

Heparin contamination is a very common cause of an unexplained prolonged PTT. Heparin neutralization with heparinase may be needed to rule out this possibility.

PTT may be falsely prolonged if anticoagulant volume is not adjusted for increased hematocrit (eg, polycythemia vera) or if the specimen tube is not fully filled.

Aarab R et al. Monitoring of unfractionated heparin in critically ill patients. Neth J Med 2013;71:466. [PMID: 24218420]

Harter K et al. Anticoagulation drug therapy: a review. West J Emerg Med 2015;16:11. [PMID: 25671002]

Warkentin TE. Anticoagulant failure in coagulopathic patients: PTT confounding and other pitfalls. Expert Opin Drug Saf 2014;13:25. [PMID: 23971903]

Wool GD et al. Pathology consultation on anticoagulation monitoring: factor X-related assays. Am J Clin Path 2013;140:623. [PMID: 24124140] |

(Continued)

pH

Test/Range/Collection	Physiologic Basis	Interpretation	Comments
pH, whole blood Arterial: 7.35–7.45 Venous: 7.31–7.41 Heparinized syringe $$$ Specimen must be collected in heparinized syringe and immediately transported on ice to lab without exposure to air.	pH assesses the acid–base status of blood, an extremely useful measure of integrated cardiorespiratory function. The essential relationship between pH, PCO_2, and bicarbonate (HCO_3^-) is expressed by the Henderson–Hasselbalch equation (at 37°C): Arteriovenous pH difference is 0.01–0.03 but is greater in patients with CHF and shock.	**Increased in:** *Respiratory alkalosis:* Hyperventilation (eg, anxiety), sepsis, liver disease, fever, early salicylate poisoning, and excessive artificial ventilation. *Metabolic alkalosis:* Loss of gastric HCl (eg, vomiting), potassium depletion, excessive alkali administration (eg, bicarbonate, antacids), diuretics, volume depletion. **Decreased in:** *Respiratory acidosis:* Decreased alveolar ventilation (eg, COPD, respiratory depressants), neuromuscular diseases (eg, myasthenia gravis). *Metabolic acidosis* (bicarbonate deficit): Increased formation of acids (eg, ketosis [diabetes mellitus, alcohol, starvation], lactic acidosis); decreased H^+ excretion (eg, renal failure, renal tubular acidosis, Fanconi syndrome); increased acid intake (eg, ion-exchange resins, salicylates, ammonium chloride, ethylene glycol, methanol); and increased loss of alkaline body fluids (eg, diarrhea, fistulas, aspiration of gastrointestinal contents, biliary drainage).	If pH is < 7.35, the patient is considered to have acidosis. If pH is > 7.45, the patient is said to have alkalosis. The pH of a standing sample decreases because of cellular metabolism. The correction of pH (measured at 37°C), based on the patient's temperature, is not clinically useful. See acid–base disturbances (Figure 9–1, Table 8–1). Singh V et al. Blood gas analysis for bedside diagnosis. Natl J Maxillofac Surg 2013;4:136. [PMID: 24665166] Wagner PD. The physiological basis of pulmonary gas exchange: implications for clinical interpretation of arterial blood gases. Eur Respir J 2015;45:227. [PMID: 25323225] Whittier WL et al. Primer on clinical acid-base problem solving. Dis Mon 2004;50:122. [PMID: 15069420]

(Continued)

Phosphorus			
Phosphorus, serum or plasma 2.5–4.5 mg/dL [0.8–1.45 mmol/L] **Panic:** <1.0 mg/dL [<0.32 mmol] SST, green $ Avoid hemolysis.	The plasma concentration of inorganic phosphate is determined by parathyroid gland function, action of vitamin D, intestinal absorption, renal function, bone metabolism, and nutrition. Serum phosphorus concentrations have a circadian rhythm (highest level in late morning, lowest in evening) and are subject to rapid change secondary to environmental factors such as diet (carbohydrate), phosphate-binding antacids, and fluctuations in GH, insulin, and renal function. There is also a seasonal variation with maximum levels in May and June (low levels in winter). During first decade of menopause, values increase ~0.2 mg/dL (~0.06 mmol/L). Bedrest causes increase up to 0.5 mg/dL (0.16 mmol/L). Ingestion of food may cause a transient decrease in blood levels. Low values are also seen during menstruation.	**Increased in:** Renal failure, calcific arteriolopathy (calciphylaxis), tumor lysis syndrome, massive blood transfusion, hypoparathyroidism, sarcoidosis, neoplasms, adrenal insufficiency, acromegaly, hypervitaminosis D, osteolytic metastases to bone, leukemia, milk-alkali syndrome, healing bone fractures, pseudohypoparathyroidism, diabetes mellitus with ketosis, malignant hyperpyrexia, cirrhosis, lactic acidosis, respiratory acidosis. Drugs: phosphate infusions or enemas, anabolic steroids, ergocalciferol, furosemide, hydrochlorothiazide, clonidine, verapamil, potassium supplements, and others. Thrombocytosis may cause spurious elevation of serum phosphate, but plasma phosphate levels are normal. **Decreased in:** Hyperparathyroidism, hypovitaminosis D (rickets, osteomalacia), malabsorption (steatorrhea), malnutrition, starvation or cachexia, refeeding syndrome, bone marrow transplantation, renal phosphate wasting due to autosomal dominant or X-linked dominant hypophosphatemic rickets, GH deficiency, chronic alcoholism, severe diarrhea, vomiting, nasogastric suction, acute pancreatitis, severe hypercalcemia (any cause), acute gout, osteoblastic metastases to bone, severe burns (diuretic phase), respiratory alkalosis, hyperalimentation with inadequate phosphate repletion, carbohydrate administration (eg, intravenous D_{50} W glucose bolus), renal tubular acidosis and other renal tubular defects, diabetic ketoacidosis (during recovery), acid-base disturbances, hypokalemia, pregnancy, hypothyroidism, hemodialysis. Drugs: acetazolamide, phosphate-binding antacids, anticonvulsants, β-adrenergic agonists, catecholamines, estrogens, isoniazid, oral contraceptives, prolonged use of thiazides, glucose infusion, insulin therapy, salicylates (toxicity).	A major role of the kidneys is to maintain phosphorus homeostasis. Serum or plasma phosphorus level is largely determined by renal tubular phosphate handling. Maintenance of a normal serum phosphorus level depends upon regulation of phosphorus reabsorption by the kidney. Most of this reabsorption (80%) occurs in the proximal tubule and is mediated by the type II sodium–phosphate cotransporter (NaPi-II). Parathyroid hormone, via a variety of intracellular signaling cascades leading to NaPi-IIa internalization and downregulation, is the main regulator of renal phosphate reabsorption. In renal insufficiency, phosphorus excretion declines and hyperphosphatemia develops. The body's homeostatic mechanisms cause secondary hyperparathyroidism and renal osteodystrophy. Shift of phosphorus from extracellular to intracellular compartments, decreased gastrointestinal absorption, and increased urinary losses, are the primary mechanisms of hypophosphatemia. Hypophosphatemia has been implicated as a cause of rhabdomyolysis, respiratory failure, hemolysis, and left ventricular dysfunction. Lee JY et al. The changing face of hypophosphatemic disorders in the FGF-23 era. Pediatr Endocrinol Rev 2013;10(Suppl 2):367. [PMID: 23858620] Nadkami GN et al. Phosphorus and the kidney: what is known and what is needed. Adv Nutr 2014;5:98. [PMID: 24425728] Wilson FP et al. Tumor lysis syndrome: new challenges and recent advances. Adv Chronic Kidney Dis 2014;21:18. [PMID: 24359983]

	Platelet antibodies

Test/Range/Collection	Physiologic Basis	Interpretation	Comments
Platelet antibodies, whole blood, plasma/serum Negative Lavender, yellow, or SST (methodology-dependent) $$$$	Clinically significant platelet antibodies (platelet-associated IgG) include autoimmune platelet antibodies that cause idiopathic thrombocytopenic purpura (ITP), platelet-specific alloantibodies that cause neonatal alloimmune thrombocytopenia (NATP) and posttransfusion purpura (PTP), and class I HLA alloantibodies that are associated with refractoriness to platelet transfusions. Platelet-specific alloantibodies are most commonly directed at the human platelet antigen referred to as HPA-1a (also known as Pl^A1), while ITP autoantibodies typically target platelet glycoproteins IIb/IIIa and/or Ib/IX. Several methods with variable sensitivity and specificity are available, and no method detects all antibodies. A combination of a sensitive binding assay such as a direct platelet immunofluorescence test along with an antigen capture immunoassay is useful. Enzyme-linked immunosorbent assay (ELISA) kits are available that detect specific antibodies against platelet glycoproteins or HLA class I antigens. Flow cytometry–based indirect and direct platelet antibody tests are also available.	**Positive in:** Chronic ITP (90–95%), autoimmune thyroid disease (51%), antiphospholipid syndrome, NATP, PTP. Testing serum/plasma for NATP should be performed using a maternal sample.	Routine testing for platelet antibodies is generally not recommended. In selected cases (eg, refractory ITP, NATP, PTP), the testing may be of value. An assay for platelet-bound antibody (direct) is more informative than detection of unbound antibodies in plasma or serum (indirect). For patients who have repeatedly failed to respond to random donor platelet transfusions (eg, multiple platelet transfusion refractoriness), detection and characterization of the specific HLA antibody may permit HLA-matched and crossmatched platelet transfusion. Hayashi T et al. Advances in alloimmune thrombocytopenia: perspectives on current concepts of human platelet antigens, antibody detection strategies, and genotyping. Blood Transfus 2015;13:380. [PMID: 26057488] Heikal NM et al. Laboratory testing for platelet antibodies. Am J Hematol 2013;88:818. [PMID: 23757218] Yehudai D et al. Autoimmunity and novel therapies in immune-mediated thrombocytopenia. Semin Hematol 2013;50(Suppl 1):S100. [PMID: 23664506]

Platelet count		
Platelet count, whole blood (Plt) 150–450 × 10³/mcL [× 10⁹/L] ***Panic:*** <25 × 10³/mcL [× 10⁹/L] Lavender $	Platelets are released from megakaryocytes in bone marrow and are important for normal hemostasis. Platelet counting is performed as part of the complete blood cell count (CBC) panel. It is typically obtained by automated hematology analyzers, which may also provide reticulated or immature platelet count. An estimated platelet count may be obtained from blood smear by multiplying the number of platelets per 100 × oil immersion field by 10,000.	**Increased in:** Myeloproliferative disorders (polycythemia vera, chronic myeloid leukemia, essential thrombocythemia, primary myelofibrosis), some myelodysplastic disorders (eg 5q- syndrome), acute blood loss, postsplenectomy, preeclampsia, reactive thrombocytosis secondary to inflammatory disorders, infection, tissue injury, iron deficiency, malignancies (paraneoplastic thrombocytosis). **Decreased in:** Decreased production: bone marrow suppression or replacement/infiltration, myelodysplasia, chemotherapy, drugs, alcohol, infection (eg, HIV), congenital marrow failure (eg, Fanconi anemia, Wiskott-Aldrich syndrome, thrombocytopenia with absent radius [TAR] syndrome, etc); increased destruction or excessive pooling: hypersplenism, DIC, TTP, platelet antibodies (idiopathic thrombocytopenic purpura, Evans syndrome, posttransfusion purpura, neonatal isoimmune thrombocytopenia, drugs [eg, quinidine, cephalosporins, clopidogrel, HIT]).	Platelet counts are determined in patients with suspected bleeding disorders, purpura or petechiae, leukemia/lymphoma, or DIC, and in patients on chemotherapy, and to determine the response to platelet transfusions. There is little tendency to bleed until the platelet count falls below 20,000/mcL. Bleeding due to low platelet counts typically presents as petechiae, epistaxis, and gingival bleeding. For invasive procedures, platelet counts > 50,000/mcL are desirable. HIV infection may result in both decreased platelet production and decreased platelet survival. Reticulated or immature platelet counts are useful for the differential diagnosis of thrombocytopenia and for monitoring bone marrow recovery after chemotherapy or stem cell transplantation. Please also see platelet antibodies, heparin-associated antibody, and complete blood cell count entries, as well as the diagnostic algorithms for thrombocytopenia and thrombocytosis (Figures 9–32 & 9–33). Hoffmann JJ. Reticulated platelets: analytical aspects and clinical utility. Clin Chem Lab Med 2014;52:1107. [PMID: 24807169] Lin RJ et al. Paraneoplastic thrombocytosis: the secrets of tumor self-promotion. Blood 2014;124:184. [PMID: 24868077] Neunert CE. Current management of immune thrombocytopenia. Hematology Am Soc Hematol Educ Program 2013;2013:276. [PMID: 24319191]

(Continued)

Test/Range/Collection	Physiologic Basis	Interpretation	Comments
Platelet function assay (PFA-100 closure time), blood CEPI: 70–170 seconds CADP: 50–110 seconds (laboratory-specific) Blue $$ Specimen must be kept at room temperature and the test should be performed within 4 hours of collection.	The PFA (platelet function assay)-100 closure time (CT) measures the time taken for blood to block a membrane aperture coated with collagen and epinephrine (CEPI) or collagen and ADP (CADP). The test is a combined measure of platelet adhesion and aggregation. PFA-100 CT serves as an alternative to the bleeding time in assessing primary hemostasis. Compared with bleeding time, the PFA-100 CT test is more reproducible, less invasive, rapid, and technically more appealing.	**Increased in:** Inherited or acquired abnormality of platelet function, von Willebrand disease (vWD), valvular heart disease, renal insufficiency, aspirin. **Increases in both CEPI CT and CADP CT:** Abnormal platelet function, vWD. **Increase in CEPI CT only:** Aspirin.	Normal PFA-100 CT can help exclude some severe platelet defects (eg, Glanzmann thrombasthenia and Bernard-Soulier syndrome) and moderate-severe vWD (eg, types 3, 2A, 2M, and severe type 1) with high negative predictive value. It is less sensitive to mild platelet disorders such as primary secretion defects or dense granule deficiencies and mild type 1 vWD. There is no evidence that a preoperative PFA-100 CT test can predict bleeding during a surgical procedure. The role of PFA-100 CT in therapeutic monitoring (eg, DDAVP and factor concentrates in vWD) also remains to be established. Patients with thrombocytopenia (platelets <100,000/mcL) and/or anemia (hematocrit <28%) may exhibit a prolonged PFA-100 CT. The newly available and updated PFA-200 has similar clinical utilities. Gorog DA et al. Platelet function tests in clinical cardiology: unfulfilled expectations. J Am Coll Cardiol 2013;61:2115. [PMID: 23541972] Paniccia R et al. Platelet function tests: a comparative review. Vasc Health Risk Manag 2015;11:133. [PMID: 25733843]
Porphobilinogen, urine (PBG) Negative (<8.8 mmol/L or <11 mmol/24 hr) $$ Protect from light.	Porphyrias are characterized clinically by neurologic and cutaneous manifestations and chemically by overproduction of porphyrin and other precursors of heme production by the liver or bone marrow. PBG is a water-soluble precursor of heme whose urinary excretion is increased in symptomatic hepatic porphyrias, including acute intermittent porphyria (AIP) and other acute attack types of porphyrias associated with neurologic and/or psychiatric symptoms. PBG is detected qualitatively by a color reaction with Ehrlich reagent and confirmed by extraction into chloroform (Watson-Schwartz test).	**Positive in:** Acute intermittent porphyria, variegate porphyria, coproporphyria, hereditary coproporphyria. **Negative in:** 20–30% of patients with hepatic porphyria between attacks.	Positive qualitative urinary PBG tests should be followed up by quantitative measurements, because there are frequent false positives with the Watson-Schwartz test. More than a 5-fold elevation of urinary PBG excretion, along with typical symptoms of an acute porphyria attack, is sufficient to justify treatment. A screening PBG test is insensitive, and a negative test does not rule out porphyria between attacks or in the carrier state. Specific porphyrias can be better defined by quantitative measurement of urine PBG, 5-aminolevulinic acid and total porphyrin levels and by measurement of erythrocyte PBG deaminase (rarely used). Currently, no rapid test for urinary PBG is available in the urgent-care setting. Bissell DM et al. Acute hepatic porphyria. J Clin Transl Hepatol 2015;3:17. [PMID: 26357631] Pischik E et al. An update of clinical management of acute intermittent porphyria. Appl Clin Genet 2015;8:201. [PMID: 26366103]

Potassium		
Potassium (K$^+$), serum or plasma 3.5–5.0 meq/L [mmol/L] **Panic:** <3.0 or > 6.0 meq/L SST, green $ Avoid hemolysis.	Potassium is predominantly an intracellular cation whose plasma level is regulated by renal excretion. Plasma potassium concentration determines neuromuscular irritability. Elevated or depressed potassium concentrations interfere with muscle contraction.	**Increased in:** Massive hemolysis, severe tissue damage, rhabdomyolysis, acidosis, dehydration, acute or chronic renal failure, Addison disease, renal tubular acidosis type IV (hyporeninemic) hypoaldosteronism, (hyperkalemic) familial periodic paralysis, pseudo-hypoaldosteronism (types I and II), congenital adrenal hyperplasia (salt-wasting form), exercise (transient). Drugs: potassium salts, potassium-sparing diuretics (eg, spironolactone, triamterene, eplerenone), nonsteroidal anti-inflammatory drugs, β-blockers, ACE inhibitors, ACE-receptor blockers, high-dose trimethoprim-sulfamethoxazole, pentamidine, verapamil. **Decreased in:** Low potassium intake, prolonged vomiting or diarrhea, renal tubular acidosis types I and II, hyperaldosteronism, Cushing syndrome, osmotic diuresis (eg, hyperglycemia), alkalosis, (hypokalemic) familial periodic paralysis, trauma (transient), subarachnoid hemorrhage, genetic hypokalemic salt-losing tubulopathies such as Gitelman syndrome (familial hypokalemia-hypocalciuria-hypomagnesemia). Drugs: adrenergic agents (isoproterenol), diuretics.	Spurious hyperkalemia can occur with hemolysis of sample, delayed separation of serum from erythrocytes, prolonged fist clenching during blood drawing, and prolonged tourniquet placement. Very high white blood cell or platelet counts may cause spurious elevation of serum potassium, but plasma potassium levels are normal. Ben Salem C et al. Drug-induced hyperkalemia. Drug Saf 2014;37:677. [PMID: 25047526] Jain G et al. Genetic disorders of potassium homeostasis. Semin Nephrol 2013;33:300. [PMID: 23953807] Lee Hamm L et al. Acid-base and potassium homeostasis. Semin Nephrol 2013;33:257. [PMID: 23953803] Medford-Davis L et al. Derangements of potassium. Emerg Med Clin North Am 2014;32:329. [PMID: 24766936]

(Continued)

Test/Range/Collection	Physiologic Basis	Interpretation	Comments
Procalcitonin, serum or plasma <0.10 ng/mL [<0.10 mcg/L] SST, PST $$$$	Procalcitonin is a 116 amino acid peptide precursor of calcitonin, produced by the parafollicular cells of the thyroid gland and by the neuroendocrine cells of the lung and intestine. Increased production by lung, intestine, and other tissues occurs in response to an inflammatory stimulus, especially bacterial. The serum values of procalcitonin correlate with the severity of sepsis; they recede with its improvement and worsen with exacerbation. Serum procalcitonin has become useful as a biomarker to assist in the diagnosis of sepsis, as well as related infectious or inflammatory conditions. Its half-life is 25–30 hours.	**Increased in:** Bacteremia (sensitivity 76%, specificity 70%), systemic inflammatory response syndrome (SIRS), bacterial meningitis, bacterial peritonitis, sepsis, septic shock.	Procalcitonin is an adjunctive diagnostic marker to differentiate sepsis from severe inflammatory response syndrome (SIRS) of a noninfectious origin. When a cut-off value of > 2.0 ng/mL is used for sepsis diagnosis, the reported sensitivity and specificity are 65–95% and 70–90%, respectively. Procalcitonin levels > 2.00 ng/mL on the first day of ICU admission indicate a high risk for progression to severe sepsis and/or septic shock. Procalcitonin levels < 0.50 ng/mL on admission indicate a low risk for such progression. Procalcitonin has also been proposed as a guide to antibiotic therapy in bacterial infections, ie, levels < 0.25 ng/mL would indicate that antibiotics are not needed; levels > 0.5 ng/mL would indicate that antibiotics are needed. Continuously declining procalcitonin levels indicate an improving prognosis, even if the peak procalcitonin values are very high. A persistent increase (or failure to decline) of the procalcitonin levels has been associated with higher mortality rates. Antibodies that neutralize the harmful effects of procalcitonin might be therapeutic in sepsis. Biron BM et al. Biomarkers for sepsis: what is and what might be? Biomark Insights 2015;10(Suppl 4):7. [PMID: 26417200] Carr JA. Procalcitonin-guided antibiotic therapy for septic patients in the surgical intensive care unit. J Intensive Care 2015;3:36. [PMID: 26244096] Meisner M. Update on procalcitonin measurements. Ann Lab Med 2014;34:263. [PMID: 24982830]

Procollagen type I N-terminal propeptide (PINP)		
Procollagen type-I intact N-terminal propeptide (PINP), serum 20–100 mcg/L Gold SST, red $$$ Serum should be separated from cells quickly (within 2 hours) and kept refrigerated or frozen.	PINP is derived from the precursor of type I collagen (type I procollagen) in mineralized bone. The level of circulating PINP reflects the synthesis rate of collagen type I primarily by osteoblasts. Serum PINP is mostly affected by changes in bone metabolism. It is considered the most sensitive marker of bone formation. It is useful for monitoring bone formation and antiresorption therapies. PINP is mostly metabolized in the liver.	**Increased in:** Paget disease, bone metastasis (eg, breast or prostate cancer). **Decreased in:** Osteogenesis imperfecta (children). **Increased from baseline in:** Bone formation therapy (eg, teriparatide). **Decreased from baseline in:** Antiresorptive therapies (eg, bisphosphonates, hormone replacement therapy with estrogen or its analogs).	PINP reference interval is broad due to considerable inter-individual variation. Baseline PINP should be obtained before starting osteoporosis therapy. A change of >20% or >10mcg/L from baseline PINP levels 3–6 months after initiation of therapy indicates an adequate therapeutic response. For therapy monitoring, serial measurements should be done using the same PINP immunoassay. Blood specimens should be collected at the same time of day for serial measurements because there is a diurnal variation of PINP and its levels are higher at night. It should not be used as a screening test for osteoporosis. Cundy T et al. Paget's disease of bone. Clin Biochem 2012;45:43. [PMID: 22024254] Krege JH, et al. PINP as a biological response marker during teriparatide treatment for osteoporosis. Osteoporos Int 2014;25:2159. [PMID: 24599274] Koivula MK et al. Measurement of aminoterminal propeptide of type I procollagen (PINP) in serum. Clin Biochem 2012;45:920. [PMID: 22480789]

(Continued)

	Prolactin		
Test/Range/Collection	**Physiologic Basis**	**Interpretation**	**Comments**
Prolactin, serum or plasma (PRL) <25 ng/mL [mcg/L] SST, PPT, green $$$	Prolactin is a polypeptide hormone secreted by the anterior pituitary. It functions in the initiation and maintenance of lactation in the postpartum period. PRL secretion is inhibited by hypothalamic secretion of dopamine. Prolactin levels increase with renal failure, hypothyroidism, and drugs that are dopamine antagonists.	**Increased in:** Sleep, nursing, nipple stimulation (breast feeding), pregnancy, exercise, hypoglycemia, stress, hypothyroidism, pituitary tumors (prolactinomas and others), hypothalamic/pituitary stalk lesions, renal failure, cirrhosis. HIV infection, CHF, SLE, advanced multiple myeloma, Rathke cyst. Drugs: phenothiazines, haloperidol, antipsychotics (eg, risperidone, clozapine, aripiprazole), reserpine, metoclopramide, methyldopa, estrogens, opiates, cimetidine. **Decreased in:** Drugs: levodopa.	Hyperprolactinemia is associated with symptoms of galactorrhea, menstrual disorders (usually amenorrhea), and infertility. Serum PRL is used primarily in work-up of suspected pituitary tumor (60% of pituitary adenomas secrete PRL). Clinical presentation is usually amenorrhea and galactorrhea in women and impotence in men. (See Amenorrhea algorithm, Figure 9–4.) In patients with macroadenoma, PRL is frequently > 500 ng/mL; in microadenoma, PRL is usually > 150 ng/mL. When there is a discrepancy between a very large pituitary tumor and a normal or mildly elevated prolactin level (eg, < 200 ng/mL), serial dilution of serum samples is recommended to eliminate an artifact that can occur with some immunometric assays leading to a falsely low prolactin value ("hook effect"). Screening for macroprolactin (dimeric or polymeric prolactin) with IgG, especially when anti-prolactin autoantibodies form) is suggested in investigation of asymptomatic hyperprolactinemic patients. Lake MG et al. Pituitary adenomas: an overview. Am Fam Physician 2013;88:319. [PMID: 24010395] Molitch ME. Endocrinology in pregnancy: management of the pregnant patient with a prolactinoma. Eur J Endocrinol 2015;172:R205. [PMID: 25805896] Vilar L et al. Challenges and pitfalls in the diagnosis of hyperprolactinemia. Arq Bras Endocrinol Metabol 2014;58:9. [PMID: 24728159]

Prostate-specific antigen		
Prostate-specific antigen, total (PSA) 0–4 ng/mL [mcg/L] SST, red, PPT, lavender, green $$$	PSA is a glycoprotein produced by cells of the prostatic ductal epithelium and is present in the serum of all men. It is absent from the serum of women.	**Increased in:** Prostate carcinoma (sensitivity ~20%; specificity ~60–70% at a 4.0 ng/mL cutoff), biochemical recurrence after localized treatment, benign prostatic hypertrophy (BPH), prostatitis. **Decreased in:** Metastatic prostate carcinoma treated with antiandrogen therapy, postprostatectomy, 5α-reductase inhibitor therapy.	PSA is used both for the early detection of prostate cancer and as a tumor marker to assess response and monitor recurrence of treated prostate cancer. There is still no consensus on whether PSA measurement should be used as a screening test for early detection of prostate cancer. A decrease in mortality rates resulting from use for cancer screening is unproven, and the risks of early therapy are significant. As a result, the United States Preventive Services Task Force discourages use of the test for healthy men in all age groups. The American Cancer Society guideline states that asymptomatic men who have less than a 10-year life expectancy should not be offered prostate cancer screening, and that men who have at least a 10-year life expectancy should have an opportunity to make an informed decision about whether to be screened for prostate cancer with PSA testing. The American Urological Association does not recommend PSA screening in men ages 70 years and older or in men who do not have a 10- to 15-year life expectancy. The PSA nadir (the lowest PSA level achieved after therapeutic intervention) appears to correlate with the likelihood of remaining disease-free. Three consecutive PSA rises are interpreted as an indicator of treatment (biochemical) failure. PSA is often increased in BPH, and the positive predictive value in healthy older men is low. Use of the free/total PSA ratio or the complexed PSA test and prostate volume can improve the diagnostic accuracy for prostate cancer. Using PSA velocity as a guide for biopsy in prostate cancer detection is not recommended. Cuzick J et al. Prevention and early detection of prostate cancer. Lancet Oncol 2014;15:e484. [PMID: 25281467] Smith RA et al. Cancer screening in the United States, 2015: a review of current American Cancer Society guidelines and current issues in cancer screening. CA Cancer J Clin 2015;65:30. [PMID: 25581023]

(Continued)

	Protein C	
Test/Range/Collection	**Physiologic Basis**	**Interpretation**	**Comments**

Test/Range/Collection	Physiologic Basis	Interpretation	Comments
Protein C, plasma 70–170% (functional) 65–150% (antigenic) Blue $$$ Transport to lab on ice. Plasma must be separated and frozen in a polypropylene tube within 2 hours.	Protein C is a vitamin K-dependent proenzyme synthesized in the liver. It is activated at the endothelial surface when thrombin binds to thrombomodulin. In the presence of its cofactor protein S, activated protein C (APC) inactivates Va and VIIIa, thereby impeding further thrombin generation. APC also has cytoprotective effects such as anti-inflammatory, anti-apoptotic, and endothelial barrier protective effects, which are mediated by the endothelial cell protein C receptor. The functional assay detects both quantitative (type I) and qualitative (type II) deficiency of protein C. The antigenic assay detects patients with quantitative protein C deficiency, but does not detect patients with qualitative abnormalities. Deficiency is inherited in an autosomal dominant fashion with incomplete penetrance or is acquired. Deficient patients may present with a hypercoagulable state, with recurrent thrombophlebitis or pulmonary embolism.	**Decreased in:** Congenital deficiency, liver disease, cirrhosis (13–25%), warfarin use (28–60%), vitamin K deficiency, DIC, thrombosis (acute). **Interfering factors:** Artifactually decreased functional protein C values may be seen in patients with abnormally elevated levels of factor VIII. Artifactually increased levels of functional protein C values may be seen in patients on heparin therapy.	Homozygous deficiency of protein C (<1% activity) is associated with fatal neonatal purpura fulminans and massive venous thrombosis at birth. Heterozygous patients (1 in 200–300 of the population, with levels 25–50% of normal) may be at risk for venous thrombosis. Kindreds with dysfunctional protein C of normal quantity have been identified. Interpretation of an abnormally low protein C must be related to the clinical setting. Anticoagulant therapy, DIC, and liver disease must not be present. There is overlap between lower limits of normal values and values found in heterozygotes. Patients should be off oral anticoagulant therapy for 2 weeks for accurate measurement of functional protein C levels. See recommended testing for venous thrombosis (Figure 9–34). Hamasaki N et al. Activated protein C anticoagulant system dysfunction and thrombophilia in Asia. Ann Lab Med 2013;33:8. [PMID: 23301217] MacCallum P et al. Diagnosis and management of heritable thrombophilias. BMJ 2014;349:g4387. [PMID: 25035247]

(Continued)

Test / Specimen	Physiologic Basis	Interpretation	Comments
Protein electrophoresis, serum (SPEP) Adults: Albumin: 3.3–5.7 g/dL α_1: 0.1–0.4 g/dL α_2: 0.3–0.9 g/dL β_2: 0.7–1.5 g/dL γ: 0.5–1.4 g/dL SST $$	Electrophoresis of serum separates serum proteins into albumin, α_1, α_2, β_2, and γ fractions. Albumin is the principal serum protein (see Albumin, p. 42). The term globulin generally refers to the nonalbumin fraction of serum protein. The α_1 fraction contains α_1-antitrypsin (90%), α_1-lipoprotein, and α_1-acid glycoprotein. The α_2 fraction contains α_2-macroglobulin, haptoglobin, and ceruloplasmin. The β fraction contains transferrin, hemopexin, complement C3, and β-lipoproteins. The γ fraction contains immunoglobulins G, A, D, E, and M (see Immunoglobulins, p. 137). The conventional agarose gel and immunofixation electrophoresis (SPEP/IFE) are being replaced by automated capillary zone electrophoresis and immunotyping (known as CZE/IT).	↑ α_1: inflammatory states (α_1-antiprotease), pregnancy. ↑ α_2: nephrotic syndrome, inflammatory states, oral contraceptives, corticosteroid therapy, hyperthyroidism. ↑ β: hyperlipidemia, hemoglobinemia, iron deficiency anemia. ↑ γ: polyclonal gammopathies (liver disease, cirrhosis [associated with β–γ "bridging"], chronic infections, autoimmune disease), plasma cell neoplasms including myeloma and monoclonal gammopathy of undetermined significance (MGUS), Waldenström macroglobulinemia, lymphoid malignancies). ↓ α_1: α_1-antiprotease deficiency. ↓ α_2: in vivo hemolysis, liver disease. ↓ β: hypo-β-lipoproteinemias. ↓ γ: immune deficiency.	Presence of "spikes" in α_2, β_2, or γ regions necessitates the use of IFE (p. 136) or CZE immunotyping to verify the presence of a monoclonal gammopathy. SPEP/IFE (or CZE/IT) in combination with serum free light-chain (FLC) assay are highly sensitive for the detection of myeloma and related plasma cell neoplasms. If Bence Jones proteins (light chains) are suspected, UPEP followed by IFE can be done for follow-up purposes. Test is insensitive for detection of decreased levels of immunoglobulins and α_1-antitrypsin (see Immunoglobulins, p. 137, and α_1-Antitrypsin, p. 50). If plasma is used, fibrinogen will be detected in the α–γ region. The acute-phase reactant protein pattern seen with acute illness, surgery, infarction, or trauma is characterized by an ↑ α_2 (haptoglobin) and ↑ α_1 (α_1-antitrypsin). Jenner E. Serum free light chains in clinical laboratory diagnostics. Clin Chim Acta 2014;427:15. [PMID: 23999048] Mathur G et al. Streamlined sign-out of capillary protein electrophoresis using middleware and an open-source macro application. J Pathol Inform 2014;5:36. [PMID: 25337433] Vincent Rajkumar S. Multiple myeloma: 2014 Update on diagnosis, risk-stratification, and management. Am J Hematol 2014;89:999. [PMID: 25223428]
Protein S (total antigen), plasma 55–155% Blue $$$ Transport to lab on ice. Plasma must be separated and frozen in a polypropylene tube within 2 hours.	Protein S is a vitamin K-dependent glycoprotein, synthesized in the liver. It has an anticoagulant function and acts as the cofactor of activated protein C (APC), with which it forms a stoichiometric complex. This complex inactivates Va and VIIIa. There are two forms of protein S: free and bound. Free protein S represents about 40% of the total and is the functional form that acts as the cofactor for APC. Bound protein S, attached to C4b-binding protein, does not possess any anticoagulant activity. Deficiency is associated with recurrent venous thrombosis and/or thromboembolism before age 45.	**Decreased in:** Congenital protein S deficiency, liver disease, thrombosis (acute), warfarin therapy, DIC, vitamin K deficiency, nephrotic syndrome.	This immunoassay measures the total protein S antigen, not biologic activity of protein S. Functional protein S clotting assay (APC cofactor activity) and free protein S antigen immunoassay are available to differentiate subtypes of congenital protein S deficiency (type I: decreased antigen and functional levels; type II: decreased functional levels, but normal total and free antigen levels; type IIa or type III: decreased functional and free antigen levels, but normal total antigen levels). Hamasaki N et al. Activated protein C anticoagulant system dysfunction and thrombophilia in Asia. Ann Lab Med 2013;33:8. [PMID: 23301217] MacCallum P et al. Diagnosis and management of heritable thrombophilias. BMJ 2014;349:g4387. [PMID: 25035247]

Protein, total			
Test/Range/Collection	Physiologic Basis	Interpretation	Comments
Protein, total, plasma or serum 6.0–8.0 g/dL [60–80 g/L] SST, green, PPT, lavender ≤ Avoid prolonged venous stasis during collection.	Plasma protein concentration is determined by nutritional state, hepatic function, renal function, hydration, and various disease states. Plasma protein concentration determines the colloidal osmotic pressure.	**Increased in:** Polyclonal or monoclonal gammopathies, marked dehydration. Drugs: anabolic steroids, androgens, corticosteroids, epinephrine. **Decreased in:** Protein-losing enteropathies, acute burns, nephrotic syndrome, severe dietary protein deficiency, chronic liver disease, malabsorption syndrome, agammaglobulinemia, cancer cachexia.	Serum total protein consists primarily of albumin and globulin. Serum globulin level is calculated as total protein minus albumin. Hypoproteinemia usually indicates hypoalbuminemia, because albumin is the major serum protein. Hypoalbuminemia is associated with higher in-hospital mortality among surgical patients. Fanali G et al. Human serum albumin: from bench to bedside. Mol Aspects Med 2012;33:209. [PMID: 22230555] Gatta A et al. Hypoalbuminemia. Intern Emerg Med 2012;7:S193. [PMID: 23073857] Nakayama H et al. Management before hepatectomy for hepatocellular carcinoma with cirrhosis. World J Hepatol 2015;7:2292. [PMID: 26380653]

Prothrombin time			
Prothrombin time, whole blood (PT) 11–15 seconds (laboratory specific) Blue $ Fill tube completely.	PT evaluates the extrinsic and common coagulation pathways. It is measured by adding calcium and tissue thromboplastin to a sample of citrated, platelet-poor plasma. The time required for fibrin clot formation is determined. It is most sensitive to deficiencies in the vitamin K-dependent clotting factors II, VII, IX, and X. It is also sensitive to deficiency of factor V. It is less sensitive to fibrinogen deficiency and heparin. PT is the most commonly used test for monitoring warfarin therapy. In addition to results reported in seconds, the International Normalized Ratio (INR) is calculated. INR = [Patient PT/Normal mean PT][ISI] Point-of-care PT/INR tests are increasingly being used for monitoring warfarin therapy.	**Increased in:** Warfarin, liver disease, DIC, vitamin K deficiency, hereditary deficiency in factors VII, X, V and II, fibrinogen abnormality (eg, hypofibrinogenemia, afibrinogenemia, dysfibrinogenemia), circulating anticoagulant affecting the PT system (rarely lupus anticoagulant), massive transfusion. **Decreased in:** Recombinant factor FVII (Novoseven) treatment.	Routine preoperative measurement of PT is unnecessary unless there is clinical history of a bleeding disorder (see Figure 9–7 and Table 8–8). The INR was introduced in the early 1980s to improve PT reporting and standardization. An International Sensitivity Index (ISI) is assigned to each thromboplastin by the reagent manufacture. The ISI is a measure of a reagent's responsiveness to low levels of vitamin K-dependent factors compared with the WHO International Reference Preparation. Despite the improvement with INR reporting, significant variation in INR results between laboratories persists. These differences in INR reflect local variables (eg, reagent and/or instrument system). A high-sensitivity, low ISI thromboplastin reagent is recommended to improve precision and accuracy of the INR. Warfarin therapeutic range is INR 2.0–3.0. Bleeding has been reported to be significantly more common in patients with INRs of 3.0–4.5 than in patients with INRs of 2.0–3.0. PT/INR are used in prognostic scoring systems in chronic liver disease, but whole blood viscoelastic tests provide clinically more relevant information in patients with liver disease. Dusse LM et al. Point-of-care test (POCT) INR: hope or illusion? Rev Bras Cir Cardiovasc 2012;27:296. [PMID: 22996982] Mallett SV et al. Clinical utility of viscoelastic tests of coagulation in patients with liver disease. Liver Int 2013;33:961. [PMID: 23638693] Pollack CV Jr. Coagulation assessment with the new generation of oral anticoagulants. Emerg Med J 2016;33:423. [PMID: 25987596] Wool GD et al. Pathology consultation on anticoagulation monitoring: factor X-related assays. Am J Clin Pathol 2013;140:623. [PMID: 24124140]

(Continued)

	Q fever antibody		
Test/Range/Collection	Physiologic Basis	Interpretation	Comments
Q fever antibody, serum <1:8 titer SST $$$ Submit paired sera, one collected within 1 week of illness and another 2–3 weeks later. Avoid hemolysis.	*Coxiella burnetii* is a rickettsial organism that is the causative organism for Q fever. Most likely mode of transmission is inhalation of aerosols from exposure to common reservoirs, sheep, and cattle. Tick bites (ixodid ticks) may also be a mode of transmission. Antibodies to the organism can be detected by the presence of agglutinins, by complement fixation (CF), by immunofluorescent antibody testing (IFA), or by enzyme-linked immunosorbent assay (ELISA). Agglutinin titers are found 5–8 days after infection. IgM can be detected at 7 days (IFA, ELISA) and may persist for up to 32 weeks (ELISA). IgG (IFA, ELISA) appears after 7 days and peaks at 3–4 weeks. Phase I and phase II antibodies are produced in response to the organism, phase II antibodies appearing first and phase I antibodies weeks to months later. Diagnosis of Q fever is usually confirmed by serologic findings of anti-phase II antigen IgM titers of ≥1:50 and IgG titers of ≥ 1:200. The finding of elevated levels of both IgM and IgA by ELISA has both high sensitivity and high specificity for acute Q fever. In chronic Q fever, phase I antibodies, especially IgG and IgA, are predominant.	**Increased in:** Acute or chronic Q fever (CF antibodies are present by the second week in 65% of cases and by the fourth week in 90%, acute and convalescent titers [immunofluorescent antibody testing, IFA, or enzyme-linked immunosorbent assay, ELISA] detect infection with 89–100% sensitivity and 100% specificity), and recent vaccination for Q fever.	Clinical presentation is similar to that of severe influenza. Typically, there is no rash. Test acute and convalescent sera for evidence of current or recent *C. burnetii* infection. Occasionally, titers do not rise for 4–6 weeks, especially if antimicrobial therapy has been given. Initial testing may not be helpful; treatment should be based on clinical and other laboratory assessment. As with any serologic procedure, demonstration of seroconversion or a fourfold increase in titer between acute and convalescent sera suggests current or recent infection. Patients with Q fever have a high prevalence of antiphospholipid antibody (81%), especially as measured by lupus anticoagulant test or measurement of antibodies to cardiolipin. These tests may be useful in diagnosing patients presenting with fever alone. Antibodies to Q fever do not cross-react with other rickettsial antibodies; a rise in titer is considered diagnostic for recent infection in the absence of prior vaccination. If chronic disease (endocarditis) suspected, order phase I antibodies; if acute disease suspected, order phase II antibodies. Jorgensen JH et al (editors): *Manual of Clinical Microbiology*, 11th ed. ASM Press, 2015. Vanderburg S et al. Epidemiology of *Coxiella burnetii* infection in Africa: a OneHealth systematic review. PLoS Negl Trop Dis 2014;8:e2787. [PMID: 24722554]

QuantiFERON-TB (Interferon-gamma releasing assay)		
QuantiFERON-TB (Interferon-gamma releasing assay), whole blood Negative Green top (must be delivered to test laboratory within 12 hr) or unique QFT-G blood collection tubes (Nil, TB Antigen, Mitogen) $$$	QuantiFERON-TB Gold (QFT-G) is an indirect test for *Mycobacterium tuberculosis* infection. It measures a cell-mediated immune response in infected persons. The T lymphocytes of infected persons are sensitized to *M. tuberculosis* proteins. When whole blood is incubated with the *M. tuberculosis* specific antigens used in the test, the T lymphocytes produce and secrete interferon-gamma (IFN-γ), which is measured via a sensitive enzyme-linked immunosorbent assay (ELISA). The test does not distinguish between active tuberculosis disease and latent tuberculosis infection and is intended for use in conjunction with risk assessment, chest radiograph, and other medical and diagnostic evaluations. Compared with the conventional tuberculin skin test, QFT-G is a simpler and more accurate, specific, and convenient TB diagnostic tool. Another equivalent interferon-gamma release assay is the T-SPOT.TB, which is based on enzyme-linked immunospot assay (ELISpot).	**Positive:** Active *M. tuberculosis* infection, latent tuberculosis infection. **Negative:** No active or latent *M. tuberculosis* infection. **Indeterminate:** Test error or patient anergy.	QFT-G is highly specific; a positive test result is strongly predictive of *M. tuberculosis* infection. QFT-G test is completely unaffected by BCG vaccination status or by sensitization due to most nontuberculous mycobacteria, with the exception of *M. kansasii, M. marinum,* and *M. szulgai.* The QFT-G sensitivity for tuberculosis is 70–85%. There are suggestions that combined use of QFT-G and tuberculin skin test may help increase the sensitivity to above 90%. The ability of QFT-G to predict the risk of latent tuberculosis infection progression to active tuberculosis has not been determined. Risk may be different from that of those with a positive tuberculin skin test. Due to HIV-associated immunosuppression (low CD4 T-cell count), the sensitivity and specificity of QFT-G in HIV-infected individuals are suboptimal. Test should not be used alone to diagnose or exclude active tuberculosis. Santin M et al. Interferon-γ release assays for the diagnosis of tuberculosis and tuberculosis infection in HIV-infected adults: a systematic review and meta-analysis. PLoS One 2012;7:e32482. [PMID: 22403663] Sollai S et al. Systematic review and meta-analysis on the utility of Interferon-gamma release assays for the diagnosis of *Mycobacterium tuberculosis* infection in children: a 2013 update. BMC Infect Dis 2014;14:S6. [PMID: 24564486]

(Continued)

Test/Range/Collection	Physiologic Basis	Interpretation	Comments
Rapid plasma reagin, serum (RPR) Nonreactive SST $	Measures nontreponemal antibodies that are produced when *Treponema pallidum* interacts with host tissue. The card test is a flocculation test performed by using a cardiolipin–lecithin–cholesterol carbon-containing antigen reagent mixed on a card with the patient's serum. A positive test (presence of antibodies) is indicated when black carbon clumps produced by flocculation are seen by the naked eye.	**Increased in:** Syphilis: primary (78%), secondary (97%), symptomatic late (74%). Biologic false positives occur in a wide variety of conditions, including leprosy, malaria, intravenous drug abuse, aging, infectious mononucleosis, HIV infection (≤15%), autoimmune diseases (SLE, rheumatoid arthritis), *Streptococcus pyogenes* infection, pregnancy.	RPR is historically used as a screening test and in suspected primary and secondary syphilis. Because the test lacks specificity (false-positive rates 5–20%), positive tests should be confirmed with the specific treponemal antibody tests (FTA-ABS or TP-PA, p. 101 and p. 211). RPR titers can be used to follow infection activity and serologic response to treatment. (See Table 8–21.) The incidence of syphilis has been on the rise and there is a high coinfection rate with HIV. A "reverse" syphilis testing algorithm using treponemal tests for screening and nontreponemal serologic tests for confirmation has been (see Syphilis Serological Testing, p. 200, and Figure 9–31, p. 211) proposed. Kaur G et al. Syphilis testing in blood donors: an update. Blood Transfus 2015;13:197. [PMID: 25545876] Morshed MG et al. Recent trends in the serologic diagnosis of syphilis. Clin Vaccine Immunol 2015;22:137. [PMID: 25428245]
Red blood cell count (RBC or erythrocyte count), whole blood Males: $4.3–6.0 \times 10^6$/mcL Females: $3.5–5.5 \times 10^6$/mcL [$\times 10^{12}$/L] Lavender $	Red blood cells (erythrocytes) are counted by automated instruments using electrical impedance or light scattering.	**Increased in:** Secondary polycythemia, hemoconcentration (dehydration), polycythemia vera. Spurious increase with increased white blood cells. **Decreased in:** Anemias. Spurious decrease with autoagglutination (eg, cold agglutinins).	In patients with cold agglutinins, the spurious lowering of the RBC count is disproportionately greater than the false elevation of MCV, so the calculated hematocrit is falsely depressed and the calculated MCH and MCHC are falsely elevated. RBC count, along with mean red blood cell volume (MCV) and reticulocyte count, can help differentiate between iron deficiency anemia and thalassemia in patients with microcytic erythropoiesis. Schoorl M et al. Application of innovative hemocytometric parameters and algorithms for improvement of microcytic anemia discrimination. Hematol Rep 2015;7:5843. [PMID: 26331001] Swiecicki PL et al. Cold agglutinin disease. Blood 2013;122:1114. [PMID: 23757733]

Test/Range/Collection	Physiology	Interpretation	Comments
Renin activity, plasma (PRA) Lavender Salt-depleted, upright: 3.0–15 ng/mL/hr Salt-replete, upright: 0.6–3.0 ng/mL/hr (age-dependent) $$	The renal juxtaglomerular apparatus generates renin, an enzyme that converts angiotensinogen to angiotensin I. Renin secretion by the kidney is stimulated by a decrease in glomerular blood pressure, decreased sodium at the renal distal tubule, or renal vascular disease. The inactive angiotensin I is then converted to angiotensin II, which is a potent vasopressor. Renin activity is measured by the ability of a patient's plasma to generate angiotensin I from substrate (angiotensinogen), and expressed as ng/mL/hr. Normal values depend on the patient's hydration, posture, and salt intake.	**Increased in:** Dehydration, some hypertensive states (eg, renal artery stenosis), edematous states (cirrhosis, nephrotic syndrome, heart failure), hypokalemic states (gastrointestinal sodium and potassium loss, Bartter syndrome), adrenal insufficiency, chronic renal failure, left ventricular hypertrophy. Drugs: ACE inhibitors, estrogen, hydralazine, nifedipine, minoxidil, oral contraceptives. **Decreased in:** Hyporeninemic hypoaldosteronism, some hypertensive states (eg, primary aldosteronism, severe preeclampsia). Drugs: β-blockers, aspirin, clonidine, prazosin, reserpine, methyldopa, indomethacin.	An elevated ratio of plasma aldosterone concentration (in ng/dL) to plasma renin activity (aldosterone-to-renin ratio or ARR) of 20 or higher is an effective screening test for primary aldosteronism (sensitivity, 95%). It has a high negative predictive value even during antihypertensive therapy. Because of a low specificity of the ratio, autonomous aldosterone production must be confirmed by demonstration of high and autonomous secretion of aldosterone (using an aldosterone suppression test). The ARR should be interpreted along with the actual values of aldosterone and plasma renin activity. Plasma renin activity is also useful in evaluation of hypoaldosteronism (low-sodium diet, patient standing) (see Aldosterone, serum, p. 44). Weiner ID. Endocrine and hypertensive disorders of potassium regulation: primary aldosteronism. Semin Nephrol 2013;33:265. [PMID: 23953804] Zennaro MC et al. An update on novel mechanisms of primary aldosteronism. J Endocrinol 2015;224:R63. [PMID: 25424518]
Reticulocyte count, whole blood 20–125 × 10³/mcL [× 10⁹/L] Lavender $	Reticulocytes are young red blood cells that contain cytoplasmic RNA. A reticulocyte count measures how rapidly reticulocytes are produced by the bone marrow and then released into the bloodstream. Reticulocyte count reflects the erythropoietic activity of the bone marrow and is thus useful in both the diagnosis of anemias and in monitoring bone marrow response to therapy.	**Increased in:** Hemolytic anemia, blood loss (before development of iron deficiency), recovery from iron, B_{12} or folate deficiency, or from drug-induced hemolytic anemia. **Decreased in:** Iron deficiency anemia, aplastic anemia, anemia of chronic disease, megaloblastic anemia, sideroblastic anemia, pure red cell aplasia, renal disease, bone marrow suppression or infiltration (tumor, infection, etc), myelodysplastic syndrome.	This test is indicated for the evaluation of anemia to distinguish hypoproliferative from hemolytic anemia or blood loss. See anemia evaluation (Figure 9–5; Tables 8–2 & 8–3). The old method of measuring reticulocytes (manual staining and counting) has poor reproducibility. It has been replaced by automated methods (eg, flow cytometry-based), which are more precise and provide absolute reticulocyte counts. Method-specific reference ranges must be used. Koury MJ et al. How to approach chronic anemia. Hematology Am Soc Hematol Educ Program 2012;2012:183. [PMID: 23233579] Meier ER et al. Absolute reticulocyte count acts as a surrogate for fetal hemoglobin in infants and children with sickle cell anemia. PLoS One 2015;10:e0136672. [PMID: 26366562] Schoorl M et al. Application of innovative hemocytometric parameters and algorithms for improvement of microcytic anemia discrimination. Hematol Rep 2015;7:5843. [PMID: 26331001]

(Continued)

	Rh(D) typing	
Test/Range/Collection	**Physiologic Basis**	**Interpretation**	**Comments**

Test/Range/Collection	Physiologic Basis	Interpretation	Comments
Rh typing, red cells (Rh) Red, lavender/pink $ Proper identification of specimen is critical.	The Rhesus blood group system is second in importance only to the ABO system for transfusion practice. Anti-Rh antibodies are the leading cause of hemolytic disease of the newborn and may also cause hemolytic transfusion reactions. Although there are other Rhesus antigens, only tests for the D antigen are performed routinely in pretransfusion testing because the D antigen is the most immunogenic. The terms Rh-positive and Rh-negative refer to the presence and absence of the D antigen on the red cell surface, respectively. Persons whose red cells lack D do not regularly have anti-D in their serum. Formation of anti-D almost always results from exposure through transfusion or pregnancy to red cells possessing the D antigen.	83% of US non-Hispanic whites are Rh(D)-positive, 17% negative; 93% of Hispanic-Americans are Rh(D)-positive, 7% negative; 93% of African Americans are Rh(D)-positive, 7% negative; 98% of Asian Americans are Rh(D)-positive, 2% negative; 90% of North American Indians are Rh(D)-positive; 10% negative.	Of D-reactive⁻ persons receiving a single D-positive⁺ blood unit, 50–75% will develop anti-D. The blood of all donors and recipients is therefore routinely tested for D, so that D-negative recipients can be given D-negative blood. Donor units must also be tested for a weak form of D antigen, previously called Dᵘ, and must be labeled D-positive if "weak D" is detected. It is not required to test recipient blood specimen for weak D. *Technical Manual of the American Association of Blood Banks,* 18th ed. American Association of Blood Banks, 2014. Wagner FF et al. The Rhesus site. Transfus Med Hemother 2014;41:357. [PMID: 25538538]

Test / Range / Collection	Physiologic Basis	Interpretation	Rheumatoid factor / Ribonucleoprotein antibody — Comments
Rheumatoid factor, serum (RF) Negative (<1:16) SST $	RF consists of heterogeneous autoantibodies usually of the IgM class that react against the Fc region of human IgG. Most methods detect only IgM-class RF.	**Positive in:** Rheumatoid arthritis (75–90%), Sjögren syndrome (80–90%), scleroderma, dermatomyositis, SLE (30%), sarcoidosis, Waldenström macroglobulinemia, chronic infection. Drugs: methyldopa, others. Low-titers of RF (eg, ≤ 1:80) are questionable and can be found in healthy older patients (20%), in 1–4% of normal individuals, and in a variety of acute immune responses (eg, viral infections, including infectious mononucleosis and viral hepatitis), chronic bacterial infections (tuberculosis, leprosy, subacute infective endocarditis), and chronic active hepatitis.	Rheumatoid factor can be useful in differentiating rheumatoid arthritis from other chronic inflammatory arthritides. However, a positive RF test is only one of several criteria needed to make the diagnosis of rheumatoid arthritis. RF, along with cyclic citrullinated protein antibody (anti-CCP), has been included in the current Rheumatoid Arthritis Classification Criteria. (See also Autoantibodies, Table 8–7.) RF must be ordered selectively because its predictive value is low (34%) if it is used as a screening test. The test has poor positive predictive value because of its lack of specificity. The subset of patients with seronegative rheumatic disease limits its sensitivity and negative predictive value. Castelar-Pinheiro Gda R et al. The spectrum and clinical significance of autoantibodies in rheumatoid arthritis. Front Immunol 2015;6:320. [PMID: 26150818] Mohan C et al. Biomarkers in rheumatic diseases: how can they facilitate diagnosis and assessment of disease activity? BMJ 2015;351:h5079. [PMID: 26612523] Schneider M et al. Rheumatoid arthritis—early diagnosis and disease management. Dtsch Arztebl Int 2013;110:477. [PMID: 23964304]
Ribonucleoprotein antibody, serum (anti-RNP) Negative SST $$	This is an antibody to a ribonucleoprotein-extractable nuclear antigen. The presence of high-titer antibodies to U1-RNP are associated with mixed connective tissue disease (MCTD), and may also be present in systemic erythematosus (SLE) and systemic sclerosis.	**Increased in:** Scleroderma (20–30% sensitivity, low specificity), mixed connective tissue disease (MCTD) (95–100% sensitivity, low specificity), SLE (38–44%), Sjögren syndrome, rheumatoid arthritis (10%), discoid lupus (20–30%). Anti-RNP is present in 2.7% of patients with positive ANA.	RNP antibodies play a role in the pathogenesis of systemic autoimmune diseases by inducing neurotoxic inflammatory mediators. A negative test essentially excludes MCTD. (See also Autoantibodies, Table 8–7.) Cozzani E et al. Serology of lupus erythematosus: correlation between immunopathological features and clinical aspects. Autoimmune Dis 2014;2014:321359. [PMID: 24649358] Fujii T. Direct and indirect pathogenic roles of autoantibodies in systemic autoimmune diseases. Allergol Int 2014;63:515. [PMID: 25339435] Wolin S. RNPs and autoimmunity: 20 years later. RNA 2015;21:548. [PMID: 25780132]

(Continued)

Test/Range/Collection	Physiologic Basis	Interpretation	Comments
Ribosomal DNA (16S rDNA)		**Ribosomal DNA (16S rDNA) sequencing**	

Test/Range/Collection	Physiologic Basis	Interpretation	Comments
Ribosomal DNA (16S rDNA) sequencing for organism identification Collect and freeze (−70°C) unidentifiable culture isolate, tissue, or body fluid. $$$$	16S ribosomal RNA (rRNA) gene sequencing is the current gold standard in bacterial and other pathogenic microorganism identification and classification. Tests use universal PCR primers that bind to conserved regions of microbial rRNA (16s, and 18s/26s) genes and amplify adjacent hyper-variable segments that are species-specific.	**Indicated when**: Culture-negative sample is suspected (eg, prior antibiotics, potential for atypical or rare organisms); establishing a definitive microbiologic diagnosis will change long-term antimicrobial plan (eg, culture-negative infective endocarditis, culture-negative prosthetic joint infection)	Identification of bacteria in clinical microbiology laboratories is typically performed by phenotypic tests such as Gram stain and bio-chemical tests, along with culture requirements and growth charac-teristics. These methods have limitations, eg, they can not identify bacteria with unusual or rare phenotypic profiles, slow-growing bacteria, uncultivable bacteria, and culture-negative infections. In addition, phenotypic tests may not be available for many newly described pathogenic microorganisms. In these clinical situations, 16S rDNA sequencing can help establish a definitive microbiologic diagnosis, that is, to rule in (with positive identification) or rule out an infection. Tests are available for identification of bacterial, fungal and mycobac-terial organisms. Lasken RS et al. Recent advances in genomic DNA sequencing of microbial species from single cells. Nat Rev Genet 2014;15:577. [PMID: 25091868] Lluch J et al. The characterization of novel tissue microbiota using an optimized 16S metagenomic sequencing pipeline. PLoS One 2015;10:e0142334. [PMID: 26544956] Tremblay J et al. Primer and platform effects on 16S rRNA tag sequencing. Front Microbiol 2015;6:771. [PMID: 26300854]

Rubella antibody			
Rubella antibody, serum <1:8 titer SST $ For diagnosis of a recent infection, submit paired sera, one collected within 1 week of illness and another 2–4 weeks later.	Rubella (German measles) is a viral infection that causes fever, malaise, coryza, lymphadenopathy, fine maculopapular rash, and congenital birth defects when infection occurs in utero. Antibodies to rubella can be detected by hemagglutination inhibition, complement fixation, indirect hemagglutination, enzyme-linked immunosorbent assay (ELISA), or latex agglutination. Tests can detect IgG and IgM antibody. Titers usually appear as rash fades (1 week) and peak at 10–14 days for hemagglutination inhibition and 2–3 weeks for other techniques. Baseline titers may remain elevated for life. Serologic tests are used to determine the immune status of the individual, to diagnose postnatal rubella, and occasionally to support the diagnosis of rubella. IgM antibody disappears within 4–5 weeks; IgG antibody remains for life.	**Increased in:** Recent rubella infection, congenital rubella infection, previous rubella infection, or vaccination (immunity). Spuriously increased IgM antibody occurs in the presence of rheumatoid factor or cross-reacting antibodies to other viral infections or autoimmune illnesses.	Rubella titers of ≤1:8 indicate susceptibility and need for immunization to prevent infection during pregnancy. Titers of > 1:32 indicate immunity from prior infection or vaccination. Demonstration of a 4-fold rise in titer between acute and convalescent sera may be indicative of a recent infection. Single titers, even > 1:256, cannot be interpreted as evidence of recent infection, since they are more likely to indicate immune status. The recent resurgence of congenital rubella can largely be prevented with improved rubella testing and vaccination programs. Cesaro S et al. Guidelines on vaccinations in paediatric haematology and oncology patients. Biomed Res Int 2014;2014:707691. [PMID: 24868544] Jorgensen JH et al (editors): *Manual of Clinical Microbiology*, 11th ed. ASM Press, 2015.

(Continued)

Test/Range/Collection	Physiologic Basis	Interpretation	Comments
Russell viper venom time (dilute, dRVVT), plasma 24–37 seconds (laboratory-specific) Blue $$	Russell viper venom is extracted from a pit viper (*Vipera russelli*), which causes a rapidly fatal syndrome of consumptive coagulopathy with hemorrhage, shock, rhabdomyolysis, and renal failure. Approximately 70% of the protein content of the venom is phospholipase A_2, which activates factor X in the presence of phospholipid, bypassing factor VII. dRVVT is used in detection of antiphospholipid antibodies (so-called lupus anticoagulant, LAC). It should be noted that the 'anticoagulant' detected *in vitro* may be associated with vascular thrombosis and pregnancy-related morbidity *in vivo*.	**Increased in:** Circulating lupus anticoagulants (LAC) (sensitivity 96%, specificity 50–70%), severe fibrinogen deficiency (<50 mg/dL), deficiencies in prothrombin, factor V, factor X, and high-dose heparin therapy. **Normal in:** Factor VII deficiency and all intrinsic pathway factor deficiencies.	The test is sensitive to phospholipid, and if heparin is not present, a prolonged dRVVT may indicate the presence of LAC (antiphospholipid antibodies). An abnormally prolonged result is followed by a dRVVT confirmatory test, in which an excess of phospholipid is added to the assay. The clotting times of both the initial dRVVT and confirmatory test are normalized and then used to calculate a ratio (ie, dRVVT-screen/dRVVT-confirm). In general, a ratio of >1.2 is considered a positive result, which implies the presence of LAC. Results should be interpreted with caution if a patient is receiving anticoagulation (eg, warfarin or direct thrombin inhibitor) therapy. Activated partial thromboplastin time (aPTT)–based hexagonal phase phospholipid test is also used for LAC detection. More than one antibody is associated with LAC activity. As examples, both anticardiolipin and antibodies to beta2-glycoprotein-I can have LAC activity. See Figure 9–28 for its use in evaluating isolated prolongation of PTT. Dusse LM et al. Antiphospholipid syndrome: a clinical and laboratorial challenge. Rev Assoc Med Bras 2014;60:181. [PMID: 24919006] Krilis SA et al. Laboratory methods to detect antiphospholipid antibodies. Hematology Am Soc Hematol Educ Program 2014;2014:321. [PMID: 25696873] Levy RA et al. Antiphospholipid antibodies and antiphospholipid syndrome during pregnancy: diagnostic concepts. Front Immunol 2015;6:205. [PMID: 25999948]

Russell viper venom time (dRVVT)

Test / Range / Specimen	Physiologic Basis	Interpretation	Comments
Salicylate, serum (aspirin) 20–30 mg/dL [200–300 mg/L] *Panic:* > 35 mg/dL [> 350 mg/L] Red $$	At high concentrations, salicylate stimulates hyperventilation, uncouples oxidative phosphorylation, and impairs glucose and fatty acid metabolism. Salicylate toxicity is thus marked by respiratory alkalosis and metabolic acidosis.	**Increased in:** Acute or chronic salicylate intoxication.	The potential toxicity of salicylate levels after acute ingestion can be determined by using a salicylate toxicity nomogram (eg, see Done reference below). Nomograms have become less valid with the increasing popularity of enteric-coated slow-release aspirin preparations. Routine testing may not be required for fully conscious asymptomatic adult patients who deny ingesting salicylate. Acute toxicity can be readily diagnosed if an ingestion history is provided. Done AK. Salicylate intoxication. Significance of measurements of salicylate in blood in cases of acute ingestion. Pediatrics 1960;26:800. Juurlink DN et al. Extracorporeal treatment for salicylate poisoning: systematic review and recommendations from the EXTRIP Workgroup. Ann Emerg Med 2015;66:165. [PMID: 25986310]
Scleroderma-associated antibody (Scl-70 antibody), serum Negative SST $$	This antibody reacts with a nuclear antigen (DNA topoisomerase 1, or topo-I) that is responsible for the relaxation of super-coiled DNA.	**Increased in:** Scleroderma (systemic sclerosis), SLE (5%).	Scl-70 antibody is seen in 20–50% of patients with scleroderma and is considered diagnostic and specific for scleroderma if it is the only antibody present. Predictive value of a positive test is >95% for scleroderma. Scl-70 antibodies are associated with diffuse cutaneous scleroderma and a higher risk of severe interstitial lung disease. Low levels of Scl-70 antibody are also present in approximately 5% of patients with systemic lupus erythematosus. 50–70% of patients with limited scleroderma (CREST syndrome) have detectable anti-centromere antibody. (See also Autoantibodies, Table 8–7.) Gelpi C et al. Efficiency of a solid-phase chemiluminescence immunoassay for detection of antinuclear and cytoplasmic autoantibodies compared with gold standard immunoprecipitation. Auto Immun Highlights 2014;5:47. [PMID: 26000155] Kayser C et al. Autoantibodies in systemic sclerosis: unanswered questions. Front Immunol 2015;6:167. [PMID: 25926833] Sticherling M. Systemic sclerosis-dermatological aspects. Part 1: Pathogenesis, epidemiology, clinical findings. J Dtsch Dermatol Ges 2012;10:705. [PMID: 22913330]

(Continued)

Test/Range/Collection	Physiologic Basis	Interpretation	Comments
Semen analysis, ejaculate Sperm count: > 20 × 10⁶/mL [10⁹/L] Motility score: > 60% motile Volume: 2–5 mL Normal morphology: > 60% $$$ Semen is collected in a urine container after masturbation following 3 days of abstinence from ejaculation. Specimen must be examined promptly.	Semen analysis is the first step in identifying cause of male infertility. Conventional semen analysis includes the determination of sperm count, semen volume, sperm motility (qualitative and quantitative), and sperm morphology. Sperm are viewed under the microscope for motility and morphology. In addition to sperm count, sperm morphology and motility may have the most predictive utility. Infertility can be associated with low counts or with sperm of abnormal morphology or decreased motility.	**Decreased in:** Primary or secondary testicular failure, cryptorchidism, following vasectomy, drugs.	A low sperm count should be confirmed by sending two other appropriately collected semen specimens for evaluation. The usefulness of conventional semen analysis parameters as predictors of fertility is somewhat limited. Therefore, alternative tests based on more functional aspects (sperm penetration, capacitation, acrosome reaction) have been developed. Flow cytometer-based sperm chromatin structure assay (SCA) can provide an assessment of DNA integrity as another parameter of sperm quality. Esteves SC. Clinical relevance of routine semen analysis and controversies surrounding the 2010 World Health Organization criteria for semen examination. Int Braz J Urol 2014;40:443. [PMID: 25254609] Wang C et al. Limitations of semen analysis as a test of male fertility and anticipated needs from newer tests. Fertil Steril 2014;102:1502. [PMID: 25458617]
Smith (anti-Sm) antibody, serum Negative SST $$	This antibody to Smith antigen (an extractable nuclear antigen) is a marker antibody for SLE.	**Positive in:** SLE (30–40% sensitivity, 90–95% specificity).	Anti-Sm is highly specific for SLE and is one of the few autoantibodies commonly seen in SLE, including anti-Sm/RNP, anti-dsDNA and anti-Ro/La. A positive test substantially increases posttest probability of SLE. Test rarely needed for the diagnosis of SLE. (See also Autoantibodies, Table 8–7.) Cozzani E et al. Serology of lupus erythematosus: correlation between immunopathological features and clinical aspects. Autoimmune Dis 2014;2014:321359. [PMID: 24649358] Fu SM et al. Anti-dsDNA antibodies are one of the many autoantibodies in systemic lupus erythematosus. F1000Res 2015;4(F1000 Faculty Rev):939. [PMID: 26594353] Han S et al. Mechanisms of autoantibody production in systemic lupus erythematosus. Front Immunol 2015;6:228. [PMID: 26029213]

Smooth muscle antibodies		
Smooth muscle antibodies, serum Negative SST $$	Antibodies against smooth muscle proteins are found in patients with type 1 chronic active hepatitis, primary biliary cirrhosis, and the overlap syndrome of autoimmune hepatitis and primary biliary cirrhosis.	**Positive in:** Autoimmune chronic active hepatitis (40–70%, predominantly IgG antibodies), lower titers in primary biliary cirrhosis (50%, predominantly IgM antibodies), viral hepatitis, infectious mononucleosis, cryptogenic cirrhosis (28%), HIV infection, vitiligo (25%), endometriosis, Behçet disease (<2% of normal individuals).	The presence of high titers of smooth muscle antibodies (>1:80) is useful in distinguishing autoimmune chronic active hepatitis from other forms of hepatitis. Two types of autoimmune hepatitis are recognised, based on the serological autoantibody profile: type 1 is defined by positivity for anti-smooth muscle antibody and/or ANA, whereas type 2 is characterized by the presence of anti-liver kidney microsomal type 1 antibody or anti-liver cytosol type 1 antibody. Liberal R et al. Update on autoimmune hepatitis. J Clin Transl Hepatol 2015;3:42. [PMID: 26357634] Muratori L et al. Autoantibodies in autoimmune hepatitis. Dig Dis 2015;33(Suppl 2):65. [PMID: 26642213] Zhao P et al. Low incidence of positive smooth muscle antibody and high incidence of isolated IgM elevation in Chinese patients with autoimmune hepatitis and primary biliary cirrhosis overlap syndrome: a retrospective study. BMC Gastroenterol 2012;12:1. [PMID: 22214224]

(Continued)

Test/Range/Collection	Physiologic Basis	Interpretation	Comments
Sodium, serum or plasma (Na⁺) 135–145 meq/L [mmol/L or mM] **Panic:** <125 or > 155 meq/L SST, green $	Sodium homeostasis is crucial for life, and the Na⁺ level of blood is strictly maintained at a range of 135–145 mM. Sodium is the predominant extracellular cation. The serum sodium level is primarily determined by the volume status of the individual. Hyponatremia can be divided into hypovolemia, euvolemia, and hypervolemia categories. (See Hyponatremia algorithm, Figure 9–18.) Sodium is commonly measured by ion-selective electrode.	**Increased in:** Dehydration (excessive sweating, severe vomiting, or diarrhea), polyuria (diabetes mellitus, diabetes insipidus), hyperaldosteronism, inadequate water intake (coma, hypothalamic disease). Drugs: steroids, licorice, oral contraceptives. **Decreased in:** CHF, cirrhosis, vomiting, diarrhea, exercise, excessive sweating (with replacement of water but not salt, eg, marathon running), salt-losing nephropathy, adrenal insufficiency, nephrotic syndrome, water intoxication, syndrome of inappropriate antidiuretic hormone (SIADH), AIDS. Drugs: thiazides, diuretics, ACE inhibitors, chlorpropamide, carbamazepine, antidepressants (selective serotonin reuptake inhibitors), antipsychotics.	Spurious hyponatremia may be produced by severe lipemia or hyperproteinemia if sodium analysis involves a dilution step. Many guidelines recommend a correction factor, whereby the serum sodium concentration decreases by 1.6 meq/L for every 100 mg/dL (5.56 mmol/L) rise in plasma glucose above normal, but there is evidence that the decrease may be greater when patients have more severe hyperglycemia (> 400 mg/dL or 22.2 mmol/L) and/or volume depletion. One group has suggested that, when the serum glucose is > 200 mg/dL, the serum sodium concentration decreases by at least 2.4 meq/L. Hyponatremia in a normovolemic patient with urine osmolality higher than serum (or plasma) osmolality suggests the possibility of SIADH, myxedema, hypopituitarism, or reset osmostat. Treatment of disorders of sodium balance relies on clinical assessment of the patient's extracellular fluid volume rather than the serum sodium. Noda M et al. Sodium sensing in the brain. Pflugers Arch 2015;467:465. [PMID: 25491503] Overgaard-Steensen C et al. Clinical review: practical approach to hyponatraemia and hypernatraemia in critically ill patients. Crit Care 2013;17:206. [PMID: 23672688] Sam R et al. Understanding hypernatremia. Am J Nephrol 2012; 36:97. [PMID: 22739333]
Somatostatin, plasma <25 pg/mL [<25 ng/L] (laboratory-specific) Lavender $$$$ Specimen should be collected in pre-chilled lavender tube and refrigerated.	Somatostatin is a peptide hormone produced by the hypothalamus and digestive system (stomach, intestine, and pancreas). It has 2 active forms produced by alternative cleavage of a single preproprotein, one of 14 amino acids, the other of 28 amino acids. Somatostatin is a physiologic regulator of islet cell and gastrointestinal functions and is an inhibitor of the release of many pituitary hormones including growth hormone, prolactin, and thyrotropin.	**Increased in:** Somatostatinoma and other somatostatin-producing neuroendocrine tumors.	Useful as a tumor marker for diagnosis and follow-up of somatostatinomas and other somatostatin-producing neuroendocrine tumors. Test is not widely available and is typically performed by reference laboratories. Results obtained with different somatostatin assays can differ substantially. Serial measurements should therefore always be performed using the same assay. Cloyd JM et al. Non-functional neuroendocrine tumors of the pancreas: advances in diagnosis and management. World J Gastroenterol 2015; 21:9512. [PMID: 26327759] Ito T et al. Pancreatic neuroendocrine tumors: clinical features, diagnosis and medical treatment: advances. Best Pract Res Clin Gastroenterol 2012;26:737. [PMID: 23582916]

Sodium	Somatostatin

	SS-A/Ro antibody	SS-B/La antibody
Test / Specimen	SS-A/Ro antibody, serum	SS-B/La antibody, serum
Reference range	Negative	Negative
	SST	SST
	$$	$$
Physiologic basis	Sjögren syndrome (SS) is a chronic autoimmune inflammatory disease that primarily involves the exocrine glands, resulting in their functional impairment. Anti-Ro and anti-La antibodies are considered the classical hallmark of SS. Antibodies to Ro (SSA or SS-associated antigen A) cellular ribonucleoprotein complexes are found in connective tissue diseases such as Sjögren syndrome (SS), SLE, neonatal lupus (particularly with congenital heart block), rheumatoid arthritis (RA), and vasculitis. There are two types of anti-Ro/SSA antibodies, anti-SSA-52 kDa and anti-SSA-60 kDa, each specific for different antigens encoded by different genes.	Sjögren syndrome (SS) is a chronic autoimmune inflammatory disease that primarily involves the exocrine glands, resulting in their functional impairment. Anti-Ro and anti-La antibodies are considered the classical hallmark of SS. Antibodies to La (SSB or SS-associated antigen B) cellular ribonucleoprotein complexes are found in Sjögren syndrome and appear to be relatively more specific for Sjögren syndrome than are antibodies to SSA. They are quantitated by immunoassay.
Interpretation	**Increased in:** Sjögren syndrome (60–70% sensitivity, low specificity), SLE (30–40%), RA (10%), subacute cutaneous lupus, vasculitis.	**Increased in:** Sjögren syndrome (40–50% sensitivity, higher specificity than anti-SSA), SLE (10%).
Comments	Useful in counseling women of childbearing age with known connective tissue disease, because a positive test is associated with a small but real risk of neonatal SLE and congenital heart block. The few (<10%) patients with SLE who do not have a positive ANA commonly have antibodies to SS-A. Circulating levels of anti-Ro/La do not correlate with disease activity. Anti-Ro/La-positive patients with SS may have severe hypergammaglobulinemia, cryoglobulins, and a high risk of developing lymphoma, when compared with seronegative Sjögren syndrome cases. (See also Autoantibodies, Table 8–7.) Brandt JE et al. Sex differences in Sjögren's syndrome: a comprehensive review of immune mechanisms. Biol Sex Differ 2015;6:19. [PMID: 26535108] Tincani A et al. Novel aspects of Sjögren's syndrome in 2012. BMC Med 2013;11:93. [PMID: 23556533]	Direct pathogenicity and usefulness of autoantibody test in predicting disease exacerbation not proven. Circulating levels of anti-Ro/La do not correlate with disease activity. Anti-Ro/La-positive patients with SS may have severe hypergammaglobulinemia, cryoglobulins, and elevated risk for lymphoma. (See also Autoantibodies, Table 8–7.) Brandt JE et al. Sex differences in Sjögren's syndrome: a comprehensive review of immune mechanisms. Biol Sex Differ 2015;6:19. [PMID: 26535108] Tincani A et al. Novel aspects of Sjögren's syndrome in 2012. BMC Med 2013;11:93. [PMID: 23556533]

(Continued)

	Syphilis, serologic testing	
Test/Range/Collection	**Physiologic Basis**	**Interpretation**	**Comments**

Test/Range/Collection	Physiologic Basis	Interpretation	Comments
Syphilis, serologic testing, serum Negative SST $$	Syphilis is a sexually transmitted infection caused by *Treponema pallidum*. It can cause long-term complications if not treated properly. Symptoms in adults are divided into stages: primary, secondary, latent and late syphilis. Serologic tests remain the mainstay of syphilis diagnosis. Non-treponemal tests (NTT) (ie, rapid plasma reagin test, RPR; Venereal Disease Research Laboratory test, VDRL) measure non-specific antibodies to treponemal infection. Both RPR and VDRL are manual flocculation tests, which detect both IgM and IgG antibodies that are detectable as early as 6 days postinfection. The RPR test is mainly used to test serum samples, while the VDRL test is used primarily for testing cerebrospinal fluid samples. Treponemal tests (TT) detect antibodies that are specific to *T pallidum* whole cells or antigens, and are designed to detect either IgM or IgG antibodies. Common TT include the *T pallidum* hemagglutination assay (TPHA), the *T pallidum* particle agglutination assay (TPPA), and fluorescent treponemal antibody absorption assay (FTA-ABS), Western blotting (WB) and an alternate line immunoassay (LIA), and automated or semiautomated assays (eg, ELISA, CLIA, EIA) using recombinant *T pallidum* antigens are available. The sensitivity and specificity of both NTT and TT vary with the type of test as well as the stage of syphilis infection.	**Positive in:** Syphilis. Traditional testing algorithms (NTT as the screening test, and TT as the confirmatory test): sensitivity ~75%, specificity >99%; "Reverse" testing algorithms (TT as the screening and NTT as the confirmatory test): sensitivity >99%, specificity >99%.	Traditionally, syphilis serologic testing has been performed using a manual NTT such as the RPR or VDRL test, with positive results then confirmed using a specific TT such as TPPA or FTA-ABS. Antibodies detected by specific treponemal assays arise earlier than those detected by NTT, and typically remain detectable for life, even after successful treatment. Although this algorithm is still used by many laboratories, limitations include the manual nature of NTT, subjective interpretation, and low sample throughput. The "reverse" screening algorithm, on the other hand, starts with an automated or semiautomated specific TT, such as an EIA- or CLIA-based test. Positive samples are then confirmed with a quantitative NTT (often the RPR with titers). If the RPR is positive, active infection is confirmed. If the test results disagree (ie, a reactive treponemal test and negative RPR) and there is no documented previous syphilis treatment, the specimen is then tested using a second, different specific TT (eg, TPPA). If the second TT result is positive, this is considered to confirm previous syphilis infection, regardless of whether the patient has been adequately treated for active or late latent syphilis. Rarely, if the second TT result is negative, a third TT may be performed, if clinically indicated. The "reverse" testing algorithm allows automation, increased sample throughput, and objective interpretation of screening results. The reverse algorithm is currently endorsed by the Association of Public Health Laboratories and the International Union against Sexually Transmitted Infections. The decision to use a treponemal or nontreponemal assay as the first screening test should be based on a combination of factors: local syphilis prevalence, expected testing volume and workload (laboratory and clinical), requirement for automation, and available budget for labor and consumables. Once active syphilis infection is confirmed, an NTT (eg, RPR) with titers is recommended for determining serological activity and following up the effect of syphilis treatment. Point-of-care tests for syphilis are available. Kaur G et al. Syphilis testing in blood donors: an update. Blood Transfus 2015;13:197. [PMID: 25545876] Morshed MG et al. Recent trends in the serologic diagnosis of syphilis. Clin Vaccine Immunol 2015;22:137. [PMID: 25428245]

Test / Specimen / Reference range	Description	Interpretation	Comments
T-cell receptor (TCR) gene rearrangement, whole blood, bone marrow, frozen or paraffin-embedded tissue Lavender $$$$	In general, the percentage of T lymphocytes with identical T-cell receptors is very low; in malignancies, however, the clonal expansion of one population leads to a large number of cells with identical T-cell receptor gene rearrangement. T-cell clonality can be assessed by flow cytometry (TCR V-β expression), restriction fragment Southern blot hybridization or polymerase chain reaction (PCR) and DNA sequencing.	**Positive in:** T-cell neoplasms such as T-cell prolymphocytic leukemia, Sézary syndrome, peripheral T-cell lymphoma, angioimmunoblastic T-cell lymphoma (monoclonal T-cell proliferation).	The diagnostic sensitivity and specificity are heterogeneous and laboratory- and method-specific. Results of the test must always be interpreted in the context of morphologic and other relevant data (eg, flow cytometry), and should not be used alone for a diagnosis of T-cell malignancy. The test is primarily for initial diagnosis, but is also used to detect minimal residual disease. Schrappe M. Detection and management of minimal residual disease in acute lymphoblastic leukemia. Hematology Am Soc Hematol Educ Program 2014; 244. [PMID: 25696862] Van Dongen JJ et al. Minimal residual disease diagnostics in acute lymphoblastic leukemia: need for sensitive, fast, and standardized technologies. Blood 2015; 125:3996. [PMID: 25999452] Vasile D et al. Peripheral T and NK cell non-Hodgkin lymphoma a challenge for diagnosis. Maedica (Buchar) 2014;9:104. [PMID: 25553137]
Testosterone, total, serum or plasma Males: 3.0–10.0 ng/mL [Males: 10–35 nmol/L] Females: 0.3–0.7 ng/mL [Females: 1.0–2.4 nmol/L] SST, green $$$	Testosterone is the principal male sex hormone, produced by the Leydig cells of the testes. Dehydroepiandrosterone (DHEA) is produced in the adrenal cortex, testes, and ovaries and is the main precursor for serum testosterone in women. In normal males after puberty, the testosterone level is twice as high as all androgens in females. In serum, it is largely bound to albumin (38%) and to a specific steroid hormone–binding globulin (SHBG) (60%), but it is the free hormone (2%) that is physiologically active. The total testosterone level measures both bound and free testosterone in the serum (by immunoassay). Free or bioavailable testosterone may be calculated or measured.	**Increased in:** Idiopathic sexual precocity (in boys, levels may be in adult range), adrenal hyperplasia (boys), adrenocortical tumors, trophoblastic disease during pregnancy, idiopathic hirsutism, virilizing ovarian tumors, arrhenoblastoma, virilizing luteoma, testicular feminization (normal or moderately elevated), cirrhosis (through increased SHBG), hyperthyroidism. Drugs: anticonvulsants, barbiturates, estrogens, oral contraceptives (through increased SHBG). **Decreased in:** Hypogonadism (primary and secondary), orchidectomy, Klinefelter syndrome, uremia, hemodialysis, hepatic insufficiency, ethanol [men]). Drugs: digoxin, spironolactone, acarbose.	The diagnosis of male hypogonadism is based on clinical symptoms and signs plus laboratory confirmation of low AM total testosterone levels on two different occasions. Levels <3.0 ng/mL should be treated. Free testosterone level is rarely needed and should only be measured in symptomatic patients with normal total testosterone levels near the lower limit of normal or if alterations of SHBG are suspected. Obtain serum luteinizing hormone and FSH levels to distinguish between primary (hypergonadotropic) and secondary (hypogonadotropic) hypogonadism. Hypogonadism associated with aging (andropause) may present a mixed picture, with low testosterone levels and low to low–normal gonadotropin levels. In men, there is a diurnal variation in serum testosterone with a 20% elevation in levels in the evenings. Kelly DM et al. Testosterone: a vascular hormone in health and disease. J Endocrinol 2013;217:R47. [PMID: 23549841] Morales A et al. A critical appraisal of accuracy and cost of laboratory methodologies for the diagnosis of hypogonadism: the role of free testosterone assays. Can J Urol 2012;19:6314. [PMID: 22704323] Tsujimura A. The relationship between testosterone deficiency and men's health. World J Mens Health 2013;31:126. [PMID: 24044107]

(Continued)

Thrombin time

Test/Range/Collection	Physiologic Basis	Interpretation	Comments
Thrombin time, plasma (TT) 17–23 seconds (laboratory-specific) Blue ↺	The thrombin time (TT) is a clot-based assay that measures the conversion of fibrinogen to fibrin. The TT is therefore affected by the level of fibrinogen and the presence of thrombin inhibitor (eg, heparin) and/or fibrin degradation products (FDPs). Because it bypasses all other coagulation reactions, it is not influenced by deficiencies of other coagulation factors.	**Increased in:** Low fibrinogen (<50 mg/dL), abnormal fibrinogen (dysfibrinogenemia), increased FDPs (eg, DIC), heparin, fibrinolytic agents (streptokinase, urokinase, tissue plasminogen activator), direct thrombin inhibitors (eg, dabigatran), liver disease.	The TT is very sensitive to heparin and has been used to monitor unfractionated heparin therapy, although this use has declined. Can be used to qualitatively assess anticoagulation status of patients receiving direct thrombin inhibitors (eg, dabigatran). A dilute TT is adequately responsive to dabigatran and has become available and may be used for monitoring dabigatran therapy. Heparin contamination is a common cause of an unexplained significantly prolonged TT. If suspected, heparin neutralization can be performed. Functional fibrinogen assay has largely replaced TT for evaluating fibrinogen. See evaluation for bleeding disorders (Figure 9–7 and Table 8–8). Cuker A et al. Laboratory measurement of the anticoagulant activity of the non-vitamin K oral anticoagulants. J Am Coll Cardiol 2014;64:1128 [PMID: 25212648] Tripodi A. The laboratory and the direct oral anticoagulants. Blood 2013;121:4032. [PMID: 23564912]

Thyroglobulin		
Thyroglobulin, serum or plasma (Tg) 3–42 ng/mL [mcg/L] SST, green $$$	Tg is a large protein specific to the thyroid gland from which thyroxine is synthesized and cleaved. Serum thyroglobulin is the primary biochemical tumor marker used to monitor differentiated thyroid cancer. Highly sensitive immunometric assays for Tg are available. Tg autoantibodies (TgAb) can interfere with the measurement of Tg, causing underestimation that could mask the presence of disease. Heterophile antibodies (eg, human anti-mouse antibodies) can cause Tg overestimation.	**Increased in:** Hyperthyroidism, subacute thyroiditis, untreated thyroid carcinomas (except medullary carcinoma): follicular cancer (sensitivity 72%, specificity 81%), Hürthle cell cancer (sensitivity 56%, specificity 84%). **Decreased in:** Factitious hyperthyroidism, presence of thyroglobulin autoantibodies, after (> 25 days) total thyroidectomy.	Follow-up of patients with differentiated thyroid cancers who are apparently disease-free after surgery and radioiodine therapy involves periodic measurement of serum Tg. Patients with detectable serum Tg during thyroid-stimulating hormone (TSH) suppression by thyroxine therapy or Tg that rises higher than 2 ng/mL after TSH stimulation are highly likely to harbor residual tumor. Undetectable serum Tg during TSH suppressive therapy does not exclude persistent disease. Therefore, serum Tg should be measured after TSH stimulation achieved either by thyroxine withdrawal or by administration of recombinant human TSH (rhTSH). Results are equivalent in detecting recurrent thyroid cancer, but use of rhTSH helps to prevent symptomatic hypothyroidism. Follow-up based on serial measurements of basal (ie, unstimulated) Tg may be superior to the single Tg measurement after TSH stimulation. Tg is typically measured together with Tg antibody. In patients with positive TgAb, the Tg level should be interpreted with caution. TgAb itself may also serve as a surrogate marker of persistent or recurrent disease. In patients with persistent or rising TgAb, neck ultrasound, along with other imaging, should be considered. Ringel MD et al. Approach to follow-up of the patient with differentiated thyroid cancer and positive anti-thyroglobulin antibodies. J Clin Endocrinol Metab 2013;98:3104. [PMID: 23922347] Spencer C et al. How sensitive (second-generation) thyroglobulin measurement is changing paradigms for monitoring patients with differentiated thyroid cancer, in the absence or presence of thyroglobulin autoantibodies. Curr Opin Endocrinol Diabetes Obes 2014;21:394. [PMID: 25122493]

(Continued)

Test/Range/Collection	Physiologic Basis	Interpretation	Comments
Thyroglobulin antibody, serum or plasma <1:10 (highly method-dependent) SST, green $$	Antibodies against thyroglobulin are produced in autoimmune diseases of the thyroid and other organs. Of the normal population, 10% have slightly elevated titers (especially women and the elderly).	**Increased in:** Hashimoto thyroiditis (> 90%), thyroid carcinoma (45%), thyrotoxicosis, pernicious anemia (50%), SLE (20%), subacute thyroiditis, Graves disease. **Not increased in:** Multinodular goiter, thyroid adenomas, and some carcinomas.	The thyroid peroxidase antibody test is more sensitive than the thyroglobulin antibody test in autoimmune thyroid disease. (See Thyroperoxidase Antibody, below.) There is limited use for this test, ie, monitoring of patients with thyroid carcinoma after treatment. (See Thyroglobulin, above.) Khan FA et al. Thyroid dysfunction: an autoimmune aspect. Int J Clin Exp Med 2015;8:6677. [PMID: 26221205] Ringel MD et al. Approach to follow-up of the patient with differentiated thyroid cancer and positive anti-thyroglobulin antibodies. J Clin Endocrinol Metab 2013;98:3104. [PMID: 23922347] Spencer C et al. How sensitive (second-generation) thyroglobulin measurement is changing paradigms for monitoring patients with differentiated thyroid cancer, in the absence or presence of thyroglobulin autoantibodies. Curr Opin Endocrinol Diabetes Obes 2014;21:394. [PMID: 25122493]
Thyroid peroxidase antibody (TPO Ab), serum or plasma Negative SST, lavender, green $$	TPO is a membrane-bound glycoprotein. This enzyme mediates the oxidation of iodide ions and incorporation of iodine into tyrosine residues of thyroglobulin. Its synthesis is stimulated by thyroid-stimulating hormone (TSH). TPO is the major antigen involved in thyroid antibody-dependent cell-mediated cytotoxicity. TPO Ab can be measured by enzyme-linked immunosorbent assay (ELISA) or automated immunoassay.	**Increased in:** Hashimoto thyroiditis (> 99%), idiopathic myxedema (> 99%), Graves disease (75–85%), Addison disease (50%), and Riedel thyroiditis. Low titers are present in approximately 10% of normal individuals and patients with nonimmune thyroid disease.	TPO antibody is an antibody to the main autoantigenic component of microsomes and is a more sensitive and specific test than hemagglutination assays for microsomal antibodies in the diagnosis of autoimmune thyroid disease. TPO antibody testing alone is often sufficient to detect autoimmune thyroid disease. TPO antibody titers correlate with TSH levels; their presence may herald impending thyroid failure. See thyroid disorders (Figures 9–16 and 9–19). Brown RS. Autoimmune thyroiditis in childhood. J Clin Res Pediatr Endocrinol 2013;5(Suppl 1):45. [PMID: 23154164] Khan FA et al. Thyroid dysfunction: an autoimmune aspect. Int J Clin Exp Med 2015;8:6677. [PMID: 26221205] Pyzik A et al. Immune disorders in Hashimoto's thyroiditis: what do we know so far? J Immunol Res 2015;2015:979167. [PMID: 26000316]

Test/Range/Collection	Physiologic Basis	Interpretation	Comments
Thyroid-stimulating hormone, serum or plasma (TSH; thyrotropin) 0.35–3.0 mcdU/mL [mIU/L] (assay-dependent) SST, PPT, green $$	TSH is an anterior pituitary hormone that stimulates the thyroid gland to produce thyroid hormones. Secretion is stimulated by thyrotropin-releasing hormone from the hypothalamus. There is negative feedback on TSH secretion by circulating thyroid hormone.	**Increased in:** Hypothyroidism, mild increases in recovery phase of acute illness, subclinical hypothyroidism. **Decreased in:** Hyperthyroidism, subclinical hyperthyroidism, acute medical or surgical illness (euthyroid sick syndrome), pituitary hypothyroidism. Drugs: dopamine, high-dose corticosteroids.	TSH assays are used for screening thyroid function, aiding the diagnosis of hyperthyroidism and hypothyroidism, and monitoring thyroid replacement therapy. The currently used TSH immunoassays are very sensitive, typically with functional sensitivity of ≤0.02 mIU/L. Measurement of serum TSH is the best initial laboratory test of thyroid function. It should be followed by measurement of free thyroxine (FT_4) if the TSH value is low and by measurement of anti-thyroperoxidase antibody (TPO Ab) if the TSH value is high. Most experts recommend against routine screening of asymptomatic patients, but screening is recommended for high-risk populations. See also Thyroid function tests and thyroid disorders (Figures 9–16 and 9–19). Test is also useful for following patients taking anti-thyroid medication. Baumgartner C et al. Subclinical hypothyroidism: summary of evidence in 2014. Swiss Med Wkly 2014;144:w14058. [PMID: 25536449] Mullur R et al. Thyroid hormone regulation of metabolism. Physiol Rev 2014;94:355. [PMID: 24692351] Papi G et al. Clinical concepts on thyroid emergencies. Front Endocrinol (Lausanne) 2014;5:102. [PMID: 25071718] Rugge JB et al. Screening for and treatment of thyroid dysfunction: an evidence review for the U.S. Preventive Services Task Force [Internet]. Rockville (MD): Agency for Healthcare Research and Quality (US); 2014 Oct. Report No.: 15-05217-EF-1. [PMID: 25927133]

(Continued)

	Thyroid stimulating immunoglobulin	
Test/Range/Collection	**Physiologic Basis**	**Interpretation**	**Comments**

Test/Range/Collection	Physiologic Basis	Interpretation	Comments
Thyroid stimulating immunoglobulin (TSI), serum Negative (TSI index <1.3, or <130% basal activity) SST, red $$$	TSIs are autoimmune immunoglobulins (IgG type) that can bind to thyroid-stimulating hormone (TSH) receptors in the thyroid gland. TSIs mimic the action of TSH, causing excess secretion of thyroxine (T4) and triiodothyronine (T3). The level of the TSIs detected in this test is abnormally high in hyperthyroidism due to Graves disease. TSIs can cross the placental barrier, causing transient hyperthyroidism in the neonates of mothers with Graves disease. TSIs are typically detected by a bioassay measuring the ability of the patient's serum (or IgG) to stimulate cyclic AMP production in tissue cultures, using cell lines carrying the human TSH receptor. This assay detects only stimulating TSH receptor antibody. Alternatively, TSIs can also be detected by measuring the ability of patient's serum (or IgG) to compete with binding of reagent TSH (or monoclonal anti-TSH-R antibody) to the solubilized TSH receptor. This test is often referred to as TSH receptor antibody (TRAb test). The TSH-R antibody (TRAb) test is less expensive and has a shorter turnaround time than bioassay. It is often used instead of the TSI bioassay, but cannot differentiate between stimulating TRAb and non-stimulating (inhibiting or neutral) TRAb.	Positive in: Graves disease (adults, 80–90%; children, 50–60%), toxic multinodular goiter (15–20%), transient neonatal thyrotoxicosis.	Although TSI is a marker for Graves disease, the test is not necessary for its diagnosis in most cases. It is helpful in confirming subclinical disease in euthyroid patients presenting with exophthalmos. Since none of the treatments for Graves disease are aimed at the underlying pathophysiologic mechanism, but rather ablate thyroid tissue or block thyroid hormone synthesis, TSI may be detectable after apparent cure. Pregnant women with history of Graves disease should be tested for TSI; if present, it may predict neonatal thyrotoxicosis. Gestational thyrotoxicosis, which is due to a combination of hCG cross-reactivity (binding to the TSH receptor) and to transient changes in thyroid hormone protein binding, is not associated with TSI. Finding an elevated TSI in pregnancy suggests underlying Graves disease. Barbesino G et al. Clinical utility of TSH receptor antibodies. J Clin Endocrinol Metab 2013;98:2247. [PMID: 23539719] Dong YH et al. Autoimmune thyroid disease: mechanism, genetics and current knowledge. Eur Rev Med Pharmacol Sci 2014;18:3611. [PMID: 25535130] McLachlan SM et al. Thyrotropin-blocking autoantibodies and thyroid-stimulating autoantibodies: potential mechanisms involved in the pendulum swinging from hypothyroidism to hyperthyroidism or vice versa. Thyroid 2013;23:14. [PMID: 23025526]

(Continued)

Thyroxine, total		
Thyroxine, total, serum or plasma (T4) 5.0–11.0 mcg/dL [64–142 nmol/L] SST, light green PPT, green $	Thyroid hormones (T3, T4) are essential for survival, due to their roles in development, growth, and metabolism. Total T4 is a measure of thyroid gland secretion of T4, bound and free, and thus is influenced by levels of thyroid hormone–binding proteins. Only free T4 is biologically active.	**Increased in:** Hyperthyroidism, increased thyroid-binding globulin (TBG) (eg, pregnancy, drug). Drugs: amiodarone, high-dose β-blockers (especially propranolol). **Decreased in:** Hypothyroidism, low TBG due to illness or drugs, congenital absence of TBG. Drugs: phenytoin, carbamazepine, androgens.

Total T4 should be interpreted with the TBG level, TSH and free T4 measurements.

Mullur R et al. Thyroid hormone regulation of metabolism. Physiol Rev 2014;94:355. [PMID: 24692351]

Papi G et al. Clinical concepts on thyroid emergencies. Front Endocrinol (Lausanne) 2014;5:102. [PMID: 25071718]

Rugge JB et al. Screening for and treatment of thyroid dysfunction: an evidence review for the U.S. Preventive Services Task Force [Internet]. Rockville (MD): Agency for Healthcare Research and Quality (US); 2014 Oct. Report No.: 15-05217-EF-1. [PMID: 25927133]

Schroeder AC et al. Thyroid hormones, T3 and T4, in the brain. Front Endocrinol (Lausanne) 2014;5:40. [PMID: 24744751]

Thyroxine, free		
Thyroxine, free, serum or plasma (free T4 or FT4) 0.8–1.7 ng/dL [10–22 pmol/L] (method-dependent) SST, light green PPT, green $$	FT4 is a direct measure of the free T4 hormone concentration (biologically available hormone). It can be measured by equilibrium dialysis/HPLC–mass spectrometry, although immunoassays are equally effective.	**Increased in:** Hyperthyroidism, nonthyroidal illness, especially psychiatric. Drugs: amiodarone, β-blockers (high-dose). **Decreased in:** Hypothyroidism, nonthyroidal illness. Drugs: phenytoin.

The free thyroxine is used along with sensitive TSH assays for detecting clinical hyperthyroidism and hypothyroidism. The TSH assay detects subclinical thyroid dysfunction (normal FT4) and monitors levothyroxine treatment better, whereas the free thyroxine test detects central hypothyroidism and monitors rapidly changing function status better.

Baumgartner C et al. Subclinical hypothyroidism: summary of evidence in 2014. Swiss Med Wkly 2014;144:w14058. [PMID:25536449]

Kim YA et al. Prevalence and risk factors of subclinical thyroid disease. Endocrinol Metab (Seoul) 2014;29:20. [PMID: 24741450]

	Toxoplasma **antibody**		
Test/Range/Collection	**Physiologic Basis**	**Interpretation**	**Comments**
Toxoplasma antibodies, serum or CSF IgG: <1:16 titer IgM: Infant <1:2 titer Adult <1:8 titer SST (serum) or CSF $$$ Submit paired sera, one collected within 1 week of illness and another 2–3 weeks later.	*Toxoplasma gondii* is an obligate intracellular protozoan that causes human infection via ingestion, transplacental transfer, blood products, or organ transplantation. Cats are the definitive hosts of *T. gondii* and pass oocysts in their feces. Human infection occurs through ingestion of sporulated oocysts or via the transplacental route. In the immunodeficient host (eg, HIV/AIDS), acute infection may progress to lethal meningoencephalitis, pneumonitis, or myocarditis. Chemoprophylaxis should be considered for patients who have a CD4 count < 200/mcL. In acute primary infection, IgM antibodies develop 1–2 weeks after onset of illness, peak in 6–8 weeks, and then decline. IgG antibodies develop on a similar time-course but persist for years. In adult infection, the disease usually represents a reactivation, not a primary infection. Therefore, the IgM test is less useful. Approximately 30% of all US adults have antibodies to *T. gondii*.	**Increased in:** Acute or congenital toxoplasmosis (IgM), previous toxoplasma exposure (IgG), and false-positive (IgM) reactions (SLE, HIV infection, rheumatoid arthritis).	Single IgG titers of > 1:256 are considered diagnostic of active infection; titers of > 1:128 are suspicious. Titers of 1:16–1:64 may merely represent past exposure. If titers subsequently rise, they probably represent early disease. An IgM titer > 1:16 is very important in the diagnosis of congenital toxoplasmosis. High titer IgG antibody results should prompt an IgM test. IgM, however, is generally not detected in adult AIDS patients because toxoplasmosis usually represents a reactivation. Some recommend ordering baseline toxoplasma IgG titers in all asymptomatic HIV-positive patients because a rising toxoplasma titer can help diagnose CNS toxoplasmosis in the future. Culture of the *T. gondii* organism is difficult, and most laboratories are not equipped for the procedure. For immunocompromised patients, diagnosis of acute toxoplasmosis may rely on the demonstration of tachyzoites in fluids or tissues by PCR or microscopic examination. (See also Brain abscess, Chapter 5.) Oz HS. Maternal and congenital toxoplasmosis, currently available and novel therapies in horizon. Front Microbiol 2014;5:385. [PMID: 25104952] Robert-Gangneux F et al. Epidemiology of and diagnostic strategies for toxoplasmosis. Clin Microbiol Rev. 2012; 25:264. [PMID: 22491772] Torgerson PR et al. The global burden of congenital toxoplasmosis: a systematic review. Bull World Health Organ. 2013;91:501 [PMID: 23825877]

Transferrin		
Transferrin (Tf), serum or plasma 200–400 mg/dL SST, PPT, green $	Transferrin is the major plasma transport protein for iron. Only a small amount of transferrin is required for normal homeostasis. The presence of moderate amounts of unsaturated transferrin may be important in control of infections and infestations by iron-requiring organisms. Immunochemical assays of transferrin are more accurate than chemical assays of total iron-binding capacity (TIBC). Assuming a molecular weight for transferrin of 89,000 daltons, 1 mg of transferrin binds 1.25 mcg of iron. Therefore, a serum transferrin level of 300 mg/dL is equal to a TIBC of 375 mcg/dL. The utility of TIBC in addition to serum iron is to calculate the percent saturation of transferrin: $$\% \text{ saturation of } Tf = \frac{\text{serum iron}}{TIBC} \times 100$$ In healthy state, about 33% of the circulating iron binding sites are occupied (interval: 20–50%). % saturation is decreased in iron deficiency and increased in iron overload (eg, hemochromatosis).	**Increased in:** Pregnancy, oral contraceptives, iron deficiency. **Decreased in:** Inherited atransferrinemia (rare), disorders associated with inflammation or necrosis, chronic inflammation or malignancy, generalized malnutrition, nephrotic syndrome, iron overload states.	Indications for transferrin quantitation include screening for nutritional status and differential diagnosis of anemia. To control for effects of estrogens and acute-phase responses, other acute-phase reactant proteins should be assayed at the same time. Iron deficiency and iron overload are best diagnosed using assays of serum levels of iron, transferrin, transferrin saturation, soluble transferrin receptor and ferritin in combination. Transferrin in CSF appears in its desialated form, the Tau protein (β_2-transferrin). This form can be identified electrophoretically by immunofixation with antitransferrin antibody. The clinical application for identification of the Tau protein is in the investigation of rhinorrhea or otorrhea suspected to be of CSF origin. Miller JL. Iron deficiency anemia: a common and curable disease. Cold Spring Harb Perspect Med 2013;3:a011866. [PMID: 23613366] Urrechaga E et al. Biomarkers of hypochromia: the contemporary assessment of iron status and erythropoiesis. Biomed Res Int. 2013;2013:603786. [PMID: 23555091] Wood JC. Guidelines for quantifying iron overload. Hematology Am Soc Hematol Educ Program. 2014;2014:210. [PMID: 25696857]

(Continued)

Transferrin receptor, soluble		
Test/Range/Collection	**Physiologic Basis**	**Interpretation**	**Comments**
Transferrin receptor, soluble (sTfR), serum or plasma Males: 2.2–5 mg/L Females: 1.9–4.4 mg/L (laboratory-specific) SST or green $$	The transferrin receptor (TfR) is expressed on the surface of human cells that require iron and acts as an iron transporting molecule. The expression of TfR depends on the concentration of iron in the cellular cytoplasm. The concentration of soluble TfR (sTfR) has been reported to be proportional to the total amount of cell–associated TfR. Measurement of sTfR is used as a surrogate marker of the status of body iron stores. Iron deficiency causes an elevation of sTfR, whereas iron repletion results in a decrease of sTfR level.	**Increased in:** Iron deficiency anemia, conditions of high red cell turnover (eg, hemolytic anemia), thalassemia.	Soluble TfR is not an acute-phase reactant. The use of sTfR improves the clinical diagnosis of iron deficiency anemia, especially in the presence of coexisting chronic inflammatory diseases, infections or gastrointestinal malignancies. A patient with ferritin ≤10 mcg/L is considered to be iron deficient in all cases regardless of sTfR level. A patient with ferritin ≥220 mcg/L is not considered to be iron deficient. For ferritin values between 10 and 220 mcg/L, levels of sTfR may be used to help identify iron–deficient patients. When assessing iron deficiency, the combination of both ferritin and sTfR levels minimizes false positives due to hemolytic anemia that elevates sTfR and false negatives due to acute–phase reactant elevation of ferritin. Ferritin index (sTfR/ferritin) can also be calculated and helps to improve the diagnostic efficiency in detecting depleted iron stores. Khatami S et al. Evaluation and comparison of soluble transferrin receptor in thalassemia carriers and iron deficient patients. Hemoglobin 2013;37:387. [PMID: 23581600] Lorenz L et al. A review of cord blood concentrations of iron status parameters to define reference ranges for preterm infants. Neonatology 2013;104:194. [PMID: 23989077]

Treponema pallidum antibody		
Treponema pallidum antibody by TP-PA, serum Nonreactive SST $$	The TP-PA test measures specific antibody against *T. pallidum* in a patient's serum by agglutination of *T. pallidum* antigen–coated erythrocytes. Antibodies to nonpathogenic treponemes are first removed by binding to nonpathogenic treponemal antigens.	**Increased in:** Syphilis: primary (64–87%), secondary (96–100%), late latent (96–100%), tertiary (94–100%), infectious mononucleosis, collagen vascular diseases, hyperglobulinemia, and dysglobulinemia.

Historically, the test was used to confirm reactive nontreponemal serologic tests for syphilis (RPR or VDRL). A new "reverse" syphilis testing algorithm using specific treponemal tests for screening and nontreponemal serologic tests for confirmation has been adopted (see Syphilis Serological Testing, p. 200).

Compared with FTA-ABS (p. 101), TP-PA is slightly less sensitive in early primary syphilis (See Table 8–21.)

Because the test usually remains positive for long periods of time regardless of whether adequate therapy has been given, it is not useful in assessing the effectiveness of therapy.

In one study, 36 months after treatment of syphilis, 13% of patients had nonreactive TP-PA tests.

The TP-PA, like the FTA-ABS, is not recommended for CSF specimens. VDRL is the preferred test for CSF.

Kaur G et al. Syphilis testing in blood donors: an update. Blood Transfus 2015;13:197. [PMID: 25545876]

Morshed MG et al. Recent trends in the serologic diagnosis of syphilis. Clin Vaccine Immunol 2015;22:137. [PMID: 25428245]

(Continued)

Test/Range/Collection	Physiologic Basis	Interpretation	Comments
Triglycerides, serum or plasma (TG) <1.65 mmol/L [<1.65 g/L] SST, green, PPT $ Fasting specimen required.	Dietary fat is hydrolyzed in the small intestine, absorbed and resynthesized by mucosal cells, and secreted into lacteals as chylomicrons. Triglycerides in the chylomicrons are cleared from the blood by tissue lipoprotein lipase. Endogenous triglyceride production occurs in the liver. These triglycerides are transported in association with β-lipoproteins in very-low-density lipoproteins (VLDL).	**Increased in:** Hypothyroidism, diabetes mellitus (diabetic dyslipidemia), nephrotic syndrome, chronic alcoholism (fatty liver), biliary tract obstruction, stress, familial lipoprotein lipase deficiency, familial dysbetalipoproteinemia, familial combined hyperlipidemia, obesity, the metabolic syndrome, viral hepatitis, cirrhosis, pancreatitis, chronic renal failure, gout, pregnancy, glycogen storage diseases types I, III, and VI, anorexia nervosa, dietary excess. Drugs: β-blockers, cholestyramine, corticosteroids, diazepam, diuretics, estrogens, oral contraceptives. **Decreased in:** Tangier disease (α-lipoprotein deficiency), hypo- and abetalipoproteinemia, malnutrition, malabsorption, parenchymal liver disease, hyperthyroidism, intestinal lymphangiectasia. Drugs: ascorbic acid, clofibrate, nicotinic acid, gemfibrozil.	If serum is clear, the serum triglyceride level is generally <350 mg/dL. Elevated triglycerides are now considered an independent risk factor for coronary artery disease and a major risk factor for acute pancreatitis, particularly when serum triglyceride levels are > 1000 mg/dL. However, screening is not currently recommended. Triglycerides > 1000 mg/dL can be seen when a primary lipid disorder is exacerbated by alcohol or fat intake or by corticosteroid or estrogen therapy. Berglund L et al. Treatment options for hypertriglyceridemia: from risk reduction to pancreatitis. Best Pract Res Clin Endocrinol Metab. 2014;28:423. [PMID: 24840268] Parhofer KG. Interaction between glucose and lipid metabolism: more than diabetic dyslipidemia. Diabetes Metab J 2015;39:353. [PMID: 26566492] Pirillo A et al. Update on the management of severe hypertriglyceridemia—focus on free fatty acid forms of omega-3. Drug Des Devel Ther 2015;9:2129. [PMID: 25914523]
Triiodothyronine, total, serum or plasma (T$_3$) 95–190 ng/dL [1.5–2.9 nmol/L] SST, light green PPT, green $$	T$_3$ is the primary active thyroid hormone. Approximately 80% of T$_3$ is produced by extrathyroidal deiodination of T$_4$ and the rest by thyroid gland. Total T$_3$ is influenced by levels of thyroxine binding proteins. Thyroid hormones (T$_3$, T$_4$) are essential for survival, due to their essential roles in development, growth, and metabolism.	**Increased in:** Hyperthyroidism (some), increased thyroid-binding globulin. **Decreased in:** Hypothyroidism, nonthyroidal illness, decreased thyroid-binding globulin. Drugs: amiodarone.	T$_3$ may be increased in approximately 5% of hyperthyroid patients in whom free T$_4$ is normal (T$_3$ toxicosis). Therefore, test is indicated when hyperthyroidism is suspected and free T$_4$ value is normal. Test is of no value in the diagnosis and treatment of primary hypothyroidism. T$_3$ levels are typically low in sick or hospitalized euthyroid patients. Mullur R et al. Thyroid hormone regulation of metabolism. Physiol Rev 2014;94:355. [PMID: 24692351] Papi G et al. Clinical concepts on thyroid emergencies. Front Endocrinol (Lausanne) 2014;5:102. [PMID: 25071718] Rugge JB et al. Screening for and treatment of thyroid dysfunction: an evidence review for the U.S. Preventive Services Task Force [Internet]. Rockville (MD): Agency for Healthcare Research and Quality (US); 2014 Oct. Report No.: 15-05217-EF-1. [PMID: 25927133] Schroeder AC et al. Thyroid hormones, T3 and T4, in the brain. Front Endocrinol (Lausanne) 2014;5:40. [PMID: 24744751]

Troponin-I, cardiac			
Troponin-I, cardiac, serum or plasma (cTnI) <0.05 ng/mL (method-dependent) PPT, SST, red $$	Troponin is the contractile regulatory protein of striated muscle. It contains three subunits: T, C, and I. Subunit I consists of three forms, which are found in slow-twitch skeletal muscle, fast-twitch skeletal muscle, and cardiac muscle, respectively. Troponin I is predominantly a structural protein and is released into the circulation after cellular necrosis. Cardiac troponin I (cTnI) is expressed only in cardiac muscle, and thus its presence in serum can distinguish between myocardial injury and skeletal muscle injury. cTnI is measured by immunometric assays using monoclonal antibodies. Between-method variation is 2- to 5-fold due to lack of calibration standard. Sensitive cTnI immunoassays with diagnostic thresholds of 0.02–0.05 ng/mL are routinely used. Although point-of-care cTnI assays are also used, they are less sensitive.	**Increased in:** Myocardial infarction (MI), cardiac trauma, cardiac surgery, myocardial damage following percutaneous transluminal coronary angioplasty, and other cardiac interventions, nonischemic dilated cardiomyopathy, acute and chronic heart failure, prolonged supraventricular tachycardia, acute dissection of the ascending aorta. Slight elevations (eg, <1.0 ng/mL) are sometimes noted in patients after noncardiac surgery and in patients with recent aggravated unstable angina, muscular disorders, CNS disorders, HIV infection, chronic renal failure, cirrhosis, sepsis, lung diseases, and endocrine disorders. **Not increased in:** Skeletal muscle disease (myopathy, myositis, dystrophy), external electrical cardioversion, noncardiac trauma or surgery, rhabdomyolysis, severe muscular exertion, chronic renal failure.	Cardiac troponin I is a more specific marker for MI than CK-MB and is the preferred marker for the diagnosis of MI. cTnI appears in serum approximately 4 hours after onset of chest pain, peaks at 8–12 hours, and persists for 5–7 days. This prolonged persistence gives it much greater sensitivity than CK-MB for diagnosis of MI beyond the first 36–48 hours. Given its utility in detection of acute coronary syndrome (ACS), the plasma troponin is important in the evaluation and stratification of patients with chest pain in the emergency room. Blood samples should be obtained for testing at hospital presentation and 6–9 hours later. With a clinical history suggestive of ACS, a cTnI level exceeding 0.05 ng/mL (method-dependent) on at least one occasion during the first 24 hours after the clinical event is indicative of myocardial necrosis consistent with MI. Note that cTnI elevations cannot be utilized in isolation to make a diagnosis of MI. In patients with suspected ACS, using a high-sensitivity cTnI assay (lowering the diagnostic threshold value) increases the diagnosis of MI and identifies patients at high risk of recurrent MI and death. Cardiac TnI elevation has prognostic value in patients presenting with ACS and the degree of elevation correlates with infarct size. Each assay has unique performance characteristics, but guidelines recommend using the 99th percentile value from a normal reference population for a given assay to define whether myocardial injury is present. Patients with troponin elevation after noncardiac surgery are at higher short-term and long-term risk of morbidity and mortality. Horr S et al. Troponin elevation after noncardiac surgery: significance and management. Cleve Clin J Med 2015;82:595. [PMID: 26366956] Mair J. High-sensitivity cardiac troponins in everyday clinical practice. World J Cardiol 2014;6:175. [PMID: 24772257] Mueller C. Biomarkers and acute coronary syndromes: an update. Eur Heart J 2014;35:552. [PMID: 24357507]

(Continued)

Test/Range/Collection	Physiologic Basis	Interpretation	Comments
Tularemia agglutinins, serum <1:80 titer SST $$ Specimen label must be signed by the person drawing the blood.	*Francisella tularensis* is a gram-negative bacterial organism of wild rodents (rabbits and hares) that infects humans (eg, trappers and skinners) via contact with animal tissues, by the bite of certain ticks and flies, and by consumption of undercooked meat or contaminated water. The infectious dose is very low. Agglutinating antibodies appear in 10–14 days and peak in 5–10 weeks. A 4-fold rise in titers is typically needed to prove acute infection. Titers decrease over years.	**Increased in:** Tularemia ("rabbit fever"); cross-reaction with brucella antigens and proteus OX-19 antigen (but at lower titers).	Single titers of > 1:160 are indicative of infection. Maximum titers are > 1:280. A history of exposure to rabbits, ticks, dogs, cats, or skunks is suggestive of, but not a requirement for, the diagnosis. The most common presentation is a single area of painful lymphadenopathy with low-grade fever. Initial treatment should be empiric. Culture of the organism is difficult, requiring special media, and hazardous to laboratory personnel. Serologic tests are the mainstay of diagnosis. Besides serologic testing, immunofluorescence staining and PCR can also be used for diagnosis. Adalja AA et al. Clinical management of potential bioterrorism-related conditions. N Engl J Med 2015;372:954. [PMID: 25738671] Ellis J et al. Tularemia. Clin Microbiol Rev 2002;15:631. [PMID: 12364373] Jorgensen JH et al (editors): *Manual of Clinical Microbiology*, 11th ed. ASM Press, 2015.
Type and crossmatch (T/C), serum and red cells (type and cross) Red or lavender/pink $$ A second "check" specimen is needed at some hospitals. The number of RBC units required must be specified.	A type and crossmatch involves ABO and Rh typing, antibody screen, and crossmatch. (Compare with Type and screen, below.) If the recipient's serum contains a clinically significant RBC alloantibody by antibody screen or by history, the antibody is then identified and RBC units negative for the corresponding antigen are selected. A crossmatch testing recipient serum (or plasma) against donor cells is also performed using anti-human globulin (AHG) to detect recipient antibodies to donor red cells (Coombs crossmatch). If no clinically significant antibodies are detected in current screen and there is no record of previous detection of such antibodies, only a method to detect ABO incompatibility, such as an immediate-spin or computer crossmatch, is required.	See Type and screen below.	A type and screen is adequate preparation for operative procedures unlikely to require transfusion. Unnecessary type and crossmatch orders reduce blood availability and add to labor and reagent costs. A preordering system should be in place, indicating the number of units of blood likely to be needed for each operative procedure. Genotyping is a powerful adjunct to serologic testing and in the future could enable electronic selection of units with antigen matched to recipients at multiple blood group loci and could therefore improve transfusion outcomes. Sandler SG et al. Historic milestones in the evolution of the cross-match. Immunohematol 2009;25:147. [PMID: 20406021] *Technical Manual of the American Association of Blood Banks*, 18th ed. American Association of Blood Banks, 2014.

Type and screen	Uric acid
Type and screen (T/S), serum and red cells Red or lavender/pink $$$$ Specimen label must be signed by the person drawing the blood. A second "check" specimen is needed at some hospitals.	Uric acid, serum or plasma Males: 2.4–7.4 mg/dL [Males: 140–440 mcmol/L] Females 1.4–5.8 mg/dL [Females: 80–350 mcmol/L] SST, PPT, green $
Type and screen includes ABO and Rh typing and antibody screen. (Compare with Type and crossmatch, above.) This is a procedure in which the patient's blood sample is tested for ABO, Rh(D), and unexpected antibodies, then stored in the transfusion service for future crossmatch if a unit is needed for transfusion.	Uric acid is an end product of nucleoprotein metabolism and is excreted by the kidney. An increase in serum uric acid concentration occurs with increased nucleoprotein synthesis or catabolism (blood dyscrasias, chemotherapy of leukemia or solid tumor) or decreased renal uric acid excretion (eg, thiazide diuretic therapy or renal failure).
A negative antibody screen implies that a recipient can receive uncrossmatched type-specific blood with minimal risk. If the recipient's serum contains a clinically significant alloantibody by antibody screen, a crossmatch is required if transfusion is needed.	Increased in: Renal failure, gout, myeloproliferative disorders (leukemia, lymphoma, myeloma, polycythemia vera), psoriasis, glycogen storage disease (type I), Lesch-Nyhan syndrome (X-linked hypoxanthine-guanine phosphoribosyltransferase deficiency), lead nephropathy, hypertensive diseases of pregnancy (preeclampsia and eclampsia), menopause, syndrome X (obesity, insulin resistance, hypertension, hyperuricemia, dyslipidemia). Drugs: antimetabolite and chemotherapeutic agents, diuretics, ethanol, nicotinic acid, salicylates (low-dose), theophylline. Decreased in: Syndrome of inappropriate antidiuretic hormone (SIADH), xanthine oxidase deficiency, low-purine diet, Fanconi syndrome, neoplastic disease (various, causing increased renal excretion), liver disease. Drugs: salicylates (high-dose), allopurinol or febuxostat (xanthine oxidase inhibitors) or uricase.
Type and screen is indicated for patients undergoing operative procedures unlikely to require transfusion. However, in the absence of preoperative indications, routine preoperative blood type and screen testing is not cost-effective and may be eliminated for some procedures, such as laparoscopic cholecystectomy, expected vaginal delivery, and vaginal hysterectomy. Technical Manual of the American Association of Blood Banks, 18th ed. American Association of Blood Banks, 2014.	Sex, age, and renal function affect uric acid levels. Both non-modifiable (sex, age, race, genetics) and modifiable (diet, lifestyle) risk factors have been associated with development of gout. The incidence of hyperuricemia is greater in some ethnic groups (eg, Filipinos) than others (whites). Elevated uric acid concentration is associated with cardiovascular and renal diseases, particularly hypertension. Gout with elevated uric acid levels is an independent risk factor for heart disease. Serum uric acid is a poor predictor of maternal and fetal complications in women with preeclampsia. Giordano C et al. Uric acid as a marker of kidney disease: review of the current literature. Dis Markers 2015;2015:382918. [PMID: 26106252] MacFarlane LA et al. Gout: a review of nonmodifiable and modifiable risk factors. Rheum Dis Clin North Am 2014;40:581. [PMID: 25437279] Mirrakhimov AE et al. Tumor lysis syndrome: a clinical review. World J Crit Care Med 2015;4:130. [PMID: 25938028]

(Continued)

Test/Range/Collection	Physiologic Basis	Interpretation	Comments
Vanillylmandelic acid			**Vanillylmandelic acid**
Vanillylmandelic acid, urine (VMA) <15 mg/g creatinine [age-dependent 10–35 mcmol/d] Urine container containing acetic or hydrochloric acid $$$ Collect random sample or 24-hour urine.	Catecholamines are secreted in excess by pheochromocytomas and other neural crest tumors, and are metabolized by the enzymes monoamine oxidase and catechol-*O*-methyltransferase to VMA, which is excreted in urine.	**Increased in:** Pheochromocytoma (64% sensitivity, 95% specificity), neuroblastoma, ganglioneuroma, generalized anxiety. **Decreased in:** Drugs: monoamine oxidase inhibitors (MAOIs), eg, phenelzine.	Because of its relatively low sensitivity, test is not commonly used for the diagnosis of pheochromocytoma. A urine or plasma free metanephrines test is the recommended initial test for suspected cases. (See also Pheochromocytoma algorithm, Figure 9–25.) Elevated VMA level is suggestive of pheochromocytoma, but is not diagnostic. A normal VMA level does not rule out pheochromocytoma. Test is usually ordered along with homovanillic acid (HVA) on random urine sample for screening children for catecholamine-secreting tumors (eg, neuroblastoma) and other neural crest tumors, and for monitoring patients who have had treatment for these tumors. The ratio of urinary VMA to urinary creatinine (VMA/Cr, mg/g) is typically reported. Patients on L-dopa may have falsely elevated VMA levels; the medication should be discontinued for at least 24 hours before collecting the urine sample. Barco S et al. Urinary homovanillic and vanillylmandelic acid in the diagnosis of neuroblastoma: report from the Italian Cooperative Group for Neuroblastoma. Clin Biochem 2014;47:848. [PMID: 24769278] Hori T et al. Malignant pheochromocytoma: hepatectomy for liver metastases. World J Gastrointest Surg 2013;5:309. [PMID: 24520430]
			VDRL test, serum
Venereal Disease Research Laboratory test, serum (VDRL) Nonreactive SST $	This syphilis test measures nontreponemal antibodies (both IgM and IgG) that are produced when *Treponema pallidum* interacts with host tissues. The VDRL usually becomes reactive at a titer of > 1:32 within 1–3 weeks after the genital chancre appears.	**Increased in:** Syphilis: primary (59–87%), secondary (100%), late latent (79–91%), tertiary (37–94%), collagen vascular diseases (rheumatoid arthritis, SLE), infections (mononucleosis, leprosy, malaria), pregnancy, drug abuse.	VDRL has historically been used as a syphilis screening test and in suspected cases of primary and secondary syphilis. Positive tests should be confirmed with specific treponemal tests (FTA-ABS or TP-PA). The VDRL has sensitivity and specificity similar to the rapid plasma reagin (RPR). (See Table 8–21.) New "reverse" syphilis testing algorithm using treponemal tests for screening and nontreponemal serologic tests for confirmation has been adopted (see Syphilis Serological Testing, p. 200). Test can be used for monitoring treatment efficacy in patients with active syphilitic infection. Kaur G et al. Syphilis testing in blood donors: an update. Blood Transfus 2015;13:197. [PMID: 25545876] Morshed MG et al. Recent trends in the serologic diagnosis of syphilis. Clin Vaccine Immunol 2015;22:137. [PMID: 25428245]

Vitamin B$_{12}$		
Vitamin B$_{12}$, serum or plasma 170–820 pg/mL [121–600 pmol/L] SST, red, green $$$ Serum vitamin B$_{12}$ specimens should be frozen if not analyzed immediately.	Vitamin B$_{12}$ is a necessary cofactor for three important biochemical processes: conversion of methylmalonyl-CoA to succinyl-CoA and methylation of homocysteine to methionine and demethylation of methyltetrahydrofolate to tetrahydrofolate (THF). All vitamin B$_{12}$ comes from ingestion of foods of animal origin. Vitamin B$_{12}$ in serum is protein bound, 70% to transcobalamin I (TC I) and 30% to transcobalamin II (TC II). The B$_{12}$ bound to TC II is physiologically active; that bound to TC I is not.	**Increased in:** Leukemia (acute myelocytic, chronic myelocytic, chronic lymphocytic, monocytic), marked leukocytosis, polycythemia vera. (Increased B$_{12}$ levels are not diagnostically useful.) **Decreased in:** Pernicious anemia, gastrectomy, gastric carcinoma, malabsorption (sprue, celiac disease (gluten enteropathy), steatorrhea, regional enteritis, fistulas, bowel resection, ileal disease, *Diphyllobothrium latum* [fish tapeworm] infestation, small bowel bacterial overgrowth), pregnancy, dietary deficiency, HIV infection (with or without malabsorption), chronic high-flux hemodialysis, Alzheimer disease, drugs (eg, omeprazole, metformin, carbamazepine).	The previously used Schilling test is no longer used for evaluating pernicious anemia. New testing algorithms have been developed using B$_{12}$, methylmalonic acid (MMA), intrinsic factor antibodies, parietal cell autoantibodies, and serum gastrin measurements. Different methods (chemiluminescence immunoassay, radioimmunoassay, etc) are available for B$_{12}$ measurement. Test results are very variable. In general, serum B$_{12}$ <170 pg/mL is consistent with deficiency, 170–300 pg/mL is borderline insufficiency, and > 300 pg/mL is adequate. Low serum B$_{12}$ levels warrant treatment; intermediate levels should be followed by repeated serum tests or by urine methylmalonic acid tests (see Methylmalonic acid, p. 160) as well as by serum homocysteine levels. Neurologic disorders caused by low serum B$_{12}$ level can occur in the absence of macrocytic anemia or pancytopenia. Briani C et al. Cobalamin deficiency: clinical picture and radiological findings. Nutrients 2013;5:4521. [PMID: 24248213] Green R. Anemias beyond B$_{12}$ and iron deficiency: the buzz about other B's; elementary, and nonelementary problems. Hematology Am Soc Hematol Educ Program 2012;2012:492. [PMID: 23233624] Wong CW. Vitamin B$_{12}$ deficiency in the elderly: is it worth screening? Hong Kong Med J 2015;21:155. [PMID: 25756278]

(Continued)

Vitamin D, 25-hydroxy

Test/Range/Collection	Physiologic Basis	Interpretation	Comments
Vitamin D, 25-hydroxy, serum or plasma (25[OH]D) 20–50 ng/mL [50–125 nmol/L] SST or green $$$	The vitamin D system functions to maintain serum calcium levels. Vitamin D is a fat-soluble steroid hormone. Two molecular forms exist: D_3 (cholecalciferol), synthesized in the epidermis, and D_2 (ergocalciferol), derived from plant sources. To become active, both need to be further metabolized. Two sequential hydroxylations occur: in the liver to 25(OH)D and then, in the kidney, to 1,25[OH]$_2$D. Besides consequences for bone health, vitamin D deficiency reportedly is associated with a number of conditions such as cardiovascular disease, autoimmunity and cancer; however, evidence-based cause-and-effect relationships have not been established.	**Increased in:** Heavy milk drinkers (up to 64 ng/mL), vitamin D intoxication, sun exposure. **Decreased in:** Dietary deficiency, malabsorption, rickets, osteomalacia, biliary and portal cirrhosis, nephrotic syndrome, renal failure, inadequate sun exposure, advanced age (> 70), primary hyperparathyroidism. Drugs: phenytoin, phenobarbital.	Serum or plasma total 25(OH)D is an integrated marker of vitamin D status, incorporating endogenous synthesis from solar exposure, dietary intake, fortified products and/or supplements. There is no universal or strong evidence-based consensus on the appropriate level of 25(OH)D. However, according to a 2011 US Institute of Medicine Report, a 25(OH)D level of 20–30 ng/mL is all that is needed for bone and general health, and nearly everyone (97.5%) in the general population is in that range. A 25(OH)D level above 30 ng/mL has not been consistently associated with increased health benefits, and, in fact, risks have been identified for outcomes at levels above 50 ng/mL. Routine screening for vitamin D deficiency is not necessary. Patients with the following conditions should be considered for testing: osteoporosis, osteomalacia, malabsorption, liver disease, pancreatic insufficiency, chronic kidney disease, COPD, bariatric surgery, cancer, bedridden or home-bound, obesity, taking anticonvulsants or long-term glucocorticoids, atraumatic fractures, elderly (> 70 years old), and chronic inflammatory conditions. Vitamin D toxicity can occur after taking excessive doses of vitamin D, a condition that is manifested by hypercalcemia, hyperphosphate-mia, soft tissue calcification, and renal failure. Bikle DD. Vitamin D metabolism, mechanism of action, and clinical applications. Chem Biol 2014;21:319. [PMID: 24529992] LeBlanc E et al. Screening for vitamin D deficiency: systematic review for the U.S. Preventive Services Task Force Recommendation [Internet]. Rockville (MD): Agency for Healthcare Research and Quality (US); 2014 Nov. [PMID: 25521000]

	Vitamin D, 1,25-dihydroxy	von Willebrand factor

Vitamin D, 1,25-dihydroxy, serum or plasma (1,25[OH]₂D)

20–76 pg/mL

SST or green

$$$$

Vitamin D, either produced in the skin or absorbed from the diet, must be activated first to 25[OH]D, and then to its active form, 1,25[OH]₂D.

1,25[OH]₂D is the primary regulator of calcium and phosphorus homeostasis.

The main actions of vitamin D are the acceleration of calcium and phosphate absorption in the intestine and stimulation of bone resorption.

Increased in: Primary hyperparathyroidism, idiopathic hypercalciuria, sarcoidosis, some lymphomas, 1,25[OH]₂D-resistant rickets, normal growth (children), pregnancy, lactation, vitamin D toxicity.

Decreased in: Chronic renal failure, anephric patients, hypoparathyroidism, pseudohypoparathyroidism, 1-α-hydroxylase deficiency, postmenopausal osteoporosis.

Test is rarely needed.

Measurement of 1,25[OH]₂D is only useful in distinguishing 1-α-hydroxylase deficiency from 1,25[OH]₂D-resistant rickets or in monitoring vitamin D status of patients with chronic renal failure.

Test is not useful for assessment of vitamin D intoxication because of efficient feedback regulation of 1,25[OH]₂D synthesis.

Parathyroid tissue expresses the vitamin D receptor, and it is thought that circulating 1,25[OH]₂D participates in the regulation of parathyroid cell proliferation, differentiation, and secretion. Primary hyperparathyroidism is usually associated with increased plasma 1,25[OH]₂D.

Bikle DD. Vitamin D metabolism, mechanism of action, and clinical applications. Chem Biol 2014;21:319. [PMID: 24529992]

Vojinovic J et al. Vitamin D—update for the pediatric rheumatologists. Pediatr Rheumatol Online J 2015;13:18. [PMID: 26022196]

von Willebrand factor (vWF), plasma

Blue

Antigen (vWFAg by enzyme-linked immunosorbent assay [ELISA])

Activity (ristocetin cofactor)

50–180%

$$$

vWF is an endothelium-derived multimeric plasma protein with two important functions in hemostasis: (1) promoting platelet adhesion at the site of injury; and (2) transporting and stabilizing factor VIII in plasma.

von Willebrand disease (vWD) is caused by hereditary quantitative (types 1 and 3) or qualitative (types 2A, 2B, 2M, 2N) defects of the vWF. Acquired vWD can occur but is rare.

Increased in: Inflammatory states (acute-phase reactant).

Decreased in: Hereditary or acquired vWD: type 1, decreased antigen and activity levels; type 3, undetectable antigen and activity; type 2, antigen level may be normal, but activity is impaired (normal activity in 2B).

The deficiency or abnormal function of vWF causes vWD, the most frequent inherited bleeding disorder.

In vWD, the platelet count and morphology are generally normal, and the bleeding time is usually prolonged (markedly prolonged by aspirin). The PTT may not be prolonged if factor VIII coagulant level is > 30%.

Diagnosis of vWD is suggested by bleeding symptoms and family history. Initial tests for vWD (bleeding time or PFA-100 CT, platelet count, PTT) are typically followed by the diagnostic tests: vWF antigen and activity. Further tests may be necessary to distinguish the subtypes of vWD, such as vWF multimer analysis, factor VIII assay, vWF propeptide to vWF antigen ratio, platelet aggregation studies (low-dose ristocetin), etc.

Castaman G et al. Laboratory aspects of von Willebrand disease: test repertoire and options for activity assays and genetic analysis. Haemophilia 2014;20(Suppl 4):65. [PMID: 24762278]

Springer TA. von Willebrand factor, Jedi knight of the bloodstream. Blood 2014;124:1412. [PMID: 24928861]

(Continued)

	White blood cell count and differential			Zinc protoporphyrin (ZPP)

Test/Range/Collection	Physiologic Basis	Interpretation	Comments
White blood cell (WBC) count and differential, blood Reference ranges are age- and laboratory-specific Adult ranges: WBC 4.5–11.0 × 10³/mcL; differential: segmented neutrophils 50–70%; band neutrophils 0–5%; lymphocytes 20–40%; monocytes 2–6%; eosinophils 1–4%; basophils 0–1%. *Panic:* WBC <1.5 × 10³/mcL and/or ANC <0.5 × 10³/mcL Lavender $	The WBC count and differential determine the total number of white blood cells as well as the percentage and absolute number of each type of white cell in a blood sample. It is typically generated by an automated laboratory hematology analyzer as part of the CBC panel. The basic principles used for WBC count and differential are instrument-dependent (eg, Beckman Coulter, Siemens, Abbott, Sysmex). If indicated, manual differential is also performed by examining a blood smear under a microscope.	**Increased in:** Acute infections, inflammatory disorders, acute and chronic leukemias, myeloproliferative disorders, solid tumor (paraneoplastic reaction), circulating lymphoma, tissue injury/necrosis, G-CSF stimulation, various drugs, corticosteroids, allergies, hypersensitivity reactions, stress, smoking. **Decreased in:** Infections, constitutional and acquired myeloid hypoplasia, myelosuppression (eg, chemotherapy, radiation, various drugs), myelodysplasia, collagen vascular diseases, hypersplenism, cyclic neutropenia, autoimmune neutropenia, alcoholism.	There are five types of white cells, each with different functions: neutrophils, lymphocytes, monocytes, eosinophils, and basophils. Absolute counts for individual cell populations can be calculated from a combination of the WBC count and the percentage of each cell type from the differential. It is important to perform a manual differential in certain conditions such as presence of blasts, immature granulocytes, nucleated red blood cells, leukemia or lymphoma cells, plasma cells, or myelodysplasia. Automated imaging systems for manual differential are now routinely available. Elliott MA et al. Chronic neutrophilic leukemia 2014: update on diagnosis, molecular genetics, and management. Am J Hematol 2014;89:651. [PMID: 24845374] Templeton AJ et al. Prognostic role of neutrophil-to-lymphocyte ratio in solid tumors: a systematic review and meta-analysis. J Natl Cancer Inst 2014;106:dju124. [PMID: 24875653]
Zinc protoporphyrin (ZPP), whole blood 0–69 μmol/mol hem (method-dependent) Lavender $$$	Protoporphyrin is produced in the next-to-last step of heme biosynthesis. In the last step, iron is incorporated into protoporphyrin to produce heme. Enzyme deficiencies (ferrochelatase deficiency or inhibition), lack of iron, or presence of interfering substances (lead) can disrupt this process. A zinc ion is alternatively incorporated, thereby increasing the concentration of zinc protoporphyrin (APP) in red blood cells.	**Increased in:** Decreased iron incorporation into heme (iron deficiency, anemia of chronic inflammation or infection, and chronic lead poisoning), erythropoietic protoporphyria.	ZPP can be used to screen for lead poisoning in children provided that iron deficiency has been ruled out. It is also used to help diagnose iron deficiency and anemia of chronic inflammation. Cameron BM et al. Estimating the prevalence of iron deficiency in the first two years of life: technical and measurement issues. Nutr Rev 2011;69(Suppl 1):S49. [PMID: 22043883] Dapul H et al. Lead poisoning in children. Adv Pediatr 2014;61:313. [PMID: 25037135]

4

Therapeutic Drug Monitoring & Pharmacogenetic Testing: Principles & Test Interpretation

Diana Nicoll, MD, PhD, MPA, and Chuanyi Mark Lu, MD

UNDERLYING ASSUMPTIONS

The basic assumptions underlying therapeutic drug monitoring (see Table 4–1) are that drug metabolism varies from patient to patient and that the plasma level of a drug is more closely related to the drug's therapeutic effect or toxicity than is the dosage. For certain drugs that are intended for long-term use (see Table 4–2), close monitoring with appropriate routine hematology and chemistry tests may be necessary to avoid or minimize drug-associated adverse events.

The basic principle underlying pharmacogenetics testing (see Table 4–3) is that the identification of genetic factors that influence drug absorption, metabolism, or action at the target level may allow for individualized therapy and thereby help optimize drug efficacy and minimize drug toxicity.

INDICATIONS FOR DRUG MONITORING

Drug monitoring involves direct measurement of plasma drug level or routine laboratory testing. Drugs with **a narrow therapeutic index** (where therapeutic drug levels do not differ greatly from levels associated with serious toxicity) should have drug level monitoring. *Example:* Lithium.

Patients who have **impaired clearance of a drug with a narrow therapeutic index** are candidates for drug level monitoring. The clearance mechanism of the drug involved must be known. *Example:* Patients with renal failure have decreased clearance of gentamicin and therefore are at a higher risk for gentamicin toxicity.

Drugs whose **toxicity is difficult to distinguish from a patient's underlying disease** may require drug level monitoring. *Example:* Theophylline in patients with chronic obstructive pulmonary disease.

Drugs whose efficacy is **difficult to establish clinically** may require monitoring of plasma drug levels. *Example:* Phenytoin.

Drugs that may cause significant **side effects or adverse events if used for an extended period of time** may require monitoring with routine laboratory tests. *Example:* Clozapine (which can cause severe neutropenia, requiring long-term monitoring of the white blood cell count).

221

SITUATIONS IN WHICH DRUG MONITORING MAY NOT BE USEFUL

Drugs that can be given in extremely high doses before toxicity is apparent are not candidates for monitoring. *Example:* Penicillin.

If better means of assessing drug effects are available, drug level monitoring may not be appropriate. *Example:* Warfarin (which is typically monitored by prothrombin time and International Normalized Ratio (INR) determinations, not by serum levels).

Drug level monitoring to assess compliance is limited by the inability to distinguish noncompliance from rapid metabolism without direct inpatient scrutiny of drug administration.

Drug toxicity cannot be diagnosed with drug levels alone; it is a clinical diagnosis. Drug levels within the usual therapeutic range do not rule out drug toxicity in a given patient. *Example:* Digoxin (where other physiologic variables such as hypokalemia affect drug toxicity).

In summary, therapeutic drug monitoring may be useful to guide dosage adjustment of certain drugs in certain patients. Patient compliance is essential if drug monitoring data are to be correctly interpreted.

OTHER INFORMATION REQUIRED FOR EFFECTIVE DRUG MONITORING

Reliability of the Analytic Method

The analytic **sensitivity** of the drug monitoring method must be adequate. For some drugs, plasma levels are in the nanogram per milliliter range. *Example:* Tricyclic antidepressants, digoxin.

The **specificity** of the method must be known, because the drug's metabolites or other drugs may interfere. Interference by metabolites, which may or may not be pharmacologically active, is of particular concern in immunologic assay methods using antibodies to the parent drug.

The **precision** of the method must be known to assess whether changes in levels are caused by method imprecision or by clinical changes.

Reliability of the Therapeutic Range

Establishing the therapeutic range for a drug requires a reliable clinical assessment of its therapeutic and toxic effects, together with plasma drug level measurements by a particular analytic method. In practice, as newer, more specific analytic methods are introduced, the therapeutic ranges for those methods are estimated by comparing the old and new methodologies—without clinical correlation.

PHARMACOKINETIC PARAMETERS

Five pharmacokinetic parameters that are important in therapeutic drug monitoring include:

1. *Bioavailability.* The bioavailability of a drug depends in part on its formulation. A drug that is significantly metabolized as it first passes through the liver exhibits a marked "first-pass effect," reducing the effective oral absorption of the drug. A reduction in this first-pass effect (eg, because of decreased hepatic blood flow in heart failure) could cause a clinically significant increase in effective oral drug absorption.

2. *Volume of distribution and distribution phases.* The volume of distribution of a drug determines the plasma concentration reached after a loading dose. The distribution phase is the time taken for a drug to distribute from the plasma to the periphery. Drug levels drawn before completion of a long distribution phase may not reflect levels of pharmacologically active drug at sites of action. *Examples:* Digoxin, lithium.

3. *Clearance.* Clearance is either renal or nonrenal (usually hepatic). Whereas changes in renal clearance can be predicted on the basis of serum creatinine or creatinine clearance,

there is no routine liver function test for assessment of hepatic drug metabolism. For most therapeutic drugs measured, clearance is independent of plasma drug concentration, so that a change in dose is reflected in a similar change in plasma level. If, however, clearance is dose dependent, dosage adjustments produce disproportionately large changes in plasma levels and must be made cautiously. *Example:* Phenytoin.

4. *Half-life.* The half-life of a drug depends on its volume of distribution and its clearance and determines the time taken to reach a steady state level. In three or four half-lives, the drug level will be 87.5–93.75% of the way to steady state. Patients with decreased drug clearance and therefore increased drug half-lives will take longer to reach a higher steady-state level. In general, because non–steady-state drug levels are potentially misleading and can be difficult to interpret, it is recommended that most clinical monitoring be done at steady state.

5. *Protein binding of drugs.* All routine drug level analysis involves assessment of both protein-bound and free drug. However, pharmacologic activity depends on only the free drug level. Changes in protein binding (eg, in uremia or hypoalbuminemia) may significantly affect interpretation of reported levels for drugs that are highly protein-bound. *Example:* Phenytoin. In cases in which the ratio of free to total measured drug level is increased, the usual therapeutic range based on total drug level does not apply.

Drug Interactions

For patients receiving several medications, the possibility of drug interactions affecting drug elimination must be considered. *Example:* Quinidine, verapamil, and amiodarone decrease digoxin clearance.

Time to Draw Levels

In general, the specimen should be drawn after steady state is reached (at least three or four half-lives after a dosage adjustment) and just before the next dose (trough level).

Peak and trough levels may be indicated to evaluate the dosage of drugs whose half-lives are much shorter than the dosing interval. *Example:* Gentamicin.

GENETIC INFLUENCES ON THERAPEUTIC DRUG RESPONSE

Genetic influences on drug response can be divided into four categories:

1. *Altered pharmacokinetics, ie, drug absorption, distribution, tissue localization, biotransformation, and excretion.* Examples include genetic polymorphisms in cytochrome P450 oxidase (CYP), thiopurine S-methyltransferase (TPMT) enzyme, and uridine diphosphate glucuronosyltransferase (UGT) enzyme.

2. *Altered pharmacodynamics, ie, the effect of a drug at its therapeutic target and at other non-target sites.* Genetic variations can modulate drug response by affecting the drug target itself or one of the downstream components in the target's mechanistic pathway. An example is the effect of polymorphisms in the gene encoding the vitamin K epoxide reductase complex (VKORC1) on response to the oral anticoagulant, warfarin.

3. *Effect on idiosyncratic drug reactions.* An idiosyncratic reaction is an adverse drug reaction (ADR) that cannot be anticipated based on the known drug target. An example is the association of HLA-B*5701 with a hypersensitivity reaction to the antiretroviral nucleoside analog, abacavir.

4. *Effect on disease pathogenesis, ie, certain genetic variations can influence a disease pathogenesis by altering the disease severity or the response to specific therapy.* For example, vemurafenib, an inhibitor of kinase B-Raf, significantly improves survival in patients with unresectable or metastatic melanoma with the V600E mutation in the *BRAF* gene.

CLINICAL USE OF PHARMACOGENETIC TESTING

Pharmacogenetic testing may help in the selection of certain drugs and their dosages. However, integration of pharmacogenetic testing into clinical care has been generally slow and prospective randomized trials have not yet demonstrated improved clinical outcomes in cases in which drug therapy and specific dosage have been selected based on genotyping results.

Table 4–3 lists drugs for which genetic testing has been suggested.

REFERENCES

NIH Pharmacogenetics Research Network. Pharmacogenomics Knowledge Base. http://www
.pharmgkb.org
Kisor DF et al. *Pharmacogenetics, Kinetics, and Dynamics for Personalized Medicine.* Jones & Bartlett
Publishers, 2013.

TABLE 4–1. THERAPEUTIC DRUG MONITORING.¹

Drug	Effective Concentrations	Half-Life (hours)	Dosage Adjustments	Comments
Amikacin	**Conventional dosing:** Peak: 20–30 mg/L; trough: <10 mg/L **High dose once daily:** Peak: 60 mg/L; trough: <5 mg/L	2–3; ↑ in uremia	↓ in renal dysfunction	Concomitant kanamycin or tobramycin therapy may give falsely elevated amikacin results by immunoassay.
Amitriptyline	95–250 ng/mL	9–25		Drug is highly protein-bound. Patient-specific decrease in protein binding may invalidate quoted therapeutic reference interval for effective concentration.
Carbamazepine	4–12 mg/L	10–15	↓ in severe renal or hepatic disease	Induces its own metabolism. Metabolite 10,11-epoxide exhibits 13% cross-reactivity by immunoassay and is pharmacologically active. Adverse reactions: skin reactions, myelosuppression.
Cyclosporine	100–300 mcg/L (ng/mL) whole blood	6–12	↓ in renal dysfunction, liver disease	Cyclosporine is lipid-soluble (20% bound to leukocytes; 40% to erythrocytes; 40% in plasma, highly bound to lipoproteins); the binding is temperature-dependent *in vitro* and concentration-dependent *in vivo*. HPLC and LC-tandem mass spectrometry methods are highly specific for parent drug and considered the gold standard assays. Monoclonal fluorescence polarization immunoassay (FPIA) and monoclonal chemiluminescence immunoassay also measure cyclosporine reliably; polyclonal immunoassays are less specific owing to cross-reaction with drug metabolites. Anticonvulsants and rifampin increase metabolism. Erythromycin, ketoconazole, and calcium channel blockers decrease metabolism. The main adverse reaction is concentration-related nephrotoxicity.
Desipramine	100–250 ng/mL	13–23		Drug is highly protein-bound. Patient-specific decrease in protein binding may invalidate quoted therapeutic reference interval for effective concentration.
Digoxin	HF: 0.5–0.9 ng/mL Atrial fibrillation: 0.5–2 ng/mL	36–42; ↑ in uremia, HF	↓ in renal dysfunction, HF, hypothyroidism; ↑ in hyperthyroidism	Bioavailability of digoxin tablets is 50–90%. Specimen must not be drawn within 4 hours of an intravenous dose or 6 hours of an oral dose. Dialysis does not remove a significant amount. Hypokalemia potentiates toxicity. Digitalis toxicity is a clinical and *not* a laboratory diagnosis. Digibind (digoxin-specific antibody) therapy of digoxin overdose can interfere with measurement of digoxin levels depending on the digoxin assay. Elimination reduced by amiodarone, quinidine, and verapamil.

(Continued)

TABLE 4–1. THERAPEUTIC DRUG MONITORING.[1] (*CONTINUED*)

Drug	Effective Concentrations	Half-Life (hours)	Dosage Adjustments	Comments
Ethosuximide	40–100 mg/L	Child: 30–40 Adult: 50–60		Levels used primarily to assess clinical response and compliance. Toxicity is rare and does not correlate well with plasma concentrations.
Gentamicin	**Conventional dosing:** Peak: 4–8 mg/L; trough: <2 mg/L **High dose once daily:** Peak: 20 mg/L; trough: undetectable	2–3; ↑ in uremia (7.3 during dialysis)	↓ in renal dysfunction	Draw peak specimen (conventional dosing) 30 minutes after end of 30- to 60-min infusion. Draw trough just before next dose. In uremic patients, some penicillins (eg, carbenicillin, ticarcillin, piperacillin) may decrease gentamicin half-life from 46 hours to 22 hours, posing a risk of reduced antibacterial efficacy. The main adverse reactions are CNS, otic, and renal toxicities.
Imipramine	180–350 ng/mL	10–16		Drug is highly protein-bound. Patient-specific decrease in protein binding may invalidate quoted therapeutic reference interval for effective concentration.
Lidocaine	1–5 mg/L	1–2; unchanged in uremia, HF; ↑ in cirrhosis	↓ in HF, liver disease	Levels increased with cimetidine therapy. CNS toxicity common in the elderly.
Lithium	0.5–1.2 mmol/L	10–35; ↑ in uremia	↓ in renal dysfunction	Thiazides and loop diuretics may increase serum lithium levels.
Methotrexate	Protocol dependent	3–10 low dose; 8–15 high dose; ↑ in uremia	↓ in renal dysfunction	Therapeutic concentrations depend on the treatment protocol (low versus high dose) and time of specimen collection. 7-Hydroxymethotrexate cross-reacts 1.5% in immunoassay. To minimize toxicity, leucovorin or glucarpidase should be continued if methotrexate level is >0.1 mcmol/L at 48 hours after start of therapy. Methotrexate >1 mcmol/L at >48 hours requires an increase in rescue therapy.
Nortriptyline	50–140 ng/mL	18–44	↓ in liver disease	Drug is highly protein-bound. Patient-specific decrease in protein binding may invalidate quoted therapeutic reference interval for effective concentration.
Phenobarbital	10–40 mg/L	Child: 37–73; Adult: 53–140; ↑ in cirrhosis	↓ in liver disease	Metabolized primarily by the hepatic microsomal enzyme system. Many drug-drug interactions.

Drug	Therapeutic range	Half-life (hours)	Decreased in	Comments
Phenytoin	10–20 mg/L; 5–10 mg/L in uremia and severe hypoalbuminemia	Dose/concentration-dependent	See comments: renal, liver dysfunction	Drug metabolite cross-reacts in immunoassays; the cross-reactivity may be of significance only in the presence of advanced chronic kidney disease. Metabolism is capacity-limited. Increase dose cautiously when level approaches therapeutic reference interval, since new steady-state level may be disproportionately higher. Drug is very highly protein-bound; protein binding is decreased in uremia and hypoalbuminemia. Monitoring free (unbound) drug level (pharmacologically active fraction, target range 0.5–2.0 mg/L) is recommended in renal failure and severe hepatic impairment.
Sirolimus	Trough: 4–12 ng/mL when used in combination with cyclosporine A; 12–20 ng/mL if used alone	57–63	↓ in liver dysfunction and with drugs inhibiting CYP3A4 activity	Sirolimus is an immunosuppressant used in combination with cyclosporine and corticosteroids for prophylaxis of organ rejection after kidney transplantation. It has also been used in liver and heart transplantation. When used in combination with cyclosporine, careful monitoring of kidney function is required. Once the initial dose titration is complete, monitoring sirolimus trough concentrations weekly for the first month and every 2 weeks for the second month appears to be appropriate. The optimal time for specimen collection is 24 hours after the previous dose or 0.5 to 1 hour before the next dose (trough level).
Tacrolimus	Trough: 8–12 ng/mL	8.7–11.3	↓ in liver dysfunction and with drugs inhibiting CYP3A4 activity	Tacrolimus is used for prophylaxis of organ rejection in adult patients undergoing liver or kidney transplantation and in pediatric patients undergoing liver transplantation. It has also been used to prevent rejection in heart, small bowel, and allogeneic bone marrow transplant patients and to treat autoimmune diseases. Antacid or sucralfate administration should be separated from tacrolimus by at least 2 hours. The optimal time for specimen collection is 12 hours after the previous dose or 0.5 to 1 hour before the next dose (trough level).
Theophylline	5–15 mg/L	4–9	↓ in HF, cirrhosis, and with cimetidine	Caffeine cross-reacts 10%. Elimination is increased by 1.5–2 times in smokers. 1,3-Dimethyl uric acid metabolite increased in uremia and, because of cross-reactivity, may cause an apparent slight increase in serum theophylline.

(Continued)

TABLE 4–1. THERAPEUTIC DRUG MONITORING.[1] (*CONTINUED*)

Drug	Effective Concentrations	Half-Life (hours)	Dosage Adjustments	Comments
Tobramycin	**Conventional dosing:** Peak: 5–10 mg/L; trough: <2 mg/L **High dose once daily:** Peak: 20 mg/L; trough: undetectable	2–3; ↑ in uremia	↓ in renal dysfunction	Tobramycin, kanamycin, and amikacin may cross-react in immunoassay. Some antibiotics may decrease tobramycin half-life in uremic patients, causing reduced antibacterial efficacy.
Valproic acid (Valproate), total	50–100 mg/L; 50–125 mg/L for bipolar disorder	Child: 6–8 Adult: 10–12	Contraindicated in severe hepatic impairment. Not recommended during pregnancy.	Significant fraction of the drug is protein-bound *in vivo* (concentration-dependent). Decreased binding in uremia and liver disease. Can produce hepatoxicity.
Vancomycin	Trough: 10–20 mg/L	6; ↑ in uremia	↓ in renal dysfunction	Trough concentrations are recommended for monitoring vancomycin efficacy. Ototoxicity in uremic patients may lead to irreversible deafness.

[1]Serum from plain red-top tube is typically used for therapeutic drug monitoring except for cyclosporine, which requires whole blood sample in a lavender (EDTA) tube. In general, the specimen should be drawn just before the next dose (trough).

↑, increased; ↓, decreased; CNS, central nervous system; CYP, cytochrome P450; HF, heart failure; HPLC, high-performance liquid chromatography.

TABLE 4–2. SELECTED DRUGS REQUIRING LABORATORY MONITORING.

Drugs	Main Use	Tests	Suggested Frequency
Acarbose	Diabetes mellitus, type 2	LFT, KFT	Every 3 months during the first year, then periodically as clinically indicated
ACE inhibitors	Hypertension, heart failure	Electrolytes, KFT	Every 3–6 months
Adalimumab	Rheumatoid arthritis, ankylosing spondylitis, inflammatory bowel disease	CBC, KFT, LFT	Every 2 months
Adefovir	Chronic hepatitis B	CBC, LFT, KFT	Every 3 months
Alpha 1-antiproteinase (antitrypsin) inhibitor	Emphysema related to alpha 1-antiproteinase (antitrypsin) deficiency	LFT, KFT	Annually
Amiodarone	Cardiac arrhythmias	TSH, LFT	Every 6 months
Anakinra	Neonatal-onset multisystem inflammatory disease, refractory rheumatoid arthritis, juvenile idiopathic arthritis	CBC, LFT, KFT	Every 3 months
Azathioprine	Immunosuppression for various conditions	CBC, LFT	Every other week for the first 8 weeks, then every 3 months
Clozapine and other atypical antipsychotics (risperidone, olanzapine, quetiapine, ziprasidone, aripiprazole)	Schizophrenia	CBC/diff, LFT, HbA₁꜀ or fasting glucose, fasting lipid profile	Annually, except for CBC/diff which should be weekly for the first 6 months, then every other week or monthly
Cyclosporine	Organ transplant (kidney, liver, heart), rheumatoid arthritis and other rheumatic diseases	CBC/diff, CMP, magnesium	Every 3 months
Darbepoetin	Anemia (chronic kidney disease, chemotherapy, myelodysplasia)	CBC	Every 3 months
Entecavir	Chronic hepatitis B, HIV/HBV coinfection	CBC, LFT, KFT	Every 3–6 months
Etanercept	Rheumatoid arthritis, other rheumatic diseases	CBC, LFT, KFT	Every 2 months
Interferon beta-1α	Multiple sclerosis	CBC/diff, LFT	Every 6 months
Lamivudine	Chronic hepatitis B, HIV infection (in combination with other agents)	CBC, LFT, KFT, amylase	Every 3 months
Lithium	Bipolar disorder	TSH, KFT	Every 3–6 months

(Continued)

TABLE 4–2. SELECTED DRUGS REQUIRING LABORATORY MONITORING. (*CONTINUED*)

Drugs	Main Use	Tests	Suggested Frequency
Mercaptopurine	Acute lymphoblastic leukemia (in combination with other agents)	CBC/diff, LFT	Every 3 months
Mesalamine	Ulcerative colitis, Crohn disease	LFT, KFT, CBC	Every 6 months
Metformin	Diabetes mellitus, type 2	CBC, KFT	Every 6–12 months
Methotrexate	Acute leukemia, lymphoma, cancer, rheumatic diseases	CBC/diff, LFT, KFT	Every 3 months
NSAIDS (chronic use)	Chronic conditions with inflammation, pain and/or fever	KFT	Annually
Oxcarbazepine	Seizures	Electrolytes	Every 6 months
Prednisone (oral >10 mg daily)	Allergic conditions, dermatitis, endocrine conditions, inflammatory bowel disease, autoimmune disorders, leukemia/lymphoma, other conditions	HbA$_{1C}$ or fasting glucose, electrolytes	Annually
Riluzole	Amyotrophic lateral sclerosis	LFT	Every 3 months
Sirolimus	Organ transplant (kidney, heart)	CBC/diff, CMP, magnesium	Every 3 months
Statins	Prevention of cardiovascular disease, treatment of hypercholesterolemia and dyslipidemia	Fasting lipid profile	Every 6–12 months
Sulfasalazine	Rheumatoid arthritis, ulcerative colitis	CBC, LFT, KFT	Every 3 months
Tacrolimus	Organ transplant (kidney, heart, liver)	CBC/diff, CMP, magnesium	Every 3 months
Tenofovir	HIV infection	KFT	Every 3 months for one year, then every 6 months
Tizanidine	Muscle spasticity, acute low back pain	LFT	Every 6 months
Topiramate	Seizures, migraine headache	Electrolytes, KFT	Annually
Valproate (valproic acid)	Seizures, mania in bipolar disorder, migraine prophylaxis	CBC, LFT, PT/PTT	Every 6 months
Warfarin	Prophylaxis and treatment of thromboembolic disorders	PT/INR	Frequency varies as clinically indicated
Zafirlukast	Asthma, chronic urticaria	LFT	Every 6 months

CBC/diff, complete blood count with white cell differential; CMP, comprehensive metabolic panel; LFT, liver function tests; KFT, kidney function tests; PT/INR, prothrombin time/International Normalized Ratio; PTT, partial thromboplastin time; TSH, thyroid-stimulating hormone.

TABLE 4–3. SELECTED PHARMACOGENETIC TESTS: CLINICAL RELEVANCE.[1]

Pharmacogenetic Biomarker	Selected Variants (Mutant Allele, Enzyme Activity)	Allele Frequency	Drugs	Clinical Relevance
BRAF gene	BRAF V600E mutation	40–60% of advanced melanomas	Vemurafenib (Zelboraf)	Activating mutations in BRAF (a serine–threonine protein kinase) are present in 40–60% of advanced melanomas. Most (80–90%) of the mutations are the substitution of glutamic acid for valine at amino acid 600 (V600E mutation). This mutation is associated with a more aggressive clinical course. Vemurafenib, a potent inhibitor of the mutant BRAF, has a high level of therapeutic activity against advanced melanomas containing the V600E mutation.
Cystic fibrosis transmembrane conductance regulator (CFTR)	CFTR G551D (defective)	CFTR G551D is present in about 4% of patients with cystic fibrosis (CF)	Ivacaftor (Kalydeco)	CFTR protein forms a channel that allows chloride ions to cross the membrane. In CF patients with the CFTR G551D mutation, the channel fails to open. Ivacaftor corrects the effects of this mutation and is approved for persons with CF age > 6 years who have at least one copy of the G551D mutation.
Cytochrome P450 (CYP) 2C9 variants	2C9*2 (430C>T, ↓); 2C9*3 (1075A>C, ↓↓)	2C9*2 and 2C9*3 are present in 9–20% of whites, 1–3% of blacks, and <1% of Asians	Warfarin (Coumadin)	Hepatic CYP2C9 is responsible for the metabolic inactivation and clearance of the anticoagulant warfarin. Patients carrying 2C9*2 or 2C9*3 (or both) (heterozygote, homozygote, or compound heterozygote) require reduced maintenance dose to reach a therapeutic INR. Although INR remains the standard for monitoring warfarin therapy, CYP2C9 genotyping can be an important aid to dosing strategy for warfarin-naïve patients, particularly whites.
CYP 2C19 variants	2C19*2 (681G>A, none); 2C19*3 (636G>A, none); 2C19*4 (1A>G, none); 2C19*5 (1297C>T, none)	The mutant variants are present in 12–25% of Asians, and 2–7% of whites and blacks	Clopidogrel (Plavix)	Clopidogrel, an antiplatelet drug, must be metabolized in the liver by CYP isoenzymes, principally CYP2C19, to become active. When treated with clopidogrel at recommended dosage, patients who metabolize the drug poorly exhibit higher rates of cardiovascular events than those of patients with normal CYP2C19 function. Alternative drug or intervention strategies should be considered for patients identified as poor metabolizers. CYP2C19*17 carrier status (25% of whites) is associated with increased enzyme activity and an increased risk of bleeding.
DPD variants	DPYD*2A (1905+1G>A, none); DPYD*13 (1679T>G, ↓↓); DPYD rs67376798 (2846A>T, ↓↓)	These non-functional variants are present in 0.1–1% of whites (eg, French Caucasians)	5-fluorouracil (5-FU), capecitabine (Xeloda)	Fluoropyrimidines (ie, 5-fluorouracil, capecitabine) are metabolized by dihydropyrimidine dehydrogenase (DPD) enzyme, encoded by the DPYD gene. To avoid severe or even fatal drug toxicity, an alternative drug should be selected for patients who are homozygous for DPYD non-functional variants (*2A, *13, or rs67376798). Consider a 50% reduction in starting dose for heterozygous patients who have low DPD activity (30–70% of normal).

(Continued)

TABLE 4–3. SELECTED PHARMACOGENETIC TESTS: CLINICAL RELEVANCE.[1] (CONTINUED)

Pharmacogenetic Biomarker	Selected Variants (Mutant Allele, Enzyme Activity)	Allele Frequency	Drugs	Clinical Relevance
HER2	HER2 gene amplification	HER2 gene amplification is present in about 20% of breast cancers	Trastuzumab (Herceptin)	Patients with HER2 gene amplification are candidates for treatment with trastuzumab. Patients without HER2 amplification will not benefit from adjuvant trastuzumab treatment. FISH with labeled DNA probes to the pericentromeric region of chromosome 17 and to the HER2 locus are used to determine if a patient's breast cancer has HER2 gene amplification. IHC stains are also used to determine if the tumor exhibits HER2 protein overexpression.
HLA-B*1502 allele	HLA-B*1502	10–15% of Asians; 1–2% of whites	Carbamazepine (Tegretol, Epitol)	Carbamazepine is associated with serious or even fatal idiosyncratic skin reactions, eg, Stevens-Johnson syndrome and toxic epidermal necrolysis. The reactions are significantly more common in patients who carry the HLA-B*1502 allele. This allele occurs almost exclusively in patients with ancestry across broad areas of Asia, including South Asian Indians. HLA-B*1502 genotyping may be useful for risk stratification in patients of Asian descent. Patients carrying the HLA-B*1502 allele should not be given carbamazepine unless the expected benefit clearly outweighs the increased risk of serious skin reactions.
HLA-B*B5701 allele	HLA-B*5701	6–8% of whites and 1–2% of blacks and East Asians	Abacavir (Ziagen)	Abacavir is a nucleoside analog reverse transcriptase inhibitor used for HIV treatment. The major treatment-limiting toxicity for abacavir use is drug hypersensitivity, occurring in 5–8% of recipients within 6 weeks of commencing therapy. There is an established association between carriage of the HLA-B*5701 allele and abacavir hypersensitivity reactions. HLA-B*5701-positive patients should not be prescribed abacavir or an abacavir-containing regimen.
HLA-B*5801 allele	HLA-B*5801	6–8% of Southeast Asians; < 1% of Western Europeans	Allopurinol (Zyloprim)	The urate-lowering drug, allopurinol, is associated with rare but severe hypersensitivity reactions (eg, toxic epidermal necrolysis and Stevens-Johnson syndrome), which are strongly associated with HLA-B*5801 alleles. Patients of Korean, Han Chinese, Japanese, or Thai origin should be screened for HLA-B*5801 allele, and if present, an alternative drug therapy is needed.
K-ras gene	K-ras mutations (in codons 12 and 13)	30–40% of colorectal cancer; 20–25% of non-small cell lung cancer	For colorectal cancer: Cetuximab (Erbitux), Panitumumab (Vectibix) For non-small cell lung cancer: Gefitinib (Iressa), Erlotinib (Tarceva)	The K-ras gene, a human proto-oncogene, encodes one of the proteins in the EGFR (epidermal growth factor receptor) signaling pathway critical in the development and progression of cancer, particularly colorectal cancer and non-small cell lung cancer. Cancer patients with mutated K-ras are not likely to respond to drugs targeting the EGFR pathway. To avoid unnecessary toxicity and cost, all patients being considered for anti-EGFR therapy should undergo K-ras mutation testing of their tumors.

Thiopurine methyl-transferase (TPMT) variants	TPMT*2 (238G>C, ↓); TPMT*3A (460G>A and 719A>G, ↓↓); TPMT*3B (460G>A, ↓); TPMT*3C (719A>G, ↓)	About 10–12% of whites and blacks have reduced enzyme activity because they are heterozygous for one of the mutant alleles. About 1 in 300 whites is homozygous for a mutant allele.	AZA is a prodrug that is metabolized to 6-MP, which is then further metabolized to active 6-thioguanine (6-TG) and inactive 6-methylmercaptopurine (6-MMP) by hypoxanthine phosphoribosyltransferase and TPMT, respectively. Variation in the *TPMT* gene can result in functional inactivation of the enzyme and an increased risk of life-threatening 6-TG–associated myelosuppression. TPMT genotyping before instituting AZA or 6-MP can help prevent toxicity by identifying individuals with low or absent TPMT enzyme activity. Patients with homozygous or compound heterozygous mutant alleles ("poor metabolizers") should not be given AZA or 6-MP, whereas heterozygotes with a single mutant allele should be treated with lower doses.
Azathioprine (AZA), 6-mercaptopurine (6-MP)			
Uridine diphospho-glucuronosyltransferase 1A1 (UGT 1A1) variants	UGT1A1*28 (7 TA repeats in promoter, ↓)	Homozygosity in 9–23% of whites, blacks, and in 1–2% of east Asians.	Irinotecan is used in the treatment of metastatic colorectal cancer. It is metabolized to active SN-38, a topoisomerase I inhibitor. SN-38 is further glucuronidated to inactive SN-38G by UGT1A1 and excreted. Heterozygous and homozygous UGT1A1*28 genotypes show a 25% and 70% decrease in the enzyme activity, respectively. The presence of the UGT1A1*28 allele is a risk factor for adverse drug reactions (eg, neutropenia, severe diarrhea). Testing for the allele can prevent drug toxicity at high doses of irinotecan.
Irinotecan (Camptosar)			
Vitamin K epoxide reductase complex (VKORC1) variants	VKORC1 (−1639G>A)	The homozygous (−1639G>A) allele (−1639AA genotype) is present in approximately 15% of whites and 80% of Chinese.	The primary therapeutic target of the anticoagulant warfarin is VKOR. Polymorphisms in the VKOR encoding gene (VKORC1) explain about 30% of the phenotypic variability in drug effect. Patients carrying the VKORC1 (−1639G>A) allele require a lower warfarin maintenance dose to reach a therapeutic INR.
Warfarin (Coumadin)			

Testing of these genetic biomarkers before instituting drug therapy is now recommended per US Food and Drug Administration-approved drug labels. Note, however, that these tests are not yet mandated as standard practice.
↓, decreased; ↓↓, markedly decreased; >, single wild-type to variant nucleotide switch at the specific gene location; CYP, cytochrome P450 oxidase; FISH, fluorescence in-situ hybridization; IHC, immunohistochemistry; INR, International Normalized Ratio.

5

Microbiology: Test Selection

Barbara Haller, MD, PhD

HOW TO USE THIS SECTION

This section displays information about clinically important infectious diseases in tabular form. Included in these tables are the *Organisms* involved in the disease/syndrome listed, *Specimens/Diagnostic Tests* that are useful in the evaluation, and *Comments* regarding the tests and diagnoses discussed. Topics are listed by body area/organ system: Central Nervous System, Eye, Ear, Sinus, Upper Airway, Lung, Heart and Vessels, Abdomen, Genitourinary, Bone, Joint, Muscle, Skin, and Blood.

Thereafter is a short section on emerging and re-emerging pathogens (viral and bacterial) and antibiotic resistance in bacterial pathogens.

Organisms

This column lists organisms that are known to cause the stated illness. Scientific names are abbreviated according to common usage (eg, *Streptococcus pneumoniae* as *S. pneumoniae* or pneumococcus) if appropriate. Specific age or risk groups are listed in order of increasing age or frequency (eg, Infant, Child, Adult, HIV).

When bacteria are listed, Gram stain characteristics follow the organism name in parentheses—eg, "*S. pneumoniae* (GPDC)." The following abbreviations are used:

AFB	Acid-fast bacilli
GPDC	Gram-positive diplococci
GPR	Gram-positive rods
GNC	Gram-negative cocci
GNCB	Gram-negative coccobacilli
GPC	Gram-positive cocci
GPCB	Gram-positive coccobacilli
GVCB	Gram-variable coccobacilli
GNDC	Gram-negative diplococci
GNR	Gram-negative rods

When known, the frequency of the specific organism's involvement in the disease process is also provided in parentheses—eg, "*S. pneumoniae* (GPDC) (50%)."

Specimen Collection/Diagnostic Tests

This column describes the collection of specimens, laboratory processing, useful radiographic procedures, and other diagnostic tests. Culture or test sensitivities with respect to the diagnosis in question are placed in parentheses immediately following the test when known—eg, "Gram stain (60%)." Pertinent serologic tests are also listed. Keep in mind that few infections can be identified by definitive diagnostic tests and that clinical judgment is critical to making difficult diagnoses when test results are equivocal.

Comments

This column includes general information about the utility of the tests and may include information about patient management. Appropriate general references are also listed.

Syndrome Name/Body Area

In the last two columns, the syndrome name and body area are placed perpendicular to the rest of the table to allow for quick referencing.

Organization

The table comprising the bulk of this chapter appears in two parts. The first table (Part I) is organized by body areas and concerns common infections with established pathogens or infectious agents. The second table (Part II) concerns emerging (new) and re-emerging viral and bacterial pathogens and antibiotic resistance in bacterial pathogens.

PART I. COMMON INFECTIONS WITH ESTABLISHED PATHOGENS/INFECTIOUS AGENTS.

CENTRAL NERVOUS SYSTEM

Brain abscess

(Continued)

Organism	Specimen/Diagnostic Tests	Comments
Brain abscess Often polymicrobial (14–28% of cases). Child: anaerobes (40%), aerobic and anaerobic viridans streptococci (GPC in chains), *S. aureus* (GPC), *S. pneumoniae* (GPDC), *S. pyogenes* (GPC in chains); less common: Enterobacteriaceae (GNR), *P. aeruginosa* (GNR), *H. influenzae* (GNCB), *N. meningitidis* (GNDC). Adults: Viridans streptococci (anaerobic *Streptococcus anginosus* [*milleri*] group) (70%). Enterobacteriaceae (GNR) (23–33%), *S. aureus* (GPC) (10–15%), *N. meningitidis, Listeria* sp., anaerobes (20–40%) including bacteroides (GNR), prevotella (GNR), fusobacterium (GNR), eubacterium (GPR), and propionibacterium (GPR). More rarely identified: *S. pneumoniae, Rhodococcus* sp., Group B streptococci (GPC in chains), nocardia (GPR), actinomyces (GPR), parasites, *T. solium* (cysticerci), *Entamoeba histolytica, Schistosoma* sp., and fungi (1%). Immunocompromised: *T. gondii, Cryptococcus neoformans,* nocardia (GPR), *Listeria* sp. (GPR), mycobacteria (AFB), *Aspergillus* sp., *C. albicans,* coccidioides, Zygomycetes (mucor, rhizopus), *E. histolytica.* Posttraumatic: *S. aureus* (GPC), viridans streptococci (GPC in chains), Enterobacteriaceae (GNR), coagulase-negative staphylococci (GPC), *Propionibacterium acnes* (GPR).	Blood for bacterial and fungal cultures. Brain abscess aspirate for Gram stain (82%), bacterial (88%), AFB, fungal cultures, and cytology. Lumbar puncture is dangerous and contraindicated. Sources of infection in the ears, sinuses, lungs, or bloodstream should be sought for culture when brain abscess is found. CT scan and MRI are the most valuable imaging procedures (see Chapter 6) and can guide brain biopsy if a specimen is needed. Serum toxoplasma antibody in HIV-infected patients may not be positive at initiation of presumptive therapy. If negative or if no response to empiric therapy, biopsy may be needed to rule out lymphoma, fungal infection, or tuberculosis. Biopsy material should be sent for toxoplasma antigen (detected by direct fluorescent antibody, DFA). Detection of toxoplasma DNA in CSF samples by PCR techniques is ~50% sensitive, 96–100% specific. PCR for toxoplasma is not useful once therapy has been started. A positive PCR result must be interpreted in the context of the clinical presentation. If cultures are negative, 16S rRNA gene sequencing of apirate specimen is an important new tool. (See also *Toxoplasma* antibody, Chapter 3.)	Occurs from direct extension of adjacent infection, hematogenous seeding, trauma, or surgery. In children, 50% of cases are secondary to sinusitis, otitis media or dental infections. Hematogenous spread from bacterial endocarditis or chronic pulmonary disease in 25%. Most occur in the first 2 decades of life. Predisposing factors: immunosuppression, congenital heart disease (patent foramen ovale). Clinical: seizures occur in 30–50%. Mortality rate is 4–12%. In adults, contiguous spread occurs in 50%, hematogenous spread in 33% of cases; and unknown mechanism is responsible for the remainder. Predisposing factors: underlying disease (HIV), immunosuppressive drugs, endocarditis or bacteremia, disruption of protective barrier around brain. Clinical: fever, headache, nausea and vomiting, altered consciousness, focal neurologic deficits, seizures. Mortality rate is 8–25%. Most toxoplasmosis abscesses are multiple and are seen on MRI in the basal ganglia, parietal and frontal lobes (ring-enhancing lesions with contrast on CT scan). Stereotactic CT-guided aspiration of abscess material facilitates microbiologic diagnosis. Treatment: long-term antimicrobial therapy and surgical drainage. Bonfield CM et al. Pediatric intracranial abscesses. J Infect 2015;71:S42. [PMID: 25917804] Brouwer MC et al. Brain abscess. N Engl J Med 2014;371:447. [PMID: 25075836] Brouwer MC et al. Clinical characteristics and outcome of brain abscess: systematic review and meta-analysis. Neurology 2014;82:806. [PMID: 24477107]

CENTRAL NERVOUS SYSTEM

Encephalitis

Organism	Specimen/Diagnostic Tests	Comments
Encephalitis Arboviruses (California encephalitis group, St. Louis encephalitis, eastern and western equine encephalitis, West Nile virus, Japanese encephalitis virus in summer and fall), enteroviruses (coxsackie, echo, polio), HSV (10–20%), *Bartonella henselae*, lymphocytic choriomeningitis virus, tick-borne encephalitis virus, measles, rubella, VZV, HHV-6, rabies (Central and South America, India, Africa), Nipah virus (Malaysia), Chikungunya virus (India and Nepal), Creutzfeldt-Jakob. Immunocompromised: CMV, VZV, EBV, West Nile virus, JC virus, HIV, *Toxoplasma gondii*. Note the increasing recognition of antibody-mediated autoimmune encephalitis as cause of acute encephalitis. In studies of acute encephalitis, 40–50% of patients had infectious cause, 20% had immune-mediated cause including anti-NMDAR (N-methyl-D-asparte receptor) encephalitis and anti-voltage-gated potassium channel (VGKC) encephalitis, and 30% remained of unknown cause.	MRI to detect patterns of abnormalities suggestive of infectious cause, eg, temporal and limbic abnormalities for HSV or HHV-6 encephalitis. CSF for pressure (elevated), cell count (WBCs elevated but variable [10–2000/mcL], mostly lymphocytes), protein (elevated, especially IgG fraction), glucose (normal), RBCs (suggestive of herpesvirus or other necrotizing virus). Repeat examination of CSF after 24 hours often useful. (See CSF [enteroviruses, HSV-2, mumps] profiles, Table 8–9). CSF cultures for viruses or fastidious bacteria like *Bartonella sp.* low yield, no longer recommended. CSF PCR for CMV (33%), HSV (98%), VZV, EBV, JC virus, enterovirus, and West Nile virus recommended based on patient age and immune status. Identification of HSV DNA in CSF by real-time PCR techniques is now the definitive diagnostic test. HSV DNA by PCR may not be detectable early in course of illness. New PCR microarray assay detects a panel of viral pathogens in CSF. Diagnosis of autoimmune encephalitis is demonstration of specific antineuronal antibodies in serum and/or CSF. Stool culture for enterovirus (2–5 days), which is frequently shed for weeks (especially in children) or in late illness. For rabies, direct fluorescent antibody staining of skin biopsy from nape of neck (50% positive in first week) or RT-PCR on CSF or saliva. Single serum for *Bartonella* (cat-scratch disease) IgM and IgG, or PCR on CSF. Test single serum for West Nile virus IgM antibody or CSF IgM antibody, or PCR of serum or CSF. Paired sera for arboviruses and other viruses should be drawn immediately (acute specimen) and after 1–3 weeks of illness (convalescent specimen); send to reference laboratory or Public Health Laboratory.	Occurs most frequently in infants younger than age 1 year and elderly patients older than 65 years. All patients with suspected encephalitis should undergo MRI and CSF analysis unless contraindicated. Polyradiculopathy is highly suggestive of CMV in AIDS. Early, empiric high-dose therapy with acyclovir warranted to treat potential HSV encephalitis pending diagnostic testing. Consult with laboratory regarding availability of serological tests and tests for antibodies associated with autoimmune encephalitis. Mortality rate in encephalitis is 5–15%, with marked physical and cognitive morbidity for survivors. Kleinschmidt-DeMasters et al. West Nile virus encephalitis 16 years later. Brain Pathol 2015;25:625. [PMID: 26276026] Singh TD et al. The spectrum of acute encephalitis: causes, management, and predictors of outcome. Neurology 2015;84:359. [PMID: 25540320] Venkatesan A. Epidemiology and outcomes of acute encephalitis. Curr Opin Neurol 2015;28:277. [PMID: 25887770]

CENTRAL NERVOUS SYSTEM

Aseptic meningitis

(Continued)

Organism/Disease	Specimen/Diagnostic Tests	Comments
Aseptic meningitis Acute: Enteroviruses (coxsackie, echo, polio) (90%), mumps, HSV, HIV (primary HIV seroconversion), VZV, lymphocytic choriomeningitis virus, adenovirus, parainfluenza virus 3, West Nile virus, St. Louis encephalitis virus and California group encephalitis viruses (rare). Recurrent benign lymphocytic meningitis: HSV-2 (Mollaret meningitis).	CSF for pressure (elevated), cell count (WBCs 10–100/mcL, polomorphonuclear neutrophils (PMNs early, lymphocytes later), protein (normal or slightly elevated), and glucose (normal). On repeat CSF after 24–48 hours, an increase in lymphocytes is seen. (See CSF profiles, Table 8–9.) CSF viral culture can be negative despite active viral infection. Enteroviruses can be isolated from the CSF in the first few days after onset (positive in 40–80%) but only rarely after the first week. Detection of enteroviral RNA, HSV DNA, or VZV DNA in CSF by PCR from specialized or reference laboratories. Paired sera (acute and convalescent) for antibody titers: mumps, West Nile virus, and VZV. Consult with laboratory regarding availability of diagnostic tests for other viruses. CT or MRI of head should be performed before lumbar puncture to evaluate for mass lesions or hydrocephalus if focal neurologic signs or papilledema are present.	Aseptic meningitis is acute meningeal inflammation in the absence of pyogenic bacteria or fungi. Diagnosis is usually made by examination of the CSF, PCR of CSF, or serologic assays and by ruling out other infectious causes of acute mental status changes or seizures (eg, toxoplasmosis, Lyme disease, neurosyphilis, tuberculosis, Rocky Mountain spotted fever, ehrlichiosis, fungal infection, and parasitic infection). Consider noninfectious causes such as nonsteroidal anti-inflammatory drugs and other medications. Enteroviral aseptic meningitis is rare after age 40. 10–30% of patients with primary genital HSV-2 infection can have stiff neck, headache, and photophobia suggestive of recurrent meningitis. De Crom SC et al. Characteristics of pediatric patients with enterovirus meningitis and no cerebral fluid pleocytosis. Eur J Pediatr 2012;171:795. [PMID: 22102153] Patriquin G et al. Clinical presentation of patients with aseptic meningitis: factors influencing treatment and hospitalization, and consequences of enterovirus cerebrospinal fluid polymerase chain reaction testing. Can J Infect Dis Med Microbiol 2012;23:e1. [PMID: 23348849] Putz K et al. Meningitis. Prim Care Clin Office Pract 2013;40:707. [PMID: 23958365]

CENTRAL NERVOUS SYSTEM

Bacterial meningitis

Organism	Specimen/Diagnostic Tests	Comments
Bacterial meningitis Neonate: Group B streptococci (GPC) (70%), *L. monocytogenes* (GPR) (20%), *S. pneumoniae* (GPC) (10%), *E. coli* (GNR) and *Klebsiella* sp. (GNR) (1%), and other streptococci. Infant: *S. pneumoniae* (GPC) (47%), *N. meningitidis* (GNDC) (30%), group B streptococci (GPC) (18%), *Listeria monocytogenes* (GPR), *H. influenzae* (GNCB) (due to vaccination, now very rare). Child: *N. meningitidis* (60%), *S. pneumoniae* (25%), *H. influenzae* (now very rare), and other streptococci. Adult: *S. pneumoniae* (60%), *N. meningitidis* (20%), *L. monocytogenes* (6%), group B streptococci (4%), other *Hemophilus* sp., and staphylococci (1%), *Ehrlichia chaffeensis* (rare). Postneurosurgical: *S. aureus* (GPC), *S. pneumoniae*, *P. acnes* (GPR), coagulase-negative staphylococci (GPC), pseudomonas (GNR), *E. coli* (GNR), other Enterobacteriaceae, *Acinetobacter* (GNR). Alcoholic patients and the elderly: In addition to the adult organisms, Enterobacteriaceae, pseudomonas, *H. influenzae*. Immunocompromised: as above, *L. monocytogenes*.	CSF for pressure (>180 mm H$_2$O), cell count and differential (WBCs 5000–20,000/mcL, >50% PMNs), protein (150–500 mg/dL), glucose (low <40 mg/dL). (See CSF profiles, Table 8–9.) CSF for Gram stain of cytocentrifuged material (positive in 70–80%). CSF culture for bacteria (positive in 70–85%). HIV antibody/antigen test. Blood culture positive in 40–60% of patients with pneumococcal, meningococcal, and *H. influenzae* meningitis. CSF antigen tests are no longer considered useful because of their low sensitivity and false-positive results.	The first priority in the care of the patient with suspected acute meningitis is therapy, then diagnosis. Start antimicrobial agents based on Gram stain, or if no bacteria are seen, start empiric antibiotics immediately based on patient age and any underlying disease process. Adjunctive dexamethasone therapy has proved beneficial, especially for pneumococcal meningitis. If lumbar puncture is performed, administer antimicrobial therapy with dexamethasone immediately after CSF collection. The mortality rate for pneumococcal meningitis is about 20%, with 25–50% of patients having long-term neurologic complications. With recurrent *N. meningitidis* meningitis, suspect a terminal complement component deficiency. With other recurrent bacterial meningitides, suspect a CSF leak; *S. pneumoniae* is most likely pathogen. Therapy usually includes a 3rd generation cephalosporin plus vancomycin until culture results return. This will cover the most common pathogens as well as *H. influenzae*. Add ampicillin if *L. monocytogenes* is suspected. Therapy can be narrowed once the pathogen is identified and susceptibility results are determined. For *S. pneumoniae*, there has been an increase in prevalence of penicillin- and cephalosporin-resistant strains, so susceptibility testing of pneumococcal strains is very important to guide therapy. Vaccines against *H. influenza* and meningococcal serogroups have been critical for prevention of invasive disease. Recent approval of vaccines for meningococcal serogroup B will offer further protection for at-risk populations, such as young adults, military personnel, and laboratory workers. Brouwer MC et al. What's new in bacterial meningitis. Intensive Care Med 2016;42:415. [PMID: 26424682] Putz K et al. Meningitis. Prim Care Clin Office Pract 2013;40:707. [PMID: 23958365] Richie MB et al. A practical approach to meningitis and encephalitis. Semin Neurol 2015;35:611. [PMID: 26595861]

(Continued)

CENTRAL NERVOUS SYSTEM

Fungal meningitis

Organism/Diagnosis	Specimen/Diagnostic Test	Comments
Fungal meningitis *C. neoformans* (spherical, budding yeast), *C. immitis* (spherules), *H. capsulatum*. Immunocompromised: *Aspergillus* sp., *Pseudallescheria boydii*, *Candida* sp., sporothrix, blastomyces.	CSF for pressure (normal or elevated), cell count (WBCs 50–1000/mcL, mostly lymphocytes), protein (elevated), and glucose (normal or decreased). Serum cryptococcal antigen (CrAg) test (latex agglutination) for *C. neoformans* (>90% sensitive and specific. (This test can be performed on CSF specimens.) For other fungi, collect at least 5 mL of CSF for fungal culture. Initial cultures are positive in 40% of coccidioides cases and 27–65% of histoplasma cases. Repeat cultures are frequently needed. Cultures of blood, bone marrow, skin lesions, or other involved organs, if clinically indicated. CSF India ink preparation for cryptococcus is not recommended. Cytospin Gram stain procedure concentrates CSF and can demonstrate round, budding yeast. Serum coccidioidal serology is a serum immunodiffusion test for antibodies against the organism (75–95%). CSF serologic testing is rarely necessary. (See Coccidioides serology, Chapter 3.) Complement fixation tests for coccidioides or histoplasma antibodies are available from reference laboratories or public health department laboratories (see Chapter 3) and can give titers that can be used to follow treatment. Histoplasma antigen can be detected in urine (90%), blood (70%), or CSF (61%) in cases of histoplasma meningitis.	The clinical presentation of fungal meningitis in non-immunocompromised and immunocompromised patients is that of an indolent chronic meningitis. Before AIDS, cryptococcal meningitis was seen both in patients with cellular immunologic deficiencies and in patients who lacked obvious defects (about 50%). In AIDs patients, cryptococcus is the most common cause of meningitis and may present with normal CSF findings. Titer of CSF CrAg can be used to monitor therapeutic success (falling titer) or failure (unchanged or rising titer) or to predict relapse during suppressive therapy (rising titer) in immunocompetent patients, though not in patients with AIDS. Baldwin K et al. Chronic meningitis: simplifying a diagnostic challenge. Curr Neurol Neurosci Rep 2016;16:30. [PMID: 26888190] Baldwin KJ et al. Evaluation and treatment of chronic meningitis. Neurohospitalist 2014;4:185. [PMID: 25360204] Kassis C et al. Role of *Coccidioides* antigen testing in the cerebrospinal fluid for the diagnosis of coccidioidal meningitis. Clin Infect Dis 2015;61:1521. [PMID: 26209683]

CENTRAL NERVOUS SYSTEM

Spirochetal meningitis/neurologic diseases

Organism	Specimen/Diagnostic Tests	Comments
Spirochetal meningitis/ neurologic diseases *B. burgdorferi* (neuroborreliosis), *T. pallidum* (neurosyphilis), leptospira, other borreliae	**Neuroborreliosis:** CSF for pressure (normal or elevated), cell count (WBCs elevated, mostly lymphocytes), protein (may be elevated), and glucose (normal). Serum and CSF for serologic testing for antibody by ELISA or IFA. False-positive serologic tests may occur. Western blots should be used to confirm borderline or positive results. CSF serology for anti–*B. burgdorferi* IgM (90%). PCR is very specific for detecting *Borrelia* DNA, but sensitivity is variable owing to stage of disease and type of body fluid tested. (See Lyme disease serologies, Chapter 3.) **Acute syphilitic meningitis:** CSF for pressure (elevated), cell count (WBCs 25–2000/mcL, mostly lymphocytes), protein (elevated), and glucose (normal or low). (See CSF profiles, Table 8–9.) Serum VDRL. (See VDRL, serum, Chapter 3.) CSF VDRL is the preferred test (see Chapter 3), but is only 66% sensitive for acute syphilitic meningitis. **Neurosyphilis:** CSF for pressure (normal), cell count (WBCs normal or slightly increased, mostly lymphocytes), protein (normal or elevated), glucose (normal), and positive CSF VDRL. Serum RPR or VDRL with confirmatory FTA-ABS, or TP PA testing should be done with a positive serum result before CSF VDRL is performed. Traditionally, nontreponemal serologic tests (RPR or VDRL) are used as screening tests for detection of syphilis. Because of the lack of specificity for these tests, positive screening tests must be confirmed with FTA-ABS or TP PA treponemal-specific assays. A new syphilis testing algorithm (reverse algorithm; see Chapters 3 and 9) using treponemal tests for screening followed by a nontreponemal serology test has been implemented in some laboratories. **Leptospirosis:** CSF cell count (WBCs <500/mcL, mostly monocytes), protein (slightly elevated), and glucose (normal). Urine for dark-field examination of sediment to detect leptospira organisms. Blood and CSF dark-field examination positive only in acute phase prior to meningitis. Serum for serology for IgM by EIA (93% specificity).	Neurosyphilis is a late stage of infection and can present with meningovascular (hemiparesis, seizures, aphasia), parenchymal (general paresis, tabes dorsalis), or asymptomatic (latent) disease. In HIV-infected patients, neurosyphilis can present in secondary syphilis. Because there is no single highly sensitive or specific test for neurosyphilis, the diagnosis must depend on a combination of clinical and laboratory data. Therapy of suspected neurosyphilis should not be withheld on the basis of a negative CSF VDRL if clinical suspicion is high. In HIV neurosyphilis, treatment failures may be common. Lyme disease can present as a lymphocytic meningitis, facial palsy, or painful radiculitis. Leptospirosis follows exposure to urine of infected rodents, small animals, or livestock. Ghanem KG. Management of adult syphilis: key questions to inform the 2015 Centers for Disease Control and Prevention Sexually Transmitted Diseases Treatment Guidelines. Clin Infect Dis 2015;61:S818. [PMID: 26602620] Harding AS et al. The performance of cerebrospinal fluid treponemal-specific antibody tests in neurosyphilis: a systematic review. Sex Transm Dis 2012;39:291. [PMID: 22421696] van Samkar A et al. Suspected leptospiral meningitis in adults: report of four cases and review of the literature. Neth J Med 2015;73:464. [PMID: 26687262]

(Continued)

CENTRAL NERVOUS SYSTEM

Parasitic meningoencephalitis

Organism	Specimen/Test	Comments
Parasitic meningo-encephalitis *T. gondii, Plasmodium falciparum* (cerebral malaria), *Naegleria fowleri, T. solium* (cysticerci), *Acanthamoeba* (granulomatous amebic encephalitis GAE), *Balamuthia* sp. (GAE), *Angiostrongylus* (eosinophilic meningoencephalitis), *Trypanosoma* sp.	CSF for pressure (normal or elevated), cell count (WBCs 100–1000/mcL, chiefly monocytes, lymphocytes), protein (elevated), glucose (normal to low). Serum serology to detect antibodies for *T. gondii, E. chaffeensis, A. phagocytophilum*. **Toxoplasmosis:** CT or MRI of brain, serology. Giemsa-stained touch prep of brain tissue, CSF PCR. ***Plasmodium falciparum:*** Thick and thin blood smear films stained with Giemsa stain demonstrate *P. falciparum* parasite. CSF for cell count (mild pleocytosis) and protein (elevated). CT and MRI abnormal in 15–20% of infected patients. ***Naegleria:*** CSF wet mount for amebic trophozoites, or hematoxylin and eosin stain of brain tissue. Serologic tests not helpful. **Neurocysticercosis:** Characteristic findings on CT and MRI are diagnostic. Serology is less sensitive. **Balamuthia:** Culture not helpful. Indirect immunofluorescence or PCR of brain tissue to detect organism. **Angiostrongyliasis:** CSF pressure (normal or elevated), cell count (WBC eosinophilic pleocytosis), protein (elevated), glucose (normal). CSF wet mount, ELISA serology. **Trypanosomiasis:** Blood-Giemsa stain on thick and thin smears. CSF wet mount. Serologic tests by ELISA, IFA have 93–98% sensitivity and 99% specificity in acute stages. Serologic tests may be negative in chronic stages.	Toxoplasmosis in HIV-infected patients: Clinically, headache, focal neurological deficit, seizures, and altered mental status. CT shows ring-enhancing lesions in brain. Cerebral malaria: Clinically, 5–28% of children develop permanent neurological deficits including epilepsy, hypertonia, cortical blindness, and ataxia. *Naegleria* follows exposure to warm, fresh, and polluted water (eg, swimming pools, sewers, fresh-water lakes). Neurocysticercosis: Worldwide prevalence estimate in 2010 of 1.4 million cases. Greatest burden in pig-raising areas with poor sanitation. Capewell LG et al. Diagnosis, clinical course, and treatment of primary amoebic meningoencephalitis in the United States, 1937–2013. J Pediatric Infect Dis Soc 2015;4:e68. [PMID: 26582886] Garcia HH et al. Clinical symptoms, diagnosis, and treatment of neurocysticercosis. Lancet Neurol 2014;13:1202. [PMID: 25453460] John CC et al. Global research priorities for infections that affect the nervous system. Nature 2015;527:S178. [PMID: 26580325] Kodym P et al. Incidence, immunological and clinical characteristics of reactivation of latent *Toxoplasma gondii* infection in HIV-infected patients. Epidemiol Infect 2015;143:600. [PMID: 24850323] Misra UK et al. Cerebral malaria and bacterial meningitis. Ann Indian Acad Neurol 2011;14:535. [PMID: 21847328]

CENTRAL NERVOUS SYSTEM
Tuberculous meningitis

Organism	Specimen/Diagnostic Tests	Comments
Tuberculous meningitis *M. tuberculosis* (MTb)	CSF for pressure (elevated), cell count (WBCs 100–500/mcL, PMNs early, lymphocytes later), protein (elevated), glucose (decreased). (See CSF profiles, Table 8–9.) CSF for AFB stain. Stain is positive in only 10–30%; culture may be negative in 15–25% of cases. Cytocentrifugation and repeat smears may increase yield. CSF for AFB culture (sensitivity 60–70%). Repeated sampling of the CSF during the first week of therapy is recommended; ideally, 3 or 4 specimens of 5–10 mL each should be obtained (87% yield with 4 specimens). Key is to examine and culture large volumes of CSF. CSF PCR available but sensitivity of most assays is low (50%). Newer real-time PCR assays claim 60–90% sensitivity where CSF culture is positive for MTb. Positive CSF PCR is helpful with appropriate clinical manifestations, but negative PCR does not rule out tuberculous meningitis. Tuberculin test or gamma interferon release assays on CSF may be helpful for diagnosis if positive. Imaging (eg, MRI) may show lesions.	Most severe form of tuberculosis; approximately 1/3 of patients die soon after presentation and many survivors have severe neurological sequelae. Children with tuberculosis have highest risk of sequelae and mortality. Early diagnosis and treatment for tuberculous meningitis is the best predictor of survival. Tuberculous meningitis is usually secondary to rupture of a subependymal tubercle into subarachnoid space or may be a consequence of miliary tuberculosis. Because CSF stain and culture are not sensitive for tuberculous meningitis, diagnosis and treatment should be based on a combination of clinical and microbiologic data. Evidence of inactive or active extrameningeal tuberculosis, especially pulmonary, is seen in 75% of patients. Empiric therapy recommended for high fever and rapid decline of consciousness for high risk groups (immigrants, household exposures). Miftode EG et al. Tuberculous meningitis in children and adults: a 10-year retrospective comparative analysis. PLoS One 2015;10:e0133477. [PMID: 26186004] Nhu NT et al. Evaluation of GeneXpert MTB/RIF for diagnosis of tuberculous meningitis. J Clin Microbiol 2014;52:226. [PMID: 24197880] Qin L et al. Diagnostic value of T-cell interferon-γ Release assays on cerebrospinal fluid for tuberculous meningitis. PLoS One 2015;10 (11): e0141814. [PMID: 26545256] Thwaites GE et al. Tuberculous meningitis: more questions, still too few answers. Lancet Neurol 2013;12:999. [PMID: 23972913]

(Continued)

EYE	EYE
Conjunctivitis	**Keratitis**
Conjunctivitis Neonate (ophthalmia neonatorum): C. trachomatis (15–50%), N. gonorrhoeae (GNDC), HSV. Children and adults: adenovirus, staphylococci (GPC), HSV, H. influenzae (GNCB), S. pneumoniae (GPDC), S. pyogenes (GPC), VZV, N. gonorrhoeae (GNDC), M. lacunata (GNCB), M. catarrhalis, Bartonella sp. (Parinaud oculoglandular syndrome). Adult inclusion conjunctivitis/trachoma: C. trachomatis. Acute hemorrhagic conjunctivitis (acute epidemic kerato-conjunctivitis): enterovirus, coxsackievirus.	**Keratitis** Bacteria: P. aeruginosa (GNR), staphylococci (GPC), S. pneumoniae (GPDC), Haemophilus sp. (GNCB), Moraxella sp. Virus: HSV (dendritic pattern on fluorescein slit-lamp examination), VZV. Contact lens: Acanthamoeba, Enterobacteriaceae (GNR). Fungus: Candida, fusarium, aspergillus, rhodotorula, other filamentous fungi. Parasite: O. volvulus (river blindness), microsporidia (HIV).
Conjunctival Gram stain is especially useful if gonococcal infection is suspected. Bacterial culture for severe cases (routine bacterial culture) or suspected gonococcal infection. Conjunctival scrapings or smears by direct immunofluorescent monoclonal antibody staining for C. trachomatis. Cell culture for chlamydia. Detection of chlamydial DNA on ocular swabs by PCR techniques may be available in reference laboratories. Ocular HSV and VZV PCR may be available in research laboratories. Adenovirus conjunctivitis: cell culture, antigen detection, DNA detection. Rapid test has been approved for detection of adenovirus antigen in tear sample in the clinic.	Corneal scrapings for Gram stain, KOH, and culture. Routine bacterial culture is used for most bacterial causes, viral tissue culture for herpes, and special media for Acanthamoeba culture. Treatment depends on Gram stain appearance and culture. Corneal biopsy may be needed if initial cultures are negative. Ocular viral DFA for HSV and VZV.
The causes of conjunctivitis change with the season. Adenovirus occurs mainly in the fall, H. influenzae in the winter. Gonococcal conjunctivitis is an ophthalmologic emergency. Cultures are usually unnecessary unless chlamydia or gonorrhea is suspected or the case is severe. Consider noninfectious causes (eg, allergy, contact lens deposits, trauma). Alfonso SA et al. Conjunctivitis. Prim Care 2015;42:325. [PMID: 26319341] Narayana S et al. Bedside diagnosis of the 'red eye': a systematic review. Am J Med 2015;128:1220. [PMID: 26169885]	Prompt ophthalmologic consultation is mandatory. Acanthamoeba infection occurs in soft contact (extended-wear) lens wearers and may resemble HSV infection on fluorescein examination (dendritic ["branching"] ulcer). Bacterial keratitis is usually caused by contact lens use or trauma. Fungal (i.e., Fusarium sp.) keratitis is usually caused by trauma. Increased resistance noted among all bacterial isolates (eg, coagulase-negative staphylococci) to ciprofloxacin (20–38%) and cefazolin (19–40%). Resistance to bacitracin, trimethoprim-sulfamethoxazole and vancomycin remains unchanged. Ghebremedhin B. Human adenovirus: viral pathogen with increasing importance. Eur J Microbiol Immunol 2014;4:26. [PMID: 24678403] Ong HS et al. Corneal infections in the 21st century. Postgrad Med J 2015;91:565. [PMID: 26354125] Slowik M et al. Mycotic infections of the eye. Adv Clin Exp Med 2015;24:1113. [PMID: 26771986]

EYE
Endophthalmitis

Organism	Specimen/Diagnostic Tests	Comments
Endophthalmitis Spontaneous or postoperative: Coagulase-negative staphylococci (70%) (GPC), *S. aureus* (10%) (GPC), viridans group streptococci (5%) (GPC in chains), *S. pneumoniae* (5%) (GPDC), gram–negative rods (6%) (eg, *E. coli*, *Klebsiella* sp., *Pseudomonas* sp.), and other gram–positive organisms (4%) (eg, group B streptococci, *Listeria* sp.). Trauma: *Bacillus* sp. (GPR), fungi, coagulase negative staphylococci (GPC), streptococci (GPC), and gram–negative rods. Postfiltering bleb created to control glaucoma: Viridans group streptococci (57%) (GPC in chains), *S. pneumoniae* (GPDC), *H. influenzae* (GNCB), *M. catarrhalis* (GNCB), *S. aureus* (GPC), *S. epidermidis* (GPC), enterococci (GPC), gram–negative rods. IV drug abuse: Add *Bacillus cereus*.	Culture material from anterior chamber, vitreous cavity, and wound abscess for bacteria, mycobacteria, and fungi. Traumatic and postoperative cases should have aqueous and vitreous aspiration for culture and smear (56%). Conjunctival cultures are inadequate and misleading.	Endophthalmitis is an inflammatory process of the ocular cavity and adjacent structures caused by a bacterial or fungal infection. Rapid diagnosis is critical, because vision may be compromised. Bacterial endophthalmitis usually occurs as a consequence of ocular surgery (cataract surgery), 75% within first postoperative week. Prophylactic antibiotics are of unproven benefit, though topical antibiotics are widely used. Also consider retinitis in immunocompromised patients, caused by CMV, HSV, VZV, and toxoplasma (retinochoroiditis), which is diagnosed by retinal examination. Assaad D et al. Bacterial endophthalmitis: 10-year review of the culture and sensitivity patterns of bacterial isolates. Can J Ophthalmol 2015;50:433. [PMID: 26651302] Durand ML. Endophthalmitis. Clin Microbiol Infect 2013;19:227. [PMID: 23438028] Vaziri K et al. Endophthalmitis: state of the art. Clin Ophthalmol 2015;9:95. [PMID: 25609911]

(Continued)

EAR		
Otitis media		
Otitis media Infant, child, and adult: *S. pneumoniae* (23%) (GPDC), *H. influenzae* (36%) (GNCB), *M. catarrhalis* (3%) (GNDC), *S. aureus* (GPC), *S. pyogenes* (GPC in chains), viruses (eg, respiratory syncytial virus [RSV], influenza virus, rhinovirus, enteroviruses, human metapneumovirus), *M. pneumoniae*, *C. trachomatis* or *C. pneumoniae*, anaerobes, fungi (eg, *Blastomyces dermatitidis*, *Candida* sp., *Aspergillus* sp.). Neonate: Same as above plus Enterobacteriaceae (GNR), group B streptococcus (GPC). Endotracheal intubation: *Pseudomonas* sp. (GNR), *Klebsiella* (GNR), Enterobacteriaceae (GNR). Chronic: *P. aeruginosa* (GNR), anaerobes, *M. tuberculosis* (AFB).	Tympanocentesis aspirate for Gram stain and bacterial culture in the patient who has a toxic appearance. Otherwise, microbiologic studies of effusions are so consistent that empiric treatment is acceptable. CSF examination if clinically indicated. Nasopharyngeal swab may be substituted for tympanocentesis. Blood culture in the toxic patient.	Peak incidence of otitis media occurs in the first 3 years of life, especially between 6 and 24 months of age. In neonates, predisposing factors include cleft palate, hypotonia, mental retardation (Down syndrome). Tympanocentesis is indicated if the patient fails to improve after 48 hours or develops fever. It may hasten resolution and decrease sterile effusion. Persistent middle ear effusion may require placement of ventilating or tympanostomy tubes. Bullous myringitis suggests mycoplasma. Emerging antibiotic resistance should be considered in choice of empiric antibiotic therapy. There is emerging resistance of *S. pneumoniae* to macrolides, to erythromycin and to penicillin, so appropriate therapy should rely on local antibiograms. *M. catarrhalis* organisms produce β-lactamase (90%), as do *H. influenzae* organisms (~33–50%). This lessens usefulness of amoxicillin, the usual drug of choice. Ngo CC et al. Predominant bacteria detected from the middle ear fluid of children experiencing otitis media: a systematic review. PLoS One 2016;11(3):e0150949. [PMID: 26953891] Rosenfeld RM et al. Clinical practice guideline: otitis media with effusion (update). Otolaryngol Head Neck Surg 2016;154:S1. [PMID: 26832942]
Otitis externa	**EAR** **Otitis externa**	
Otitis externa Acute localized: *S. aureus* (15%) (GPC), anaerobes (32%), *S. pyogenes* (GPC in chains), *H. influenzae*, other gram-positive cocci. "Swimmer's ear": *Pseudomonas* sp. (40%) (GNR), fungi (6%) (eg, *Aspergillus* sp., *Candida* sp.). Chronic: Usually secondary to seborrhea or eczema. Diabetes mellitus, AIDS ("malignant otitis externa"): *P. aeruginosa* (GNR), *Aspergillus* sp., *Candida* sp. Furuncle of external canal: *S. aureus*.	Ear drainage for Gram stain and bacterial culture, especially in malignant otitis externa. CT or MRI can aid in diagnosis by demonstrating cortical bone erosion or meningeal enhancement.	Infection of the external auditory canal is similar to infection of skin and soft tissue elsewhere. If malignant otitis externa is present, exclusion of associated osteomyelitis and surgical drainage may be required. Hobson CE et al. Malignant otitis externa: evolving pathogens and implications for diagnosis and treatment. Otolaryngol Head Neck Surg 2014;151:112. [PMID: 24675790] Rosenfeld RM et al. Clinical practice guideline: acute otitis externa. Otolaryngol Head Neck Surg 2014;150:S1. [PMID: 24491310]

SINUS

Sinusitis

Organism	Specimen/Diagnostic Tests	Comments
Sinusitis Acute: *S. pneumoniae* (GPDC) (20–43%), *H. influenzae* (GNCB) (21–35%), *M. catarrhalis* (GNDC) (2–10%), other streptococci (3–9%) (GPC), anaerobes (1–9%), viruses (4%) (adenovirus, influenza, parainfluenza), *S. aureus* (GPC) (1–8%). Chronic (child): Viridans and anaerobic streptococci (GPC in chains) (23%), *S. aureus* (19%), *S. pneumoniae*, *H. influenzae*, *M. catarrhalis*, *P. aeruginosa* (GNR) in cystic fibrosis. Chronic (adult): Coagulase-negative staphylococci (GPC) (36%), *S. aureus* (GPC) (25%), viridans streptococci (GPC in chains) (8%), corynebacteria (GPR) (5%), anaerobes (6%), including *Bacteroides* sp., *Prevotella* sp. (GNR), peptostreptococcus (GPC), *Fusobacterium* sp. (GNR). Hospitalized with nasogastric tube or nasotracheal intubation: Enterobacteriaceae (GNR), *Pseudomonas* sp. (GNR). Fungal: Zygomycetes (rhizopus), aspergillus, *P. boydii*, other dematiaceous mold. Immunocompromised: *P. aeruginosa* (GNR), CMV, *Aspergillus* sp. and other filamentous fungi plus microsporidia, *Cryptosporidium parvum*, *Acanthamoeba* in HIV-infected patients.	Clinical diagnosis. Nasal aspirate for bacterial culture is not usually helpful due to respiratory flora contamination of aerobes and anaerobes. Maxillary sinus aspirate for bacterial culture may be helpful in severe or atypical cases.	Diagnosis and treatment of sinusitis are usually based on clinical and radiologic features. Microbiologic studies can be helpful in severe or atypical cases. Sinus CT scan (or MRI) is better than plain x-ray for diagnosing sinusitis, particularly if sphenoid sinusitis is suspected. However, sinus CT scans should be interpreted cautiously, because abnormalities are also seen in patients with the common cold. Acute and chronic sinusitis occur frequently in HIV-infected patients, may be recurrent or refractory, and may involve multiple sinuses (especially when the CD4 cell count is <200/mcL). Acute sinusitis often results from bacterial superinfection following viral upper respiratory infection. Chen PG et al. A golden experience: fifty years of experience managing the frontal sinus. Laryngoscope 2016;126:802. [PMID: 26393824] Rosenfeld RM et al. Clinical practice guideline (update): adult sinusitis. Otolaryngol Head Neck Surg 2015;152:S1. [PMID: 25832968]

(Continued)

UPPER AIRWAY	UPPER AIRWAY
Pharyngitis	Laryngitis

Pharyngitis

Exudative: *S. pyogenes* (GPC) (15–30%), viruses (rhinovirus, coronavirus, adenovirus) (30%), group C and G streptococci (GPC) (5%), herpes simplex virus (HSV) (4%), parainfluenza and influenza virus A and B (2–4%), Epstein-Barr virus (mononucleosis) (1%), HIV (1%), *N. gonorrhoeae* (GNDC) (1%), *C. diphtheriae* (GPR) (≤1%), *Arcanobacterium hemolyticum* (GPR) (≤1%), *M. pneumoniae*, *C. pneumoniae*.

Membranous: *C. diphtheriae* (GPR), *C. pseudodiphtheriticum* (GPR), HSV, Epstein-Barr virus.

Throat swab for culture. Place in sterile tube or transport medium. If *N. gonorrhoeae* is suspected, use chocolate agar or Thayer-Martin media. If *C. diphtheriae* is suspected, use Tinsdale or blood agar. Throat swabs are routinely cultured for group A streptococcus only. If other organisms are suspected, this must be stated.

Throat culture has about 70–90% sensitivity and 95% specificity for group A streptococcus.

"Rapid" tests for group A streptococcus can speed diagnosis and aid in the treatment of family members. However, false-negative results may lead to under-diagnosis and failure to treat. Back-up throat cultures are recommended so group A streptococcus is not missed. Sequelae of group A streptococcus infection, such as rheumatic fever, post-streptococcal glomerulonephritis, can be severe. New rapid molecular assays for group A streptococcus are now available with high sensitivity and specificity.

Controversy exists over how to evaluate patients with sore throat, although some authors suggest culturing all patients and then treating only those with positive cultures.

Most laboratories only report group A streptococcus from throat culture. Many CLIA-waived tests are now available for use in doctors' offices.

In patients with compatible histories, be sure to consider pharyngeal abscess or epiglottitis, both of which may be life-threatening.

Complications include pharyngeal abscess and Lemierre syndrome (infection with *Fusobacterium* sp.), which can progress to sepsis and multi-organ failure.

Herath VC et al. Sore throat: is it such a big deal anymore? J Infect 2015;71:S101. [PMID: 25917806]

Lean WL et al. Rapid diagnostic tests for group A streptococcal pharyngitis: a meta-analysis. Pediatrics 2014;134:771. [PMID: 25201792]

Van Brusselen D et al. Streptococcal pharyngitis in children: to treat or not to treat? Eur J Pediatr 2014;173:1275. [PMID: 25113742]

Laryngitis

Virus (90%) (influenza, rhinovirus, adenovirus, parainfluenza, Epstein-Barr virus), *S. pyogenes* (GPC) (10%), *M. catarrhalis* (GNDC), *H. influenzae* (GNCB), *M. tuberculosis*, fungus (cryptococcosis, histoplasmosis).

Immunocompromised: *Candida* sp., CMV, HSV.

Diagnosis is made by clinical picture of upper respiratory infection with hoarseness.

Laryngitis usually occurs with common cold or influenza syndromes.

Fungal laryngeal infections occur most commonly in immunocompromised patients (AIDS, cancer, organ transplants, corticosteroid therapy, diabetes mellitus).

Chronic laryngitis is associated with one or more chronic irritants such as gastric acid, chronic sinusitis, chronic alcohol use, inhaled toxins.

Hah JH et al. Evaluation of the prevalence of and factors associated with laryngeal diseases among the general population. Laryngoscope 2015;125:2536. [PMID: 26154733]

Wood JM et al. Laryngitis. BMJ 2014;349:g5827. [PMID: 25300640]

	UPPER AIRWAY	UPPER AIRWAY
	Laryngotracheobronchitis	Epiglottitis
Organism	**Specimen/Diagnostic Tests**	**Comments**
Laryngotracheobronchitis Infant/child: RSV (50–75%) (bronchiolitis), adenovirus, parainfluenza virus (HPIV types 1, 2, 3) (80%) (croup), B. pertussis (GNCB) (whooping cough), other viruses, including rhinovirus, coronavirus, influenza, bocavirus, human metapneumovirus. Adolescent/adult: Usually viruses, M. pneumoniae, C. pneumoniae, B. pertussis. Chronic adult: S. pneumoniae (GPDC), H. influenzae (GNCB), M. catarrhalis (GNDC), Klebsiella (GNR), other Enterobacteriaceae (GNR), viruses (eg, influenza), aspergillus (allergic bronchopulmonary aspergillosis). Chronic obstructive airway disease: Viral (25–50%), S. pneumoniae (GPC), H. influenzae (GNCB), S. aureus (GPC), Enterobacteriaceae (GNR), anaerobes (<10%).	Nasopharyngeal aspirate or swab for respiratory virus DFA, for viral culture (rarely indicated), and for PCR for B. pertussis. PCR for pertussis is test of choice; culture and DFA are less sensitive. Cellular examination of early morning sputum will show many PMNs in chronic bronchitis. Sputum Gram stain and culture for ill adults. In chronic bronchitis, mixed flora are usually seen with oral flora or colonized H. influenzae or S. pneumoniae on culture. Paired sera for mycoplasmal antibody assays can help make a diagnosis retrospectively in infants and children but are not clinically useful except for seriously ill patients.	Chronic bronchitis is diagnosed when sputum is coughed up on most days for at least 3 consecutive months for more than 2 successive years. Bacterial infections are usually secondary infections of initial viral or mycoplasma-induced inflammation. Airway endoscopy can aid in the diagnosis of bacterial tracheitis in children. Delany DR et al. Role of direct laryngoscopy and bronchoscopy in recurrent croup. Otolaryngol Head Neck Surg 2015;152:159. [PMID: 25389322] Tibballs J et al. Symptoms and signs differentiating croup and epiglottitis. J Paediatr Child Health 2011;47:77. [PMID: 21091577]
Epiglottitis Child: H. influenzae type B (GNCB), H. parainfluenzae (GCNB), S. pneumoniae (GPC), S. aureus (GPC), other streptococci (groups A, B, C). Adult: S. pyogenes (GPC), S. pneumoniae (GPC), Klebsiella sp. (GNR), H. influenzae (GNCB), Pseudomonas sp. (GNR), HSV, viruses (parainfluenza and influenza). HIV: Candida (fungi) and Pseudomonas sp. (GNR).	Blood for bacterial culture: positive in 50–100% of children with H. influenzae. Lateral neck x-ray may show an enlarged epiglottis but has a low sensitivity (31%).	Acute epiglottitis is a rapidly moving cellulitis of the epiglottis and represents an airway emergency. Epiglottitis can be confused with croup, a viral infection of gradual onset that affects infants and causes inspiratory and expiratory stridor. Airway management is the primary concern, and an endotracheal tube should be placed or tracheostomy performed as soon as the diagnosis of epiglottitis is made in children. A tracheostomy set should be at the bedside for adults. Chroboczek T et al. Long-term outcome of critically ill adult patients with acute epiglottitis. PLoS One 2015;10:e125736. [PMID: 25945804] Richards AM. Pediatric respiratory emergencies. Emerg Med Clin North Am 2016;34:77. [PMID: 26614243] Westerhuis B et al. Acute epiglottitis in adults: an under-recognized and life-threatening condition. S D Med 2013;66:309. [PMID: 24175495]

LUNG		
Community-acquired pneumonia		

Community-acquired pneumonia

Neonate: *E. coli* (GNR), group A or B streptococcus (GPC), *S. aureus* (GPC), *Pseudomonas* sp (GNR), *C. trachomatis.*

Infant/child (<5 years): Virus, *S. pneumoniae* (GPC), *H. influenzae* (GNCB), *S. aureus.*

Age 5−40 years: Virus, *M. pneumoniae, C. pneumoniae* (formerly known as TWAR strain), *C. psittaci, S. pneumoniae, Legionella* sp.

Age >40 years without other disease: *S. pneumoniae* (GPDC), *H. influenzae* (GNCB), *S. aureus* (GPC), *M. catarrhalis* (GNDC), *C. pneumoniae, Legionella* sp. (GNR), *S. pyogenes* (GPC), *K. pneumoniae* (GNR), Enterobacteriaceae (GNR), viruses (eg, influenza).

Cystic fibrosis: *P. aeruginosa* (GNR), *Burkholderia cepacia.*

Elderly: *S. pneumoniae* (GPDC), *H. influenzae* (GNCB), *S. aureus* (GPC), Enterobacteriaceae (GNR), *M. catarrhalis* (GNDC), group B streptococcus (GPC), legionella (GNR), nocardia (GPR), influenza.

Aspiration: *S. pneumoniae* (GPDC), *K. pneumoniae* (GNR), Enterobacteriaceae (GNR), *Bacteroides* sp. and other oral anaerobes.

Fungal: *H. capsulatum, C. immitis, B. dermatitidis.*

Exposure to birthing animals, sheep: *C. burnetii* (Q fever), rabbits: *F. tularensis* (tularemia), deer mice: hantavirus, birds: *C. psittaci.*

Sputum for Gram stain desirable; culture, if empiric therapy fails or patient is seriously ill. An adequate specimen should have <10 epithelial cells and >25 PMNs per low-power field. Special sputum cultures for legionella are available.

Legionella urine antigen test is 70−80% sensitive, but only detects *Legionella pneumophila* serogroup 1 (90% of cases of Legionaire disease), so test may be falsely negative.

Blood for bacterial cultures (2 sets); obtain before antibiotic treatment, especially in ill patients.

Pleural fluid for bacterial culture if significant effusion is present.

Bronchoalveolar lavage or brushings for bacterial, fungal, and viral antigen tests and AFB culture in immunocompromised patients and atypical cases.

Paired sera for *M. pneumoniae* EIA testing can diagnose infection retrospectively.

Serologic tests for Q fever and for hantavirus (IgM and IgG) are available. Culture of respiratory specimens for *C. pneumoniae, C. psittaci* strains.

Other special techniques (bronchoscopy with telescoping plugged catheter and protected brush, transtracheal aspiration, transthoracic fine-needle aspiration, or, rarely, open-lung biopsy) can be used to obtain specimens for culture in severe cases, in immunocompromised patients, or in cases with negative conventional cultures and progression despite empiric antibiotic therapy.

About 60% of cases of community-acquired pneumonia have an identifiable microbial cause. Pneumatoceles suggest *S. aureus* but are also reported with pneumococcus, group A streptococcus, *H influenzae,* and Enterobacteriaceae (in neonates).

An "atypical pneumonia" presentation (diffuse pattern on chest x-ray with lack of organisms on Gram stain of sputum) should raise suspicion of mycoplasma, legionella, or chlamydial infection. Consider hantavirus pulmonary syndrome if pulmonary symptoms follow afebrile illness.

Aspiration pneumonias are most commonly associated with stroke, alcoholism, drug abuse, sedation, and periodontal disease.

Approval and widespread use of pneumococcal conjugate vaccine (PCV13) for at-risk populations has been effective prevention strategy.

Irfan M et al. Community-acquired pneumonia. Curr Opin Pulm Med 2013;19:198. [PMID: 23422417]

Sharma D et al. Pneumococcal carriage and invasive disease in children before introduction of the 13-valent conjugate vaccine: comparison with the era before 7-valent conjugate vaccine. Pediatr Infect Dis J 2013;32:e45. [PMID: 23080290]

Viasus D et al. Community-acquired *Legionella pneumophila* pneumonia: a single-center experience with 214 hospitalized sporadic cases over 15 years. Medicine (Baltimore) 2013;92:51. [PMID: 23266795]

(*Continued*)

	LUNG	LUNG
	Anaerobic pneumonia	**Hospital-acquired pneumonia**

Organism	Specimen/Diagnostic Tests	Comments
Anaerobic pneumonia/lung abscess Usually polymicrobial: Anaerobes: *Bacteroides* sp. (15% *B. fragilis*), *Peptostreptococcus, Prevotella* sp., *Porphyromonas* sp., *Fusobacterium* sp., micro-aerophilic streptococcus, veillonella, and facultative anaerobes; *S. aureus, P. aeruginosa, S. pneumoniae* (rare), Klebsiella (rare), *H. influenzae* type B, legionella, nocardia, actinomyces, fungi, parasites.	Sputum Gram stain and culture for anaerobes are of little value because of contaminating oral flora. Bronchoalveolar sampling (brush or aspirate or biopsy) for Gram stain and culture will usually make an accurate diagnosis. Percutaneous transthoracic needle aspiration may be useful for culture and for cytology to demonstrate coexistence of an underlying carcinoma. Blood cultures are usually (80%) negative.	Aspiration is the most important underlying cause of lung abscess. Without clear-cut risk factors such as alcoholism, coma, or seizures, bronchoscopy is often performed to rule out neoplasm. Bartlett JG. Anaerobic bacterial infection of the lung. Anaerobe 2012;18:235. [PMID: 22209937] Bartlett JG. How important are anaerobic bacteria in aspiration pneumonia: when should they be treated and what is optimal therapy. Infect Dis Clin North Am 2013;27:149. [PMID: 23398871] DiBardino DM et al. Aspiration pneumonia: a review of modern trends. J Crit Care 2015;30:40. [PMID: 25129577]
Hospital-acquired pneumonia *P. aeruginosa* (GNR), Klebsiella (GNR), *S. aureus* (GPC), *Acinetobacter* (GNR), Enterobacteriaceae (GNR). *S. pneumoniae* (GPDC), *H. influenzae* (GNCB), influenza virus, RSV, parainfluenza virus, adenovirus, oral anaerobes, *S. maltophilia* (GNR), *B. cepacia* (GNR). Mendelson syndrome (see Comments): No organisms initially, then pseudomonas, Enterobacteriaceae, *S. aureus, S. pneumoniae*.	Sputum Gram stain and culture for bacteria (aerobic and anaerobic) and fungus (if suspected). Blood cultures for bacteria are often negative (80%). Endotracheal aspirate or bronchoalveolar sample for bacterial and fungal culture in selected patients. Ventilator-associated pneumonia (VAP) is difficult to diagnose. Suspect VAP in a patient with fever, leukocytosis, purulent respiratory secretions or a progressive radiographic pulmonary infiltrate.	Most cases are related to aspiration. Hospital-acquired aspiration pneumonia is associated with intubation and the use of broad-spectrum antibiotics. A strong association between aspiration pneumonia and swallowing dysfunction is demonstrable by video fluoroscopy. Mendelson syndrome is due to acute aspiration of gastric contents (eg, during anesthesia or drowning). Hospital-acquired pneumonia is the second most common nosocomial infection, accounting for 25% of all ICU infections. Moreover, there has been a dramatic increase in multidrug-resistant bacteria. Montravers P et al. Current and future considerations for the treatment of hospital-acquired pneumonia. Adv Ther 2016;33:151. [PMID: 26861846] Nair GB et al. Ventilator-associated pneumonia: present understanding and ongoing debates. Intensive Care Med 2015;41:34. [PMID: 25427866] Quartin AA et al. A comparison of microbiology and demographics among patients with healthcare-associated, hospital-acquired, and ventilator-associated pneumonia: a retrospective analysis of 1184 patients from a large, international study. BMC Infect Dis 2013;13:561. [PMID: 24279701]

(Continued)

LUNG		
Pneumonia in immunocompromised host		
Pneumonia in the immunocompromised host AIDS: *M. avium* (31%), *P. jirovecii* (13%), CMV (11%), *H. capsulatum* (7%), *S. pneumoniae* (GPDC), *H. influenzae* (GNCB), *P. aeruginosa* (GNR), Enterobacteriaceae (GNR), *C. neoformans*, *M. tuberculosis* (AFB), other mycobacteria, *C. immitis*, *P. marneffei*, *Rhodococcus equi* (GPR). Neutropenic: *S. aureus* (GPC), *Pseudomonas* sp. (GNR), *Klebsiella* sp., enterobacter (GNR), *Bacteroides* sp. and other oral anaerobes, legionella, candida, aspergillus, mucor. Transplant recipients: CMV (60–70%), *P. aeruginosa* (GNR), *S. aureus* (GPC), *S. pneumoniae* (GPDC), legionella (GNR), RSV, influenza virus, *P. jirovecii*, aspergillus, *P. boydii*, nocardia, strongyloides.	Expectorated sputum for Gram stain and bacterial culture, if purulent. AFB and fungal cultures of respiratory specimens. Sputum induction or bronchiolar lavage for Giemsa or methenamine silver staining or DFA for *P. jirovecii* trophozoites or cysts; for mycobacterial, fungal staining and culture, for legionella culture, and for CMV culture. Nasal washings or swab for viral respiratory direct fluorescent antibody (DFA), viral culture, or molecular assays. Urine for legionella and histoplasma antigen test. Blood for CMV quantitative PCR, or fungal galactomannan antigen test or beta-D-glucan assay. Blood, respiratory specimen, or bone marrow fungal culture for histoplasmosis (positive in 50%), coccidioidomycosis (positive in 30%). Blood culture for bacteria. Blood cultures are more frequently positive in HIV-infected patients with bacterial pneumonia and often are the only source where a specific organism is identified; bacteremic patients have higher mortality rates. Histoplasma urine antigen positive in 90% of AIDS patients with disseminated histoplasmosis. Immunodiffusion is useful for screening for antibodies, and complement fixation for antibody titers for suspected histoplasmosis or coccidioidomycosis. Serum cryptococcal antigen or culture of respiratory specimens when pulmonary cryptococcosis is suspected. Serum lactate dehydrogenase (LDH) levels are elevated in 63% and hypoxemia with exercise (PaO$_2$ <75 mm Hg) occurs in 57% of PCP cases.	In pneumocystis pneumonia (PCP), the sensitivities of the various diagnostic tests are: sputum induction 80% (in experienced labs), bronchoscopy with lavage 90–97%, transbronchial biopsy 94–97%. In PCP, chest x-ray may show interstitial (36%) or alveolar (25%) infiltrates or may be normal (39%), particularly if leukopenia is present. Recurrent episodes of bacterial pneumonia are common. Kaposi sarcoma of the lung is a common neoplastic process that can imitate infection in homosexual and African HIV-infected patients. Crotty MP et al. Epidemiology, co-infections, and outcomes of viral pneumonia in adults: an observational cohort study. Medicine (Baltimore) 2015;94:e2332. [PMID: 26683973] Schmiedel Y et al. Common invasive fungal diseases: an overview of invasive candidiasis, aspergillosis cryptococcosis, and *Pneumocystis* pneumonia. Swiss Med Wkly 2016;146:w14281. [PMID: 26901377]

	LUNG	LUNG
	Mycobacterial pneumonia	**Empyema**

Organism	Specimen/Diagnostic Tests	Comments
Mycobacterial pneumonia M. tuberculosis (MTb, AFB, acid-fast beaded rods), M. kansasii, M. avium-intracellulare complex (MAC), other mycobacteria (M. abscessus, M. xenopi, M. fortuitum, M. chelonei).	Sputum for acid-fast bacilli (AFB) stain and culture. First morning samples are best, and at least three samples are required. Culture systems detect mycobacterial growth in as little as several days to 8 weeks. Bronchoalveolar lavage for AFB stain and culture or gastric washings for AFB culture can be used if sputum tests are negative or if unable to obtain sputum (children). Sputum for amplification assays to detect MTb available for confirmation of smear positive (99%), less sensitive for smear negative (75%). Once AFB has been detected on solid media or in broth culture, nucleic acid hybridization probes or high-performance liquid chromatography can be used to identify the mycobacterial species. CT- or ultrasound-guided transthoracic fine-needle aspiration cytology can be used if clinical or radiographic features are nonspecific or if malignancy is suspected. Blood culture for MTb (15%) or MAC. Pleural fluid culture for MTb (25%).	AFB organisms found on sputum stain do not necessarily make the diagnosis of tuberculosis, because they could represent nonpathogenic mycobacteria. Tuberculosis is very common in HIV-infected patients, in whom the chest x-ray appearance may be atypical and occasionally (4%) may mimic PCP (especially in patients with CD4 cell counts <200/mcL). Consider HIV testing if MTb is diagnosed. Delayed diagnosis of pulmonary tuberculosis is common (up to 20% of cases), especially among patients who are older or who do not have respiratory symptoms. In any patient with suspected tuberculosis, respiratory isolation is required. Multi-drug resistant and extensively drug-resistant tuberculosis are now a major concern in many countries. Aksamit TR et al. Nontuberculosis mycobacteria (NTM) lung disease: the top ten essentials. Respir Med 2014;108:47. [PMID: 24484653] Horsburgh CR Jr et al. Treatment of tuberculosis. N Engl J Med 2015;373:2149. [PMID: 26605929]
Empyema Neonate: E. coli (GNR), group A or B streptococcus (GPC), S. aureus (GPC), Pseudomonas sp. (GNR). Infant/child (<5 years): S. aureus (60%) (GPC), S. pneumoniae (27%) (GPC), H. influenzae (GNCB), anaerobes. Child (>5 years)/adult, acute: S. pneumoniae (GPC), group A streptococcus (GPC), S. aureus (GPC), H. influenzae (GNCB), legionella, coagulase-negative staphylococci, viridans streptococci (GPC in chains). Child (>5 years)/adult, chronic: Anaerobic streptococci, Bacteroides sp., Prevotella sp., Porphyromonas sp., Fusobacterium sp. (anaerobes 36–76%), Enterobacteriaceae, E. coli, Klebsiella pneumoniae, M. tuberculosis, Actinomyces sp.	Pleural fluid for cell count (WBCs 25,000–100,000/mcL, mostly PMNs), protein >50% of serum), glucose (<serum, often very low), pH (<7.20), LDH (>60% of serum). (See Pleural fluid profiles, Table 8–16.) Blood cultures for bacteria. Sputum for Gram stain and bacterial culture. Special culture can also be performed for legionella when suspected. Pleural fluid for Gram stain and bacterial culture (aerobic and anaerobic).	Chest tube drainage is paramount. The clinical presentation of empyema is nonspecific. Chest CT with contrast is helpful in demonstrating pleural fluid accumulations due to mediastinal or subdiaphragmatic processes and can identify loculated effusions, bronchopleural fistulae, and lung abscesses. Some 40–60% of empyema develop following pneumonia. About 25% of cases result from trauma or surgery. Bronchoscopy is indicated when the infection is unexplained. Occasionally, multiple thoracenteses may be needed to diagnose empyema. Bender MT et al. Current surgical management of empyema thoracis in children: a single-center experience. Am Surg 2015;81:849. [PMID: 26350659] McCauley L et al. Pneumonia and empyema: causal, casual or unknown. J Thorac Dis 2015;7:992. [PMID: 26150912]

(Continued)

HEART AND VESSELS	HEART AND VESSELS
Pericarditis	**Tuberculous pericarditis**

Pericarditis

Viruses: Enteroviruses (coxsackie A and B, echovirus), influenza, Epstein-Barr, HSV, mumps, HIV, CMV, varicella-zoster, rubella, hepatitis B.

Bacteria: *S. aureus* (GPC), *S. pyogenes* (GPC), Enterobacteriaceae (GNR), *N. meningitidis* (GNDC), *N. gonorrhoeae* (GDNC), *Haemophilus* sp., anaerobic bacteria, mycobacteria (HIV and AIDS).

Fungi: *Aspergillus* sp., *Candida* sp., histoplasma, coccidioides, blastomyces, Cryptococcus (immunocompromised).

Parasites: *E. histolytica, T. gondii, Schistosoma* sp.

In acute pericarditis, specific bacterial diagnosis is made in only 19%.

Pericardial fluid aspirate for Gram stain and bacterial culture (aerobic and anaerobic). In acute pericarditis, only 54% have pericardial effusions.

Virus isolation from stool or throat can be attempted, but frequently fails to identify the pathogenic agent. PCR may be available in reference laboratories.

Surgical pericardial drainage with biopsy of pericardium for culture (22%) and histologic examination.

Acute and convalescent sera can be tested for antibodies (coxsackie B viruses and other enteroviruses and mycoplasma).

Viral pericarditis is usually diagnosed clinically (precordial pain, muffled heart sounds, pericardial friction rub, cardiomegaly). The diagnosis is rarely aided by microbiologic tests.

CT and MRI may demonstrate pericardial thickening.

Bacterial pericarditis is usually secondary to surgery, immunosuppression (including HIV), esophageal rupture, endocarditis with ruptured ring abscess, extension from lung abscess, aspiration pneumonia or empyema, or sepsis with pericarditis.

Imazio M et al. Evaluation and treatment of pericarditis: a systematic review. JAMA 2015;314:1498. [PMID: 26461998]

Yusuf SW et al. Pericardial disease: a clinical review. Expert Rev Cardiovasc Ther 2016;14:525. [PMID: 26691443]

Tuberculous pericarditis

Mycobacterium tuberculosis (MTb). MAC, *M. kansasii* (acid-fast beaded rods).

PPD skin testing or interferon-gamma release assays should be performed (negative in a sizable minority). The interferon gamma release assays are unaffected by BCG vaccination.

Pericardial fluid obtained by needle aspiration can show AFB by smear (rare) or culture (low yield).

Pericardial biopsy for culture and histologic examination for granulomatous inflammation has highest diagnostic yield.

Pericardial fluid may show markedly elevated levels of adenosine deaminase.

Pericardial fluid for cell count, protein (elevated), PMN (elevated).

Major cause of heart disease in Africa and in patients with AIDS.

Spread from nearby caseous mediastinal lymph nodes or pleurisy is the most common route of infection. Acutely, serofibrinous pericardial effusion develops with substernal pain, fever, and friction rub. Tamponade may occur.

Tuberculosis accounts for 4% of cases of acute pericarditis, 7% of cases of cardiac tamponade, and 6% of cases of constrictive pericarditis. One-third to one-half of patients develop constrictive pericarditis despite drug therapy. Constrictive pericarditis can occur 2–4 years after acute infection.

Lazaros G et al. Tuberculous pericarditis: a complex puzzle to put together. EBioMedicine 2015;2:1570. [PMID: 26870768]

Ntsekhe M et al. Tuberculous pericarditis with and without HIV. Heart Fail Rev 2013;18:367. [PMID: 2242006]

| HEART AND VESSELS | | HEART AND VESSELS | |
| Infectious myocarditis | | Infective endocarditis | |
Organism	Specimen/Diagnostic Tests	Comments
Infectious myocarditis Viruses: Enteroviruses (especially coxsackie A and B), Epstein-Barr, adenovirus, influenza virus, HIV, CMV. Bacteria: *Borrelia burgdorferi* (Lyme disease), scrub typhus, *Rickettsia rickettsii* (Rocky Mountain spotted fever), *Coxiella burnetii* (Q fever), *Mycoplasma pneumoniae*, *Chlamydophila pneumoniae*, *C. diphtheriae* (GPR). Parasites: *Trichinella spiralis* (trichinosis), *Trypanosoma cruzi* (Chagas disease), *T. gondii*.	Endomyocardial biopsy for pathologic examination, PCR, and culture in selected cases. Indium-111 antimyosin antibody imaging is more sensitive than endomyocardial biopsy. MRI techniques are improving. Stool or throat swab for enterovirus culture. Acute and convalescent sera for coxsackie B, *M. pneumoniae*, *C. pneumoniae*, scrub typhus, *R rickettsii*, *C. burnetii*, toxoplasma. Serum for antibodies against HIV, *B. burgdorferi*.	In most cases, no definitive cause is established. Viruses are most important infectious causes in U.S. and western Europe. Acute infectious myocarditis should be suspected in a patient with dynamically evolving changes in ECG, echocardiography, and serum CK levels and symptoms of an infection. The value of endomyocardial biopsy in such cases has not been established. In contrast, an endomyocardial biopsy is needed to diagnose lymphocytic inflammatory response with necrosis or giant cell myocarditis. The incidence of myocarditis in AIDS may be as high as 46%. Many patients with acute myocarditis progress to dilated cardiomyopathy. Fung G et al. Myocarditis. Circ Res 2016;118:496. [PMID: 26846643] Kindermann I et al. Update on myocarditis. J Am Coll Cardiol 2012;59:779. [PMID: 22361396]
Infective endocarditis *S. aureus* (GPC), coagulase-negative staphylococci (GPC), viridans group streptococci (GPC in chains), enterococci (GPC), *Abiotrophia* sp., nutritionally deficient streptococcus (GPC), *S. pneumoniae* (GPC), other β-hemolytic streptococci (GPC), *Erysipelothrix rhusiopathiae* (GPR), brucella (GVCB), other gram-negative bacilli, *Coxiella burnetii*, *C. pneumoniae*, bartonella, yeast. Slow-growing fastidious GNRs: HACEK (*H. aphrophilus*, *Aggregatibacter actinomycetemcomitans*, *Cardiobacterium hominis*, *Eikenella corrodens*, *Kingella kingae*).	Blood cultures for bacteria are positive in 97%, if two to three sets are drawn from peripheral venous sites and before start of antibiotic therapy. Blood cultures are frequently positive with gram-positive organisms but can be negative (5%) with gram-negative or anaerobic organisms, fungi, HACEK, and organisms that grow slowly. Request that the laboratory hold blood cultures 10–14 days to detect slow-growing organisms. Echocardiography can identify valvular vegetations in 50% of cases. Transesophageal echocardiography (TEE) can help in diagnosis by demonstrating the presence of valvular vegetations (sensitivity >90%), prosthetic valve dysfunction, valvular regurgitation, secondary "jet" or "kissing" lesions, and paravalvular abscess. TEE has greater sensitivity than transthoracic echocardiography (TTE) (see Chapter 7).	Patients with congenital or valvular heart disease, or prosthetic valves should receive prophylaxis before dental procedures or surgery of the upper respiratory, genitourinary, or gastrointestinal tract. In left-sided endocarditis, patients should be watched carefully for development of valvular regurgitation or ring abscess. The size and mobility of valvular vegetations on TEE can help to predict the risk of arterial embolization. Streptococci account for 60–80% of infective endocarditis cases and currently *S. aureus* and coagulase negative staphylococci account for 20–35% of cases. Fungi (2–4%) and mixed infections (1–2%) can also be etiologic agents. Almost any structural heart disease can predispose to infective endocarditis, especially if there is increased turbulence of blood flow. Prosthetic valve endocarditis and intravascular infections due to cardiac devices (pacemakers, defibrillators) have been increasing. Colville T et al. Infective endocarditis in intravenous drug users: a review article. Postgrad Med J 2016;92:105. [PMID: 26719453] El Rafei A et al. Beta-haemolytic streptococcal endocarditis: clinical presentation management and outcomes. Infect Dis 2016;48:373. [PMID: 26950685] Keynan Y et al. Infective endocarditis in the intensive care unit. Crit Care Clin 2013;29:923. [PMID: 24094385] Pierce D et al. Infectious endocarditis: diagnosis and treatment. Am Fam Physician 2012;85:981. [PMID: 22612050]

HEART AND VESSELS

Infectious thrombophlebitis

(Continued)

Infectious thrombophlebitis		
Infectious thrombophlebitis Associated with venous catheters: *S. aureus* (GPC) (65–78%), coagulase-negative staphylococci (GPC), *Candida* sp. (yeast), *Pseudomonas* sp. (GNR), Enterobacteriaceae (GNR), streptococci (GPC), enterococci (GPC), anaerobes. Hyperalimentation with catheter: *Candida* sp., *Malassezia furfur* (yeast). Indwelling venous catheter (eg, Broviac, Hickman): *S. aureus*, coagulase-negative staphylococci, diphtheroids (GPR), *Pseudomonas* sp., Enterobacteriaceae, *Candida* sp. Postpartum or postabortion pelvic thrombophlebitis: Bacteroides (GNR), Enterobacteriaceae, clostridium (GPR), streptococcus (GPC).	Blood cultures for bacteria are positive in 97%, if three sets are drawn from peripheral venous sites and before start of antibiotic therapy. Catheter tip for bacterial culture to document etiology. More than 15 colonies (CFUs) suggests colonization or infection. CT and MRI are the studies of choice in the evaluation of puerperal septic pelvic thrombophlebitis.	Thrombophlebitis is an inflammation of the vein wall. Infectious thrombophlebitis with microbial invasion of the vessel is associated with bacteremia and thrombosis. Risk of infection from an indwelling peripheral venous catheter goes up significantly after 4 days. Heit JA. Epidemiology of venous thromboembolism. Nat Rev Cardiol 2015;12:464. [PMID: 26076949] Heit JA et al. Predictors of venous thromboembolism recurrence, adjusted for treatments and interim exposures: a population-based case–cohort study. Thromb Res 2015;136:298. [PMID: 26143712] Wong AP et al. Internal jugular vein septic thrombophlebitis (Lemierre syndrome) as a complication of pharyngitis. J Am Board Fam Med 2015;28:425. [PMID: 25957375]

ABDOMEN		
Organism	Specimen/Diagnostic Tests	Comments
Gastritis *Helicobacter pylori.*	Serology: Serum for antibody testing used for initial screening because test is noninvasive with no false negative results for patients on treatment (56–100% sensitivity, specificity 60–98%). Stool for antigen detection: Test is noninvasive (94% sensitivity, 97% specificity) and can be used to monitor therapy. [^{13}C] or [^{14}C] urea breath tests: Tests (88–95% sensitive, 95–100% specific) are relatively noninvasive, safe, and accurate for initial diagnosis. Performance in children not established. Endoscopy: Gastric mucosal biopsy for detection of *H. pylori* with histology (91% sensitivity, 100% specificity). Rapid urease test based on production of large amounts of urease enzyme by *H. pylori* (85–95% sensitivity, 95–100% specificity). Culture (very difficult given the fastidious nature of the bacterium, but may be attempted to evaluate potential antibiotic resistance for patients failing therapy).	Also associated with duodenal ulcer, gastric carcinoma, and gastroesophageal reflux disease. Proton pump inhibitors may cause false-negative urea breath tests and stool antigen tests, and should be withheld for at least 2 weeks before collecting specimens for testing. Lopes AI et al. *Helicobacter pylori* infection—recent developments in diagnosis. World J Gastroenterol 2014;20:9299. [PMID: 25071324] Mentis A et al. Epidemiology and diagnosis of *Helicobacter pylori* infection. Helicobacter 2015;20(Suppl 1):1. [PMID: 26372818] Wang YK et al. Diagnosis of *Helicobacter pylori* infection: current options and developments. World J Gastroenterol 2015;21:11221. [PMID: 26523098]
Infectious esophagitis Fungal: *Candida albicans, Candida glabrata,* (rare organisms are Aspergillus, Blastomyces, Cryptococcus). Viral: CMV, HSV, (rarer are HPV, VZV, Epstein-Barr viruses). Bacterial: Viridans streptococci, staphylococci, Mycobacteria.	Rule out noninfectious causes of esophagitis, especially gastroesophageal reflux. Definitive diagnosis requires esophagoscopy with biopsy for histological and microbiologic examinations. Barium esophagram may reveal abnormalities in cases of candidal esophagitis.	Most common in immunosuppressed individuals. Most common cause is *Candida albicans* infection. Thrush (25%) and odynophagia (50%) in an immunocompromised patient warrant empiric therapy for candida. Factors predisposing to infectious esophagitis include HIV infection, exposure to radiation, cytotoxic chemotherapy, recent antibiotic therapy, corticosteroid therapy, and neutropenia. Ahuja NK et al. Evaluation and management of infectious esophagitis in immunocompromised and immunocompetent individuals. Curr Treat Options Gastroenterol 2016;14:28. [PMID: 26847359] O'Rourke A. Infective oesophagitis: epidemiology, cause, diagnosis and treatment options. Curr Opin Otolaryngol Head Neck Surg 2015;23:459. [PMID: 26371605] Patel NC et al. Esophageal infections: an update. Curr Opin Pediatr 2015;27:642. [PMID: 26208233]

ABDOMEN

Infectious colitis/dysentery

(Continued)

Infectious colitis/dysentery

Infant: *E. coli* (enteropathogenic), rotavirus.

Child/adult without travel, afebrile, diarrhea with no gross blood or WBCs in stool: Rotavirus, norovirus and other caliciviruses, *E. coli* (GNR).

Child/adult with acute watery diarrhea, low-grade fever: *E. coli* (GNR) (enterotoxigenic (ETEC), entero-invasive (EIEC), *Clostridium difficile* (GPR), norovirus.

Child/adult with fever and dysentery (WBC in stool): *E. coli* (EIEC), shigella (GNR), *Campylobacter* sp. (GNR).

Child/Adult with diarrhea, bloody stool or history of travel to subtropics/tropics (or elsewhere) (varies with epidemiology): *E. coli* (GNR), enterohemor-rhagic (EHEC, 0157:H7, STEC 0104:H4), and other shiga-toxin-producing *E. coli* serotypes).

Other causes of acute diarrhea: salmonella (GNR), *Yersinia enterocolitica* (GNR), aeromonas (GNR), plesiomonas (GNR), vibrio (GNR), cryptosporidium, *Entamoeba histolytica, Giardia lamblia*, cyclospora, strongyloides, microsporidia (in HIV infection).

Child/adult with diarrhea and vomiting: *E. coli* (EPEC, enteropathogenic), norovirus.

Stool cultures routinely done for salmonella, shigella, and campylobacter.

Special stool culture techniques are needed for detection of yersinia, *E. coli* 0157:H7, vibrio, aeromonas, plesiomonas.

Stool cultures for salmonella, shigella, and campylobacter are not helpful for patients who have been hospitalized for >3 days.

Sensitivity of stool culture is 72%, but its specificity is 100%. For patients who have been hospitalized for >3 days, test for toxigenic *C. difficile* or its toxins.

Stool ova and parasite exam or antigen EIAs (minimum 3 stool specimens over 10 days) for detection of parasites.

Modified trichrome stain for microsporidia.

Shiga toxin EIA for suspected hemorrhagic *E. coli* infection.

RT-PCR on stool for diagnosis of norovirus infection. Highly contagious.

Proctosigmoidoscopy is indicated in patients with chronic or recurrent diarrhea or in diarrhea of unknown cause for smears of aspirates and biopsy. Culture of a biopsy specimen has a slightly higher sensitivity than routine stool culture.

Obtain rectal and jejunal biopsies from HIV-infected patients, culture for bacterial pathogens and Mycobacteria (eg, MAC), and perform modified acid-fast stains for cryptosporidium, isospora, and cyclospora.

Acute dysentery is diarrhea with bloody, mucoid stools, tenesmus, and pain on defecation and implies an inflammatory invasion of the colonic mucosa. BUN and serum electrolytes may be indicated for supportive care.

Severe dehydration is a medical emergency.

Necrotizing enterocolitis is a fulminant disease of premature newborns; cause is unknown, but human breast milk is protective. Air in the intestinal wall (pneumatosis intestinalis), in the portal venous system, or in the peritoneal cavity seen on plain x-ray can confirm diagnosis. 30–50% of these infants will have bacteremia or peritonitis.

Risk factors for infectious colitis include poor hygiene and immune compromise (infancy, advanced age, corticosteroid or immunosuppressive therapy, HIV infection).

Aboutaleb N et al. Emerging infectious colitis. Curr Opin Gastroenterol 2014;30:106. [PMID: 24275672]

Ayukekbong JA et al. Role of noroviruses as aetiological agents of diarrhoea in developing countries. J Gen Virol 2015;96:1983. [PMID: 26002299]

Lübbert C. Antimicrobial therapy of acute diarrhoea: a clinical review. Expert Rev Anti Infect Ther 2016;14:193. [PMID: 26641310]

Steffen R et al. Traveler's diarrhea: a clinical review. JAMA 2015;313:71. [PMID: 25562268]

	ABDOMEN
	Antibiotic-associated colitis

Organism	Specimen/Diagnostic Tests	Comments
Antibiotic-associated pseudomem-branous colitis *Clostridium difficile* (GPR) (90%), *Clostridium perfringens* (GPR) (8%), *Candida albicans* (yeast) in elderly, hospitalized patients.	*C. difficile* produces two toxins: Toxin A is an enterotoxin and toxin B is a cytotoxin. Send stool for detection of *C. difficile* cytotoxin B by tissue culture (test takes >48 hours with sensitivity 60–80%, specificity 99%). Stool for rapid EIA to detect toxin A or toxin A and B takes only 2–4 hours (sensitivity 70–90%, specificity 99%), but these assays are no longer recommended for primary testing. New molecular assays (>90% sensitive) that detect the gene for toxin B are more sensitive and specific and can give rapid results to aid in patient contact isolation procedures. Test only one watery stool specimen and do not repeat testing unless relapse infection is suspected. Colonoscopy and visualization of characteristic 1–5 mm raised yellow plaques provides a definitive diagnosis. Antibiotic-associated diarrhea may include uncomplicated diarrhea, colitis, or pseudomembranous colitis. Only 10–20% of cases are caused by infection with *C. difficile*. Most clinically mild cases are due to functional disturbances of intestinal carbohydrate or bile acid metabolism, to allergic and toxic effects of antibiotics on intestinal mucosa, or to their pharmacologic effects on motility.	Antibiotics cause changes in normal intestinal flora, allowing overgrowth of *C. difficile* and elaboration of toxins. Other risk factors for *C. difficile*-induced colitis are GI manipulations, advanced age, female sex, inflammatory bowel disease, HIV, chemotherapy, and renal disease. Over the past 10 years, the incidence of *C. difficile* disease has increased and the disease has become more severe. Hospital-acquired *C. difficile* infection can be controlled by hand washing with soap and water. Note that alcohol gels do not kill *C. difficile* spores on hands or in the environment. Calls for increased control of antibiotic usage, use of new molecular assays and tighter infection control practices have been put forward to prevent spread and outbreaks of *C. difficile* disease. Emerging therapeutic options for treating *C. difficile* infection include a new drug, fidaxomicin, and fecal microbiota transplantation to restore intestinal microbiota. Kociolek LK et al. Breakthroughs in the treatment and prevention of *Clostridium difficile* infection. Infect Dis Clin North Am 2015;29:109. [PMID: 25677705] Rao K et al. Fecal microbiota transplantation for the management of *Clostridium difficile* infection. Infect Dis Clin North Am 2015;29:109. [PMID: 26860266] Zhanel GG et al. Fidaxomicin: a novel agent for the treatment of *Clostridium difficile* infection. Can J Infect Dis Med Microbiol 2015;26:305. [PMID: 26744587]

ABDOMEN
Diarrhea in HIV

(Continued)

Diarrhea in the HIV-infected host
Same as child–adult infectious colitis with addition of CMV, adenovirus, cryptosporidium, *Isospora belli*, microsporidia (*Enterocytozoon bieneusi* and *E. intestinalis*), *C. difficile*, *Giardia intestinalis*, *M. avium-intracellulare* complex (MAC, [AFB]), HSV, *Entamoeba histolytica*, *Balantidium coli*, *Sarcocystis* sp.

Stool for culture (especially for salmonella, shigella, yersinia, and campylobacter), *C. difficile* tissue culture or molecular assays, ova and parasite examination. Multiple samples are often needed.

Proctosigmoidoscopy with fluid aspiration and biopsy is indicated in patients with chronic or recurrent diarrhea or in diarrhea of unknown cause for smears of aspirates (may show organisms) and histologic examination and culture of tissue.

Rectal and jejunal biopsies may be necessary, especially in patients with tenesmus or bloody stools. Need modified acid-fast stain for cryptosporidium, isospora, and cyclospora. Intranuclear inclusion bodies on histologic examination suggest CMV.

Immunodiagnosis of giardia, cryptosporidium, and *E. histolytica* cysts in stool is highly sensitive and specific.

Most patients with HIV infection develop diarrhea at some point, which can be difficult to diagnose and treat. Antiretroviral therapy decreases disease incidence.

Cryptosporidium causes a chronic debilitating diarrheal infection that rarely remits spontaneously and is still without effective treatment. Diarrhea seems to be the result of malabsorption and produces a cholera-like syndrome.

Between 15% and 50% of HIV-infected patients with diarrhea have no identifiable pathogen.

De A. Current laboratory diagnosis of opportunistic enteric parasites in human immunodeficiency virus-infected patients. Trop Parasitol 2013;3:7. [PMID: 23961436]

Dikman AE et al. Human immunodeficiency virus-associated diarrhea: still an issue in the era of antiretroviral therapy. Dig Dis Sci 2015;60:2236. [PMID: 25772777]

Haines CF et al. *Clostridium difficile* in a HIV-infected cohort: incidence, risk factors, and clinical outcomes. AIDS 2013;27:2799. [PMID: 23842125]

Pavlinac PB et al. High-risk enteric pathogens associated with HIV infection and HIV exposure in Kenyan children with acute diarrhoea. AIDS 2014;28:2287. [PMID: 25028987]

	ABDOMEN
	Peritonitis

Organism	Specimen/Diagnostic Tests	Comments
Peritonitis Primary or spontaneous (associated with nephrosis or cirrhosis) (SBP): Enterobacteriaceae (GNR) (69%), enterococci (GPC), viridans streptococci (GPC in chains), *S. pneumoniae* (GPC), group A streptococcus (GPC), *S. aureus* (GPC), anaerobes (5%). Secondary (bowel perforation, hospital acquired, or antecedent antibiotic therapy): Enterobacteriaceae, enterococcus (GPC), *Bacteroides fragilis* group (GNR), *Pseudomonas aeruginosa* (GNR) (3–15%). Chronic ambulatory peritoneal dialysis (CAPD): Coagulase-negative staphylococci (GPC) (43%), *S. aureus* (14%), *Streptococcus* sp. (12%), Enterobacteriaceae (14%), *Pseudomonas aeruginosa*, *Corynebacterium* sp. (GPR), candida (2%), aspergillus (rare), cryptococcus (rare).	Peritoneal fluid sent for WBC (>1000/mcL in SPB, >100/mcL in CAPD) with PMN (>250/mcL in SBP and secondary peritonitis, 50% PMN in CAPD); total protein (>1 g/dL); glucose (<0 mg/dL), and LDH (>225 units/mL) in secondary; pH (<7.35 in 57% of SBP). Gram stain (sensitivity 22–77% for SBP); submit large volumes of peritoneal fluid for bacterial culture. (See Ascitic fluid profiles, Table 8–6.) Blood cultures for bacteria positive in 85% of SBP cases. Catheter-related infection is associated with a WBC >500/mcL.	In nephrotic patients, Enterobacteriaceae and *S. aureus* are most common. In cirrhotics, 69% of cases are due to Enterobacteriaceae. Cirrhotic patients (40%) with low ascitic fluid protein levels (≤1 g/dL) and high bilirubin level or low platelet count are at high risk of developing spontaneous bacterial peritonitis. "Bacterascites," a positive ascitic fluid culture without an elevated PMN count, is seen in 8% of cases of SBP and probably represents early infection. Neutrocytic ascites can have a negative culture in 10–30% of cases. In secondary peritonitis, factors influencing the incidence of postoperative complications and death include age, presence of certain concomitant diseases, site of origin of peritonitis, type of admission, and the ability of the surgeon to eliminate the source of infection (appendicitis [with or without rupture], diverticulitis, perforated ulcer, perforated gallbladder). Alfa-Wali M et al. Treatment of uncomplicated acute appendicitis. JAMA 2015;314:1402. [PMID: 26441190] Walker A et al. KHA-CARI Guideline: peritonitis treatment and prophylaxis. Nephrology 2014;19:69. [PMID: 23944845] Wenzel RP et al. Antibiotics for abdominal sepsis. N Engl J Med 2015;372:2062. [PMID: 25992751]

ABDOMEN
Tuberculous peritonitis/enterocolitis

(Continued)

Tuberculous peritonitis/enterocolitis
Mycobacterium tuberculosis (MTb, AFB, acid-fast beaded rods).

Ascitic fluid for appearance (clear, hemorrhagic, or chylous), RBCs (can be high), WBCs (>1000/mcL, >70% lymphs), protein (>3.5 g/dL), serum/ascites albumin gradient (SAAG) (<1.1), LDH (>90 units/L), AFB culture (<50% positive). (See Ascitic fluid profiles, Table 8–6.) With coexistent chronic liver disease, protein level and SAAG are usually not helpful, but LDH >90 units/L is a useful predictor. Culture or AFB smear from other sources (especially from respiratory tract) can help confirm diagnosis.

Abdominal ultrasound may demonstrate free or loculated intra-abdominal fluid, intra-abdominal abscess, ileocecal mass, and retroperitoneal lymphadenopathy. Ascites with fine, mobile septations shown by ultrasound and peritoneal and omental thickening detected by CT strongly suggest tuberculous peritonitis.

Marked elevations of serum CA 125 have been noted; levels decline to normal with antituberculous therapy.

Diagnosis of enterocolitis rests on biopsy of colonic lesions via endoscopy if pulmonary or other extrapulmonary infection cannot be documented.

Diagnosis is best confirmed by laparoscopy with peritoneal biopsy and culture.

Operative procedure may be needed to relieve obstruction or for diagnosis.

Infection of the intestines can occur anywhere along the GI tract but occurs most frequently in the ileocecal area or mesenteric lymph nodes. It often complicates pulmonary infection. Peritoneal infection usually is an extension of intestinal disease. Symptoms may be minimal even with extensive disease.

In the United States, 29% of patients with abdominal tuberculosis have a normal chest x-ray.

Presence of AFB in the feces does not correlate with intestinal involvement.

Akhan SE et al. A deceiving disease in women for clinicians: peritoneal tuberculosis. Clin Exp Obstet Gynecol 2014;41:132. [PMID: 24779236]

Bolognesi M et al. Complicated and delayed diagnosis of tuberculous peritonitis. Am J Case Rep 2013;14:109. [PMID: 23826447]

Burke KA et al. Diagnosing abdominal tuberculosis in the acute abdomen. Int J Surg 2014;12:494. [PMID: 24560849]

Masood I et al. Multiple, pan-enteric perforation secondary to intestinal tuberculosis. Case Rep Surg 2015;2015:318678. [PMID: 26798540]

	ABDOMEN	ABDOMEN
	Diverticulitis	Liver abscess

Organism	Specimen/Diagnostic Tests	Comments
Diverticulitis Polymicrobial Enterobacteriaceae (GNR), *Bacteroides* sp. (GNR), Peptostreptococcus (GPC), enterococcus (GPC in chains), viridans streptococci (GPC in chains).	Identification of organism is not usually sought. Ultrasonography or flat and upright x-rays of abdomen can rule out perforation (free air under diaphragm) and localize abscess (air-fluid collections). CT is the diagnostic procedure of choice. CT-guided percutaneous drainage of abscesses can be performed.	Pain usually is localized to the left lower quadrant because the sigmoid and descending colon are the most common sites for diverticula. Fever, nausea, vomiting and changes in bowel habits may be present. It is important to rule out other abdominal disease (eg, colon carcinoma, Crohn disease, ischemic colitis, *C. difficile*-associated colitis, appendicitis), and gynecologic disorders (eg, ectopic pregnancy, ovarian cyst, or torsion). Collins D et al. Modern concepts in diverticular disease. J Clin Gastroenterol 2015;49:358. [PMID: 25811113] Jackson JD et al. Systematic review: outpatient management of acute uncomplicated diverticulitis. Int J Colorectal Dis 2014;29:775. [PMID: 24859874] Regenbogen SE et al. Surgery for diverticulitis in the 21st century: a systematic review. JAMA Surg 2014;149:292. [PMID: 24430164] Stollman N et al. American Gastroenterological Association Institute Guideline on the management of acute diverticulitis. Gastroenterology 2015;149:1944. [PMID: 26453777]
Liver abscess Usually polymicrobial: Enterobacteriaceae, especially *E. coli, Enterobacter* sp., *Proteus* sp., *Klebsiella* sp. (GNR), enterococcus (GPC in chains), *Bacteroides* sp. (GNR), actinomyces (GPR), *S. aureus* (GPC) (MRSA), viridans streptococci (GPC), *Candida* sp., *Entamoeba histolytica*.	CT scan with contrast and ultrasonography are the most accurate tests for the diagnosis of liver abscess. An antibody test against *E. histolytica* (95%) should be obtained on all patients. Uncomplicated amebic liver abscesses can be treated medically without drainage. *E. histolytica* invades the intestinal wall and it can be carried to the liver by the blood where it may produce abscesses. Complete removal of abscess material obtained via surgery or percutaneous aspiration is recommended for large abscesses and for culture and direct examination to distinguish pyogenic abscess from *E. histolytica* abscess. Complications of drainage or removal of *E. histolytica* abscess are rupture, amebic peritonitis, and death.	Travel to and origin in an endemic area are important risk factors for amebic liver abscess. 60% of patients have a single lesion; 40% have multiple lesions. Biliary tract disease is the most common underlying disease, accounting for 40–60% of cases, followed by malignancy (biliary tract or pancreatic), colonic disease (diverticulitis), diabetes mellitus, liver disease, and alcoholism. In mid-1980s, a syndrome of monomicrobial *K. pneumonia* pyogenic liver abscess, often in diabetics, was described in Taiwan. Infections were caused by hypermucoid strains of *K. pneumonia* of capsular K1 serotype. This is now a major health problem in Asia. Jha AK et al. Clinicopathological study and management of liver abscess in a tertiary care center. J Nat Sci Biol Med 2015;6:71. [PMID: 25810638] Shon AS et al. Hypervirulent (hypermucoviscous) *Klebsiella pneumonia*: a new and dangerous breed. Virulence. 2013;4:107. [PMID: 23302790]

(Continued)

ABDOMEN	GENITOURINARY
Cholangitis/cholecystitis	**Urinary tract infection**

Cholangitis/cholecystitis

Enterobacteriaceae (GNR) (68%), enterococcus (GPC in chains) (14%), *Pseudomonas aeruginosa* (GNR), bacteroides (GNR) (10%), *Clostridium* sp. (GPR) (7%), fusobacterium, *M. avium–intracellulare* complex (MAC) in AIDS patients.

Parasites: microsporidia (*Enterocytozoon bieneusi*) cryptosporidia, *Ascaris lumbricoides, Opisthorchis viverrini, O. felineus, Clonorchis sinensis, Fasciola hepatica, Echinococcus granulosus, E. multilocularis.*

Viruses: CMV in AIDS.

Ultrasonography is the best test to quickly demonstrate gallstones or phlegmon around the gallbladder or dilation of the biliary tree. (See Abdominal Ultrasound, Chapter 6.)

CT scanning is useful in cholangitis in detecting the site and cause of obstruction. (See Abdominal CT, Chapter 6.)

Blood cultures for bacteria.

WBC elevated (12,000–15,000 per mcL).

Serum total bilirubin elevated (1–4 mg/dL).

Serum aminotransferase and alkaline phosphatase may be elevated.

90% of cases of acute cholecystitis are calculous, 10% are acalculous. Risk factors for acalculous disease include prolonged illness, trauma, burns, sepsis, immunosuppression, diabetes mellitus, HIV infection, adenocarcinoma of the gallbladder or bile ducts (cholangiocarcinoma).

Biliary obstruction and cholangitis (inflammation or infection of common bile duct) can develop before biliary dilation is detected.

Common bile duct obstruction secondary to tumor or pancreatitis seldom results in infection (0–15%).

In the era of potent antiretroviral therapy, AIDS cholangiopathy is now rare. Most common pathogen in cholangitis in AIDS is cryptosporidium.

Halilbasic E et al. Therapy of primary sclerosing cholangitis—today and tomorrow. Dig Dis 2015;33(Suppl 2):149. [PMID: 26641242]

Kochar R et al. Infections of the biliary tract. Gastrointest Endosc Clin N Am 2013;23:199. [PMID: 23540957]

Patel PP et al. Training vs practice: a tale of opposition in acute cholecystitis. World J Hepatol 2015;7:2470. [PMID: 26483868]

Urinary tract infection (UTI)/cystitis/ pyuria-dysuria syndrome

Enterobacteriaceae (GNR, especially *E. coli* [80% of infections]), *Chlamydia trachomatis, Staphylococcus saprophyticus* (GPC) (in young women), enterococcus (GPC), group B streptococci (GPC), *Candida* sp. (yeast), *N. gonorrhoeae* (GNCB), *Corynebacterium urealyticum* (GPR), *Aerococcus urinae* (GPC), *Ureaplasma urealyticum* (lack of cell walls prevents staining by Gram stain), HSV, adenovirus.

Urinalysis and culture reveal the two most important signs: bacteriuria and pyuria (>10 WBCs/mcL). 30% of patients have hematuria. Cystitis (95%) is diagnosed by >10² CFU/mL of bacteria; other urinary infections (90%) by >10⁵ CFU/mL. Culture is generally not necessary for uncomplicated cystitis in women. Combination of current symptoms (eg, dysuria, frequency, and hematuria) and prior history yields a >90% probability of UTI. However, pregnant women should be screened for asymptomatic bacteriuria and promptly treated.

Both Gram stain for nitrite and dipstick analysis for nitrite and leukocyte esterase perform similarly in detecting UTI in children and are superior to microscopic analysis for pyuria. Nitrite or leukocyte esterase may be negative in 19% of patients with bacteremia due to enterococci and staphylococci.

DNA amplification tests for chlamydia and gonorrhea are available.

Most men with UTIs have a functional or anatomic genitourinary abnormality.

In catheter-related UTI, cure is unlikely unless the catheter is removed. In asymptomatic catheter-related UTI, antibiotics should be given only if patients are at risk for sepsis (old age, underlying disease, diabetes mellitus, pregnancy).

Up to one-third of cases of acute cystitis have "silent" upper tract involvement.

Increasing resistance of enteric bacteria causing urinary tract infection to trimethoprim-sulfamethoxazole, fluoroquinolones, and the rise of extended-spectrum beta-lactamase (ESBL) producing bacteria are major concerns.

Cardwell SM et al. Epidemiology and economics of adult patients hospitalized with urinary tract infections. Hosp Pract (1995) 2016;44:33. [PMID: 26673518]

Fan NC et al. Rise of community-onset urinary tract infection caused by extended-spectrum β-lactamase-producing *Escherichia coli* in children. J Microbiol Immunol Infect 2014;47:399. [PMID: 23834784]

Lakeman MM et al. Urinary tract infections in women with urogynaecological symptoms. Curr Opin Infect Dis 2016;29:92. [PMID: 26658649]

Tandogdu Z et al. Global epidemiology of urinary tract infections. Curr Opin Infect Dis 2016;29:73. [PMID: 26694621]

	GENITOURINARY	GENITOURINARY
	Prostatitis	**Pyelonephritis**

Organism	Specimen/Diagnostic Tests	Comments
Prostatitis Acute and chronic: *E. coli* (80%) (GNR), other Enterobacteriaceae (GNR), *Pseudomonas* sp. (GNR), enterococci (GPC in chains), CMV, *Staphylococcus* sp. (GPC), chlamydiae, mycoplasma, ureaplasma. HIV: *M. tuberculosis*, *Candida* sp., Coccidioides, Cryptococcus, Histoplasma.	Urinalysis shows pyuria, bacteriuria, and hematuria (variable). Urine culture usually identifies causative organism. Prostatic massage is useful in chronic prostatitis to retrieve organisms but is contraindicated in acute prostatitis (it may cause bacteremia). Bacteriuria is first cleared by antibiotic treatment. Then urine cultures are obtained from first-void, bladder, and postprostatic massage urine specimens. A higher organism count in the postprostatic massage specimen localizes infection to the prostate (91%) (Meares-Stamey 3-glass test).	Acute prostatitis is a severe illness characterized by fever, dysuria, and a boggy or tender prostate. Chronic prostatitis often has no symptoms of dysuria, but may present with perineal or pelvic pain and discomfort. Nonbacterial prostatitis (prostatodynia) represents 90% of prostatitis cases. Its cause is unknown, although chlamydia antigen can be found in up to 25% of patients. Coker TJ et al. Acute bacterial prostatitis: diagnosis and management. Am Fam Physician 2016;93:114. [PMID: 26926407] Gujadhur R et al. Careful assessment key in managing prostatitis. Practitioner 2015;259:15. [PMID: 26529825] Holt JD et al. Common questions about chronic prostatitis. Am Fam Physician 2016;93:290. [PMID: 26926816] Rees J et al. Diagnosis and treatment of chronic bacterial prostatitis and chronic prostatitis/chronic pelvic pain syndrome: a consensus guideline. BJU Int 2015;116:509. [PMID: 25711488]
Pyelonephritis Acute, uncomplicated (usually young women): Enterobacteriaceae (especially *E. coli*) (GNR), enterococci (GPC in chains), *Staphylococcus saprophyticus* (GPC), *S. aureus* (GPC). Complicated (older women, men; postcatheterization, obstruction, post-renal transplant): Enterobacteriaceae (especially *E. coli*), *Pseudomonas aeruginosa* (GNR), enterococcus (GPC), *S. aureus* (GPC).	Urine culture is indicated when pyelonephritis is suspected. Urinalysis will usually show pyuria (>5 WBC/hpf) and may show WBC casts. Blood cultures for bacteria if sepsis is suspected. In uncomplicated pyelonephritis, ultrasonography is not necessary. In severe cases, however, ultrasound is the optimal procedure for ruling out urinary tract obstruction, pyonephrosis, and calculi. Doppler ultrasonography (88%) has a specificity of 100% for acute pyelonephritis.	Patients usually present with fever, chills, nausea, vomiting, and costovertebral angle tenderness. 20–30% of pregnant women with untreated bacteriuria develop pyelonephritis. Major concern is antibiotic resistance of uropathogens. Hospitals should review local resistance patterns and make recommendations for empiric therapy based on the resistance patterns. Prabhu A et al. Pyelonephritis: what are the present day causative organisms and antibiotic susceptibilities? Nephrology (Carlton) 2013;18:463. [PMID: 23573984] Schneeberger C et al. Febrile urinary tract infections: pyelonephritis and urosepsis. Curr Opin Infect Dis 2016;29:80. [PMID: 26658652]

(Continued)

GENITOURINARY	GENITOURINARY
Perinephric abscess	**Urethritis**
Perinephric abscess Associated with staphylococcal bacteremia: *S. aureus* (GPC). Associated with pyelonephritis: Enterobacteriaceae (GNR), *Candida* sp. (yeast), coagulase–negative staphylococci (GPC).	**Urethritis (gonococcal and nongonococcal)** Gonococcal (GC): *Neisseria gonorrhoeae* (GNDC). Nongonococcal (NGU): *Chlamydia trachomatis* (50%), *Ureaplasma urealyticum*, *Trichomonas vaginalis*, HSV, *Mycoplasma genitalium*, adenoviruses, *Gardnerella vaginalis*.
CT scan with contrast is more sensitive than ultrasound in imaging abscess and confirming diagnosis. (See Abdominal CT, Chapter 6.) Plain films of abdomen and ultrasonography can detect stones and abscesses. Urinalysis may be normal or may show pyuria. Urine culture (positive in 60–72%). Blood cultures for bacteria (positive in 20–40%). Bacterial culture of abscess fluid via needle aspiration or drainage (percutaneous or surgical).	Urethral discharge collected with urethral swab usually shows >4 WBCs per oil-immersion field; Gram stain (identify gonococcal organisms as gram-negative intracellular diplococci), PMNs (in GC urethritis, >95% of WBCs are PMNs, in NGU usually <80% are PMNs). Urethral discharge for GC culture (80%). Bacterial culture. Special culture needed for *Ureaplasma urealyticum*. Molecular amplification assays for gonorrhea and chlamydia are the preferred diagnostic method (urine or urethral swab for men; vaginal swab (doctor-collected or self-collected), endocervical specimen or urine for women). Wet mount for *T. vaginalis*. RPR or VDRL should be checked in all patients because of high incidence of associated syphilis.
Uncommon complication of urinary tract infection. Predisposing factors are urinary tract calculi and diabetes mellitus. Most perinephric abscesses are the result of extension of an ascending urinary tract infection. Often they are very difficult to diagnose. Perinephric abscesses should be considered in patients who fail to respond to antibiotic therapy, in patients with anatomic abnormalities of the urinary tract, and in patients with diabetes mellitus. Gardiner RA et al. Perinephric abscess. BJU Int 2011;107(Suppl 3):20. [PMID: 21492371] Jacobson D et al. Perinephric abscesses in the pediatric population: case presentation and review of the literature. Pediatr Nephrol 2014;29:919. [PMID: 24389603] Rubilotta E et al. Current clinical management of renal and perinephric abscesses: a literature review. Urologia 2014;81:144. [PMID: 24474535]	About 50% of patients with GC urethritis have concomitant NGU infection. Always treat sexual partners. Recurrence may be secondary to failure to treat partners. Frequently, no pathogen can be isolated. Persistent or recurrent episodes with adequate treatment of patient and partners may warrant further evaluation for other causes (eg, prostatitis). Couldwell DL et al. *Mycoplasma genitalium* infection: current treatment options, therapeutic failure, and resistance–associated mutations. Infect Drug Resist 2015;8:147. [PMID: 26060411] Moi H et al. Management of non–gonococcal urethritis. BMC Infect Dis 2015;15:294. [PMID: 26220178] Workowski KA et al. Sexually transmitted diseases treatment guidelines, 2015. MMWR Recomm Rep 2015;64(RR-03):1. [PMID: 26042815]

	GEENITOURINARY	GENITOURINARY
	Epididymitis/orchitis	Vaginitis/vaginosis

Organism	Specimen/Diagnostic Tests	Comments
Epididymitis/orchitis Age <35 years, homosexual men: *Chlamydia trachomatis, U. urealyticum, E. coli* (GNR), *Enterococcus faecalis* (GPC), *P. aeruginosa* (GNR), brucella (GVCB). Age >35 years, or children: Enterobacteriaceae (especially *E. coli*) (GNR), *Pseudomonas* sp. (GNR), salmonella (GNR), *Haemophilus influenzae* (GNCB), VZV, mumps. Immunosuppression: *H. influenzae, Mycobacterium tuberculosis* (AFB), *Candida* sp. (yeast), CMV.	Urinalysis may reveal pyuria. Patients aged >35 years often have midstream pyuria and scrotal pain and edema. Culture urine and expressible urethral discharge when present. Prostatic secretions for Gram stain and bacterial culture are helpful in older patients. When testicular torsion is considered, Doppler ultrasound or radionuclide scan can be useful in diagnosis.	Testicular torsion is a surgical emergency that is often confused with orchitis or epididymitis. Sexual partners should be examined for signs of sexually transmitted diseases. In non-sexually transmitted disease, evaluation for underlying urinary tract infection or structural defect is recommended. Redshaw JD et al. Epididymitis: a 21-year retrospective review of presentations to an outpatient urology clinic. J Urol 2014;192:1203. [PMID: 24735936] Taylor SN. Epididymitis. Clin Infect Dis 2015;61 (Suppl 8):S770. [PMID: 26602616] Walker NA et al. Managing epididymo-orchitis in general practice. Practitioner 2013;257:21. [PMID: 23724748]
Vaginitis/vaginosis *Candida* sp. (yeast), *Trichomonas vaginalis, Gardnerella vaginalis* (GPR), bacteroides (non-*fragilis*) (GNR), mobiluncus (GPR), peptostreptococcus (GPC), *Mycoplasma hominis*, groups A and B streptococci (GPC), HSV.	Vaginal discharge for appearance (in candidiasis, area is pruritic with thick "cheesy" discharge; in trichomoniasis, copious foamy, yellow-green, or discolored discharge), pH (about 4.5 for candida; 5.0–7.0 in trichomonas; 5.0–6.0 with bacterial), saline ("wet") preparation (motile organisms seen in trichomonas; cells covered with organisms—clue cells—in gardnerella; yeast and hyphae in candida, "fishy" odor on addition of KOH with gardnerella infection). Vaginal fluid pH as a screening test for bacterial vaginosis showed a sensitivity of 74.3%, but combined with clinical symptoms and signs its sensitivity increased to 81.3%. Atrophic vaginitis is seen in postmenopausal patients, often with bleeding, scant discharge, and pH 6.0–7.0. Cultures for gardnerella are not useful and are not recommended. Culture for *T. vaginalis* has greater sensitivity than wet mount. Culture for groups A and B streptococci and rare causes of bacterial vaginosis may be indicated. Gram stain of discharge is more reliable than wet mount for diagnosis of bacterial vaginosis (93% vs. 70%, respectively).	Bacterial vaginosis results from massive overgrowth of anaerobic vaginal bacterial flora (especially gardnerella). New research suggests bacterial vaginosis results from biofilm formation. Serious infectious sequelae associated with bacterial vaginosis include abscesses, endometritis and pelvic inflammatory disease. There is also a danger of miscarriage, premature rupture of the membranes, and premature labor. Kenyon CR et al. Recent progress in understanding the epidemiology of bacterial vaginosis. Curr Opin Obstet Gynecol 2014;26:448. [PMID: 25304606] Machado A et al. Influence of biofilm formation by *Gardnerella vaginalis* and other anaerobes on bacterial vaginosis. J Infect Dis 2015;212:1856. [PMID: 26080369] Meites E et al. A review of evidence-based care of symptomatic Trichomoniasis and asymptomatic *Trichomonas vaginalis* infections. Clin Infect Dis 2015;61(Suppl 8):S837. [PMID: 26602621] van Schalkwyk J et al. Vulvovaginitis: screening for and management of trichomoniasis, vulvovaginal candidiasis, and bacterial vaginosis. J Obstet Gynaecol Can 2015;37:266. [PMID: 26001874]

GENITOURINARY		
Cervicitis		
Cervicitis, mucopurulent *Chlamydia trachomatis* (50%), *N. gonorrhoeae* (GNDC) (8%), HSV, *Mycoplasma genitalium*.	Cervical swab specimen for appearance (yellow or green purulent material), cell count (>10 WBCs per high-power oil immersion field) and culture (58–80%) or nucleic acid assay (93%) for GC; urine for nucleic acid assay (93%) for GC; urine (80–92%), vaginal swab (97%), or cervical swab (97%) for detection of *C. trachomatis* by nucleic acid amplification. Culture (52%) or nonamplified assays (50–80%) are considerably less sensitive for diagnosis of *C. trachomatis*.	Because of the danger of false-positive amplified nucleic acid assays, culture is the preferred method in cases of suspected child abuse. In one study of pregnant women, a wet mount preparation of endocervical secretions with <10 PMNs per high-power field had a negative predictive value of 99% for gonococcus-induced cervicitis and of 96% for *C trachomatis*-induced cervicitis. In family planning clinics, however, a mucopurulent discharge with >10 PMNs/hpf had a low positive predictive value of 29.2% for *C. trachomatis*-related cervicitis. Mucopurulent discharge may persist for 3 months or more even after appropriate therapy. Lusk MJ et al. Cervicitis aetiology and case definition: a study in Australian women attending sexually transmitted infection clinics. Sex Transm Infect 2016;92:175. [PMID: 26586777] Taylor SN. Cervicitis of unknown etiology. Curr Infect Dis Rep 2014;16:409. [PMID: 24859465] Workowski KA et al. Sexually transmitted diseases treatment guidelines, 2015. MMWR Recomm Rep 2015;64 (RR-03):1. [PMID: 26042815]

(Continued)

GENITOURINARY		
Salpingitis		**Chorioamnionitis/endometritis**

Organism	Specimen/Diagnostic Tests	Comments
Salpingitis/pelvic inflammatory disease (PID) Usually polymicrobial: *N. gonorrhoeae* (GNDC), *Chlamydia trachomatis*, bacteroides, peptostreptococcus, *G. vaginalis*, and other anaerobes, Enterobacteriaceae (GNR), streptococci (GPC in chains), *Mycoplasma hominis* (debatable).	Gram stain and culture or amplified nucleic acid assays of urethral or endocervical exudate. Ultrasonographic findings include thickened fluid-filled tubes, polycystic-like ovaries, and free pelvic fluid. MRI imaging findings for PID (95%) include fluid-filled tube, pyosalpinx, tubo–ovarian abscess, or polycystic-like ovaries and free fluid. Laparoscopy supplemented by microbiologic tests and fimbrial biopsy is the diagnostic standard for PID. Transvaginal ultrasonography (81%) has a lower specificity than MRI. Laparoscopy is the most specific test to confirm the diagnosis of PID. RPR or VDRL should be checked in all patients because of the high incidence of associated syphilis.	PID typically progresses from cervicitis to endometritis to salpingitis. PID is a sexually transmitted disease in some cases, not in others. All sexual partners should be examined. All IUDs should be removed. A strategy of identifying, testing, and treating women at increased risk for cervical chlamydial infection can lead to a reduced incidence of PID. All patients with diagnosis of acute PID should also be tested for HIV infection. Brunham RC et al. Pelvic inflammatory disease. N Engl J Med 2015;372:2039. [PMID: 25992748] Hafner LM. Pathogenesis of fallopian tube damage caused by *Chlamydia trachomatis* infections. Contraception 2015;92:108. [PMID: 25592078]
Chorioamnionitis/endometritis Group B streptococcus (GPC), *E. coli* (GNR), *Listeria monocytogenes* (GPR), *Mycoplasma hominis*, *M. genitalium*, *Ureaplasma urealyticum*, *Gardnerella vaginalis*, enterococci (GPC), viridans streptococci (GPC in chains), *N. gonorrhoeae* (GDNC), bacteroides (GNR), prevotella (GNR), and other anaerobic flora, *Chlamydia trachomatis*, group A streptococcus (GPC).	Diagnosis based mostly on clinical findings. Amniotic fluid for Gram stain, glucose levels <10–20 mg/dL, and aerobic and anaerobic culture, blood for culture (10–20%). Sonographic evaluation of fetus can be helpful, but findings are nonspecific.	Risk factors include bacterial vaginosis, preterm labor, duration of labor, parity, internal fetal monitoring. Ericson JE et al. Chorioamnionitis: implications for the neonate. Clin Perinatol 2015;42:155. [PMID: 25678002] Johnson CT et al. Current management and long-term outcomes following chorioamnionitis. Obstet Gynecol Clin North Am 2014;41:649. [PMID: 25454996] Kim CJ et al. Acute chorioamnionitis and funisitis: definition, pathologic features, and clinical significance. Am J Obstet Gynecol 2015;213(Suppl 4):S29. [PMID: 26428501] Kitaya K et al. Chronic endometritis: potential cause of infertility and obstetric and neonatal complications. Am J Reprod Immunol 2016;75:13. [PMID: 26478517]

BONE		
Osteomyelitis		

Osteomyelitis	Blood cultures for bacteria are positive in about 60%.	Hematogenous or contiguous infection (eg, infected prosthetic joint, chronic cutaneous ulcer) may lead to osteomyelitis in children (metaphyses of long bones) or adults (vertebrae, metaphyses of long bones).
Staphylococcus aureus (GPC) (60%).	Cultures of percutaneous needle biopsy or open bone biopsy are needed if blood cultures are negative and osteomyelitis is suspected.	Hematogenous osteomyelitis in drug addicts occurs in unusual locations (vertebrae, clavicle, ribs).
Infant: *S. aureus*, Enterobacteriaceae (GNR), groups A and B streptococci (GPC).	Imaging with bone scan or gallium plus indium scan (sensitivity 95%, specificity 60–97%) can localize areas of suspicion. Technetium methylene diphosphonate bone scan can suggest osteomyelitis days or weeks before plain bone films. Plain bone films are abnormal in acute cases after about 2 weeks of illness (33%). Indium-labeled WBC scan is useful in detecting abscesses.	In infants, osteomyelitis is often associated with contiguous joint involvement. Berbari EF et al. 2015 Infectious Diseases Society of America (IDSA) Clinical Practice Guidelines for the Diagnosis and Treatment of native vertebral osteomyelitis in adults. Clin Infect Dis 2015;61:e26. [PMID: 26229122]
Child (<3 years): *H. influenzae* (GNCB), *S. aureus*, streptococci.		Malhotra R et al. Osteomyelitis in the diabetic foot. Diabet Foot Ankle 2014;5:24445. [PMID: 25147627]
Child (>3 years) to adult: *S. aureus*, coagulase negative staphylococci, Group A streptococci, *Pseudomonas aeruginosa*.	Ultrasound to detect subperiosteal abscesses and ultrasound-guided aspiration can assist in diagnosis and management of osteomyelitis. Ultrasound can differentiate acute osteomyelitis from vaso-occlusive crisis in patients with sickle cell disease.	Martin AC et al. Predictors of outcome in pediatric osteomyelitis: five years' experience in a single tertiary center. Pediatr Infect Dis J 2016;35:387. [PMID: 26669740]
Postoperative: *S. aureus*, Enterobacteriaceae, *Pseudomonas* sp. (GNR), *Bartonella henselae* (GNR).	CT scan is useful, but MRI is more sensitive and is now the standard of care.	
Joint prosthesis: Coagulase-negative staphylococci, peptostreptococcus (GPC), *Propionibacterium acnes* (GPR), viridans streptococci (GPC in chains).	When bone x-rays and scintigraphy are negative, MRI (98%) is useful for detecting early osteomyelitis (specificity 89%), in defining extent, and in distinguishing osteomyelitis from cellulitis.	
Immunocompromised patients (eg, elderly, HIV-infected): *M. tuberculosis*, *M. avium-intracellulare* (MAC), *Candida* sp., cryptococcus, coccidioides, histoplasma.		

(Continued)

	JOINT	MUSCLE
	Bacterial/septic arthritis	**Gas gangrene**

Organism	Specimen/Diagnostic Tests	Comments
Bacterial/septic arthritis Infant (<3 months): *S. aureus* (GPC), Group A streptococci (GPC), Enterobacteriaceae (GNR), *Kingella kingae* (GNCB), *Haemophilus influenzae* (GNCB). Child (3 months to 6 years): *S. aureus* (35%), *H. influenzae*, group A streptococcus (GPC) (10%), Enterobacteriaceae (6%), *Borrelia burgdorferi* (Lyme), *S. pneumoniae* (GPC), *K. kingae*. Adult, STD not likely: *S. aureus* (40%), group A streptococcus (27%), Enterobacteriaceae (23%), *Streptobacillus moniliformis* (GNR) (rat bite fever), brucella (GVCB) (*Neisseria* sp.), *Mycobacterium marinum* (AFB). Adult, STD likely: *N. gonorrhoeae* (GNDC) (disseminated gonococcal infection [DGI]). Prosthetic joint, postoperative or following intra-articular injection: Coagulase-negative staphylococci (40%), *S. aureus* (20%), viridans streptococci (GPC in chains), enterococci (GPC), peptostreptococcus (GPC), *Propionibacterium acnes* (GPR), Enterobacteriaceae, *Pseudomonas* sp.	Joint aspiration (synovial) fluid for WBCs (in nongonococcal infection, mean WBC is 100,000/mcL). Gram stain (best on centrifuged concentrated specimen, positive in one-third of cases), culture (nongonococcal infection in adults [85–95%], disseminated gonococcal infection (DGI) [25%]). (See Arthritis: Synovial fluid profiles, Table 8–5.) Yield of culture is greatest when 10 mL of synovial fluid is inoculated onto a plate or into culture media. Blood cultures for bacteria may be useful, especially in infants, nongonococcal infection in adults (50%), DGI (13%) *B. burgdorferi* serology for Lyme disease. Genitourinary, throat, or rectal culture: DGI may be diagnosed by positive culture from a nonarticular source and by a compatible clinical picture. In difficult cases, MRI can help differentiate septic arthritis from transient synovitis.	Septic arthritis is considered a rheumatologic emergency due to potential for rapid joint destruction and loss of function. It is important to obtain synovial fluid and blood for culture before starting antimicrobial treatment. Septic arthritis is usually hematogenously acquired. Prosthetic joint and diminished host defenses secondary to cancer, HIV, liver disease, or hypogammaglobinemia are common predisposing factors. Nongonococcal bacterial arthritis is usually monarticular (and typically affects one knee joint). DGI is the most common cause of septic arthritis in urban centers and is usually polyarticular with associated tenosynovitis. Lin WT et al. High prevalence of methicillin-resistant *Staphylococcus aureus* among patients with septic arthritis caused by *Staphylococcus aureus*. PLoS One 2015;10:e127150. [PMID: 25996145] Lin WT et al. Clinical manifestations and bacteriological features of culture-proven gram-negative bacterial arthritis. J Microbiol Immunol Infect 2015 Sept 18. [Epub ahead of print] [PMID: 26455489] Peterson TC et al. Septic arthritis in intravenous drug abusers: a historical comparison of habits and pathogens. J Emerg Med 2014;47:723. [PMID: 25282119]
Gas gangrene *Clostridium perfringens* (GPR) (80–95%), other *Clostridium* sp.: *C. ramosum*, *C. bifermentans*, *C. histolyticum*, *C. septicum*, *C. sordelli*, *C. tertium*.	Diagnosis should be suspected in areas of devitalized tissue when gas is discovered by palpation (subcutaneous crepitation) or x-ray. Gram stain of foul-smelling, brown, or blood-tinged watery exudate from lesion or abscess, if present, can be diagnostic with gram-positive rods (can be gram-variable) and a remarkable absence of neutrophils. Anaerobic culture of discharge is confirmatory.	Gas gangrene occurs in the setting of a contaminated wound. *C. perfringens* produces potent exotoxins, including alpha toxin and theta toxin, which depress myocardial contractility, induce shock, and cause direct vascular injury at the site of infection. Infections with enterobacteriacae, other gram-negative rods, *S. aureus*, streptococci, and mixed aerobic and anaerobic infections can also cause gas formation. These agents cause cellulitis rather than myonecrosis. Kitterer D et al. Gas gangrene caused by *Clostridium perfringens* involving the liver, spleen, and heart in a man 20 years after an orthotopic liver transplant: a case report. Exp Clin Transplant 2014;12:165. [PMID: 23962047] Shindo Y et al. Epidemiological and pathobiological profiles of *Clostridium perfringens* infections: review of consecutive series of 33 cases over a 13-year period. Int J Clin Exp Pathol 2015;8:569. [PMID: 2575747] Simon TG et al. Massive intravascular hemolysis from *Clostridium perfringens* septicemia: a review. J Intensive Care Med 2014;29:327. [PMID: 24019300]

(Continued)

SKIN	SKIN
Impetigo	**Cellulitis**

Impetigo

Infant (impetigo neonatorum): *Staphylococcus* (GPC).

Nonbullous or "vesicular" (70% of cases): *S. pyogenes* (GPC), *S. aureus* (GPC), anaerobes. Bullous (30% of cases): *S. aureus*.

Gram stain, culture, and smear for HSV and VZV antigen detection by direct fluorescent antibody (DFA) of scrapings from lesions may be useful in differentiating impetigo from other vesicular or pustular lesions (HSV, VZV, contact dermatitis). DFA smear can be performed by scraping the contents, base, and roof of vesicle and applying to glass slide. After fixing, the slide is stained with DFA reagents for identification of HSV or VZV antigens.

Impetigo neonatorum requires prompt treatment and protection of other infants (isolation).

Polymicrobial aerobic-anaerobic infections are present in some patients. Patients with recurrent impetigo should have cultures of the anterior nares to identify and treat carriage of *S. aureus*.

Hartman-Adams H et al. Impetigo: diagnosis and treatment. Am Fam Physician 2014;90:229. [PMID: 25250996]

Ibrahim F et al. Bacterial skin infections. Prim Care 2015;42:485. [PMID: 26612370]

Rush J et al. Childhood skin and soft tissue infections: new discoveries and guidelines regarding the management of bacterial soft tissue infections, molluscum contagiosum, and warts. Curr Opin Pediatr 2016;28:250. [PMID: 26900921]

Cellulitis

Spontaneous, traumatic wound: Polymicrobial: *S. aureus* (GPC), groups A, C, and G streptococci (GPC), enterococci (GPC), Enterobacteriaceae (GNR), *Clostridium perfringens* (GPR), *Clostridium tetani*, *Pseudomonas* sp. (GNR) (if water exposure).

Postoperative wound (not GI or GU): *S. aureus*, group A streptococcus, Enterobacteriaceae, *Pseudomonas* sp.

Postoperative wound (GI or GU): Must add *Bacteroides* sp., anaerobes, enterococcus (GPC), groups B or C streptococci.

Diabetes mellitus: Polymicrobial: *S. pyogenes*, enterococcus, *S. aureus*, Enterobacteriaceae, anaerobes.

Bullous lesions, sea water contaminated abrasion, after raw seafood consumption: *Vibrio vulnificus* (GNR).

Vein graft donor site: Beta-hemolytic streptococci.

Decubitus ulcers: Polymicrobial: *S. aureus*, anaerobic streptococci, Enterobacteriaceae, *Pseudomonas* sp., *Bacteroides* sp., other anaerobes.

Necrotizing fasciitis, type 1: streptococcus, anaerobes, Enterobacteriaceae; type 2: Group A streptococcus (hemolytic streptococcal gangrene).

Immunocompromised including HIV-infected individuals: *Helicobacter cinaedi* cellulitis-associated with bacteremia.

Skin culture: In spontaneous cellulitis, isolation of the causative organism is difficult. In traumatic and postoperative wounds, Gram stain may allow rapid diagnosis of staphylococcal or clostridial infection. Culture of wound or abscess material after disinfection of the skin site almost always yields the diagnosis.

MRI can aid in diagnosis of secondary abscess formation, necrotizing fasciitis, or pyomyositis. Frozen section of biopsy specimen may be useful.

Cellulitis has long been considered to be the result of an antecedent bacterial invasion with subsequent bacterial proliferation. However, the difficulty in isolating putative pathogens from cellulitic skin has cast doubt on this theory. Predisposing factors for cellulitis include diabetes mellitus, edema, peripheral vascular disease, venous insufficiency, leg ulcer or wound, tinea pedis, dry skin, obesity, and history of cellulitis.

Consider updating anti-tetanus prophylaxis for all wounds.

In the diabetic patient, and in postoperative and traumatic wounds, consider prompt surgical debridement for necrotizing fasciitis. With abscess formation, surgical drainage is the mainstay of therapy and may be sufficient.

Hemolytic streptococcal gangrene may follow minor trauma and involves specific strains of streptococcus.

Bruun T et al. Etiology of cellulitis and clinical prediction of streptococcal disease: a prospective study. Open Forum Infect Dis 2015;3:ofv181. [PMID: 26734653]

Gunderson CG et al. A systematic review of bacteremias in cellulitis and erysipelas. J Infect 2012;64:148. [PMID: 22101078]

Kawamura Y et al. Clinical and bacteriological characteristics of *Helicobacter cinaedi* infection. J Infect Chemother 2014;20:517. [PMID: 25022901]

BLOOD

Bacteremia of unknown source

Organism	Specimen/Diagnostic Tests	Comments
Bacteremia of unknown source Neonate (<4 days): Group B streptococcus (GPC), E. coli (GNR), klebsiella (GNR), enterobacter (GNR), S. aureus (GPC), coagulase-negative staphylococci (GPC), Candida sp. Neonate (>5 days): Add H. influenzae (GNCB). Child (nonimmunocompromised): S. pneumoniae (GPDC), N. meningitidis (GNDC), S. aureus (GPC), enterococci (GPC). Adult (IV drug use): S. aureus or viridans streptococci (GPC in chains), enterococci (GPC). Adult (catheter-related, "line" sepsis): coagulase-negative staphylococci (30%), S. aureus (12%), Candida sp. (11%), enterococci (9%), other strep-tococci (9%), Klebsiella pneumoniae (9%), Entero-bacter sp. (4%), Serratia sp. (4%), Pseudomonas sp. (4%), Acinetobacter baumanii (1–4%), Corynebac-terium jeikeium (1%), other yeast (1%). Adult (splenectomized): S. pneumoniae, H. influenzae, N. meningitidis. Neutropenia (<500 PMN/mcL): Enterobacteriaceae, Pseudomonas sp., S. aureus, coagulase-negative staphylococci, viridans streptococci (GPC in chains). Immunocompromised: Bartonella sp. (GNR), Mycobacterium avium/intracellulare (AFB).	Blood cultures are mandatory for all patients with fever and no obvious source of infection. Often they are negative, especially in neonates. Cultures (2–3 sets) should be drawn from different sites before start of antibiotic therapy. Culture should not be drawn from an IV line or from a femoral site if possible. Culture and Gram stain of urine, wounds, and other potentially infected sites may provide a more rapid diag-nosis than blood cultures. Blood cultures are incubated for 5 days. New methods are being introduced that rapidly (within 3–5 hours) identify bacteria or yeast genus and species from a positive blood culture bottle (eg, peptide nucleic acid fluorescence in situ hybridization [PNA-FISH], real-time PCR assays, and microarray assays).	Occult bacteremia affects approximately 5% of febrile children ages 2–36 months. In infants, the findings of an elevated total WBC count (>15,000 mcL) and absolute neutrophil count (ANC >10,000/mcL) are equally sensitive in predicting bacteremia, but the ANC is more specific. Predisposing factors in adults include IV drug use, neutropenia, urinary tract infection, cancer, diabetes mellitus, venous catheterization, hemodialysis, and plasmapheresis. Catheter-related infection in patients with long-term venous access (Broviac, Hickman, etc.) may be treated successfully without removal of the line, but recurrence of bacteremia is frequent. Belhassen-Garcia M et al. Fever of unknown origin as the first manifestation of colonic pathology. Clin Med (Lond) 2013;13:141. [PMID: 23681860] Gil-Diaz A et al. Fever of unknown origin in a young man. Ir J Med Sci 2014;183:461. [PMID: 24852662] Manzano S et al. Markers for bacterial infection in children with fever without source. Arch Dis Child 2011;96:440. [PMID: 21278424] Ruiz-Giardin JM et al. Clinical diagnostic accuracy of suspected sources of bacteremia and its effect on mortality. Eur J Intern Med 2013;24:541. [PMID: 23768564]

... **EMERGING (NEW) AND RE-EMERGING PATHOGENS/INFECTIOUS AGENTS.**

Organism	Specimen/Diagnostic Tests	Comments
Acinetobacter *Acinetobacter* species are gram-negative rods, and important pathogens causing healthcare-associated infections.	Stool, respiratory, or blood culture. Most common in debilitated ICU patients. Organism can survive for a long period of time in the environment and on the hands of healthcare workers.	Healthcare-associated infection caused by *Acinetobacter* has increased in the last decade during which this strain has developed multidrug resistance. Multidrug-resistant strains are universally susceptible to the polymyxins (colistin, polymyxin B); however, these drugs have significant side effects. Alternative therapy is tigecycline. High morbidity and mortality rates with *Acinetobacter* infections. Kaye KS et al. Infections caused by resistant gram-negative bacteria: epidemiology and management. Pharmacotherapy 2015;35:949. [PMID: 26497481] Park SY et al. Risk factors for mortality in patients with *Acinetobacter baumannii* bacteremia. Infect Chemother 2013;45:325. [PMID: 24396634] Protic D et al. Nosocomial infections caused by *Acinetobacter baumannii*: are we losing the battle? Surg Infect (Larchmt) 2016;17:236. [PMID: 26885722] Zhou HY et al. Prior use of four invasive procedures increases the risk of *Acinetobacter baumannii* nosocomial bacteremia among patients in intensive care units: a systematic review and meta-analysis. Int J Infect Dis 2014;22:25. [PMID: 24607429]
Avian influenza A/H5N1, Avian influenza A/H7N9, and Novel H1N1 influenza A Influenza A virus subtype H5N1 has greater virulence, easier (more efficient) human-to-human transmission, and resistance to antiviral drugs, compared to seasonal influenza A viruses and other avian influenza viruses. Novel H1N1 influenza A virus caused a pandemic in 2009.	Nasopharyngeal swab specimens for viral culture (specimen from patients with suspected avian influenza should not be cultured in a routine laboratory—send specimens to CDC or State Department of Public Health Laboratory and contact local/state communicable disease group). CDC and State Public Health Laboratories perform molecular methods for strain typing. Molecular assays for influenza A and B with identification of H1N1 strain are now commercially available for clinical laboratories. These assays will identify influenza A but not the subtype, so specimens have to be sent to CDC or Public Health Laboratory for identification of H5N1 subtype. Healthcare workers who have close contact with patients with influenza-like symptoms should follow CDC guidelines for personal protective equipment (masks, etc) to prevent infection.	The first documented case of bird-to-human transmission of avian influenza A (H5N1) occurred in 1997 in Hong Kong. The H5N1 virus is carried by birds that shed the virus in saliva, nasal secretions, and feces. Other birds/fowls are infected by fecal-oral transmission through contact with contaminated surface, feed, water, grout, etc. By 2006, almost every country in the world had reported at least one case of H5N1 influenza. Clinical symptoms and signs: mild-to-severe respiratory symptoms and fever. High mortality in humans. There are fears of a future pandemic with H5N1 influenza A. Since influenza A viruses can reassort gene segments, new viruses can arise with potential to cause human disease. A recent influenza A viral strain— avian influenza A (H7N9) virus—with pandemic potential caused many cases of severe influenza in China. Novel H1N1 influenza A caused mostly mild illness except for severe illness in young children, pregnant women, and obese patients. Gautret P et al. Emerging viral respiratory tract infections—environmental risk factors and transmission. Lancet Infect Dis 2014;14:1113. [PMID: 25189350] Mubareka S et al. Influenza virus emitted by naturally-infected hosts in a healthcare setting. J Clin Virol 2015;73:105. [PMID: 26590688] Tanner WD et al. The pandemic potential of avian influenza A(H7N9) virus: a review. Epidemiol Infect 2015;143:3359. [PMID: 26205078] Trombetta C et al. Emerging influenza strains in the last two decades: a threat of a new pandemic? Vaccines (Basel) 2015;3:172. [PMID: 26344952]

(Continued)

Organism	Specimen/Diagnostic Tests	Comments
Carbapenem-resistant enterobacteriaceae (CRE) Carbapenemase production in the Enterobacteriaceae was unknown until early 2000s. Almost all carbapenem-resistant isolates were sporadic cases of hyperproduction of a beta-lactamase (AmpC or ESBL) combined with porin loss. In 2001, there was the first report of carbapenem-resistant *Klebsiella pneumoniae*; it carried a new carbapenemase, KPC enzyme. New Delhi metallo-beta-lactamase (NDM1) has been described in patients infected with *Escherichia coli* or *Klebsiella pneumoniae* during surgery in India and Pakistan. Outbreaks have been seen worldwide since 2003 of OXA-48 carbapenemase in *K. pneumoniae*, resulting in resistance to all beta-lactams.	Accurate and timely detection of CRE is of great importance to guide therapeutic decisions and start appropriate infection control measures. Susceptibility testing is done on Enterobacteriaceae isolates with MIC method (elevated MIC to certain carbapenems) or detection of hydrolysis of carbapenem by modified Hodge test or the Carba NP test. MIC testing is often used as a first screen. Genotypic tests involve amplification and detection of specific beta lactamase (*bla*) genes using PCR assay (highly sensitive and specific). Chromogenic agar and newer PCR assays are available for screening rectal swabs from high-risk groups, eg. residents in long-term care facilities.	Patients infected with CRE have higher morbidity and mortality than those not. CRE can cause urinary tract infection, abdominal infection, bacteremia, pneumonia, and skin and soft tissue infection. CRE infection is spread by the fecal-oral route and from patient to patient via contaminated hands of healthcare workers; more recently, transmission has been noted from contaminated endoscopes, sinks and drains. In addition to most beta-lactams, CRE organisms are often resistant to other antimicrobial classes of drugs. Few treatment options remain: colistin, polymyxin B, tigecycline have all shown in vitro activity, but can have side effects, eg, nephrotoxicity with colistin. Two recently released beta-lactam/beta-lactamase inhibitor combinations show promise in fighting CRE infections: ceftolozane/tazobactam and ceftazidime/avibactam. More drugs and more studies are needed. Kaye KS et al. Infection caused by resistant Gram-negative bacteria: epidemiology and management. Pharmacotherapy 2015;35:949. [PMID: 26497481] Temkin E et al. Carbapenem-resistant Enterobacteriaceae: biology, epidemiology, and management. Ann NY Acad Sci 2014;1323:22. [PMID: 25195939] Yamamoto M et al. Treatment for infections with carbapenem-resistant Enterobacteriaceae: what options do we still have? Crit Care 2014;18:229. [PMID: 25041592]
Chikungunya Virus Mosquito-borne alphavirus of the Togaviridae family. Disease characterized by fever, headache, myalgia, rash, and both acute and persistent arthralgia.	Clinical presentation (acute onset fever with severe arthralgia or arthritis) and travel to an endemic/epidemic area would be a suspected case. Confirmation of diagnosis in acute phase of illness could involve RT-PCR on serum samples. Serology to detect IgM and IgG available at most reference laboratories.	Transmitted by *Aedes* spp. mosquitoes. Since 2005, global chikungunya virus outbreaks associated with severe chronic morbidity and deaths have occurred. Endemic in tropical regions and an emerging infection in Europe, the Middle East, Indian Ocean islands, and the Caribbean islands. Polyarthralgia can be severe and debilitating. No vaccine or treatment. Burt FJ et al. Chikungunya: a re-emerging virus. Lancet 2012;379:662. [PMID: 22100854] Morrison TE. Reemergence of chikungunya virus. J Virol 2014;88:11644. [PMID: 25078691] Rougeron V et al. Chikungunya, a paradigm of neglected tropical disease that emerged to be a new health global risk. J Clin Virol 2015;64:144. [PMID: 25453326]

Clostridium difficile		
Clostridium difficile is a gram-positive anaerobic rod. *C. difficile* produces 2 toxins: toxin A, which is an enterotoxin, and toxin B, which is a cytotoxin. *C. difficile* has been found in stool in 15–25% of patients with antibiotic-associated diarrhea, 10% of patients treated with antibiotics who do not have diarrhea, and in 95% of patients with diarrhea associated with pseudomembranous colitis.	Stool for culture is a sensitive test (89–100%), but 25% of isolates recovered are nonpathogenic and test takes 72 hours. A toxin assay on the isolated organism must still be completed. Stool for cytotoxicity assay (toxin B) using tissue cultures has been considered a good test, but recent reports suggest a lower sensitivity of 60–80% for toxin detection and the test takes 48 hours. Toxigenic culture of stool (demonstrates production of toxin from a *C. difficile* isolate) has become the new "gold standard" assay, but this assay also takes several days. Stool for EIA testing for toxin A and B has 70–80% sensitivity and rapid tests are available. However, the EIA assays are no longer recommended for routine testing for the toxins. A rapid lateral flow assay that detects both toxins A and B and an enzyme, glutamate dehydrogenase (GDH), by EIA is available and useful for screening for presence of toxigenic *C. difficile* in stool. Molecular assays that detect the toxin B gene are very sensitive (95%) and specific. These assays are becoming the standard of care in many laboratories. Flexible sigmoidoscopy or colonoscopy may be performed in patients with severe symptomatology to detect plaques of pseudomembranous colitis when a rapid diagnosis is needed; sensitivity is 51%.	Clinical symptoms and signs: watery diarrhea, fever, anorexia, and abdominal pain and tenderness. Diarrhea can be mild to severe. Severe diarrhea can lead to ulceration and bleeding from the colon (colitis) and to perforation of the intestine (peritonitis). A new emerging type of *C. difficile* is ribotype 027, also known as NAP-1, which produces 16–23 times more toxin A and B and is resistant to fluoroquinolones. This emerging *C. difficile* strain causes more severe disease, increased need for surgical procedures, and death. Treatment options include metronidazole, vancomycin, or a new expensive drug, fidaxomicin. For severe, recurrent disease, fecal transplantation has been successful. Kociolek LK et al. Breakthroughs in the treatment and prevention of *Clostridium difficile* infection. Nat Rev Gastroenterol Hepatol 2016;13:150. [PMID: 26860266] Leffler DA et al. *Clostridium difficile* infection. N Engl J Med 2015;373:287. [PMID: 26176396] Lessa FC et al. Burden of *Clostridium difficile* infection in the United States. N Engl J Med 2015;372:2369. [PMID: 26061850] Zanella Terrier MC et al. Recurrent *Clostridium difficile* infections: the importance of the intestinal microbiota. World J Gastroenterol 2014;20:7416. [PMID: 24966611]

(Continued)

Organism	Specimen/Diagnostic Tests	Comments
Cryptococcus gattii While found around the world in tropical and sub-tropical areas, this yeast emerged as a human and animal pathogen in 2000 in the Pacific Northwest after being recognized on Vancouver Island, British Columbia. Unlike *Cryptococcus neoformans*, which mostly causes illness in immunocompromised individuals, *C. gattii* can cause disease in healthy, immunocompetent persons and in immunocompromised persons (HIV-infected, organ transplant, hematologic malignancy).	Diagnosed by isolation of *C. gattii* from culture of clinical samples. Biochemical characteristics same as *C. neoformans* except for reaction in special media, L-canvanine–glycine–bromothymol blue (CGB) medium. *C. gattii* produces blue coloration on this CGB agar.	*C. gattii* is associated with environmental sources, and is isolated from trees, soil, air, freshwater and seawater within the Coastal Douglas Fir climate zones in British Columbia. Transmission thought to be through inhalation of spores from the environment causing pneumonia or meningitis. Infection requires longer, more aggressive treatment than *C. neoformans*. Espinel-Ingroff A et al. Current trends in the prevalence of *Cryptococcus gattii* in the United States and Canada. Infect Drug Resist 2015;8:89. [PMID: 25999744] Harris J et al. *Cryptococcus gattii*: where do we go from here? Med Mycol 2012;50:113. [PMID: 21939343] Harris JR et al. *Cryptococcus gattii* infections in multiple states outside the US Pacific Northwest. Emerg Infect Dis 2013;19:1620. [PMID: 24050410]
Dengue Virus Single-stranded RNA virus in family Flaviviridae and genus *Flavivirus* of which there are 5 known serotypes. Arthropod-borne virus (arbovirus) spread by mosquitos of the *Aedes* genus, specifically *A. aegypti* and *A. albopictus*.	On initial presentation, thrombocytopenia and minor bleeding complications (petechiae and nose bleeds). Diagnostic tests include: ELISA tests for IgM and IgG antibodies (not serotype-specific) early in illness (most common). Acute and convalescent sera for IgG antibody by ELISA test enable later diagnosis. Dengue virus NS1 antigen detection by ELISA is available in some reference laboratories. Reverse-transcriptase PCR, real-time PCR, or isothermal amplification methods for detection of viral nucleic acid is available at reference laboratories.	Most infections with dengue virus lead to a self-limiting illness, yet stricter monitoring is needed compared to chikungunya virus infections, due to the potential for significant morbidity and mortality with dengue infection. Infection with one serotype of dengue virus confers lifelong immunity to that particular serotype, but only short-lived immunity to the other serotypes; subsequent infections with a different serotype increases the risk for severe complications like dengue hemorrhagic fever (hemorrhagic complications and/or severe organ impairment). Endemic in tropical and subtropical regions, so tourists are at risk for infection. L'Azou M et al. Symptomatic dengue in children in 10 Asian and Latin American countries. N Engl J Med 2016;374:1155. [PMID: 27007959] Mardekian SK et al. Diagnostic options and challenges for dengue and chikungunya viruses. Biomed Res Int 2015;2015 [PMID: 26509163] Simmons CP et al. Dengue. N Engl J Med 2012;366:1423. [PMID: 22494122]

Ebola virus

Ebola virus disease (EVD) caused by infection with a single-stranded RNA virus of the genus *Ebolavirus*. Zaire ebola virus (EBOV) first identified in humans in an outbreak in 1976 near the Ebola River in the Democratic Republic of the Congo (DRC, formerly Zaire). EBOV has the highest case fatality rate of all the known Ebola virus species.

EVD is diagnosed by nucleic acid amplification tests (NAAIs). Several groups have developed rapid antigen tests using lateral flow immunochromatographic assays that can detect antigen in 15–25 minutes. One assay detecting EBOV VP40 antigen in serum, plasma, or fingerstick whole blood reported a 92% sensitivity, 85% specificity. A positive result can guide isolation decisions to prevent spread to the community as well as supportive care (rehydration, electrolytes, antibiotics, antimalarial drugs).

Later in disease course or after recovery, IgM and IgG antibody testing is available. Retrospectively in deceased patients, immunohistochemistry, PCR and virus isolation can also be carried out.

Ebola testing should be conducted only for persons who have consistent symptoms ro signs and who meet epidemiological risk criteria. In the United States, testing for Ebola virus is typically done at designated laboratories in the national response network. Healthcare facilities should follow their state and/or local health department procedures for notifying and consulting about Ebola virus testing requests.

Ebola virus causes a nonspecific febrile illness associated with myalgia, progressive gastro-intestinal symptoms (abdominal pain, nausea, vomiting, and diarrhea). In second week, hemorrhagic symptoms and sepsis may develop.

Mortality from Ebola virus disease ranges from 40–88%. Human-to-human transmission of EVD is primarily through direct contact with body fluids of infected person after fever has developed or with the body of a person who has recently died.

In 2014–2015, the largest outbreak in the history of EVD due to Zaire ebola virus occurred in West Africa. Through April 2016, 28,616 EVD cases and 11,310 deaths were reported from Guinea, Sierra Leone and Liberia.

The natural reservoir for Ebola virus has not been definitively determined, but some data indicate the virus is present in frugivorous and insectivorous bats.

Beeching NJ et al. Ebola virus disease. BMJ 2014;349:g7348. [PMID: 25497512]

Benzine JW et al. Molecular diagnostic field test for point-of-care detection of Ebola virus directly from blood. J Infect Dis. 2016 Oct 15;214(suppl):S234. [PMID: 2763847]

Lyon GM et al. Clinical care of two patients with Ebola virus disease in the United States. N Engl J Med 2014;371:2402. [PMID: 25390460]

Martinez MJ et al. Ebola virus infection: overview and update on prevention and treatment. Infect Dis Ther 2015;4:365. [PMID: 26363787]

Semper AE et al. Performance of the GeneXpert Ebola assay for diagnosis of Ebola virus disease in Sierra Leone: a field evaluation study. PLoS Med. 2016 Mar 29;13(3):e1001980. [PMID: 27023868]

Stamm LV. Ebola virus disease: rapid diagnosis and timely case reporting are critical to the early response for outbreak control. Am J Trop Med Hyg 2015;93:438. [PMID: 26175026]

(*Continued*)

Organism	Specimen/Diagnostic Tests	Comments
Escherichia coli, Diarrheagenic *Escherichia coli* is a member of genus Escherichia within the family Enterobacteriaceae. *E. coli* can be characterized by shared liposaccharide (O) and flagellar (H) antigens that define serogroups (O antigen only) or serotypes (O and H antigens). More than 175 O antigens and 53 H antigens have been recognized, but only a few serotype combinations are associated with diarrheal diseases.	Stool culture, with special tests (see entries below). *E. coli* has at least 6 different mechanisms by which to cause diarrhea, and each is associated with a different pathotype and different virulence determinants. The 6 pathotypes are diffusely adherent *E. coli* (**DAEC**), Enteroaggregative *E. coli* (**EAEC**), Enterohemorrhagic *E. coli* (**EHEC**) (also known as Shiga toxin (Stx)-producing *E. coli*, **STEC**), Enteroinvasive *E. coli* (**EIEC**), Enteropathogenic *E. coli* (**EPEC**), and Enterotoxigenic *E. coli* (**ETEC**). Over 200 types of *E. coli* are known to produce shiga toxins. Approximately 1% of stool samples tested in clinical laboratories contain (STEC) shiga toxins. EIAs are available for detection of shiga toxins.	The principal reservoir of EHEC/STEC is the intestinal tract of cattle and herbivorous animals (eg, sheep, deer, goats, birds). EHEC/STEC strains are most frequently identified as diarrheagenic *E. coli* serotypes. Over 60 STEC serotypes are associated with human diseases. *E. coli* O157:H7 is the most common STEC serotype, but there was an outbreak of several thousand cases of *E. coli* O104:H4 in Western Europe in 2011. The source was thought to be contaminated raw sprouts originating from a farm in Germany, traceable to Egypt. It was associated with > 800 cases of hemolytic-uremic syndrome and >30 deaths. Several US cases and 1 HUS death were documented. Clinical symptoms and signs: Diarrhea, dysentery (bloody diarrhea). Jandhyala DM et al. Shiga toxin-producing *Escherichia coli* O104:H4: an emerging pathogen with enhanced virulence. Infect Dis Clin North Am 2013;27:631. [PMID: 24011834] Kalita A et al. Recent advances in adherence and invasion of pathogenic *Escherichia coli.* Curr Opin Infect Dis 2014;27:459. [PMID: 25023740] Smith JL et al. Shiga toxin-producing *Escherichia coli.* Adv Appl Microbiol 2014;86:145. [PMID: 24377855]
***E. coli,* Diffusely adherent (DAEC)** Organism elicits a characteristic diffuse aggregative pattern of adherence to HEP-2 cells.	Stool for tissue culture assay for diffuse adherence; test performed by State Public Health Laboratories.	Centers for Disease Control and Prevention (CDC). Diarrheagenic *Escherichia coli.* http://www.cdc.gov/ecoli/diarrheagenic-ecoli.html
***E. coli,* Enteroaggregative (EAEC)** Organism adheres to small and large bowel epithelial cells and expresses secretory enterotoxins and cytotoxins.	Stool for tissue culture adhesion assay; test performed by State Public Health Laboratories. DNA and PCR tests lack sufficient sensitivity and specificity.	Clinical symptoms and signs: intestinal colic, bloody stool, and mucus. Persistent diarrhea in children. Chronic diarrhea in HIV-infected patients/immunocompromised patients. Correlated with interleukin-8 production. Estrada-Garcia T et al. Enteroaggregative *Escherichia coli* pathotype: a genetically heterogeneous emerging foodborne enteropathogen. FEMS Immunol Med Microbiol 2012;66:281. [PMID: 22775224] Jandhyala DM et al. Shiga toxin-producing *Escherichia coli* O104:H4: an emerging pathogen with enhanced virulence. Infect Dis Clin North Am 2013;27:631. [PMID: 24011834]

Organism	Specimen/Diagnostic Test	Comments
E. coli, Enterohemorrhagic/ Shiga-toxin-producing E. coli (EHEC/STEC) Organism colonizes enterocytes of the large bowel and causes a characteristic attaching and effacing pathology. It produces Shiga toxin (Stx) 1 or 2, which inhibit protein synthesis.	Stool for bacterial culture, special media for testing O157:H7 and O104:H4. Stool for Shiga toxin by EIA.	Clinical symptoms and signs: frequently bloody diarrhea (although diarrhea without blood can occur), abdominal pain, vomiting, fever usually absent. Hemolytic uremic syndrome (HUS) develops in up to 10%. *E. coli* O157:H7 and O104:H4. EHEC/STEC cause >80% of cases of HUS. Among those with HUS, up to 30–50% will have long-term kidney damage; and up to 5–10% die. Recommendation is to not use antibiotics in these infected patients since such usage can increase risk of progression to HUS. Gould LH et al. Increased recognition of non-O157 Shiga toxin-producing *Escherichia coli* infections in the United States during 2000–2010: epidemiologic features and comparison with *E. coli* O157 infections. Foodborne Pathol Dis 2013;10:453. [PMID: 23560425] Smith JL et al. Shiga toxin-producing *Escherichia coli*. Adv Appl Microbiol 2014;86:145. [PMID: 24377855]
E. coli, Enteroinvasive (EIEC) Organism invades colonic epithelial cells, lyses the phagosome, multiplies intracellularly, and moves through the cell, exits and re-enters the basolateral plasma membrane. It is closely related to *Shigella* species genetically, biochemically and pathogenetically.	Stool for PCR or DNA probes for *inv* genes; test performed by State Public Health Laboratories or research laboratories.	Clinical symptoms and signs: watery diarrhea with a mechanism similar to shigella-related diarrhea and also related to induced apoptosis in infected macrophages, fever, abdominal cramps. Clinical symptoms and signs: mild to severe diarrhea. Martinez-Medina M et al. *Escherichia coli* in chronic inflammatory bowel diseases: an update on adherent invasive *Escherichia coli* pathogenicity. World J Gastrointest Pathophysiol 2014;5:213. [PMID: 25133024]
E. coli, Enteropathogenic (EPEC) Organism adheres to small bowel enterocytes and destroys the normal microvillar structure.	Stool for EPEC PCR or DNA probes may be offered in Public Health Laboratories or research laboratories.	Leading cause of pediatric diarrhea in developing countries. Clinical symptoms and signs: severe diarrhea, low-grade fever, vomiting. Prolonged diarrhea resulting in weight loss, malnutrition, and death. Infantile diarrhea, dehydration. Hu J et al. Enteropathogenic *Escherichia coli*: foe or innocent bystander? Clin Microbiol Infect 2015;21:729. [PMID: 25726041]
E. coli, Enterotoxigenic (ETEC) Organism adheres to small bowel enterocytes and the enterotoxin causes mild to severe watery diarrhea. Produces two types of toxin: heat-labile (LT) or heat-stable (ST) toxins.	Stool for detection of toxin-producing *E. coli*; test performed by State Public Health Laboratories. Stool does not contain WBCs, mucus, or RBCs.	Clinical symptoms and signs: watery diarrhea, usually lasting for 3–7 days, which can be prolonged or can relapse for months; abdominal cramps; occasional nausea; fever usually absent. Frequent cause of traveler's diarrhea. Bourgeois AL et al. Status of vaccine research and development for enterotoxigenic *Escherichia coli*. Vaccine 2016 Jun 3;34:2880. [PMID: 26988259]

(Continued)

Organism	Specimen/Diagnostic Tests	Comments
Human granulocytotropic anaplasmosis (HGA) Causing agent is the intracellular bacteria, *Ixodes* ticks are the vectors for *Anaplasma phagocytophilum*.	CBC, liver tests. Blood abnormalities may include leukopenia and thrombocytopenia. Transaminases may be elevated. HME: rarely, morulae (clusters of *Ehrlichia* bacteria) can be seen in the cytoplasms of peripheral blood monocytes. HGA: 20–80% of patients have ehrlichial morulae identified in peripheral blood neutrophils.	Severe complications (rare) include meningoencephalitis and toxic shock with multi-organ failure; these complications are more common in immunocompromised patients. *E. chaffeensis* is found primarily in North Atlantic and South Central states of the US. *A. phagocytophilum* is found primarily in the Northeast and upper Midwestern areas of US. Atif FA. *Anaplasma marginale* and *Anaplasma phagocytophilum*: Rickettsiales pathogens of veterinary and public health significance. Parasitol Res 2015;114:3941. [PMID: 26346451] Centers for Disease Control and Prevention (CDC). Human Ehrlichiosis. http://www.cdc.gov/ehrlichiosis/ Lotrič-Furlan S et al. Comparison of clinical and laboratory characteristics of patients fulfilling criteria for proven and probable human granulocytic anaplasmosis. Microbes Infect 2015;17:829. [PMID: 26432519] Nichols HK et al. Increasing incidence of ehrlichiosis in the United States: a summary of national surveillance of *Ehrlichia chaffeensis* and *Ehrlichia ewingii* infections in the United States, 2008–2012. Am J Trop Med Hyg 2016;94:52. [PMID: 26621561] Rikihisa Y. Molecular pathogenesis of *Ehrlichia chaffeensis* infection. Annu Rev Microbiol 2015;69:283. [PMID: 26488275]
Human metapneumovirus (huMPV) huMPV is the causative agent of infant bronchiolitis in 5–15% of cases. Accounts for 1–5% childhood upper respiratory infections and 10–15% of hospitalizations for lower respiratory tract infections. From the family of Paramyxoviridae, this RNA virus is a new metapneumovirus related to the turkey trachetitis virus and respiratory syncytial virus (RSV). The first documented case of huMPV occurred in 2001 in the US.	Isolation of huMPV in viral tissue culture is difficult since the virus replicates slowly. Reverse-transcriptase PCR of nasopharyngeal specimens is the most favored method for the identification of huMPV. Direct detection of viral antigens in respiratory specimens by IFA is commercially available, but less commonly used and, as with RSV, IFA methods are insensitive in adults due to low viral load in secretions.	huMPV is a respiratory pathogen that causes infections ranging from colds to severe bronchiolitis and pneumonia. Clinical symptoms and signs: 70–80% of infected individuals are asymptomatic, 20% have mild flu-like symptoms, 6% have symptoms indistinguishable from RSV, bronchiolitis, croup, asthma, or pneumonia. Serology shows infections with huMPV are nearly universal by age 5 years and reinfection can occur throughout life, likely due to impaired CD8+ T-cell response. Most commonly causes upper and lower respiratory tract infections in young children, but also in elderly individuals and immunocompromised patients. Haas LE et al. Human metapneumovirus in adults. Viruses 2013;5:87. [PMID: 23299785] Panda S et al. Human metapneumovirus: review of an important respiratory pathogen. Int J Infect Dis 2014;25:45. [PMID: 24841931] Schuster JE et al. Human metapneumovirus. Pediatr Rev 2013;34:558. [PMID: 24295817]

Organism/Disease	Specimen/Test	Clinical Notes
Human monkeypox virus Monkeypox virus is in the family of Orthopoxvirus, which is in the same genus as the smallpox (variola) virus. Monkeypox is a zoonotic disease endemic to central and western Africa, where it is a major public health concern. First documented case in US occurred in June 2003. The infected humans had contact with prairie dogs that had been housed with infected Gambian giant rats from Ghana. This outbreak of 72 cases, as reported to the CDC, involved patients in six states.	Respiratory samples and skin lesion specimens submitted for viral culture. Blood and/or CSF samples for monkeypox virus DNA by PCR and for IgM antibodies by ELISA. Tissue samples for immunohistochemical testing or by demonstrating virus morphologically consistent with orthopoxvirus by electron microscopy.	History: Exposure to wild mammalian pet or exotic animal. Clinical symptoms and signs: Fever, chills or sweats, headaches, backache, sore throat, cough, shortness of breath, lymphadenopathy, rash (macular, papular, vesicular or pustular, generalized or localized, discrete or confluent), encephalitis. Mortality rate in Africa: approximately 10%, higher in immunocompromised patients. Centers for Disease Control and Prevention (CDC). Monkeypox Homepage http://www.cdc.gov/poxvirus/monkeypox/ McCollum AM et al. Human monkeypox. Clin Infect Dis 2014;58:260. [PMID: 24158414] Ramdass P et al. Viral skin diseases. Prim Care 2015;42:517. [PMID: 26612372] Shchelkunov SN. An increasing danger of zoonotic orthopoxvirus infections. PLoS Pathog 2013;9:e1003756. [PMID: 24339772]
Human monocytic ehrlichiosis (HME) Causative agent is *Ehrlichia chaffeensis*. Transmitted to humans and animals by various ticks: *Dermacentor*, *Ixodes* and *Amblyomma* species.	Both HME and HGA can be diagnosed with serology or PCR tests. Blood/serum for IgM or IgG antibodies by IFA or ELISA. Blood/serum/bone marrow for ehrlichial DNA by PCR.	Clinical symptoms and signs (similar for HME and HGA): Illness is mild to fatal; most recover completely without treatment. Disease can resemble Rocky Mountain spotted fever, lasting 1–2 weeks with rash (20%), fever, headache, chills, nausea, vomiting, anorexia, myalgias, cough, diarrhea, lymphadenopathy.
Lyme disease Causative agent is *Borrelia burgdorferi*. Found primarily in the Northeast, mid-Atlantic coastal areas, and north-central US. *Borrelia burgdorferi* is transmitted primarily by the deer tick (*Ixodes* species) after it has been attached to a host for more than 24 hours.	Serum for IgM and IgG antibodies by ELISA, need confirmation by Western immunoblot (CDC recommendation).	Clinical symptoms and signs: *Acute stage:* erythema migrans (expanding rash with area of central clearing) at the site of tick bite within 10 days in 70–80%. Other symptoms: low-grade fever, headache, myalgia, arthralgia, and regional lymphadenopathy for 3–4 weeks. *Musculoskeletal symptoms:* asymmetric arthritis; may require 3–4 years to resolve (regardless of treatment). *Early neurologic involvement:* cranial neuritis, meningitis, and encephalitis. *Chronic neurologic disease:* subacute encephalopathy, axonal polyneuropathy, and leukoencephalopathy. Choi E et al. Tick-borne illnesses. Curr Sports Med Rep 2016;15:98. [PMID: 26963018] Chomel B. Lyme disease. Rev Sci Tech 2015;34:569. [PMID: 26601457] Koedel U et al. Lyme neuroborreliosis-epidemiology, diagnosis and management. Nat Rev Neurol 2015;11:446. [PMID: 26215621] Sanchez JL. Clinical manifestations and treatment of Lyme disease. Clin Lab Med 2015;35:765. [PMID 26593256]

(Continued)

Organism	Specimen/Diagnostic Tests	Comments
Methicillin-resistant *Staphylococcus aureus* (MRSA) MRSA infections are divided into two categories by source: (1) healthcare-associated (HA-MRSA) secondary to hospitalization, surgery, long-term care, dialysis, invasive device, etc; and (2) community-associated (CA-MRSA). Methicillin resistance is associated with the acquisition of the *mecA* gene, which encodes the mutant penicillin-binding protein, PBP 2a.	Cultures of skin, soft tissue, blood with isolation of *S. aureus* and susceptibility testing for methicillin resistance. Swab of anterior nares to screen for MRSA using molecular assays, chromogenic agar plates (MRSA colonies are pink or blue on chromogenic media), or standard bacterial culture and susceptibility testing.	Clinical symptoms and signs: cellulitis, erysipelas, bacteremia, endocarditis, pneumonia, death. Increasing prevalence of community-associated MRSA, which can cause severe disease in immunocompetent persons, has led to recommendations to screen for MRSA colonization in vulnerable patient populations. This includes patients in ICUs, dialysis centers, or long-term-care facilities, patients admitted for elective surgery, or patients with history of recent hospitalization. Carrel M et al. USA300 Methicillin-resistant *Staphylococcus aureus*, United States, 2000–2013. Emerg Infect Dis 2015;21:1973. [PMID: 26484389] Esposito S et al. Epidemiology and microbiology of skin and soft tissue infections. Curr Opin Infect Dis 2016;29:109. [PMID: 26779772] Rhee Y et al. Evolving epidemiology of *Staphylococcus aureus* bacteremia. Infect Control Hosp Epidemiol 2015;36:1417. [PMID: 26372679]
Middle East respiratory syndrome coronavirus (MERS-CoV) Cause of Middle East respiratory syndrome (MERS). In 2012, the first human infection with the Middle East respiratory syndrome coronavirus (MERS-CoV) was reported from Saudi Arabia. It emerged from a zoonotic reservoir and continues to be the current dominant coronavirus circulating in the human population and causing severe illness.	Molecular detection by real-time reverse transcriptase PCR to detect active disease and viral RNA in clinical specimens (performed by State Public Health Laboratories or CDC). Multiple specimens recommended: BAL, sputum, tracheal aspirate, nasopharyngeal and oropharyngeal swabs, serum, stool. Serology for antibodies can detect previous infection.	MERS-CoV enzootic in dromedary camels across the Arabian Peninsula and in parts of Africa, causing mild upper respiratory illness in camel reservoir and sporadic, rare human infections. MERS-CoV can cause mild, influenza-like illnesses, but it is most known as a lower respiratory tract pathogen causing fever, cough, dyspnea, and pneumonia. May progress to acute respiratory distress syndrome, multi-organ failure and death in 20–40% of those infected. Compared to SARS, which has essentially disappeared, MERS progresses more rapidly to respiratory failure and acute kidney injury, is more commonly reported in patients with underlying disease, and is more often fatal. As with SARS, healthcare workers have been infected due to lapses in infection control and prevention procedures. MERS cases are currently restricted to Middle Eastern countries with some cases reported in Europe, Asia, and the United States linked to travel to the Middle East. Al-Tawfiq JA et al. Coronaviruses: severe acute respiratory syndrome coronavirus and Middle East respiratory syndrome coronavirus in travelers. Curr Opin Infect Dis 2014;27:411. [PMID: 25033169] Hui DS et al. Severe acute respiratory syndrome vs. the Middle East respiratory syndrome. Curr Opin Pulm Med 2014;20:233. [PMID: 24626235] Mackay IM et al. MERS coronavirus: diagnostics, epidemiology and transmission. Virol J 2015;12:222. [PMID: 26695637]

Mumps A virus from the family Paramyxovirus. Disease is spread by respiratory droplets; infectivity precedes the symptom by 1 day and may last a week. Incubation period is 14–21 days, average 18 days.	Buccal/oral swab for viral culture (gold standard) or mumps viral RNA by RT-PCR. Blood for serologic tests for acute mumps infection (IgM) and test of immunity (IgG) antibodies using EIA assay. Blood for serologic tests for mumps include detection of virus-specific IgM in a single sample or a fourfold or greater increase in IgG antibodies between acute- and convalescent-phase specimens using indirect EIA assay. In previously vaccinated persons, serologic tests have limited use. In a recent outbreak, mumps virus IgM antibodies were detected in <15% of infected persons who were previously vaccinated; 95% had mumps virus IgG antibodies. Virus detection can also vary owing to low viral loads in immunized persons.	Clinical symptoms and signs: Acute onset of unilateral or bilateral, tender, self-limited swelling of the parotids (75%) or other salivary glands, lasting 2 or more days, without other apparent causes; fever, malaise, stiff neck, headaches. Complications include meningitis (30%), orchitis, pancreatitis, oophoritis, thyroiditis, neuritis, hepatitis, myocarditis, thrombocytopenia, arthralgias and nephritis. Barskey AE et al. Mumps outbreak in Orthodox Jewish communities in the United States. N Engl J Med 2012;367:1704. [PMID: 23113481] Gouma S et al. Severity of mumps disease is related to MMR vaccination status and viral shedding. Vaccine 2016;34:1868. [PMID: 26954106] Rubin S et al. Molecular biology, pathogenesis and pathology of mumps virus. J Pathol 2015;235:242. [PMID: 25229387]
Severe acute respiratory syndrome—coronavirus A (SARS-CoA) First reported in Southern China in 2002; by mid-2003 over 8500 cases had been reported with nearly 800 deaths. Identified in 2003 as a coronavirus; infection originates from wildlife (eg, civets and other mammals). Highly infectious, spread by close person-to-person contact. SARS-CoA virus infection rapidly spread around the world before being controlled by public health intervention strategies.	Obtain CBC, activated PTT, serum liver tests, creatine kinase (CK), lactate dehydrogenase (LDH), chest radiograph, blood cultures, pleural fluid culture, sputum for bacterial culture and respiratory virus panel (rule out influenzae A and B, and RSV). Viral culture of respiratory specimens is not recommended. Respiratory sample, stool, plasma/serum may be sent to CDC for SAR-CoA RT-PCR assay. Blood or serum for SAR-CoA antibody EIA assay performed by State Public Health Laboratories. Laboratory abnormalities: normal or low WBC with decreased lymphocytes, prolonged activated PTT, increased transaminases, increased CK, increased LDH.	Clinical symptoms and signs: Early symptoms include fever, chills, rigors, myalgias, and headaches. Respiratory symptoms appear 2–7 days after onset, with shortness of breath and/or dry cough; pneumonia in 60–100%. Healthcare workers who have close contact with patients with symptoms consistent with a respiratory viral illness should follow CDC guidelines for use of personal protective equipment (masks, etc) to prevent infection. Al-Tawfiq JA et al. Coronaviruses: severe acute respiratory syndrome coronavirus and Middle East respiratory syndrome coronavirus in travelers. Curr Opin Infect Dis 2014;27:411. [PMID: 25033169] Peck KM et al. Coronavirus host range expansion and Middle East respiratory syndrome coronavirus emergence: biochemical mechanisms and evolutionary perspectives. Annu Rev Virol 2015;2:95. [PMID: 26958908]

(Continued)

Organism	Specimen/Diagnostic Tests	Comments
Streptococcus pneumoniae, resistant *Streptococcus pneumoniae* is a gram-positive diplococcus that was generally susceptible to all classes of antimicrobial agents in the 1970s. With increased usage of antibiotics in patients with viral infections, *S. pneumoniae* has acquired genetic material that encodes resistance to many commonly used antibiotics. It has developed resistance to beta-lactamases (45%) at altered penicillin-binding protein sites, to macrolides (40%) with a macrolide efflux pump (*mef* genes) and erythromycin-ribosomal methylases (*erm* genes) sites, to lincosamines (14%), to tetracycline, to folate-inhibitors (14–21%), and to fluoroquinolones (1–2%) with mutations in genes that code for DNA gyrase and topoisomerase IV sites. Emergence of the multidrug-resistant *S. pneumoniae* serotype 19A is due in part to routine use of protein-conjugated pneumococcal vaccine in the US, since this serotype is not included in the vaccine.	Cultures of sputum, blood, cerebrospinal fluid.	Cillóniz C et al. What is the clinical relevance of drug-resistant pneumococcus? Curr Opin Pulm Med 2016;22:227. [PMID: 26901109] Marom T et al. The effect of immunization with pneumococcal conjugated vaccines on *Streptococcus pneumoniae* resistance patterns in acute otitis media. J Microbiol Immunol Infect 2015;15:832. [PMID: 26507672] Ubukata K et al. Serotype changes and drug resistance in invasive pneumococcal diseases in adults after vaccinations in children, Japan, 2010–2013. Emerg Infect Dis 2015;21:1956. [PMID: 26485679]
Transmissible spongiform encephalopathy (TSE) TSE is a progressive, fatal, incurable, neurodegenerative prion disease occurring in both animals and humans. TSEs include bovine spongiform encephalopathy (BSE) in cattle; scrapie in sheep; chronic wasting disease in deer and elk; kuru in humans; Creutzfeldt-Jakob disease (CJD) in humans; and certain genetically determined or familial disorders (eg, fatal familial insomnia and Gerstmann–Straussler–Scheinker syndrome). There is the potential for bovine spongiform encephalopathy (BSE) transmission to humans from eating infected meat or meat products. Another public health issue involves the potential transmission through blood transfusions or via corneal, dura mater, and other transplants.	Tissue from brain, spinal cord, eyes, tonsils, lymphoid tissue, spleen, pancreas, and nerves for immunohistochemical (IHC) analysis; and for conformation-dependent immunoassay (CDI), which is faster and uses specific antibodies that bind to all disease-causing prions in the brain. Use great caution when handling tissue from brain or spinal cord of a potential TSE patient.	Clinical symptoms and signs: rapidly progressive dementia, myoclonic fasciculations, ataxia, tremor, psychiatric symptoms. Diack AB et al. Variant CJD. 18 years of research and surveillance. Prion 2014;8:286. [PMID: 25495404] Huang WJ et al. Prions mediated neurodegenerative disorders. Eur Rev Med Pharmacol Sci 2015;19:4028. [PMID: 26592824] Manix M et al. Creutzfeldt-Jakob disease: updated diagnostic criteria, treatment algorithm, and the utility of brain biopsy. Neurosurg Focus 2015;39:E2. [PMID: 26646926]

West Nile virus (WNV) Although it first appeared in the U.S. in 1999, within 5 years WNV had established itself as endemic in the US. Responsible agent is a single-strand RNA virus of the family Flavivirus. Its enzootic cycle involves several species of mosquitoes and birds before infecting humans; however, it is transmitted to humans from the bite of *Culex* species of mosquitoes. Incubation period of 2–14 days.	Serum, CSF, or tissue collected within 8 days of illness for IgM antibody ELISA; test performed by State Public Health Laboratories or reference laboratories. PCR molecular tests are available in Public Health Laboratories and reference laboratories.	Clinical symptoms and signs: 80% of those infected are asymptomatic, 20% have mild flulike symptoms: fever, headache, myalgias, skin rash, and lymphadenopathy. In immunocompetent patients, illness is self-limited, lasting 3–6 days. Central nervous system infection (encephalitis or meningitis or flaccid paralysis) develops in 1%, with change in mental status, movement disorders, and focal neurologic deficits (more common with increased age). Gastrointestinal symptoms also occur. McVey DS et al. West Nile virus. Rev Sci Tech 2015;34:431. [PMID: 26601446] Montgomery RR et al. Risk factors for West Nile virus infection and disease in populations and individuals. Expert Rev Anti Infect Ther 2015;13:317. [PMID: 25637260] Tyler KL. Current developments in understanding of West Nile virus central nervous system disease. Curr Opin Neurol 2014;27:342. [PMID: 24722324]
Vancomycin-resistant *Enterococcus* (VRE) Emergence of VRE seen in both *E. faecalis* and *E. faecium* (most common) and at least 7 phenotypes (van A through van G). VRE, especially *E. faecium*, usually demonstrates intrinsic resistance to cephalosporins, aminoglycosides, and β-lactam antibiotics. Enterococci that acquire the van A gene are highly resistant to vancomycin and to teicoplanin. The location of this gene on a plasmid means that it can be spread between strains, and therefore identification of VRE may require contact isolation in the hospital by infection control. Enterococci can also pass the van A gene cluster to *S. aureus* resulting in vancomycin-resistant *S. aureus*.	Cultures of stool, blood, wound, abscesses, CSF.	De Angelis G et al. Infection control and prevention measures to reduce the spread of vancomycin-resistant enterococci in hospitalized patients: a systemic review and meta-analysis. J Antimicrob Chemother 2014;69:1185. [PMID: 24458513] Toner L et al. Vancomycin resistant enterococci in urine cultures: antibiotic susceptibility trends over a decade at a tertiary hospital in the United Kingdom. Investig Clin Urol 2016;57:129. [PMID: 26981595]

(Continued)

Organism	Specimen/Diagnostic Tests	Comments
Zika virus A flavivirus transmitted by *Aedes* mosquitoes. Zika virus was first identified in 1947 in the Zika Forest of Uganda. Virus spread slowly from Africa to Southeast Asia, then to French Polynesia with large outbreaks. Since 2015, there has been an explosive outbreak of cases of microcephaly and other congenital abnormalities seen in infants of women pregnant when infected. Zika virus and cases of Guillain-Barre syndrome following Zika virus infection throughout South America, Central America, and the Caribbean.	Reverse transcriptase-polymerase chain reaction (RT-PCR) is used to detect viral RNA during period of viremia. RT-PCR test is indicated for serum and urine samples collected from symptomatic patients within 2 weeks post onset of symptoms or from asymptomatic pregnant women presenting within 2 weeks of exposure, if epidemiological criteria are met. If PCR test is negative, serum should be tested for anti-Zika IgM. Serological testing for anti-Zika IgM is indicated for serum samples collected from patients presenting 2-12 weeks post onset of symptoms or from asymptomatic pregnant women first presenting 2-12 weeks following exposure, if epidemiological criteria are met. If anti-Zika IgM is positive or equivocal, then either perform serum plaque reduction neutralization test (PRNT) to confirm IgM result (for non-pregnant symptomatic patients) or perform RT-PCR test on serum and urine (for pregnant women, symptomatic or asymptomatic). For the latter, if RT-PCR test is negative, PRNT should be performed to confirm IgM result. Occasionally, cerebrospinal fluid (CSF) or amniotic fluid can also be used for RT-PCR test if clinically indicated, but timing is critical.	Most infections are mild or even asymptomatic. Main concern is potential association of Zika virus infection in pregnant women and microcephaly and other neurologic abnormalities (eg, hearing loss, blindness) in their newborns. Two studies have detected Zika virus in fetal brain and tissues of infants with microcephaly, strengthening the association. Cases of Guillain-Barre syndrome have also been associated with Zika infection. Male-to-female and female-to-male sexual transmission has been documented even among asymptomatic individuals. Current outbreak of Zika virus infection was first recognized in Northeastern Brazil in early 2015. By September, 2015, there was a sharp increase in number of reported cases of microcephaly in infants. By January 2016, a total of 3,530 suspected microcephaly cases had been reported in Brazil, many of which occurred in infants born to women who lived in or visited areas where Zika virus transmission has been occurring. Rash and fever during 1st trimester is associated with increased risk of microcephaly. In the United States, as of September 2016, more than 2300 confirmed and probable cases has been reported to CDC and State Public Health Laboratories. In February 2016, the WHO declared the current Zika outbreak a Public Health Emergency and guidelines for travel restrictions and avoidance of mosquitoes were issued. CDC. Zika Virus for Health Care Providers. https://www.cdc.gov/zika/hc-providers/index.html Petersen EE et al. Update: Interim guidance for preconception counseling and prevention of sexual transmission of Zika virus for persons with possible Zika virus exposure—United States, September 2016. MMWR 2016 Oct 7;65:1077. [PMID: 27711033] Rubin EJ et al. Zika virus and microcephaly. N Engl J Med 2016;374:984. [PMID: 26862812]

[1]Nearly 70% of emerging infectious disease outbreaks during the last 10 years have been zoonotic diseases transmitted from animals to humans. Controlling the diseases caused by new/re-emerging infectious agents is difficult owing to the diversity of geographic sources, the potential for rapid global dissemination from the source, and ecologic and social/economic influences.

6

Diagnostic Imaging: Test Selection & Interpretation

Zhen Jane Wang, MD, and Benjamin M. Yeh, MD

HOW TO USE THIS SECTION

Information in this chapter is arranged anatomically from superior to inferior. It would not be feasible to include all available imaging tests in one chapter in a book of this size, but we have attempted to summarize the essential features of those examinations that are most frequently ordered in modern clinical practice or those that may be associated with difficulty or risk. Indications, advantages and disadvantages, contraindications, and patient preparation are presented. Costs of the studies are approximate and represent averages reported from several large medical centers.

$$\$ = <\$250$$
$$\$\$ = \$250–\$750$$
$$\$\$\$ = \$750–\$1000$$
$$\$\$\$\$ = >\$1000$$

RISKS OF IODINATED CT INTRAVENOUS CONTRAST AGENTS

Although iodinated CT intravenous contrast is an important tool in radiology, it is not without risks. Minor reactions (nausea, vomiting, hives) occur with an overall incidence between 1% and 12%. Major reactions (laryngeal edema, bronchospasm, cardiac arrest) occur in 0.16–1 cases per 1000 patients. Deaths have been reported in 1:40,000 to 1:170,000 cases. Patients with an allergic history (asthma, hay fever, allergy to foods or drugs) have a slightly increased risk. A history of allergic-type reaction to contrast material is associated with an increased risk of a subsequent severe reaction. Prophylactic measures that may be required in such cases include corticosteroids and H_1 and H_2 blockers.

In addition, there is a risk of iodinated contrast-induced nephropathy, which is usually mild and reversible. Recent data suggests the risk of contrast-induced nephropathy is lower than previously estimated. Persons at increased risk for potentially irreversible renal damage include patients with preexisting renal disease (particularly diabetics with renal dysfunction), multiple myeloma, and severe hyperuricemia. Iodinated CT contrast materials are generally contraindicated in patients with severe renal insufficiency (ie, estimated glomerular filtration rate < 30 mL/min/1.73 m^2). In patients with mild to moderate renal insufficiency (ie, estimated glomerular filtration rate between 30 and 60 mL/min/1.73 m^2), minimizing the dose of contrast and increasing hydration are suggested.

RISKS OF GADOLINIUM-BASED MRI INTRAVENOUS CONTRAST AGENTS

Contrast agents used in MRI are different from those used in most other radiology studies. Most MRI contrast agents are gadolinium-based and are teratogenic and thus contraindicated in pregnancy. Rarely, patients with severe renal dysfunction, particularly if on dialysis, or those with acute renal failure may develop irreversible nephrogenic systemic fibrosis after receiving gadolinium-based intravenous contrast. Gadolinium-based contrast is contraindicated in these patients. In patients with mild to moderate renal insufficiency, the dose of gadolinium-based contrast material should be minimized. Immediate contrast reactions are rare (minor reactions in approximately 0.07% and major reactions in 0.001%). Contrast-induced renal failure is generally not associated with MRI intravenous contrast.

In summary, intravenous contrast agents should be viewed in the same manner as other medications—that is, risks and benefits must be balanced before any examination using these pharmaceuticals is ordered.

	HEAD	BRAIN
	CT	CTA

Test	Indications	Advantages	Disadvantages/Contraindications	Preparation
HEAD **Computed tomography** (CT) $$$	Evaluation of acute craniofacial trauma, acute neurologic dysfunction (<72 hours) from suspected intracranial or subarachnoid hemorrhage. Further characterization of intracranial masses identified by MRI (presence or absence of calcium or involvement of the bony calvarium). Evaluation of sinus disease and temporal bone disease.	Rapid acquisition makes it the modality of choice for trauma. Superb spatial resolution. Superior to MRI in detection of hemorrhage within the first 24–48 hours.	Artifacts from bone may interfere with detection of disease at the skull base and in the posterior fossa. Generally limited to transaxial views. Direct coronal images of paranasal sinuses and temporal bones are routinely obtained if patient can lie prone. **Contraindications and risks:** Caution in pregnancy because of the potential harm of ionizing radiation to the fetus. Also see Risks of Iodinated CT Intravenous Contrast Agents, p. 289.	Normal hydration. Sedation of agitated patients. Recent estimated glomerular filtration rate determination if intravenous contrast is to be used.
BRAIN **CT angiography** (CTA) $$$	Evaluation of cerebral arteriovenous malformations, intracranial aneurysm, and in cases of suspected stroke, evaluation of intracranial vessels for dissections or occlusions.	Rapid acquisition makes it an excellent choice for evaluation of blood vessels in stroke. Can cover a large territory, including down to the heart. Superb spatial resolution.	Artifacts from bone may interfere with detection of disease at the skull base and in the posterior fossa. **Contraindications and risks:** Caution in pregnancy because of the potential harm of ionizing radiation to the fetus. Also see Risks of Iodinated CT Intravenous Contrast Agents, p. 289.	Normal hydration. Sedation of agitated patients. Recent estimated glomerular filtration rate determination prior to intravenous contrast administration.

(Continued)

Test	Indications	Advantages	Disadvantages/Contraindications	Preparation
BRAIN				
MRI				
HEAD **Magnetic resonance imaging** (MRI) $$$$	Evaluation of essentially all intracranial disease, except in the setting of acute trauma or suspected acute bleed where CT is preferred.	Provides excellent tissue contrast resolution, multiplanar capability. Can detect flowing blood and cryptic vascular malformations. Can detect demyelinating and dysmyelinating disease. No ionizing radiation.	Subject to motion artifacts. Inferior to CT in the setting of acute trauma because it is insensitive to acute hemorrhage, incompatible with traction devices, inferior in detection of bony injury and foreign bodies, and requires longer image acquisition time. **Contraindications:** Patients with cardiac pacemakers, intraocular metallic foreign bodies, intracranial aneurysm clips, cochlear implants, and some artificial heart valves.	Sedation of agitated patients. Screening CT or plain radiograph images of orbits if history suggests possible metallic foreign body in the eye.
MRA/MRV				
BRAIN **Magnetic resonance angiography/venography** (MRA/MRV) $$$$	Evaluation of cerebral arteriovenous malformations, intracranial aneurysm, and blood supply of vascular tumors as aid to operative planning. Evaluation of intracranial vascular stenosis/occlusion/dissection in patients with symptoms of cerebral vascular disease or transient ischemic attack. Evaluation of dural sinus thrombosis (MRV).	No ionizing radiation. No iodinated contrast needed.	Subject to motion artifacts. Special instrumentation required for patients on life support. **Contraindications:** Patients with cardiac pacemakers, intraocular metallic foreign bodies, intracranial aneurysm clips, cochlear implants, and some artificial heart valves.	Sedation of agitated patients. Screening CT or plain radiograph images of orbits if history suggests possible metallic foreign body in the eye.

(*Continued*)

BRAIN			
	Brain scan	**Brain PET/SPECT**	**Cisternography**
BRAIN **Brain scan** (radionuclide) $$	Confirmation of brain death.	Confirmation of brain death not impeded by hypothermia or barbiturate coma. Can be portable.	Limited resolution. Delayed imaging required with some agents. Cannot be used alone to establish diagnosis of brain death. Must be used in combination with clinical examination or cerebral angiography to establish diagnosis. **Contraindications and risks:** Caution in pregnancy because of the potential harm of ionizing radiation to the fetus.
			Premedication with potassium perchlorate when using TcO_4 to block choroid plexus uptake.
BRAIN **Positron emission tomography (PET)/ Single Photon Emission Computed Tomography (SPECT) brain scan with** [18F]**fluorodeoxyglucose (FDG)** $$$	Evaluation of suspected dementia. Evaluation of medically refractory seizures.	Provides functional information. Can localize seizure focus prior to surgical excision. Can improve the early diagnosis of Alzheimer disease and the differential diagnosis of dementia. Provides cross-sectional images and therefore improved lesion localization compared with planar imaging techniques.	PET has limited resolution compared with MRI and CT. Combined PET/CT or PET/MRI examination can improve anatomic resolution. Limited application in work-up of dementia due to low specificity of images and fact that test results do not alter clinical management. **Contraindications and risks:** Caution in pregnancy because of potential harm of ionizing radiation to the fetus.
			NPO for 6 hours. Sedation of agitated patients. Diabetic patients may need to adjust their insulin or other diabetic medication doses to ensure proper fasting glucose level at the time of the examination.
BRAIN **Myelography and cisternography** $$$$	Evaluation of cerebrospinal fluid leak, symptoms of spontaneous intracranial hypotension, surgical planning especially in regard to the nerve roots.	Provides anatomic and functional information. Can detect CSF leaks.	**Contraindications:** Patients with increased intracranial pressure, coagulopathy, and history of adverse reaction to iodinated contrast media and /or gadolinium-based MRI contrast material. Caution in pregnancy because of the potential harm of ionizing radiation to the fetus.
			Check coagulation tests prior to procedure. Must follow strict sterile precautions for intrathecal injection.

	NECK		
	MRI	**MRA**	**CT**
Test	**Indications**	**Advantages**	**Disadvantages/Contraindications**	**Preparation**

Test	Indications	Advantages	Disadvantages/Contraindications	Preparation
NECK **Magnetic resonance imaging** (MRI) $$$$	Evaluation of upper aerodigestive tract. Staging of neck masses. Differentiation of lymphadenopathy from blood vessels. Evaluation of head and neck malignancy, thyroid nodules, parathyroid adenoma, lymphadenopathy, retropharyngeal abscess, brachial plexopathy.	Provides excellent tissue contrast resolution. Tissue differentiation of malignancy or abscess from benign tumor often possible. Sagittal and coronal planar imaging possible. Multiplanar capability especially advantageous for brachial plexus. No iodinated contrast needed to distinguish lymphadenopathy from blood vessels.	Subject to motion artifacts, particularly those of carotid pulsation and swallowing. Special instrumentation required for patients on life support. **Contraindications:** Patients with cardiac pacemakers, intraocular metallic foreign bodies, intracranial aneurysm clips, cochlear implants, and some artificial heart valves.	Sedation of agitated patients. Screening CT or plain radiograph images of orbits if history suggests possible metallic foreign body in the eye.
NECK **Magnetic resonance angiography** (MRA) $$$$	Evaluation of carotid bifurcation atherosclerosis, cervicocranial arterial dissection.	No ionizing radiation. No iodinated contrast needed. MRA of the carotid arteries can be a sufficient preoperative evaluation regarding critical stenosis when local expertise exists.	Subject to motion artifacts, particularly from carotid pulsation and swallowing. Special instrumentation required for patients on life support. **Contraindications:** Patients with cardiac pacemakers, intraocular metallic foreign bodies, intracranial aneurysm clips, cochlear implants, and some artificial heart valves.	Sedation of agitated patients. Screening CT or plain radiograph images of orbits if history suggests possible metallic foreign body in the eye.
NECK **Computed tomography** (CT) $$$	Evaluation of the upper aerodigestive tract. Staging of neck masses for patients who are not candidates for MRI. Evaluation of suspected abscess.	Rapid. Superb spatial resolution. Can guide percutaneous fine-needle aspiration of possible tumor or abscess.	Inferior soft tissue contrast compared to MRI. **Contraindications and risks:** Caution in pregnancy because of the potential harm of ionizing radiation to the fetus. See Risks of Iodinated CT Intravenous Contrast Agents, p. 289.	Normal hydration. Sedation of agitated patients. Recent estimated glomerular filtration rate determination.

(Continued)

	NECK	THYROID	
	Ultrasound	Ultrasound	Thyroid uptake and scan
NECK **Ultrasound** (US) $$	Patency and morphology of arteries and veins. Evaluation of thyroid and parathyroid. Guidance for percutaneous fine-needle aspiration biopsy of neck lesions.	Can detect and monitor atherosclerotic stenosis of carotid arteries noninvasively and without iodinated contrast. Can guide percutaneous fine-needle aspiration.	Operator-dependent. **Contraindications and risks:** None.	None.
THYROID **Ultrasound** (US) $$	Evaluation of thyroid nodules. Assessment of response to suppressive therapy. Screening patients with a history of radiation to the head and neck. Guidance for biopsy.	Noninvasive. No ionizing radiation. Can be portable. Can image in all planes. Can guide percutaneous fine-needle aspiration.	Operator-dependent. **Contraindications and risks:** None.	None.
THYROID **Thyroid uptake and scan** (radionuclide) $$	Evaluation of clinical hypothyroidism, hyperthyroidism, thyroiditis, effects of thyroid-stimulating and thyroid-suppressing medications, and for calculation of therapeutic radiation dosage. Evaluation of palpable nodules, mediastinal mass. Total body scanning used for postoperative evaluation of thyroid cancer metastases.	Demonstrates both morphology and function. Can identify ectopic thyroid tissue and "cold" nodules that have a greater risk of malignancy. Imaging of whole body with one dose (^{131}I).	Substances interfering with test include iodides in vitamins and medicines, antithyroid drugs, corticosteroids, and intravascular contrast agents. Delayed imaging is required with iodides (^{123}I, 6 hours and 24 hours; ^{131}I total body, 72 hours). Test may not visualize thyroid gland in subacute thyroiditis. **Contraindications and risks:** Not advised in pregnancy because of the risk of ionizing radiation to the fetus (iodides cross placenta and concentrate in fetal thyroid). Significant radiation exposure occurs in total body scanning with ^{131}I; patients should be instructed about precautionary measures by nuclear medicine personnel.	Administration of dose after a 4- to 6-hour fast aids absorption. Discontinuation of all interfering substances prior to test, especially thyroid-suppressing medications: T_3 (1 week), T_4 (4–6 weeks), propylthiouracil (2 weeks).

| | THYROID | | | PARATHYROID |
| | Radionuclide therapy | | | Radionuclide scan |
Test	**Indications**	**Advantages**	**Disadvantages/Contraindications**	**Preparation**
THYROID **Thyroid therapy** (radionuclide) $$$	Hyperthyroidism and some thyroid carcinomas (papillary and follicular types are amenable to treatment, whereas medullary and anaplastic types are not).	Noninvasive alternative to surgery.	Rarely, radiation thyroiditis may occur 1–3 days after therapy. Hypothyroidism occurs commonly as a long-term complication. Higher doses that are required to treat thyroid carcinoma may result in pulmonary fibrosis. **Contraindications and risks:** Contraindicated in pregnancy and lactation. Contraindicated in patients with metastatic thyroid cancer to the brain, because treatment may result in brain edema and subsequent herniation, and in those < 20 years of age with hyperthyroidism because of possible increased risk of thyroid cancer later in life. After treatment, a patient's activities are restricted to limit total exposure of any member of the general public until radiation level is ≤ 0.5 rem.	After treatment, patients must isolate all bodily secretions from household members. High doses for treatment of thyroid carcinoma may necessitate hospitalization.
PARATHYROID **Parathyroid scan** (radionuclide) $$	Evaluation of suspected parathyroid adenoma.	Identifies hyperfunctioning tissue, which is useful when planning surgery.	Small adenomas (< 500 mg) may not be detected. **Contraindications and risks:** Caution in pregnancy is advised because of the risk of ionizing radiation to the fetus.	Requires strict patient immobility during scanning.

(Continued)

CHEST				
			Chest radiograph	**CT**
CHEST **Chest radiograph** $	Evaluation of pleural and parenchymal pulmonary disease, mediastinal disease, cardiogenic and noncardiogenic pulmonary edema, congenital and acquired cardiac disease. Screening for traumatic aortic rupture (though CT is playing an increasing role). Evaluation of possible pneumothorax (expiratory upright film) or pleural effusion.	Inexpensive. Widely available.	Difficult to distinguish between causes of hilar and mediastinal enlargement (ie, vasculature versus adenopathy). Not sensitive for small pulmonary nodules. **Contraindications and risks:** Caution in pregnancy because of the potential harm of ionizing radiation to the fetus.	None.
CHEST **Computed tomography** (CT) $$$	Evaluation of thoracic trauma. Evaluation of mediastinal and hilar tumor. Evaluation and staging of primary and metastatic lung neoplasm. Characterization of pulmonary nodules. Differentiation of parenchymal versus pleural process (ie, lung abscess versus empyema). Evaluation of interstitial lung disease (1-mm thin sections), aortic dissection, and aneurysm. Screening for lung cancer in high-risk populations (can use low radiation dose techniques).	Rapid. Superb spatial resolution. Can guide percutaneous fine-needle aspiration of possible tumor or abscess.	Patient cooperation required for appropriate breath-holding. **Contraindications and risks:** Caution in pregnancy because of the potential harm of ionizing radiation to the fetus. See Risks of Iodinated CT Intravenous Contrast Agents, p. 289.	Normal hydration. Sedation of agitated patients. Recent estimated glomerular filtration rate determination if intravenous contrast is administered. Intravenous contrast is not necessary for lung parenchyma evaluation.

	CHEST	
	MRI	**PET/CT**

Test	Indications	Advantages	Disadvantages/Contraindications	Preparation
CHEST **Magnetic resonance imaging** (MRI) $$$$	Evaluation of mediastinal masses. Discrimination between hilar vessels and enlarged lymph nodes. Tumor staging (especially when invasion of vessels or pericardium is suspected). Evaluation of aortic dissection, aortic aneurysm, congenital and acquired cardiac disease.	Provides excellent tissue contrast resolution and multiplanar capability. No ionizing radiation.	Subject to motion artifacts. **Contraindications and risks:** Contraindicated in patients with cardiac pacemakers, intraocular metallic foreign bodies, intracranial aneurysm clips, cochlear implants, and some artificial heart valves.	Sedation of agitated patients. Screening CT of the orbits if history suggests possible metallic foreign body in the eye.
CHEST **Positron emission tomography/Computed tomography (PET/CT) with** ^{18}F**fluorodeoxyglucose (FDG)** $$$$	Evaluation for mediastinal masses and metastases. Discrimination between benign and malignant lymph nodes. Tumor staging and treatment monitoring.	Combines metabolic and anatomic information. Large area of coverage (can image whole body).	Patient cooperation required for appropriate breath-holding. **Contraindications and risks:** Contraindicated in pregnancy because of the potential harm of ionizing radiation to the fetus. See Risks of Iodinated CT Intravenous Contrast Agents, p. 289.	Normal hydration. Recent serum creatinine determination. NPO for 4–6 hours Diabetic patients may need to adjust their insulin or other diabetic medication doses to ensure proper fasting glucose level at the time of the examination.

LUNG			
Ventilation-perfusion scan	**CT**		

(Continued)

LUNG

Ventilation-perfusion scan (radionuclide)

= $$
= $$
= $$$ – $$$$

Indications	Comments	Contraindications	Preparation
Evaluation of pulmonary embolism or burn inhalation injury. However, evaluation of pulmonary embolism has largely been replaced by CT angiography of the chest. scans may be appropriate for evaluation of pulmonary embolism in patients with normal chest radiographs, and in young female patients to avoid the higher radiation dose from CT pulmonary angiography. Preoperative evaluation of patients with chronic obstructive pulmonary disease and of those who are candidates for pneumonectomy.	Noninvasive. Provides functional information in preoperative assessment. Permits determination of differential and regional lung function in preoperative assessment. Less radiation dose compared to CT angiography for the assessment of pulmonary embolism.	Patients must be able to cooperate for ventilation portion of the examination. There is a high proportion of intermediate probability studies in patients with underlying lung disease. The likelihood of pulmonary embolism ranges from 20–80% in these cases. A patient who has a low probability scan still has a chance ranging from 0–19% of having a pulmonary embolus. **Contraindications and risks:** Patients with severe pulmonary artery hypertension or significant right-to-left shunts should have fewer particles injected. Caution advised in pregnancy because of risk of ionizing radiation to the fetus.	Current chest radiograph is mandatory for interpretation.

LUNG

Computed tomography (CT) angiography

$$$

Indications	Comments	Contraindications	Preparation
Evaluation of clinically suspected pulmonary embolism.	Rapid. High sensitivity and specificity for clinically relevant pulmonary emboli. Allows determination of causes for dyspnea other than pulmonary embolism. Evaluation of pulmonary vein anatomy before electrophysiology ablation.	Respiratory motion artifacts can be a problem in dyspneic patients and older CT scanners. High-quality study requires breath-holding of approximately 10–20 seconds. **Contraindications and risks:** Caution in pregnancy because of potential harm of ionizing radiation to fetus. See Risks of Iodinated CT Intravenous Contrast Agents, p. 289.	Large-gauge intravenous access (minimum 20-gauge) required. Prebreathing oxygen may help dyspneic patients perform adequate breath hold. Normal hydration. Preferably NPO for 4 hours before study. Recent estimated glomerular filtration rate determination.

		BREAST			
		Mammogram			
Test	Indications	Advantages	Disadvantages/Contraindications	Preparation
BREAST **Mammogram and tomosynthesis** $	The US Preventive Services Task Force recommends screening asymptomatic women for breast cancer with mammograms: (1) based on individual preference in women ages 40–49; and (2) every 2 years between ages 50 and 74. In women ages 75 and older, it concluded that there is insufficient evidence to assess the benefits of screening mammograms. With a history of breast cancer, mammograms should be performed yearly at any age. Indicated at any age for symptoms (palpable mass, bloody discharge) or before breast surgery.	Newer digital and film screen techniques generate lower radiation doses (0.1–0.2 centigray (cGy) per film, mean glandular dose). Digital breast tomosynthesis is a new mammogram technique that provides multiple projection images and improves the detection and characterization of breast lesions when compared to conventional mammograms. A 23% lower mortality rate has been demonstrated in patients screened with combined mammogram and physical examination compared with physical examination alone. In a screening population, more than 40% of cancers are detected by mammography alone and cannot be palpated on physical examination.	Detection of breast masses is more difficult in patients with radiographically dense breasts. Breast compression may cause patient discomfort. In a screening population, 9% of cancers are detected by physical examination alone and are not detectable by mammography. **Contraindications and risks:** Radiation from repeated mammograms can theoretically cause breast cancer; however, the benefits of screening mammograms greatly outweigh the risks.	None.
BREAST **Ultrasound** $$	Evaluation of palpable masses. Evaluation of abnormalities detected on mammogram. Initial evaluation of palpable masses in women under age 30 who are not at high risk of breast cancer. Guidance for breast biopsy.	No ionizing radiation. Sonographic features and tissue stiffness assessment are helpful in characterizing breast masses.	Operator-dependent. **Contraindications and risks:** None.	None.

	BREAST	HEART
	Breast MRI	**Myocardial perfusion scan**
BREAST **MRI** $$$$	Screening for breast cancer in very high-risk women. Screening of the contralateral breast for occult cancer in patients with new diagnosis of breast cancer. Screening in patients with breast augmentation in whom mammography is difficult. Evaluation of the extent of the breast cancer. Evaluation of neoadjuvant therapy for breast cancer. May be used to guide breast biopsy of MRI-detected abnormalities.	Improved cancer detection, compared with mammograms, particularly for women with radiographically dense breasts. Better assessment of the extent of the cancer compared to mammography. No ionizing radiation.
		Higher rate of false positives than mammography. Utilizes intravenous contrast material. **Contraindications:** Patients with cardiac pacemakers, intraocular metallic foreign bodies, intracranial aneurysm clips, cochlear implants, and some artificial heart valves.
		Screening CT of the orbits if history suggests possible metallic foreign body in the eye. Increased breast parenchymal enhancement occurs normally during the secretory phase of the menstrual cycle, therefore MRI should be performed during the second week of the menstrual cycle for patients undergoing screening breast MRI.
HEART **Myocardial perfusion scan** (thallium scan, technetium-99m methoxyisobutyl isonitrile [sestamibi] scan, others) $–$$–$$$ (broad range)	Evaluation of atypical chest pain. Detection of presence, location, and extent of myocardial ischemia.	Highly sensitive for detecting physiologically significant coronary stenosis. Noninvasive. Able to stratify patients according to risk for myocardial infarction. Normal examination associated with average risk of cardiac death or nonfatal myocardial infarction of <1% per year.
		The patient must be carefully monitored during treadmill or pharmacologic stress—optimally, under the supervision of a cardiologist. False-positive results may be caused by exercise-induced spasm, aortic stenosis, or left bundle branch block; false-negative results may be caused by inadequate exercise, mild or distal disease, or balanced diffuse ischemia. **Contraindications and risks:** Aminophylline (inhibitor of dipyridamole) is a contraindication to the use of dipyridamole. Treadmill or pharmacologic stress carries a risk of arrhythmia, ischemia, infarct, and, rarely, death. Caution in pregnancy because of the risk of ionizing radiation to the fetus.
		In case of severe peripheral vascular disease, severe pulmonary disease, or musculoskeletal disorder, pharmacologic stress with dipyridamole or other agents may be used. Tests should be performed in the fasting state. Patient should not exercise between stress and redistribution scans.

HEART

Test	Indications	Advantages	Disadvantages/Contraindications	Preparation
HEART **Computed tomography coronary artery calcium scoring/angiography** $$–$$$	Screening evaluation for coronary artery calcification. Evaluation for coronary artery stenoses and congenital anomalies.	Noninvasive. Higher coronary artery calcium score correlates with increased risk for significant coronary artery stenosis.	Gated data acquisition may be difficult in patients with severe arrhythmias or rapid heart rate. If high calcium score or coronary artery stenosis is found, patient may need additional treatment (to reduce risk of myocardial infarction). **Contraindications and risks:** Caution in pregnancy because of potential harm of ionizing radiation to fetus. See Risks of Iodinated CT Intravenous Contrast Agents, p. 289.	May require medication with β-blocker to decrease heart rate.
HEART **Radionuclide ventriculography** (multigated acquisition [MUGA]) $$–$$$–$$$$	Evaluation of patients with ischemic heart disease and other cardiomyopathies. Evaluation of response to pharmacologic therapy and effects of cardiotoxic drugs.	Noninvasive. Ejection fraction is a reproducible index that can be used to follow course of disease and response to therapy.	Gated data acquisition may be difficult in patients with severe arrhythmias. **Contraindications and risks:** Recent infarct is a contraindication to exercise ventriculography (arrhythmia, ischemia, infarct, and, rarely, death may occur with exercise). Caution is advised in pregnancy because of the risk of ionizing radiation to the fetus.	Requires harvesting, labeling, and reinjecting the patient's red blood cells. Sterile technique required in handling of red cells.

(Continued)

	HEART	ABDOMEN	
	Cardiac MRI	KUB	Ultrasound
HEART **Cardiac MRI** $$$$	Evaluation of dynamic cardiac anatomy and ventricular function. Assessment of cardiomyopathies, myocardial fibrosis, and infarction. Assessment of chronic myocardial ischemia and viability through the use of pharmacologic agents. Characterization of cardiac masses, pericardial diseases, and valvular disease. Evaluation of congenital heart disease.	Provides both excellent anatomic and functional information in various heart diseases. No ionizing radiation.	**Contraindications:** Patients with cardiac pacemakers, intraocular metallic foreign bodies, intracranial aneurysm clips, cochlear implants, and some artificial heart valves. Patients must be carefully monitored when pharmacological stress is performed.	Sedation of agitated patients. Screening CT of the orbits if history suggests possible metallic foreign body in the eye.
ABDOMEN **Abdominal plain radiograph** (KUB [kidneys, ureters, bladder] x-ray) $	Assessment of bowel gas patterns (eg, to assess bowel obstruction). To assess pneumoperitoneum, order an upright abdomen and chest radiograph (abdominal series).	Inexpensive. Widely available.	Supine film alone is inadequate to evaluate pneumoperitoneum (see Indications). Obstipation may obscure lesions. **Contraindications and risks:** Caution in pregnancy because of the risk of ionizing radiation to the fetus.	None.
ABDOMEN **Ultrasound** (US) $$	Differentiation of cystic versus solid lesions of the liver and kidneys. Detection of intra- and extrahepatic biliary ductal dilation, cholelithiasis, gallbladder wall thickness, pericholecystic fluid, peripancreatic fluid and pseudocyst, hydronephrosis, abdominal aortic aneurysm, appendicitis (in pediatric or young patients), ascites, primary and metastatic liver carcinoma.	Noninvasive. No ionizing radiation. Can be portable. Imaging in all planes. Can guide percutaneous fine-needle aspiration of tumor or abscess.	Technique very operator-dependent. Organs (particularly pancreas and distal aorta) may be obscured by bowel gas. **Contraindications and risks:** None.	NPO for 6 hours.

			ABDOMEN	
			CT	
Test	Indications	Advantages	Disadvantages/Contraindications	Preparation
ABDOMEN **Computed tomography** (CT) $$$–$$$$	Morphologic evaluation of all abdominal and pelvic organs. Evaluation of abscess, trauma, mesenteric and retroperitoneal lymphadenopathy, bowel obstruction, obstructive biliary disease, pancreatitis, appendicitis, peritonitis, visceral infarction, and retroperitoneal hemorrhage. Characterization of masses in the abdomen. Staging and monitoring of malignancy in the liver, pancreas, kidneys, and other abdominopelvic organs and spaces. Determination of tumor resectability. Excellent screening tool for evaluation of suspected renal and ureteral stones or other cause of upper urinary tract bleeding. CT angiography evaluates the aorta and its branches. Can provide preoperative assessment of abdominal aortic aneurysm and dissection size, proximal and distal extent, relationship to renal arteries, and presence of anatomic anomalies. CT colonography useful in patients with failed colonoscopy or those unable to undergo colonoscopy.	Rapid. Complete coverage of abdomen and pelvis. Superb spatial resolution. Not limited by overlying bowel gas, as with ultrasound. Can guide fine-needle aspiration and percutaneous drainage. Noncontrast is the standard of reference for determining the extent and locations of urinary tract stone disease.	Dense barium, surgical clips, and metallic prostheses can cause artifacts and degrade image quality. **Contraindications and risks:** Generally contraindicated in pregnancy because of the potential harm of ionizing radiation to the fetus. See Risks of Iodinated CT Intravenous Contrast Studies, p. 289.	Preferably NPO for 4–6 hours. Normal hydration. Distention of gastrointestinal tract with water or positive oral contrast material. Sedation of agitated patients. Recent estimated glomerular filtration rate determination if intravenous contrast material is to be given.

ABDOMEN		
	MRI	**PET/CT**

| ABDOMEN
Magnetic resonance imaging (MRI)
$$$$ | Assessment and preoperative staging of intra-abdominal cancers. Differentiation of benign from malignant masses in the liver, pancreas, adrenals, kidney, spleen. Complementary to CT for liver lesion evaluation (especially metastatic disease and possible tumor invasion of hepatic or portal veins). | Provides excellent tissue contrast resolution which improves lesion characterization, multiplanar capability. No ionizing radiation. | Patient cooperation required for appropriate breath-holding. Subject to motion and other artifacts, degrading image quality. Much longer imaging time compared to CT of the abdomen. Special instrumentation required for patients on life support. **Contraindications:** Patients with cardiac pacemakers, intraocular metallic foreign bodies, intracranial aneurysm clips, cochlear implants, and some artificial heart valves. | Preferably NPO for 4 hours. Sedation of agitated patients. Screening CT or plain radiograph images of orbits if history suggests possible metallic foreign body in the eye. |
| ABDOMEN/PELVIS
Positron emission tomography/computed tomography (PET/CT) with ^{18}F-fluorodeoxyglucose (FDG)
$$$$ | Evaluation for abdominopelvic malignancy and metastases. Discrimination between benign and malignant masses in the abdomen and pelvis. Tumor staging and treatment monitoring. | Combines metabolic and anatomic information. Large area of coverage (can image whole body). | **Contraindications and risks:** Contraindicated in pregnancy because of the potential harm of ionizing radiation to the fetus. See Risks of Iodinated CT Intravenous Contrast Agents, p. 289. | NPO for 4–6 hours before study. Normal hydration. Sedation of agitated patients. Recent estimated glomerular filtration rate determination. In diabetic patients, adjustment of insulin and other diabetic medications needed to ensure proper glucose level at the time of FDG injection. |

(Continued)

| | | ABDOMEN | GASTROINTESTINAL |
| | | Mesenteric angiography | UGI |

Test	Indications	Advantages	Disadvantages/Contraindications	Preparation
ABDOMEN **Mesenteric angiography** $$$$	Gastrointestinal hemorrhage that does not resolve with conservative therapy and cannot be treated endoscopically. Localization of gastrointestinal bleeding site. Evaluation of possible vasculitis, such as polyarteritis nodosa. Detection of islet cell tumors not identified by other studies. Abdominal trauma.	Therapeutic embolization of gastrointestinal vessels during hemorrhage is often possible.	Invasive. Patient may need to remain supine with leg extended for 6 hours after the procedure to protect the common femoral artery at the catheter entry site. **Contraindications and risks:** Allergy to iodinated contrast material may require corticosteroid and H_1 blocker or H_2 blocker premedication. Contraindicated in pregnancy because of the potential harm of ionizing radiation to the fetus. Contrast nephrotoxicity may occur, especially with preexisting impaired renal function due to diabetes mellitus or multiple myeloma; however, any creatinine elevation following the procedure is usually reversible (see Risks of Iodinated Contrast Agents, p. 289).	NPO for 4–6 hours. Good hydration to limit possible renal insult due to iodinated contrast material. Recent estimated glomerular filtration rate determination, assessment of clotting parameters, reversal of anticoagulation. Performed with conscious sedation. Requires cardiac, respiratory, blood pressure, and pulse oximetry monitoring.
GASTROINTESTINAL **Upper GI study** (UGI) $$	Double-contrast barium technique demonstrates esophageal, gastric, and duodenal mucosa for evaluation of inflammatory disease and other mucosal abnormalities. Single-contrast technique assesses bowel motility, peristalsis, possible outlet obstruction, gastroesophageal reflux and hiatal hernia, esophageal cancer, and varices. Water-soluble contrast (Gastrografin) is suitable for evaluation of anastomotic leak or gastrointestinal perforation.	Good evaluation of mucosa with double-contrast examination. No sedation required. Less expensive than endoscopy.	Aspiration of water-soluble contrast material may occur, resulting in severe pulmonary edema. Leakage of barium from a perforation may cause granulomatous inflammatory reaction. Administration of barium delays subsequent endoscopy and body CT examination. **Contraindications and risks:** Caution in pregnancy because of the potential harm of ionizing radiation to the fetus.	NPO for 8 hours.

GASTROINTESTINAL	
CT enterography	**Small bowel follow-through**

(Continued)

GASTROINTESTINAL **CT enterography** $$$	Diagnose and assess the extent of inflammatory bowel disease. Assess small bowel tumors.	Noninvasive. Complete visualization of the small bowel. Evaluates extraluminal disease, including extent of intra-abdominal abscesses and fistulas.	Requires drinking large amounts of oral contrast material (Volumen). **Contraindications and risks:** Caution in pregnancy because of the potential harm of ionizing radiation to the fetus. Caution in repeated examinations of young patients because of cumulative radiation dose.	NPO for 4–6 hours. Distention of gastrointestinal tract with 1–1.5L of neutral oral contrast material (barium sulfate, Volumen) 45 minutes before the examination. Intravenous or intramuscular injection of glucagon to reduce bowel peristalsis.
GASTROINTESTINAL **Small bowel follow-through** $$	Barium fluoroscopic study for location of site of intermittent partial small bowel obstruction. Evaluation of small bowel inflammatory diseases.	Less expensive than CT or MRI. May be combined with UGI.	Less accurate for the detection of small bowel pathology compared to CT or MRI. Very limited evaluation of extraluminal diseases. **Contraindications and risks:** Contraindicated in pregnant women because of the potential harm of ionizing radiation to the fetus.	NPO for 8 hours.

		GASTROINTESTINAL	
		MR enterography	**Barium enema**

Test	Indications	Advantages	Disadvantages/Contraindications	Preparation
GASTROINTESTINAL **MR enterography** $$$$	Diagnose and assess the extent of inflammatory bowel disease. Assess small bowel tumors.	Provides excellent soft tissue contrast resolution, multiplanar capability. Evaluates extraluminal disease, including extent of intraabdominal abscesses and fistulas. No ionizing radiation.	Patient cooperation required for appropriate breath-holding. Subject to motion and other artifacts, degrading image quality. Much longer imaging time compared to CT. Special instrumentation required for patients on life support. **Contraindications:** Patients with cardiac pacemakers, intraocular metallic foreign bodies, intracranial aneurysm clips, cochlear implants, and some artificial heart valves.	NPO for 4–6 hours. Distention of gastrointestinal tract with 1–1.5 L of neutral oral contrast material (barium sulfate, Volumen) 45 minutes before the examination. Intravenous or intramuscular injection of glucagon to reduce bowel peristalsis. Sedation of agitated patients.
GASTROINTESTINAL **Barium enema** (BE) $$	Double-contrast technique for evaluation of colonic mucosa for suspected inflammatory bowel disease or neoplasm. Single-contrast technique for investigation of possible fistulous tracts, anastomotic leak, bowel obstruction, and for examination of debilitated patients.	Less expensive than conventional (but more optimal) colonoscopy. No sedation required.	Retained fecal material limits evaluation of mucosa. Requires patient cooperation and patient mobility. Marked diverticulosis precludes evaluation for possible neoplasm in involved area. Evaluation of right colon occasionally incomplete or limited by reflux of barium across ileocecal valve and overlapping opacified small bowel. Use of barium delays subsequent colonoscopy and body CT. **Contraindications and risks:** Contraindicated in patients with toxic megacolon and immediately after full-thickness colonoscopic biopsy.	Colon cleansing with enemas, cathartic, and clear liquid diet (1 day in young patients, 2 days in older patients).

GASTROINTESTINAL		
CT colonography	**Hypaque enema**	**Esophageal reflux study**
GASTROINTESTINAL **CT colonography** $$	GASTROINTESTINAL **Hypaque enema** $$	GASTROINTESTINAL **Esophageal reflux scintigraphy study** (radionuclide) $$
Thin section CT for evaluation of possible colonic polyps and masses.	Water-soluble contrast for fluoroscopic evaluation of colonic anatomy, anastomotic leak, or other perforation. Differentiation of colonic versus small bowel obstruction. Therapy for obstipation.	Evaluation of heartburn, regurgitation, recurrent aspiration pneumonia.
Has ability to evaluate extracolonic intraabdominal disease (ie, abdominal aneurysm, renal cell carcinoma, kidney stones). No IV contrast is necessary. Better tolerated than colonoscopy. Low radiation dose technique.	Safer than barium agents in suspected cases of bowel leaks.	Noninvasive and well tolerated. More sensitive for reflux than fluoroscopy, endoscopy, and manometry; sensitivity similar to that of acid reflux test. Permits quantitation of reflux. Can identify aspiration into the lung.
Retained fecal material may limit study. Requires patient cooperation. If polyps or masses are found, patient will still need to undergo colonoscopy or sigmoidoscopy for tissue diagnosis. **Contraindications and risks:** Caution in pregnancy because of the potential harm of ionizing radiation to the fetus.	Demonstrates only colonic anatomy and not mucosal changes. **Contraindications and risks:** Contraindicated in patients with toxic megacolon. Hypertonic solution may lead to fluid imbalance in debilitated patients and children.	Incomplete emptying of esophagus may mimic reflux. Abdominal binder—used to increase pressure in the lower esophagus—may not be tolerated in patients who have undergone recent abdominal surgery. **Contraindications and risks:** Caution in pregnancy because of the potential harm of ionizing radiation to the fetus.
Requires colonic preparation that varies from institution to institution.	Colonic cleansing is desirable but not always necessary.	NPO for 4 hours. During test, patient must be able to consume 300 mL of liquid.

(Continued)

	GASTROINTESTINAL	
	Gastric emptying study	**GI bleeding scan**
Test	GASTROINTESTINAL **Gastric emptying scintigraphy study** (radionuclide) $$	GASTROINTESTINAL **GI bleeding scan** (labeled red cell scan, radionuclide) $$–$$$
Indications	Evaluation of dumping syndrome, vagotomy, gastric outlet obstruction due to inflammatory or neoplastic disease, effects of drugs, and other causes of gastroparesis (eg, diabetes mellitus).	Evaluation of upper or lower gastrointestinal blood loss. Distinguishing hemangioma of the liver from other mass lesions of the liver.
Advantages	Gives functional information not available by other means.	Noninvasive compared with angiography. Longer period of imaging possible, which aids in detection of intermittent bleeding. Labeled red cells and sulfur colloid can detect bleeding rates as low as 0.05–0.10 mL/min (angiography can detect a bleeding rate of about 0.5 mL/min). 90% sensitivity for blood loss > 500 mL/24 h.
Disadvantages/Contraindications	Reporting of meaningful data requires adherence to standard protocol and establishment of normal values. **Contraindications and risks:** Contraindicated in pregnancy because of the potential harm of ionizing radiation to the fetus.	Bleeding must be active during time of imaging. Presence of free TcO$_4$ (poor labeling efficiency) can lead to gastric, kidney, and bladder activity that can be misinterpreted as sites of bleeding. Uptake in hepatic hemangioma, varices, arteriovenous malformation, abdominal aortic aneurysm, and bowel wall inflammation can also lead to false-positive examination. **Contraindications and risks:** Contraindicated in pregnancy because of the potential harm of ionizing radiation to the fetus.
Preparation	NPO for 4 hours. During test, patient must be able to eat a 300 g meal consisting of both liquids and solids.	Sterile technique required during in vitro labeling of red cells.

(Continued)

BLOOD				
Leukocyte scan				
BLOOD **Leukocyte scan** (indium scan, labeled white blood cell [WBC] scan, technetium-99m hexamethylpropyleneamine oxime [Tc99m-HMPAO]-labeled WBC scan, radionuclide) $$-$$$	Evaluation of fever of unknown origin, suspected abscess, pyelonephritis, osteomyelitis, inflammatory bowel disease. Examination of choice for evaluation of suspected vascular graft infection.	Highly specific (98%) for infection (in contrast to gallium). Highly sensitive in detecting abdominal source of infection. In patients with fever of unknown origin, total body imaging is advantageous compared with CT scan or ultrasound. Preliminary imaging as early as 4 hours is possible with indium but less sensitive (30–50% of abscesses are detected at 24 hours).	24-hour delayed imaging may limit the utility of indium scan in critically ill patients. False-negative scans occur with antibiotic administration or in chronic infection. Perihepatic or splenic infection can be missed because of normal leukocyte accumulation in these organs; liver and spleen scan is necessary adjunct in this situation. False-positive scans occur with swallowed leukocytes, bleeding, indwelling tubes and catheters, surgical skin wound uptake, and bowel activity due to inflammatory processes. Pulmonary uptake is nonspecific and has low predictive value for infection. Patients must be able to hold still during relatively long acquisition times (5–10 minutes). Tc99m-HMPAO WBC may be suboptimal for detecting infection involving the genitourinary and gastrointestinal tracts because of normal distribution of the agent to these organs. **Contraindications and risks:** Contraindicated in pregnancy because of the hazard of ionizing radiation to the fetus. High radiation dose to spleen.	Leukocytes from the patient are harvested, labeled in vitro, and then reinjected; process requires 12 hours. Scanning takes place 24 hours after injection of indium-labeled WBC and 1–2 hours after injection of Tc99m-HMPAO WBC. Homologous donor leukocytes should be used in neutropenic patients.

Test	Indications	Advantages	Disadvantages/Contraindications	Preparation
GALLBLADDER				
GALLBLADDER **Ultrasound** (US) $	Evaluation of right upper quadrant pain and suspected gallbladder disease. Demonstrates cholelithiasis (95% sensitive), sonographic Murphy sign, gallbladder wall thickening, pericholecystic fluid, intra- and extrahepatic biliary dilation.	Noninvasive. No ionizing radiation. Can be portable. Imaging in all planes. Can guide fine-needle aspiration, percutaneous transhepatic cholangiography, and biliary drainage procedures.	Operator-dependent. Difficult in obese patients. Administration of excessive pain medication before examination limits accuracy of diagnosing acute cholecystitis. **Contraindications and risks:** None.	Preferably NPO for 6 hours to enhance visualization of gallbladder.
GALLBLADDER **Hepatic iminodiacetic acid scan** (HIDA) $$	Ultrasound is usually the first test performed for the evaluation of gallbladder diseases. However, in patients with suspected gallbladder disease but unremarkable ultrasound, HIDA scan can be obtained. **Indications for HIDA include:** Evaluation of suspected acute cholecystitis or common bile duct obstruction. Evaluation of bile leaks, biliary atresia, and biliary enteric bypass patency.	95% sensitive and 99% specific for diagnosis of acute cholecystitis. Hepatobiliary function assessed. Defines pathophysiology underlying acute cholecystitis. Can be performed in patients with elevated serum bilirubin. No intravenous contrast used.	Does not demonstrate the cause of obstruction (eg, tumor or gallstone). Not able to evaluate biliary excretion if hepatocellular function is severely impaired. Sensitivity may be lower in acalculous cholecystitis. False-positive results can occur with hyperalimentation, prolonged fasting, and acute pancreatitis. **Contraindications and risks:** Contraindicated in pregnancy because of the potential harm of ionizing radiation to the fetus.	NPO for at least 4 hours but preferably less than 24 hours. Premedication with cholecystokinin can prevent false-positive examination in patients who are receiving hyperalimentation or who have been fasting longer than 24 hours. Avoid administration of morphine prior to examination if possible.

(Continued)

PANCREAS/BILIARY TREE		
	ERCP	**MRCP**
PANCREAS/BILIARY TREE **Endoscopic retrograde cholangiopancrea-tography** (ERCP) $$$$	Demonstrates cause, location, and extent of extra hepatic biliary obstruction (eg, choledocholithiasis). Can diagnose chronic pancreatitis. Primary sclerosing cholangitis, AIDS-associated cholangitis, and cholangiocarcinomas. Allows placement of biliary stents to relieve biliary obstruction. Allows biopsy of the biliary tract in suspected cases of cholangiocarcinoma.	Less invasive than surgery. Offers therapeutic potential (sphincterotomy and extraction of common bile duct stone, balloon dilatation of strictures, placement of stents). Finds gallstones in up to 14% of patients with symptoms but negative ultrasound.	Requires endoscopy. May cause pancreatitis (1%), cholangitis (<1%), peritonitis, hemorrhage (if sphincterotomy performed). **Contraindications and risks:** Relatively contraindicated in patients with concurrent or recent (<6 weeks) acute pancreatitis or suspected pancreatic pseudocyst. Contraindicated in pregnancy because of the potential harm of ionizing radiation to the fetus.	NPO for 6 hours. Sedation required. Vital signs should be monitored by the nursing staff. Not possible in patient who has undergone Roux-en-Y hepaticojejunostomy.
PANCREAS/BILIARY TREE **Magnetic resonance cholangiopancrea-tography** (MRCP) $$$$	Evaluation of intra- and extrahepatic biliary and pancreatic duct dilatation, and the cause of obstruction. Evaluation of biliary anatomy and variants in potential liver donors.	Noninvasive. No ionizing radiation. Imaging in all planes. Can image ducts beyond the point of obstruction. Evaluates extraluminal disease.	Requires patient cooperation for breath-holding. Motion artifact may degrade image quality. Special instrumentation required for patients on life support. **Contraindications:** Patients with cardiac pacemakers, intraocular metallic foreign bodies, intracranial aneurysm clips, cochlear implants, and some artificial heart valves.	Preferably NPO for 6 hours.

Test	Indications	Advantages	Disadvantages/Contraindications	Preparation
LIVER **Ultrasound** (US) $	Differentiation of cystic versus solid liver lesions. Evaluation of intra- and extrahepatic biliary dilation, primary and metastatic liver tumors, and ascites. Evaluation of patency and flow velocity of portal vein, hepatic arteries, and hepatic veins.	Noninvasive. No radiation. Can be portable. Imaging in all planes. Can guide fine-needle aspiration, percutaneous transhepatic cholangiography, and biliary drainage procedures.	Operator-dependent. Less sensitive for liver lesion detection and characterization compared to CT or MRI. May miss solid liver lesions, including hepatocellular carcinoma. More difficult in obese patients. The presence of fatty liver or cirrhosis can limit the sensitivity of ultrasound for focal mass lesions. **Contraindications and risks:** None.	Preferably NPO for 6 hours.
LIVER **Computed tomography** (CT) $$$–$$$$	Suspected metastatic or primary liver tumor, gallbladder carcinoma, biliary obstruction, abscess.	Excellent spatial resolution. Allows characterization of most liver masses. Can direct percutaneous fine-needle aspiration biopsy. Excellent evaluation of hepatic vasculature.	Requires iodinated contrast material administered intravenously. **Contraindications and risks:** Contraindicated in pregnancy because of the potential harm of ionizing radiation to the fetus. See Risks of Iodinated CT Intravenous Contrast Agents, p. 289.	Preferably NPO for 4–6 hours. Recent estimated glomerular filtration rate determination. Specific hepatic protocol with arterial, portal venous, and delayed images used for evaluation of neoplasm.
LIVER **Magnetic resonance imaging** (MRI) $$$$	Characterization of hepatic lesions, including suspected cyst, hepatocellular carcinoma, focal nodular hyperplasia, and metastasis. Suspected metastatic or primary tumor. Differentiation of benign from malignant tumor. Evaluation of diffuse liver disease, including hemochromatosis, hemosiderosis, fatty liver, and suspected focal fatty infiltration.	Requires no iodinated contrast material. Provides excellent tissue contrast resolution, multiplanar capability. Excellent characterization of liver lesions compared to CT. Newer hepatobiliary contrast material (ie, gadoxetate disodium) may further improve focal lesion detection and characterization.	Subject to motion artifacts, particularly those of respiration. Special instrumentation required for patients on life support. **Contraindications:** Patients with cardiac pacemakers, intraocular metallic foreign bodies, intracranial aneurysm clips, cochlear implants, some artificial heart valves.	Screening CT or plain radiograph images of orbits if history suggests possible metallic foreign body in the eye.

LIVER

Ultrasound	CT	MRI

LIVER/BILIARY TREE			
PTC			
LIVER/BILIARY TREE **Percutaneous transhepatic cholangiogram** (PTC) $$$	Evaluation of biliary obstruction in patients in whom ERCP has failed or patients with Roux-en-Y hepaticojejunostomy for whom ERCP is not possible.	Can characterize the nature of diffuse intrahepatic biliary disease such as primary sclerosing cholangitis. Provides guidance and access for percutaneous transhepatic biliary drainage and possible stent placement to treat obstruction. Assesses site and morphology of biliary obstruction	Invasive; requires special training. Performed with conscious sedation. **Contraindications and risks:** Ascites may present a contraindication.	NPO for 4–6 hours. Sterile technique, assessment of clotting parameters, correction of coagulopathy. Performed with conscious sedation.

LIVER			
Hepatic angiography			
LIVER **Hepatic angiography** $$$$	Confirmation of and potential embolization for CT signs of hepatic vascular injury in hemodynamically stable patients. Evaluation of hepatic neoplasm prior to transcatheter embolotherapy of hepatic malignancy.	Provides guidance and access for embolization in cases of injury to the hepatic vasculature and in cases of hepatic malignancies.	Invasive. Patient must remain supine with leg extended for 6 hours following the procedure to protect the common femoral artery at the catheter entry site. **Contraindications and risks:** Allergy to iodinated contrast material may require corticosteroid and H_1 blocker or H_2 blocker premedication. Contraindicated in pregnancy because of the potential harm of ionizing radiation to the fetus. Contrast nephrotoxicity may occur, especially with preexisting impaired renal function due to diabetes mellitus or multiple myeloma; however, any creatinine elevation after the procedure is usually reversible.	NPO for 4–6 hours. Good hydration to limit possible renal insult due to iodinated contrast material. Recent estimated glomerular filtration rate determination, assessment of clotting parameters, reversal of anticoagulation. Performed with conscious sedation. Requires cardiac, respiratory, blood pressure, and pulse oximetry monitoring.

	LIVER/SPLEEN	PANCREAS
	Liver, spleen scan	CT

Test	Indications	Advantages	Disadvantages/Contraindications	Preparation
LIVER-SPLEEN **Liver, spleen scan** (radionuclide) $$	Identification of functioning splenic tissue to localize an accessory spleen or evaluate suspected functional asplenia. Assessment of size, shape, and position of liver and spleen. Differentiation of hepatic hemangiomas and focal nodular hyperplasia from other liver lesions.	May detect isodense lesions missed by CT. Useful to detect location of active GI bleed (see GI bleeding scan, above).	Diminished sensitivity for small lesions (less than 1.5–2.0 cm) and deep lesions. SPECT increases sensitivity (can detect lesions of 1.0–1.5 cm). Nonspecific; unable to distinguish solid versus cystic or inflammatory versus neoplastic tissue. Lower sensitivity for diffuse hepatic tumors. **Contraindications and risks:** Caution in pregnancy advised because of the risk of ionizing radiation to the fetus.	None.
PANCREAS **Computed tomography** (CT) $$$–$$$$	Evaluation of pancreatic and biliary obstruction and possible adenocarcinoma. Staging of pancreatic carcinoma. Evaluation of complications and causes of acute pancreatitis.	Excellent spatial resolution. Allows characterization of most pancreatic lesions, and staging of pancreatic cancers. Can guide fine-needle biopsy or placement of a drainage catheter.	**Contraindications and risks:** Contraindicated in pregnancy because of the potential harm of ionizing radiation to the fetus. See Risks of Iodinated CT Intravenous Contrast Agents, p. 289.	Preferably NPO for 4–6 hours. Normal hydration. Recent estimated glomerular filtration rate determination. Optimal imaging requires special protocol, including precontrast plus arterial and venous phase contrast-enhanced images.

| | ADRENAL | GENITOURINARY | |
	MIBG scan	CT	Ultrasound
ADRENAL **MIBG (meta-iodobenzyl-guanidine)** (radionuclide) $$$	Suspected pheochromocytoma when CT is negative or equivocal. Also useful in evaluation of neuroblastoma, carcinoid, and medullary carcinoma of thyroid.		
	Test is useful for localization of pheochromocytomas. Positive scans may indicate patients that are potential candidates for ^{131}I MIBG therapy.		
	High radiation dose to adrenal gland. Delayed imaging (at 1, 2, and 3 days) necessitates return of patient. **Contraindications and risks:** Contraindicated in pregnancy because of the risk of ionizing radiation to the fetus. Because of the relatively high dose of ^{131}I, patients should receive instructions on precautionary measures by nuclear medicine personnel.		
	Administration of Lugol iodine solution (to block thyroid uptake) before and after administration of MIBG.		
GENITOURINARY **Computed tomography** (CT) $$$		Evaluation for possible kidney or ureteral stones. Evaluation of staging of renal parenchymal tumors, hydronephrosis, pyelonephritis, and perinephric abscess. CT urogram test of choice for evaluation of upper tract uroepithelium.	
		Rapid. Outstanding sensitivity for nephroureterolithiasis. Can guide percutaneous procedures. Excellent spatial resolution. CT urogram has replaced intravenous pyelogram for evaluation of upper tract uroepithelium.	
		Contraindications and risks: Caution in pregnancy because of the risk of ionizing radiation to the fetus. See Risks of Iodinated CT Intravenous Contrast Agents, p. 289.	
		Sedation of agitated patients. Hydration or administration of furosemide to distend the ureters if uroepithelial evaluation is desired.	
GENITOURINARY **Ultrasound** (US) $$			Evaluation of renal morphology, hydronephrosis, size of prostate, and residual urine volume. Differentiation of cystic versus solid renal lesions.
			Noninvasive. No radiation. Can be portable. Imaging in all planes. Can guide fine-needle aspiration or placement of drainage catheter.
			Operator-dependent. More difficult in obese patients. **Contraindications and risks:** None.
			Preferably NPO for 6 hours. Full urinary bladder required for pelvic studies.

(Continued)

	GENITOURINARY	
	MRI	**Radionuclide scan**

Test	Indications	Advantages	Disadvantages/Contraindications	Preparation
GENITOURINARY **Magnetic resonance imaging** (MRI) $$$$	Staging of cancers of the uterus, cervix, and prostate. Can provide information additional to what is obtained by CT in some cases of renal cell and bladder carcinoma.	Provides excellent tissue contrast resolution, multiplanar capability. No ionizing radiation.	Subject to motion artifacts. Special instrumentation required for patients on life support. Long imaging time compared to CT, more sensitive to motion artifact. **Contraindications:** Patients with cardiac pacemakers, intraocular metallic foreign bodies, intracranial aneurysm clips, cochlear implants, and some artificial heart valves.	Sedation of agitated patients. Screening CT or plain radiograph images of orbits if history suggests possible metallic foreign body in the eye.
GENITOURINARY **Renal scan** (radionuclide) $$	Determination of relative renal function. Evaluation of suspected renal vascular hypertension. Differentiation of a dilated but non-obstructed system from one that has a urodynamically significant obstruction. Evaluation of renal blood flow and function in acute or chronic renal failure. Evaluation of both medical and surgical complications of renal transplant. Estimation of glomerular filtration rate and effective renal plasma flow.	Provides renal functional information. Estimates glomerular filtration rate and renal plasma flow.	Finding of poor renal blood flow does not pinpoint an etiologic diagnosis. Limited utility when renal function is extremely poor. Estimation of glomerular filtration rate and renal plasma flow often is imprecise. **Contraindications and risks:** Caution in pregnancy because of the risk of ionizing radiation to the fetus.	Normal hydration needed for evaluation of suspected obstructive uropathy because dehydration may result in false-positive examination. Blood pressure should be monitored and an intravenous line started when an angiotensin-converting enzyme (ACE) inhibitor is used to evaluate renal vascular hypertension. Patient should discontinue ACE inhibitor medication for at least 48 hours before examination if possible.

PELVIS				
	Ultrasound		**MRI**	

Test	Indications	Strengths	Limitations / Contraindications	Comments
PELVIS **Ultrasound** (US) $$	Evaluation of ovarian mass, enlarged uterus, vaginal bleeding, pelvic pain, possible ectopic pregnancy, and infertility. Monitoring of follicular development. Localization of intrauterine device.	Use of a vaginal probe allows excellent visualization of female pelvic organs and pathologies without ionizing radiation. Inexpensive compared to MRI and CT.	Operator dependent. Transabdominal scan has limited sensitivity for uterine or ovarian pathology. Vaginal probe has limited field of view and therefore may miss large masses outside the pelvis. **Contraindications and risks:** None.	Distended bladder required (only in transabdominal examination).
PELVIS **Magnetic resonance imaging** (MRI) $$$$	Evaluation of gynecologic malignancies, particularly endometrial, cervical, and vaginal carcinoma. Evaluation of prostate, bladder, and rectal carcinoma. Evaluation of congenital anomalies of the genitourinary tract. Useful in distinguishing lymphadenopathy from vasculature.	Provides excellent tissue contrast resolution, multiplanar capability. No ionizing radiation. Best imaging evaluation of uterine, cervical, prostate, and bladder carcinoma. May provide metabolic and functional information on prostate cancer.	Subject to motion artifacts. Special instrumentation required for patients on life support. **Contraindications:** Patients with cardiac pacemakers, intraocular metallic foreign bodies, intracranial aneurysm clips, cochlear implants, and some artificial heart valves.	Sedation of agitated patients. Screening CT or plain radiograph images of orbits if history suggests possible metallic foreign body in the eye. An endorectal coil is preferred for prostate MRI.

(Continued)

	BONE		
	Bone scan		**Na¹⁸F bone PET/CT**
Test	**Indications**	**Advantages**	**Disadvantages/Contraindications**	**Preparation**

Test	Indications	Advantages	Disadvantages/Contraindications	Preparation
BONE **Bone scan,** whole body (radionuclide; 99mTc–methyl diphosphonate [MDP]) $$–$$$	Evaluation of primary or metastatic neoplasm, osteomyelitis, arthritis, metabolic disorders, trauma, avascular necrosis, joint prosthesis, and reflex sympathetic dystrophy. Evaluation of clinically suspected but radiographically occult fractures. Identification of stress fractures.	Can examine entire osseous skeleton or specific area of interest. Highly sensitive compared with plain film radiography for detection of bone neoplasm. In osteomyelitis, bone scan may be positive much earlier (24 hours) than plain film (10–14 days).	Nonspecific. Correlation with plain film radiographs often necessary. Limited utility in patients with poor renal function. Poor resolution in distal extremities, head, and spine; in these instances, SPECT is often useful. Sometimes difficult to distinguish osteomyelitis from cellulitis or septic joint; dual imaging with gallium or with indium-labeled leukocytes can be helpful. False-negative results for osteomyelitis can occur following antibiotic therapy and within the first 24 hours after trauma. **Contraindications and risks:** Caution in pregnancy because of the risk of ionizing radiation to the fetus.	Patient should be well hydrated and void frequently after the procedure.
BONE **Bone positron emission tomography/ Computed tomography (PET/CT), whole body, with sodium ¹⁸fluoride (Na¹⁸F)** $$$$	Detection and evaluation of bone metastases, from prostate, breast, lung, kidney, and thyroid.	Improved spatial and contrast resolution compared to conventional 99mTc-MDP bone scans. Improved accuracy compared to 99mTc-MDP bone scans. Shorter examination time compared to 99mTc-MDP bone scans.	**Contraindications and risks:** Caution in pregnancy because of the risk of ionizing radiation to the fetus.	Patient should be well hydrated and void frequently after the procedure.

(Continued)

SPINE		
	CT	**MRI**
SPINE **Computed tomography** (CT) $$$	Evaluation of structures that are not well visualized on MRI, including ossification of the posterior longitudinal ligament, tumoral calcification, osteophytic spurring, retropulsed bone fragments after trauma. Also used for patients in whom MRI is contraindicated.	Rapid. Superb spatial resolution. Can guide percutaneous fine-needle aspiration of possible tumor or abscess.	MRI unequivocally superior in evaluation of the spine nerve roots and cord, except for conditions mentioned here in indications. Artifacts from metal prostheses degrade images. **Contraindications and risks:** Pregnancy because of the potential harm of ionizing radiation to the fetus. See Risks of Iodinated CT Intravenous Contrast Agents, p. 289.	Normal hydration. Sedation of agitated patients.
SPINE **Magnetic resonance imaging** (MRI) $$$$	Diseases involving the spine and cord except where CT is superior (ossification of the posterior longitudinal ligament, tumoral calcification, osteophytic spurring, retropulsed bone fragments after trauma).	Provides excellent tissue contrast resolution, multiplanar capability. No ionizing radiation.	Less useful in detection of calcification, small spinal vascular malformations, acute spinal trauma (because of longer acquisition time, and inferior detection of bony injury). Subject to motion artifacts. Special instrumentation required for patients on life support. **Contraindications:** Patients with cardiac pacemakers, intraocular metallic foreign bodies, intracranial aneurysm clips, cochlear implants, and some artificial heart valves.	Sedation of agitated patients. Screening CT or plain radiograph images of orbits if history suggests possible metallic foreign body in the eye.

| | MUSCULOSKELETAL | VASCULATURE |
| | MRI | Ultrasound |

Test	Indications	Advantages	Disadvantages/Contraindications	Preparation
MUSCULOSKELETAL SYSTEM **Magnetic resonance imaging** (MRI) $$$$	Evaluation of joints except where a prosthesis is in place. Extent of primary or malignant tumor (bone and soft tissue). Evaluation of aseptic necrosis, bone and soft tissue infections, marrow space disease, and traumatic derangements.	Provides excellent tissue contrast resolution, multiplanar capability. No ionizing radiation.	Subject to motion artifacts. Less able than CT to detect calcification, ossification, and periosteal reaction. Special instrumentation required for patients on life support. **Contraindications:** Patients with cardiac pacemakers, intraocular metallic foreign bodies, intracranial aneurysm clips, cochlear implants, and some artificial heart valves.	Sedation of agitated patients. Screening CT or plain radiograph images of orbits if history suggests possible metallic foreign body in the eye.
VASCULATURE **Ultrasound** (US) $$	Evaluation of deep venous thrombosis, extremity grafts, patency of inferior vena cava, portal vein, and hepatic veins. Carotid Doppler indicated for symptomatic carotid bruit, atypical transient ischemic attack, monitoring after endarterectomy, and baseline prior to major vascular surgery. Surveillance of TIPS patency and flow.	Noninvasive. No radiation. Can be portable. Imaging in all planes.	Technique operator-dependent. May be difficult to diagnose tight stenosis versus occlusion (catheter angiography may be necessary). **Contraindications and risks:** None.	None.

AORTA				
AORTA AND ITS BRANCHES **Angiography** $$$	Noninvasive MR and CT angiography have largely replaced conventional catheter angiography for the diagnosis of diseases of the aorta and its branch vessels. However, catheter angiography is still indicated for the assessment of vascular anatomy and diseases not characterized by other imaging tests; assessment of small vessel disease (eg, vasculitis, vascular malformations) in cases in which other noninvasive imaging gives insufficient spatial resolution; assessment of direct arterial supply to tumors.	Excellent spatial resolution. Provides access and can guide intervention.	Invasive. Patient must remain supine with leg extended for 6 hours following the procedure to protect the common femoral artery at the catheter entry site. **Contraindications and risks:** Allergy to iodinated contrast material may require corticosteroid and H_1 blocker or H_2 blocker premedication. Contraindicated in pregnancy because of the potential harm of ionizing radiation to the fetus. Contrast nephrotoxicity may occur, especially with preexisting impaired renal function due to diabetes mellitus or multiple myeloma; however, any creatinine elevation that occurs after the procedure is usually reversible.	NPO for 4–6 hours. Good hydration to limit possible renal insult due to iodinated contrast material. Recent estimated glomerular filtration rate determination, assessment of clotting parameters, reversal of anticoagulation. Performed with conscious sedation. Requires cardiac, respiratory, blood pressure, and pulse oximetry monitoring.
AORTA AND ITS BRANCHES **Computed tomography angiography** (CTA) $$$	Preoperative assessment of aortic or branch artery aneurysms and dissections. Evaluation of thoraco-abdominal trauma. Evaluation of possible aortic injury. Evaluation of mesenteric ischemia.	Rapid. Excellent spatial resolution and large territory coverage. Evaluates calcified vascular plaques.	Limited functional and hemodynamic evaluation. **Contraindications and risks:** Pregnancy because of potential harm of ionizing radiation to the fetus. See Risks of CT and Angiographic Intravenous Contrast Agents, p. 289.	Sedation of agitated patients. Hydration.

(Continued)

	AORTA	
	MRA	
Test	Indications	Advantages	Disadvantages/Contraindications	Preparation
---	---	---	---	---
AORTA AND ITS BRANCHES **Magnetic resonance angiography** (MRA) $$$$	More cost-effective and safer than conventional catheter-based angiography. Can provide preoperative assessment of thoracoabdominal aortic aneurysms and dissections to determine diseased arterial size, proximal and distal extent, relationship to major branch arteries, and presence of anatomic anomalies.	No ionizing radiation. No iodinated contrast needed. Non-gadolinium MRA options available for patients with renal insufficiency.	Subject to motion artifacts. Special instrumentation required for patients on life support. **Contraindications:** Patients with cardiac pacemakers, intraocular metallic foreign bodies, intracranial aneurysm clips, cochlear implants, and some artificial heart valves.	Sedation of agitated patients. Screening CT or plain radiograph images of orbits if history suggests possible metallic foreign body in the eye.

7

Basic Electrocardiography & Echocardiography

Fred M. Kusumoto, MD

I. BASIC ELECTROCARDIOGRAPHY*

How to Use This Section

This chapter includes criteria for the diagnosis of basic electrocardiographic waveforms and cardiac arrhythmias. It is intended for use as a reference and assumes a basic understanding of the electrocardiogram (ECG).

Electrocardiographic interpretation is a "stepwise" procedure, and the first steps are to study and characterize the cardiac rhythm.

Step One (Rhythm)

Categorize what you see in the 12-lead ECG or rhythm strip, using the three major parameters that allow for systematic analysis and subsequent diagnosis of the rhythm:

1. Mean rate of the QRS complexes (slow, normal, or fast).
2. Width of the QRS complexes (wide or narrow).
3. Rhythmicity of the QRS complexes (characterization of spaces between QRS complexes) (regular or irregular).

Step Two (Morphology)

Step 2 consists of examining and characterizing the morphology of the cardiac waveforms.

1. Examine for atrial abnormalities and bundle branch blocks (BBBs) (pp. 339–342).
2. Assess the QRS axis and the causes of axis deviations (pp. 342–343).
3. Examine for signs of left ventricular hypertrophy (pp. 343–344).
4. Examine for signs of right ventricular hypertrophy (pp. 344–345).
5. Examine for signs of myocardial infarction, if present (p. 346).
6. Bear in mind conditions that may alter the ability of the ECG to diagnose a myocardial infarction (p. 353).
7. Examine for abnormalities of the ST segment or T wave (pp. 354–357).
8. Assess the QT interval (pp. 357–358).
9. Examine for miscellaneous conditions (pp. 359–361).

   (bpm = beats per minute, s = second, ms = millisecond, m/s = meters per second, cm/s = centimeters per second)

---

*Several parts of this section on electrocardiography are based on the work of G. T. Evans, MD, who was the author of this chapter in the first edition of the book.

Step One: Diagnosis of the Cardiac Rhythm

A. Approach to Diagnosis of the Cardiac Rhythm

Most electrocardiograph machines display 10 seconds of data in a standard tracing. A rhythm is defined as three or more successive P waves or QRS complexes.

Categorize the patterns seen in the tracing according to a systematic method. This method proceeds in three steps that lead to a diagnosis based on the most likely rhythm producing a particular pattern:

1. What is the mean rate of the QRS complexes?

    Slow (<60 bpm): The easiest way to determine this is to count the total number of QRS complexes in a 10-second period. If there are no more than 9, the rate is slow.
    Another method for determining the rate is to count the number of large boxes (0.20 s) between QRS complexes and use the following formula:

    $$\text{Rate} = 300 \div (\text{number of large boxes between QRS complexes})$$

    A slow heart rate (<60 bpm) has more than five large boxes between QRS complexes.
    Normal (60–100 bpm): If there are 10–16 complexes in a 10-second period, the rate is normal.
    In normal heart rates, the QRS complexes are separated by 3 to 5 large boxes.
    Fast (>100 bpm): If there are ≥ 17 complexes in a 10-second period, the rate is fast. Fast heart rates have fewer than three large boxes between QRS complexes.
2. Is the duration of the dominant QRS morphology narrow (<0.12 s) or wide (≥0.12 s)? (Refer to the section on the QRS duration.)
3. What is the "rhythmicity" of the QRS complexes (defined as the spacing between QRS complexes)? Regular or irregular? (Any change in the spacing of the R-R intervals defines an irregular rhythm.)

Using the categorization above, refer to Tables 7–1 and 7–2 to select a specific diagnosis for the cardiac rhythm.

B. Normal Heart Rate

Sinus Rhythm

The sinus node is the primary pacemaker for the heart. Because the sinus node is located at the junction of the superior vena cava and the right atrium, in **sinus rhythm** the atria are activated from "right to left" and "high to low." The P wave in sinus rhythm is upright

TABLE 7–1. SUSTAINED REGULAR RHYTHMS.

Rate	Fast	Normal	Slow
Narrow QRS duration	Sinus tachycardia Atrial tachycardia Atrial flutter (2:1 AV conduction) Junctional tachycardia Orthodromic AVRT	Sinus rhythm Ectopic atrial rhythm Atrial flutter (4:1 conduction) Accelerated junctional rhythm	Sinus bradycardia Ectopic atrial bradycardia Junctional rhythm
Wide QRS duration	All rhythms listed above under narrow QRS duration, but with BBB or IVCD patterns		
	Ventricular tachycardia Antidromic AVRT	Accelerated ventricular rhythm	Ventricular escape rhythm

AV = atrioventricular; *BBB* = bundle branch blocks; *IVCD* = intraventricular conduction delay.

TABLE 7–2. SUSTAINED IRREGULAR RHYTHMS.

Rate	Fast	Normal	Slow
Narrow QRS duration	Atrial fibrillation Atrial flutter (variable AV conduction) Multifocal atrial tachycardia Atrial tachycardia with AV block (rare)	Atrial fibrillation Atrial flutter (variable AV conduction) Multiform atrial rhythm Atrial tachycardia with AV block (rare)	Atrial fibrillation Atrial flutter (variable AV conduction) Multiform atrial rhythm Sinus rhythm with 2° AV block
Wide QRS duration	All rhythms listed above under narrow QRS duration, but with BBB or IVCD patterns		
	Torsade de pointes Rarely, anterograde conduction of atrial fibrillation over an accessory pathway in patients with WPW syndrome		

AV = atrioventricular; *BBB* = bundle branch blocks; *IVCD* = intraventricular conduction delay; *WPW* = Wolff-Parkinson-White syndrome.

in lead II and inverted in lead aVR. In lead V_I, the P wave is usually biphasic with a small initial positive deflection due to right atrial activation and a terminal negative deflection due to left atrial activation.

The normal sinus rate is usually between 60 and 100 bpm but can vary significantly. During sleep, when parasympathetic tone is high, **sinus bradycardia** (sinus rates <60 bpm) is a normal finding, and during conditions associated with increased sympathetic tone (exercise, stress), **sinus tachycardia** (sinus rates >100 bpm) is common. In children and young adults, **sinus arrhythmia** (sinus rates that vary by more than 10% during 10 seconds) due to respiration is frequently observed.

Ectopic Atrial Rhythm

In some situations, the atria are activated by an ectopic atrial focus rather than the sinus node. In this case, the P wave will have an abnormal shape depending on where the ectopic focus is located. For example, if the focus arises from the left atrium, the P wave is inverted in leads I and aVL. If the depolarization rate of the ectopic focus is between 60 and 100 bpm, the patient has an **ectopic atrial rhythm.** If the rate is <60 bpm, the rhythm is defined as an ectopic atrial bradycardia.

Atrial Flutter With 4:1 Atrioventricular Conduction

In **atrial flutter**, the atria are activated rapidly (usually 300 bpm) owing to a stable reentrant circuit. Most commonly, the reentrant circuit rotates counterclockwise around the tricuspid valve. Because the left atrium and interatrial septum are activated low-to-high, "sawtooth" flutter waves that are inverted in the inferior leads (II, III, and aVF) are usually observed. If every fourth atrial beat is conducted to the ventricles (owing to slow conduction in the atrioventricular [AV] node), a relatively normal ventricular rate of 75 bpm is observed.

Accelerated Junctional Rhythm (p. 338)

Premature QRS Activity

It is common to have isolated premature QRS activity that leads to mild irregularity of the heart rhythm. A premature narrow QRS complex is most often due to a normally conducted **premature atrial complex (PAC)** or more rarely a **premature junctional complex (PJC)**. A premature wide QRS complex is usually due to a **premature ventricular complex (PVC)** or to a premature supraventricular complex (PAC or PJC) that conducts to the ventricle with aberrant conduction due to block in one of the bundle branches (p. 340). Premature supraventricular complexes (with or without aberrant conduction) are commonly observed phenomena that are not associated with cardiac disease. Although PVCs are observed in normal individuals, they are usually associated with higher risk in patients with cardiac disease.

C. Tachycardia

Tachycardias are normally classified by whether the QRS complex is narrow or wide and whether the rhythm is regular or irregular. A narrow QRS tachycardia indicates normal activation of the ventricular tissue regardless of the tachycardia mechanism. Narrow QRS tachycardias are frequently grouped together as supraventricular tachycardia (SVT) and can be due to a number of mechanisms described in the following text. This grouping also has clinical usefulness because SVTs are not usually life-threatening. In addition to QRS width, it is useful to consider the anatomic site from which the tachycardia arises: atrium, atrioventricular junction, ventricle, or utilization of an accessory pathway (Figure 7–1).

Narrow QRS Tachycardia with a Regular Rhythm: Regular SVT (Figure 7–2)

A. **Sinus Tachycardia:** Under many physiologic conditions, the sinus node discharges at a rate >100 bpm. In **sinus tachycardia**, an upright P wave can be observed in II and aVF and an inverted P wave is observed in aVR. The PR interval is usually relatively normal, because conditions associated with sinus tachycardia (most commonly sympathetic activation) also cause more rapid AV conduction.

B. **Atrial Tachycardia:** Rarely, a single atrial site other than the sinus node fires rapidly. This leads to an abnormally shaped P wave. The specific shape of the P wave depends on the specific site of **atrial tachycardia.** The PR interval depends on how quickly atrioventricular conduction occurs. As the atrial tachycardia rate increases, the AV node conduction slows (decremental conduction) and the PR interval increases; decremental conduction properties of the AV node prevent rapid ventricular rates in the presence of rapid atrial rates.

C. **Atrial Flutter:** The mechanism for **atrial flutter** is described above. Most commonly atrioventricular conduction occurs with every other flutter wave (2:1 conduction), leading to a heart rate of approximately 150 bpm. In some situations, very rapid ventricular rates can be observed due to 1:1 conduction, or slower rates observed due to 3:1 conduction.

D. **Junctional Tachycardia:** The most common type of tachycardia to arise from tissue near the atrioventricular junction is **AV nodal reentrant tachycardia (AVNRT).** In AVNRT, two separate parallel pathways of conduction are present within junctional and perijunctional tissue. Usually, one of the pathways has relatively rapid conduction properties but a long refractory period ("fast pathway"), and the other has slow conduction and a short refractory period ("slow pathway"). In some cases, a premature atrial contraction can block one of the pathways (usually the fast pathway), conduct down the slow pathway, and activate the fast pathway retrogradely, initiating a reentrant circuit. In rare circumstances, a site within the AV node fires rapidly as a result of increased automaticity.

Regardless of the mechanism, because the tachycardia originates within the AV junction, the atria and ventricles are activated simultaneously. Most commonly (in approximately 50% of cases), the P wave is buried in the QRS complex and is not seen. In approximately 40% of cases, the retrograde P wave is observed in the terminal portion of the QRS complex. The easiest place to see the retrograde P wave is in lead V_1, where a low-amplitude terminal positive deflection (pseudo-R' wave) is seen (Figure 7–2). In addition, a terminal negative deflection (pseudo-S wave) is seen in the inferior leads (II, III, and aVF). Finally, in about 10% of cases, the P wave is observed in the initial portion of the QRS complex. The location of the P wave

Atrial tachycardias

Atrial flutter   Atrial fibrillation   Atrial tachycardia   Atrial tachycardia (MAT)

Junctional tachycardias

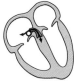

Atrioventricular node   Atrioventricular node
reentrant tachycardia   automatic tachycardia

Ventricular tachycardias

 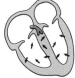

Ventricular tachycardia   Ventricular fibrillation

Accessory pathway-mediated tachycardias

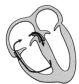 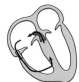

Orthodromic   Antidromic   Atrial fibrillation
atrioventricular   atrioventricular   with activation of the
reentrant tachycardia   reentrant tachycardia   ventricles via an
                                                    accessory pathway
                                                    and the AV node

Figure 7–1. Anatomic classification of tachycardias. (*Adapted with permission from Kusumoto FM: Arrhythmias. In*: Cardiovascular Pathophysiology, *FM Kusumoto [editor], Hayes Barton Press, 2004.*)

depends on the relative speeds of retrograde activation of the atria and anterograde activation of the ventricles via the His-Purkinje system.

E. **Accessory Pathway–Mediated Tachycardia:** Usually, the AV node and His bundle provide the only path for AV conduction. In approximately 1 in 1000 individuals, an additional AV connection called an **accessory pathway** is present. The presence of two parallel pathways (the accessory pathway and the AV node-His bundle) for AV conduction increases the likelihood that reentrant tachycardia will occur. The most common tachycardia is a reentrant narrow QRS tachycardia in which the ventricles are activated via the His-Purkinje system and the atria are activated via retrograde activation

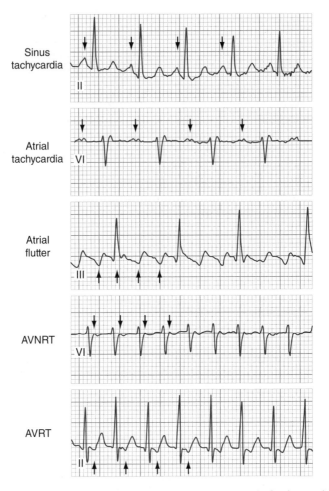

Figure 7–2. ECG appearance of different forms of regular SVTs. Arrows show the first four atrial deflections in each SVT. In *sinus tachycardia,* the P wave has a normal morphology, and the PR interval is normal. In *atrial tachycardia,* the P wave is abnormal (positive in V_1, and the PR interval is prolonged because of decremental conduction in the AV node). In *atrial flutter,* inverted "saw-tooth" waves are observed in lead III. In *AVNRT,* a pseudo-R wave due to retrograde atrial activation is observed in lead V_1. In *AVRT,* a retrograde P wave is observed in the ST segment because the atria and ventricles are activated sequentially. The P wave is usually located relatively close to the preceding QRS complex because the accessory pathway conducts rapidly.

from the accessory pathway (Figure 7–3). This type of tachycardia is frequently called **orthodromic atrioventricular reentrant tachycardia (AVRT)** because conduction through the AV node and His-Purkinje fibers occurs normally (*ortho* is Greek for straight or normal). Orthodromic AVRT is one cause of SVT; the QRS complexes are narrow and normal-appearing because the ventricles are activated via the AV node and His-Purkinje system, ventricular tissue, an accessory pathway, and atrial tissue. Because the ventricles and atria are activated sequentially, the P wave is most often observed within the ST segment (Figure 7–2). As discussed later, accessory pathways can also be associated with regular and irregular wide complex tachycardias.

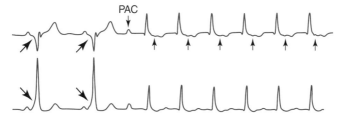

PAC
↓

Figure 7–3. Initiation of SVT in a patient with an accessory pathway. During sinus rhythm, the ventricles are activated via the accessory pathway and the AV node-His bundle. Because the accessory pathway conducts rapidly and inserts into regular ventricular myocardium, the PR interval is short and a delta wave is observed (*large arrows*). A premature atrial complex (PAC) blocks in the accessory pathway and travels only down the AV node-His bundle, leading to a narrow QRS complex. The atria are activated retrogradely by the accessory pathway (*small arrows*), and orthodromic AVRT is initiated. *(Adapted with permission from Kusumoto FM: Cardiovascular disorders: Heart disease. In: Pathophysiology of Disease: An Introduction to Clinical Medicine, 7th ed. Hammer G, McPhee SJ [editors], McGraw-Hill, 2014.)*

Narrow QRS Tachycardias with an Irregular Rhythm: Irregular SVT (Figure 7–4)

A. **Atrial Fibrillation:** Atrial fibrillation is the most common abnormal fast heart rhythm observed. Atrial fibrillation is most commonly due to multiple chaotic wandering wavelets of reentry that cause irregular activation of the atria. Because the AV node is also activated irregularly, AV conduction is variable and an irregular ventricular rhythm is observed. In atrial fibrillation, the rhythm is often called "irregularly irregular" because there is no organized atrial activity. On the ECG, continuous fibrillatory low-amplitude waves with varying morphology are observed with no easily identifiable isoelectric period. The fibrillatory waves are usually best seen in leads V_1, V_2, II, III, and aVF.

Atrial fibrillation

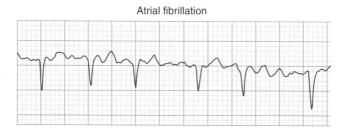

Multifocal atrial tachycardia

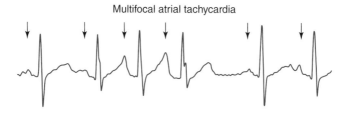

Figure 7–4. ECG appearance of atrial fibrillation and multifocal atrial tachycardia (MAT). In atrial fibrillation, continuous chaotic activation of the atria results in continuous low-amplitude fibrillatory waves. In MAT, discrete P waves (*arrows*) and an isoelectric T–P segment are observed.

B. **Multifocal Atrial Tachycardia:** In **multifocal atrial tachycardia** (often called **MAT**), several atrial sites beat due to abnormal automaticity. This leads to P waves of three or more different morphologies. The rhythm is usually irregular; the different sites fire at different rates. MAT can be distinguished from atrial fibrillation by discrete P waves and isoelectric periods between the T wave and the P wave. The most common cause of MAT is chronic obstructive pulmonary disease (approximately 60% of cases).

C. **Atrial Flutter With Variable Block:** Atrial flutter can sometimes present as an irregular rhythm because of variable AV block. In this case, although the ventricular rhythm is irregular, there are often relatively constant intervals between the QRS complexes. For example, if the atrial flutter rate is 300 bpm, the possible ventricular rates will be 300 bpm, 150 bpm, 100 bpm, or 75 bpm for 1:1, 2:1, 3:1, and 4:1 AV conduction, respectively.

Wide QRS Complex Tachycardia With a Regular Rhythm

The most common cause of **wide QRS complex tachycardia with a regular rhythm (WCT-RR)** is sinus tachycardia with either right bundle branch block (RBBB) or left bundle branch block (LBBB). However, if a patient with structural heart disease presents with WCT-RR, one assumes a worst-case scenario and the presumptive diagnosis becomes **ventricular tachycardia (VT).** Most commonly, VT originates from a rapid reentrant circuit located at the border of infarcted and normal myocardium. Because the ventricles are not activated via the bundle branches or the Purkinje system, an abnormally wide QRS complex is observed. Any atrial or junctional tachycardias associated with aberrant conduction can also cause a WCT-RR. Finally, in very rare circumstances, patients with accessory pathways present with **antidromic AVRT** in which the ventricles are activated via the accessory pathway (leading to a wide and bizarre QRS complex) and the atria are activated retrogradely via the His bundle-AV node (*anti* is Greek for against).

The ECG differentiation between regular SVTs with aberrant conduction (sinus tachycardia, atrial tachycardia, atrial flutter, junctional tachycardia, orthodromic AVRT) and VT can sometimes be difficult. Accurate diagnosis of VT is critical because this rhythm is frequently life-threatening. The two principal techniques for identifying VT are the presence of AV dissociation and abnormal QRS morphology.

A. **Atrioventricular Dissociation:** In **AV dissociation,** the atria and ventricles are not related in one-to-one fashion. AV dissociation can be due to several conditions:

1. Atrioventricular conduction block (pp. 338–339).
2. Slowing of the primary pacemaker, most commonly due to sinus bradycardia or sinus pauses with junctional escape rhythm (pp. 338–339).
3. Acceleration of a subsidiary pacemaker, most commonly due to VT or much less commonly due to junctional tachycardia.

The most important reason to identify AV dissociation is in wide complex tachycardia for the differentiation of SVT with aberrancy from VT. In VT, the rapid ventricular rate is often associated with retrograde block within the His-Purkinje system (ventriculoatrial block). This leads to P waves (from sinus node depolarization) that are not associated in 1:1 fashion with the QRS complexes (Figure 7–5). The presence of AV dissociation makes

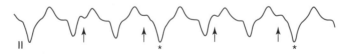

Figure 7–5. Lead II from a wide complex tachycardia. The arrows mark P waves that are not associated with every QRS complex (AV dissociation). The QRS complexes marked with an (*) are slightly narrower owing to partial activation from the preceding P wave (fusion complex).

VT the most likely diagnosis in a patient with a regular wide complex tachycardia. In some circumstances, AV dissociation can be identified by the presence of **capture beats** or **fusion beats**. Occasionally, a properly timed P wave conducts to the ventricles and a portion (fusion beat) or all (capture beat) of ventricular tissue is activated by the His-Purkinje tissue for one QRS complex. It is always easier to identify AV dissociation rather than AV association; T waves can often be confused with P waves. Always examine the entire ECG for unexpected deflections in the QRS complex, ST segment, and T waves that are dissociated P waves. The P waves are usually most obvious in the inferior leads (II, III, and aVF) or V_1.

Morphology Algorithms for Identifying VT

1. Method One: Quick Method for Diagnosis of VT (Requires Leads I, V_1, and V_2)

This method derives from an analysis of typical waveforms of RBBB or LBBB as seen in leads I, V_1, and V_2. If the waveforms do not conform to either the common or uncommon typical morphologic patterns, the diagnosis defaults to VT.

Step One

Determine the morphologic classification of the wide QRS complexes (RB type or LB type), using the criteria below.

   A. **Determination of the Morphologic Type of Wide QRS Complexes:** Use lead V_1 only to determine the type of bundle branch block morphology of abnormally wide QRS complexes.

   1. **RBBB- and RBB-type QRS complexes as seen in lead V_1:** A wide QRS complex with a net positive area under the QRS curve is called the right bundle branch "type" of QRS. This does not mean that the QRS conforms exactly to the morphologic criteria for RBBB. Typical morphologies seen in RBBB are shown in the box at left below. Atypical morphologies at the right are most commonly seen in PVCs or during VT.

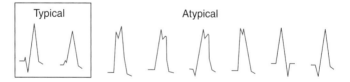

   2. **LBBB- and LBB-type QRS complexes as seen in lead V_1:** A wide QRS complex with a net negative area under the QRS curve is called a left bundle branch "type" of QRS. This does not mean that the QRS conforms exactly to the morphologic criteria for LBBB. Typical morphologies of LBBB are shown in the box at left below. Atypical morphologies at the right are most commonly seen in PVCs or during VT.

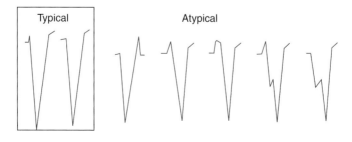

Step Two

Apply criteria for common and uncommon normal forms of either RBBB or LBBB, as described below. The waveforms may not be identical, but the morphologic descriptions must match. If the QRS complexes do not match, the rhythm is probably VT.

A. RBBB: Lead I must have a terminal broad S wave, but the R/S ratio may be <1.

Lead
I

In lead V_1, the QRS complex is usually triphasic but sometimes is notched and monophasic. The latter must have notching on the ascending limb of the R wave, usually at the lower left.

Lead
V_1

B. LBBB: Lead I must have a monophasic, usually notched R wave and may not have Q waves or S waves.

Lead
I

Both lead V_1 and lead V_2 must have a dominant S wave, usually with a small, narrow R wave. S descent must be rapid and smooth, without notching.

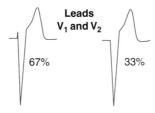

Leads
V_1 and V_2

67%   33%

2. Method Two: The Brugada Algorithm for Diagnosis of VT

(Requires all six precordial leads.)

Brugada and coworkers reported on a total of 554 patients with WC-TRR whose mechanism was diagnosed in the electrophysiology laboratory. Patients included 384 (69%) with VT and 170 (31%) with SVT with aberrant ventricular conduction.

1. **Is there absence of an RS complex in ALL precordial leads?**

   If Yes ($n = 83$), VT is established diagnosis (sensitivity 21%, specificity 100%).
   Note: Only QR, Qr, qR, QS, QRS, monophasic R, or rSR′ are present. qRs complexes were not mentioned in the Brugada study.
   If No ($n = 471$), proceed to next step.

2. **Is the RS interval >100 ms in ANY ONE precordial lead?**

   If Yes ($n = 175$), VT is established diagnosis (sensitivity 66%, specificity 98%).
   Note: The onset of R to the nadir of S is >100 ms (>2.5 small boxes) in a lead with an RS complex.

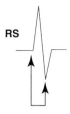

RS

If No ($n = 296$), proceed to next step.

3. Is there AV dissociation?

If Yes ($n = 59$), VT is established diagnosis (sensitivity 82%, specificity 98%). *Note:* AV block also implies the same diagnosis.

If No ($n = 237$), proceed to next step. *Note:* Antiarrhythmic drugs were withheld from patients in this study. Clinically, drugs that prolong the QRS duration may give a false-positive sign of VT using this criterion.

4. Are morphologic criteria for VT present?

If Yes ($n = 59$), VT is established diagnosis (sensitivity 99%, specificity 97%). *Note*: RBBB type QRS in V_1 versus LBBB type QRS in V_1 should be assessed as shown in the boxes below.

If No ($n = 169$)—and if there are no matches for VT in the boxes below—the diagnosis is SVT with aberration (sensitivity 97%, specificity 99%).

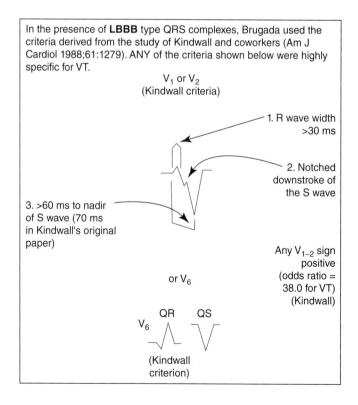

In the presence of **LBBB** type QRS complexes, Brugada used the criteria derived from the study of Kindwall and coworkers (Am J Cardiol 1988;61:1279). ANY of the criteria shown below were highly specific for VT.

V_1 or V_2
(Kindwall criteria)

1. R wave width >30 ms

2. Notched downstroke of the S wave

3. >60 ms to nadir of S wave (70 ms in Kindwall's original paper)

Any V_{1-2} sign positive (odds ratio = 38.0 for VT) (Kindwall)

or V_6

V_6 QR   QS

(Kindwall criterion)

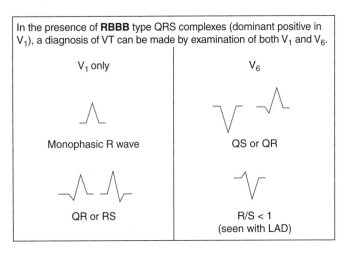

In the presence of **RBBB** type QRS complexes (dominant positive in V_1), a diagnosis of VT can be made by examination of both V_1 and V_6.

V_1 only	V_6
Monophasic R wave	QS or QR
QR or RS	R/S < 1 (seen with LAD)

3. Method Three: The Griffith Method for Diagnosis of VT (Requires Leads V_1 and V_6)

This method derives from an analysis of typical waveforms of RBBB or LBBB as seen in both leads V_1 and V_6. If the waveforms do not conform to the typical morphologic patterns, the diagnosis defaults to VT.

Step One

Determine the morphologic classification of the wide QRS complexes (RB type or LB type), using the criteria above.

Step Two

Apply criteria for normal forms of either RBBB or LBBB, as described below. A negative answer to any of the three questions is inconsistent with either RBBB or LBBB, and the diagnosis defaults to VT.

A. For QRS Complexes With RBBB Categorization:

1. Is there an rSR′ morphology in lead V_1?

V_1

2. Is there an RS complex in V_6 (may have a small septal Q wave)?

V_6

3. Is the R/S ratio in lead $V_6 > 1$?

B. For QRS Complexes With LBBB Categorization:

1. Is there an rS or QS complex in leads V_1 and V_2?

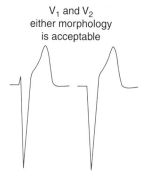

V_1 and V_2
either morphology
is acceptable

2. Is the onset of the QRS to the nadir of the S wave in lead V_1 < 70 ms?
3. Is there an R wave in lead V_6, without a Q wave?

V_6

Wide QRS Tachycardia with an Irregular Rhythm

A. **Polymorphic Ventricular Tachycardia and Ventricular Fibrillation:** In **polymor-phic ventricular tachycardia** and **ventricular fibrillation,** the ventricles are often activated continuously in chaotic fashion by disorganized wavelets of activation that produce irregular QRS complexes with no isoelectric periods. Both ventricular fibrillation and polymorphic ventricular tachycardia are life-threatening conditions that require prompt defibrillation. The distinction between ventricular fibrillation and polymorphic ventricular tachycardia is simply based on the amplitude of the QRS complexes and has very little clinical utility. The most common cause of polymorphic ventricular tachycardia and ventricular fibrillation is myocardial ischemia due to coronary artery occlusion.

B. **Torsade de Pointes:** Torsade de pointes ("twisting of the points") is a specific form of polymorphic VT that is often pause dependent, has a characteristic shifting morphology of the QRS complex, and occurs in the setting of a prolonged QT interval. Torsade de pointes is associated with drug-induced states, congenital long QT syndrome, and hypokalemia (p. 358).

C. **Atrial Fibrillation with Anterograde Accessory Pathway Activation:** If a patient with an accessory pathway develops atrial fibrillation, the ventricles are activated by both the normal AV node-His bundle axis and the accessory pathway. Because the accessory pathway does not have decremental conduction properties, it allows very rapid activation of the ventricles. The combination of an irregular wide complex rhythm with very rapid rates (250–300 bpm) should arouse suspicion of this scenario, particularly in a young, otherwise healthy patient.

D. **Bradycardia,** or slow heart rates, can be due to failure of impulse formation (sinus node dysfunction) or blocked AV conduction.

Sinus Node Dysfunction

Sinus node dysfunction is manifested in a number of ECG findings. Most commonly, there is a sinus pause with a junctional escape beat. Alternatively, sinus bradycardia can be associated with sinus node dysfunction.

A. **Sinus Bradycardia:** The normal range of sinus rates changes with age. In infants less than 12 months old, the mean heart rate is 140 bpm with a range of 100–190 bpm. In contrast, the normal range for adults is probably 50–90 bpm. Sinus rates less than 60 bpm are classified as **sinus bradycardia,** but it must be remembered that sinus rates of less than 60 bpm are commonly observed (sleep, athletes). Treatment of sinus bradycardia (usually with a pacemaker) is indicated only when it is associated with symptoms, not because of a specific heart rate.

B. **Sinus Pauses:** In some individuals, the sinus node abruptly stops firing, leading to **sinus pauses.** Usually an escape rhythm from an ectopic atrial focus or the junction prevents asystole. Sinus pauses up to 2 seconds are seen in normal adults. Patients with sinus pauses >3 seconds should be evaluated for the presence of sinus node dysfunction.

C. **Junctional Rhythm:** If the sinus node rate is very low, **sustained junctional rhythm** can sometimes be observed. In junctional rhythm, the QRS is not preceded by a P wave. A retrograde P wave can sometimes be seen in the initial portion or terminal portion of the QRS complex, but most commonly it is "buried" in the QRS complex. Normally, junctional rhythms are <60 bpm. Transient junctional rhythm can be observed in normal individuals during sleep, but sinus node dysfunction should be suspected if junctional rhythm is observed when a patient is awake.

In rare circumstances, **accelerated junctional rhythms** between 60 and 100 bpm are observed due to more rapid depolarization of AV nodal cells. If the junctional rate is faster than the sinus rate, the sinus node will be suppressed by retrograde atrial activation because of repetitive depolarization from the junction. Accelerated junctional rhythms can be present in digitalis toxicity, rheumatic fever, and after cardiac surgery.

AV Block

Because AV conduction normally occurs along a single axis, the AV node and His bundle, **atrioventricular (AV) block** most commonly is due to block at one of these two sites. Block within the His bundle is associated with a worse prognosis and should be suspected in any form of AV block associated with a wide QRS complex. Electrocardiographically, AV block is usually described as first-degree, second-degree, or third-degree AV block. In **first-degree (1°) AV block,** every P wave is conducted to the ventricles, but there is an abnormal delay between atrial activation and ventricular activation (PR interval >0.2 second). In 1° AV block, the ventricular rate is not slow unless sinus bradycardia is also present.

In **second-degree (2°) AV block,** some but not all P waves are conducted to the ventricles. This leads to an irregular ventricular rhythm. Second-degree AV block is usually subclassified as **Mobitz type I block, Wenckebach block** or **Mobitz type II block.** In type I 2° AV block, progressive prolongation of the PR interval is observed; in type II 2° AV block, the PR interval remains relatively constant before the blocked P wave. The importance of this distinction is this: type I 2° AV block usually indicates that conduction is blocked within the AV node, whereas type II AV block suggests that conduction is blocked within the His bundle (regardless of the width of the QRS complex). The simplest way to differentiate between type I and type II 2° AV block is to compare the PR intervals before and after the blocked P wave. In type I 2° AV block, the PR interval after the blocked P wave is shorter than the PR interval before the blocked P wave; in type II 2° AV block, the PR intervals are the same.

In **third-degree (3°) or complete AV block,** no P waves are conducted to the ventricles. The P-to-P and QRS-to-QRS intervals are constant and unrelated (AV dissociation). The QRS rate and morphology depend on the site of the subsidiary intrinsic pacemaker.

If the block is within the AV node, a lower AV nodal pacemaker often takes over and the rate is 40–50 bpm with a normal-appearing QRS complex (junctional rhythm). If the block is within the His bundle, a ventricular pacemaker with a rate of 20–40 bpm and a wide QRS will be noted (**ventricular escape rhythm**).

Step Two: Morphologic Diagnosis of the Cardiac Waveforms

A. The Normal ECG: Two Basic QRST Patterns

The most common pattern is illustrated below and is usually seen in leads I or II and V_6. There is a small "septal" Q wave <30 ms in duration. The T wave is upright. The normal ST segment, which is never normally isoelectric except sometimes at slow rates (<60 bpm), slopes upward into an upright T wave, whose proximal angle is more obtuse than the distal angle. The normal T wave is never symmetric.

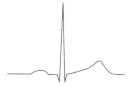

The pattern seen in the right precordial leads, usually $V_{1–3}$, is shown below. There is a dominant S wave. The J point—the junction between the end of the QRS complex and the ST segment—is usually slightly elevated, and the T wave is upright. The T wave in V_1 may occasionally be inverted as a normal finding in up to 50% of young women and 25% of young men, but this finding is usually abnormal in adult males. V_2 usually has the largest absolute QRS and T-wave magnitude of any of the 12 electrocardiographic leads.

B. Atrial Abnormalities

Right Atrial Enlargement (RAE)

Diagnostic criteria include a positive component of the P wave in lead V_1 or $V_2 \geq 1.5$ mm. Another criterion is a P-wave amplitude in lead II >2.5 mm.

Note: A tall, peaked P in lead II may represent RAE but is more commonly due to either chronic obstructive pulmonary disease (COPD) or increased sympathetic tone.

Clinical correlation: RAE is seen with right ventricular hypertrophy (RVH).

Left Atrial Enlargement (LAE)

The most sensitive lead for the diagnosis of LAE is lead V_1, but the criteria for lead II are more specific. Criteria include a terminal negative wave ≥1 mm deep and ≥40 ms wide (one small box by one small box in area) for lead V_1 and > 40 ms between the first (right) and second (left) atrial components of the P wave in lead II, or a P-wave duration >110 ms in lead II.

Clinical correlations: left ventricular hypertrophy (LVH), coronary artery disease, mitral valve disease, or cardiomyopathy.

C. Bundle Branch Block

The normal QRS duration in adults ranges from 67–114 ms (Glasgow cohort). If the QRS duration is ≥120 ms (three small boxes or more on the electrocardiographic paper), there is usually an abnormality of conduction of the ventricular impulse. The most common causes are either RBBB or LBBB (see below). However, other conditions may also prolong the QRS duration.

RBBB is defined by delayed terminal QRS forces that are directed to the right and anteriorly, producing broad terminal positive waves in leads V_1 and aVR and a broad terminal negative wave in lead I.

LBBB is defined by delayed terminal QRS forces that are directed to the left and posteriorly, producing wide R waves in leads that face the left ventricular free wall and wide S waves in the right precordial leads.

Right Bundle Branch Block

Diagnostic Criteria

The diagnosis of uncomplicated complete RBBB is made when the following criteria are met:

1. Prolongation of the QRS duration to 120 ms or more.
2. An rsr′, rsR′, or rSR′ pattern in lead V_1 or V_2. The R′ is usually greater than the initial R wave. In a minority of cases, a wide and notched R pattern may be seen.
3. Leads V_6 and I show a QRS complex with a wide S wave (S duration is longer than the R duration or >40 ms in adults).

(See common and uncommon waveforms for RBBB under Step Two, p. 334).

ST–T changes in RBBB

In uncomplicated RBBB, the ST–T segment is depressed and the T wave inverted in the right precordial leads with an R′ (usually only in lead V_1 but occasionally in V_2). The T wave is upright in leads I, V_5, and V_6.

Left Bundle Branch Block

Diagnostic Criteria

The diagnosis of uncomplicated complete LBBB is made when the following criteria are met:

1. Prolongation of the QRS duration to 120 ms or more.
2. There are broad and notched or slurred R waves in left-sided precordial leads V_5 and V_6, as well as in leads I and aVL. Occasionally, an RS pattern may occur in leads V_5 and V_6 in uncomplicated LBBB associated with posterior displacement of the left ventricle.
3. With the possible exception of lead aVL, Q waves are absent in the left-sided leads, specifically in leads V_5, V_6, and I.
4. The R peak time is prolonged to >60 ms in lead V_5 or V_6 but is normal in leads V_1 and V_2 when it can be determined.
5. In the right precordial leads V_1 and V_3, there are small initial r waves in the majority of cases, followed by wide and deep S waves. The transition zone in the precordial leads is displaced to the left. Wide QS complexes may be present in leads V_1 and V_2 and rarely in lead V_3.

(See common and uncommon waveforms for LBBB under Step Two, p. 334.)

ST–T Changes in LBBB

In uncomplicated LBBB, the ST segments are usually depressed and the T waves inverted in left precordial leads V_5 and V_6 as well as in leads I and aVL. Conversely, ST-segment elevations and positive T waves are recorded in leads V_1 and V_2. Only rarely is the T wave upright in the left precordial leads. As a general rule, ST–T changes in LBBB are usually in the direction opposite the direction of the QRS complex (inverted T waves and ST-segment depression if the QRS is upright).

D. Incomplete Bundle Branch Blocks

Incomplete LBBB

The waveforms are similar to those in complete LBBB, but the QRS duration is <120 ms. Septal Q waves are absent in I and V_6. Incomplete LBBB is synonymous with LVH and commonly mimics a delta wave in leads V_5 and V_6.

Incomplete RBBB

The waveforms are similar to those in complete RBBB, but the QRS duration is <120 ms. This diagnosis suggests RVH. Occasionally, in a normal variant pattern, there is an rSr′ waveform in lead V_1. In this case, the r′ is usually smaller than the initial r wave; this pattern is not indicative of incomplete RBBB.

Intraventricular Conduction Delay or Defect

If the QRS duration is ≥120 ms but typical waveforms of either RBBB or LBBB are not present, there is an intraventricular conduction delay or defect (IVCD). This pattern is common in dilated cardiomyopathy. An IVCD with a QRS duration of ≥170 ms is highly predictive of dilated cardiomyopathy.

E. Fascicular Blocks (Hemiblocks)

1. Left Anterior Fascicular Block (LAFB)

Diagnostic Criteria

1. Mean QRS axis from –45 degrees to –90 degrees (possibly –31 to –44 degrees).
2. A qR pattern in lead aVL, with the R peak time, that is, the onset of the Q wave to the peak of the R wave ≥45 ms (slightly more than one small box wide), as shown below.

    Clinical correlations: hypertensive heart disease, coronary artery disease, or idiopathic conducting system disease.

2. Left Posterior Fascicular Block (LPFB)

Diagnostic Criteria

1. Mean QRS axis from +90 degrees to +180 degrees.
2. A qR complex in leads III and aVF, an rS complex in leads aVL and I, with a Q wave ≥40 ms in the inferior leads.

Clinical correlations: LPFB is a diagnosis of exclusion. It may be seen in the acute phase of inferior myocardial injury or infarction or may result from idiopathic conducting system disease.

F. Determination of the Mean QRS Axis

The mean electrical axis is the average direction of the activation or repolarization process during the cardiac cycle. Instantaneous and mean electrical axes may be determined for any deflection (P, QRS, ST–T) in the three planes (frontal, transverse, and sagittal). The determination of the electrical axis of a QRS complex is useful for the diagnosis of certain pathologic cardiac conditions.

The Mean QRS Axis in the Frontal Plane (Limb Leads)

Arzbaecher developed the **hexaxial reference system** that allowed for the display of the relationships among the six frontal plane (limb) leads, which is shown on the following diagram.

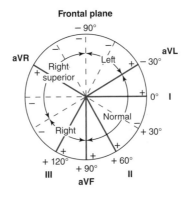

The normal range of the QRS axis in adults is –30 degrees to +90 degrees.

It is rarely important to precisely determine the degrees of the mean QRS. However, the recognition of abnormal axis deviations is critical because it leads to a presumption of disease. The mean QRS axis is derived from the net area under the QRS curves. The most efficient method of determining the mean QRS axis uses the method of Grant, which requires only leads I and II (see below). If the net area under the QRS curves in these leads is positive, the axis falls between –30 degrees and +90 degrees, which is the normal range of axis in adults. (The only exception to this rule is in RBBB, in which the first 60 ms of the QRS is used. Alternatively, one may use the maximal amplitude of the R and S waves in leads I and II to assess the axis in RBBB.) The following diagram shows abnormal axes.

Left Axis Deviation (LAD)

The four main causes of left axis deviation are as follows:

A. Left Anterior Fascicular Block (LAFB): See criteria above.

B. Inferior Myocardial Infarction: There is a pathologic Q wave ≥30 ms either in lead aVF or lead II in the absence of ventricular preexcitation.

C. Ventricular Preexcitation (WPW Pattern): LAD is seen with inferior paraseptal accessory pathway locations. This can mimic inferoposterior myocardial infarction. The classic definition of the Wolff-Parkinson-White (WPW) pattern includes a short PR interval (<120 ms); an initial slurring of the QRS complex, called a delta wave; and prolongation of the QRS complex to >120 ms. However, because this pattern may not always be present despite the presence of ventricular preexcitation, a more practical definition is an absent PR segment and an initial slurring of the QRS complex in any lead. The diagnosis of the WPW pattern usually requires sinus rhythm.

D. COPD: LAD is seen in 10% of patients with COPD.

Right Axis Deviation (RAD)

The four main causes of right axis deviation (RAD) are as follows:

A. Right Ventricular Hypertrophy: This is the most common cause (refer to diagnostic criteria, p. 344). However, one must first exclude acute occlusion of the posterior descending coronary artery, causing LPFB, and exclude also items B and C below.

B. Extensive Lateral and Apical Myocardial Infarction: Criteria include QS or Qr patterns in leads I and aVL and in leads V_{4-6}.

C. Ventricular Preexcitation (WPW Pattern): RAD seen with left lateral accessory pathway locations. This can mimic lateral myocardial infarction.

D. Left Posterior Fascicular Block (LPFB): This is a diagnosis of exclusion (see criteria above).

Right Superior Axis Deviation

This category is rare. Causes include RVH, apical myocardial infarction, VT, and hyperkalemia. Right superior axis deviation may rarely be seen as an atypical form of LAFB.

G. Ventricular Hypertrophy

1. Left Ventricular Hypertrophy

The ECG is very insensitive as a screening tool for LVH, but electrocardiographic criteria are usually specific. Echocardiography is the major resource for this diagnosis.

The best electrocardiographic criterion for the diagnosis of LVH is the Cornell voltage, the sum of the R-wave amplitude in lead aVL and the S-wave depth in lead V_3, adjusted for sex:

1. RaVL + SV_3 >20 mm (females), >25 mm (males). The R-wave height in aVL alone is a good place to start.
2. RaVL >9 mm (females), >11 mm (males).

Alternatively, application of the following criteria will diagnose most cases of LVH.

3. Sokolow-Lyon criteria: SV_1 + RV_5 or RV_6 (whichever R wave is taller) >35 mm (in patients age >35).
4. Romhilt-Estes criteria: Points are scored for QRS voltage (1 point), the presence of LAE (1 point), typical repolarization abnormalities in the absence of digitalis (1 point), and a few other findings. The combination of LAE (see above) and typical repolarization abnormalities (see below) (score ≥5 points) will suffice for the diagnosis of LVH even when voltage criteria are not met.

5. $RV_6 > RV_5$ (usually occurs with dilated LV). First exclude anterior myocardial infarction and establish that the R waves in V_5 are >7 mm tall and that in V_6 they are >6 mm tall before using this criterion.

Repolarization Abnormalities

Typical repolarization abnormalities in the presence of LVH are an ominous sign of end-organ damage. In repolarization abnormalities in LVH, the ST segment and T wave are directed opposite to the dominant QRS waveform in all leads. However, this directional rule does not apply either in the transitional lead (defined as a lead having an R-wave height equal to the S wave depth) or in the transitional zone (defined as leads adjacent to the transitional lead) or one lead to the left in the precordial leads.

Spectrum of Repolarization Abnormalities

The waveforms, as in the following illustration, usually seen in leads I, aVL, V_5, and V_6 but more specifically in leads with dominant R waves, represent hypothetical stages in the progression of LVH.

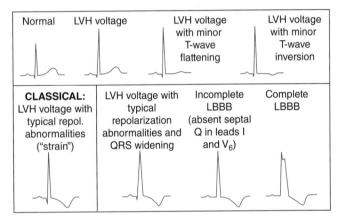

2. Right Ventricular Hypertrophy (RVH)

The ECG is insensitive for the diagnosis of RVH. In 100 cases of RVH from one echocardiography laboratory, only 33% had RAD because of the confounding effects of LV disease. Published electrocardiographic criteria for RVH are listed below, all of which have ≥97% specificity.

With rare exceptions, right atrial enlargement is synonymous with RVH.

Diagnostic Criteria

Recommended criteria for the electrocardiographic diagnosis of RVH are as follows:

1. Right axis deviation (>90 degrees), or
2. An R/S ratio ≥1 in lead V_1 (absent posterior myocardial infarction [MI] or RBBB), or
3. An R wave >7 mm tall in V_1 (not the R′ of RBBB), or
4. An rsR′ complex in V_1 (R′ ≥10 mm), with a QRS duration of <0.12 s (incomplete RBBB), or
5. An S wave >7 mm deep in leads V_5 or V_6 (in the absence of a QRS axis more negative than +30 degrees), or
6. RBBB with RAD (axis derived from first 60 ms of the QRS). (Consider RVH in RBBB if the R/S ratio in lead I is <0.5.)

A variant of RVH (type C loop) may produce a false-positive sign of an anterior myocardial infarction.

Repolarization Abnormalities

The morphology of repolarization abnormalities in RVH is identical to those in LVH, when a particular lead contains tall R waves reflecting the hypertrophied RV or LV. In RVH, these typically occur in leads V_{1-2} or V_3 and in leads aVF and III. This morphology of repolarization abnormalities due to ventricular hypertrophy is illustrated earlier (p. 344). In cases of RVH with massive dilation, all precordial leads may overlie the diseased RV and may exhibit repolarization abnormalities.

H. Low Voltage of the QRS Complex

Low-Voltage Limb Leads Only

Defined as peak-to-peak QRS voltage <5 mm in all limb leads.

Low-Voltage Limb and Precordial Leads

Defined as peak-to-peak QRS voltage <5 mm in all limb leads and <10 mm in all precordial leads. Primary myocardial causes include multiple or massive infarctions; infiltrative diseases such as amyloidosis, sarcoidosis, or hemochromatosis; and myxedema. Extracardiac causes include pericardial effusion, COPD, pleural effusion, obesity, anasarca, and subcutaneous emphysema. When there is COPD, expect to see low voltage in the limb leads as well as in leads V_5 and V_6.

I. Progression of the R Wave in the Precordial Leads

The normal R-wave height increases from V_1 to V_5. The normal R-wave height in V_5 is always taller than that in V_6 because of the attenuating effect of the lungs. The normal R-wave height in lead V_3 is usually >2 mm.

Poor R-Wave Progression

The term "poor R-wave progression" (PRWP) is a nonpreferred term because most physicians use this term to imply the presence of an anterior myocardial infarction, although it may not be present. Other causes of small R waves in the right precordial leads include LVH, LAFB, LBBB, cor pulmonale (with the type C loop of RVH), and COPD.

Reversed R-Wave Progression (RRWP)

Reversed R-wave progression is defined as a loss of R-wave height between leads V_1 and V_2 or between leads V_2 and V_3 or between leads V_3 and V_4. In the absence of LVH, this finding suggests anterior myocardial infarction or precordial lead reversal.

J. Tall R Waves in the Right Precordial Leads

Etiology

Causes of tall R waves in the right precordial leads include the following:

A. Right Ventricular Hypertrophy: This is the most common cause. There is an R/S ratio ≥1 or an R-wave height >7 mm in lead V_1.

B. Posterior Myocardial Infarction: There is an R wave ≥6 mm in lead V_1 or ≥15 mm in lead V_2. One should distinguish the tall R wave of RVH from the tall R wave of posterior myocardial infarction in lead V_1. In RVH, there is a downsloping ST segment and an inverted T wave, usually with right axis deviation. In contrast, in posterior myocardial infarction, there is usually an upright, commonly tall T wave and, because posterior myocardial infarction is usually associated with concomitant inferior myocardial infarction, a left axis deviation.

C. **Right Bundle Branch Block:** The QRS duration is prolonged, and typical waveforms are present (see pp. 333–334).

D. **The WPW Pattern:** Left-sided accessory pathway locations produce prominent R waves with an R/S ratio ≥1 in V_1, with an absent PR segment and initial slurring of the QRS complex, usually best seen in lead V_4.

E. **Rare or Uncommon Causes:** The normal variant pattern of early precordial QRS transition (not uncommon); the reciprocal effect of a deep Q wave in leads V_{5-6} (very rare); Duchenne muscular dystrophy; dextrocardia (very rare); chronic constrictive pericarditis (very rare); and reversal of the right precordial leads.

K. Myocardial Injury, Ischemia, and Infarction

Definitions

A. **Myocardial Infarction:** Pathologic changes in the QRS complex reflect ventricular activation away from the area of infarction.

B. **Myocardial Injury:** Injury always points *outward* from the surface that is injured.
    1. **Epicardial injury:** ST elevation in the distribution of an acutely occluded artery.
    2. **Endocardial injury:** Diffuse ST-segment depression, which is really reciprocal to the primary event, reflected as ST elevation in aVR.

C. **Myocardial Ischemia:** Diffuse ST-segment depression, usually with associated T-wave inversion. It usually reflects subendocardial injury, reciprocal to ST elevation in lead aVR. In ischemia, there may only be inverted T waves with a symmetric, sharp nadir.

D. **Reciprocal Changes:** Passive electrical reflections of a primary event viewed from either the other side of the heart, as in epicardial injury, or the other side of the ventricular wall, as in subendocardial injury.

Steps in the Diagnosis of Myocardial Infarction

The following pages contain a systematic method for the electrocardiographic diagnosis of myocardial injury or infarction, arranged in seven steps. Following the steps will achieve the diagnosis in most cases.

Step 1: Identify the presence of myocardial injury by ST-segment deviations.

Step 2: Identify areas of myocardial injury by assessing lead groupings.

Step 3: Define the primary area of involvement and identify the culprit artery producing the injury.

Step 4: Identify the location of the lesion in the artery to risk stratify the patient.

Step 5: Identify any electrocardiographic signs of infarction found in the QRS complexes.

Step 6: Determine the age of the infarction by assessing the location of the ST segment in leads with pathologic QRS abnormalities.

Step 7: Combine all observations into a final diagnosis.

Steps One and Two

Identify presence of and areas of myocardial injury.

The GUSTO study of patients with ST-segment elevation in two contiguous leads defined four affected areas as set out in Table 7–3.

TABLE 7–3. GUSTO STUDY DEFINITIONS.

Area of ST-Segment Elevation	Leads Defining This Area
Anterior (Ant)	V_{1-4}
Apical (Ap)	V_{5-6}
Lateral (Lat)	I, aVL
Inferior (Inf)	II, aVF, III

Two other major areas of possible injury or infarction were not included in the GUSTO categorization because they do not produce ST elevation in two contiguous standard leads. These are:

1. **Posterior Injury:** The most commonly used sign of posterior injury is ST depression in leads V_{1-3}, but posterior injury may best be diagnosed by obtaining posterior leads V_7, V_8, and V_9.
2. **Right Ventricular Injury:** The most sensitive sign of right ventricular injury, ST-segment elevation ≥1 mm, is found in lead V_4R. A very specific—but insensitive—sign of right ventricular injury or infarction is ST elevation in V_1, with concomitant ST-segment depression in V_2 in the setting of ST elevation in the inferior leads.

Step Three

Identify the primary area of involvement and the culprit artery.

Primary Anterior Area

ST elevation in two contiguous V_{1-4} leads defines a primary anterior area of involvement. The left anterior descending coronary artery (LAD) is the culprit artery. Lateral (I and aVL) and apical (V_5 and V_6) areas are contiguous to anterior (V_{1-4}), so ST elevation in these leads signifies more myocardium at risk and more adverse outcomes.

Primary Inferior Area

ST-segment elevation in two contiguous leads (II, aVF, or III) defines a primary inferior area of involvement. The right coronary artery (RCA) is usually the culprit artery. Apical (V_5 and V_6), posterior (V_{1-3} or V_{7-9}), and right ventricular (V_4R) areas are contiguous to the inferior (II, aVF, and III) area, so ST elevation in these contiguous leads signifies more myocardium at risk and more adverse outcomes.

The Culprit Artery

In the GUSTO trial, 98% of patients with ST-segment elevation in any two contiguous V_{1-4} leads, either alone or with associated changes in leads V_{5-6} or I and aVL, had LAD obstruction. In patients with ST-segment elevation only in leads II, aVF, and III, there was RCA obstruction in 86%.

Primary Anterior Process

Acute occlusion of the LAD produces a sequence of changes in the anterior leads (V_{1-4}).

Earliest Findings

A. **"Hyperacute" Changes:** ST elevation with loss of normal ST-segment concavity, commonly with tall, peaked T waves.

rS complex V_2

B. **Acute Injury:** ST elevation, with the ST segment commonly appearing as if a thumb has been pushed up into it.

rS complex V_2

Evolutionary Changes

A patient who presents to the emergency department with chest pain and T-wave inversion in leads with pathologic Q waves is most likely to be in the evolutionary or completed phase of infarction. Successful revascularization usually causes prompt resolution of the acute signs of injury or infarction and results in the electrocardiographic signs of a fully evolved infarction. The tracing below shows QS complexes in lead V_2.

A. **Development of Pathologic Q Waves (Infarction):** Pathologic Q waves develop within the first hour after onset of symptoms in at least 30% of patients.

QS complexes
V_2 shown

day 1

B. **ST-Segment Elevation Decreases:** T-wave inversion usually occurs in the second 24-hour period after infarction.

day 2

C. **Fully Evolved Pattern:** Pathologic Q waves, ST segment rounded upward, T waves inverted.

chronic

Primary Inferior Process

A primary inferior process usually develops after acute occlusion of the RCA, producing changes in the inferior leads (II, III, and aVF).

Earliest Findings

The earliest findings are of acute injury (ST-segment elevation). The J point may "climb up the back" of the R wave (a), or the ST segment may rise up into the T wave (b).

Evolutionary Changes

ST-segment elevation decreases and pathologic Q waves develop. T-wave inversion may occur in the first 12 hours of an inferior myocardial infarction—in contrast to that in anterior myocardial infarction.

Right Ventricular Injury or Infarction

With right ventricular injury, there is ST-segment elevation, best seen in lead V_4R. With right ventricular infarction, there is a QS complex.

For comparison, the normal morphology of the QRS complex in lead V_4R is shown below. The normal J point averages +0.2 mm.

Posterior Injury or Infarction

Posterior injury or infarction is commonly due to acute occlusion of the left circumflex coronary artery, producing changes in the posterior leads (V_7, V_8, V_9) or reciprocal ST-segment depression in leads V_{1-3}.

Acute Pattern

Acute posterior injury or infarction is shown by ST-segment depression in V_{1-3} and perhaps also V_4, usually with upright (often prominent) T waves.

Chronic Pattern

Chronic posterior injury or infarction is shown by pathologic R waves with prominent tall T waves in leads V_{1-3}.

Step Four

Identify the location of the lesion within the artery to risk stratify the patient.

Primary Anterior Process

Aside from an acute occlusion of the left main coronary artery, occlusion of the proximal LAD conveys the most adverse outcomes. Four electrocardiographic signs indicate proximal LAD occlusion:

1. ST elevation >1 mm in lead I, in lead aVL, or in both
2. New RBBB
3. New LAFB
4. New first-degree AV block

   If the occlusion occurs in a more distal portion of the LAD (after the first diagonal branch and after the first septal perforator), ST-segment elevation is observed in the anterior leads, but the four criteria described above are not seen. In patients with occlusion of the left main coronary artery, diffuse endocardial injury leads to ST-segment elevation in aVR, because this is the only lead that "looks" directly at the ventricular endocardium, and diffuse ST-segment depression is observed in the anterior and inferior leads.

Primary Inferior Process

Nearly 50% of patients with inferior myocardial infarction have distinguishing features that may produce complications or adverse outcomes unless successfully managed:

1. Precordial ST-segment depression in V_{1-3} (suggests concomitant posterior wall involvement);
2. Right ventricular injury or infarction (identifies a proximal RCA lesion);
3. AV block (implies a greater amount of involved myocardium);
4. The sum of ST-segment depressions in leads V_{4-6} exceeds the sum of ST-segment depressions in leads V_{1-3} (suggests multivessel disease).

Reciprocal Changes in the Setting of Acute Myocardial Infarction

ST depressions in leads remote from the primary site of injury are felt to be a purely reciprocal change. With successful reperfusion, the ST depressions usually resolve. If they persist, patients more likely have significant three-vessel disease and so-called ischemia at a distance. Mortality rates are higher in such patients.

Step Five

Identify Electrocardiographic Signs of Infarction in the QRS Complexes

The 12-lead ECG shown below contains numbers corresponding to pathologic widths for Q waves and R waves for selected leads (see Table 7–4 for more complete criteria).

One can memorize the above criteria by mastering a simple scheme of numbers that represents the durations of pathological Q waves or R waves. Begin with lead V_1 and repeat the numbers in the box below in the following order. The numbers increase from "any" to 50.

Any Q wave in lead V_1, for anterior MI
Any Q wave in lead V_2, for anterior MI
Any Q wave in lead V_3, for anterior MI
20 Q wave ≥ 20 ms in lead V_4, for anterior MI
30 Q wave ≥ 30 ms in lead V_5, for apical MI
30 Q wave ≥ 30 ms in lead V_6, for apical MI
30 Q wave ≥ 30 ms in lead I, for lateral MI
30 Q wave ≥ 30 ms in lead aVL, for lateral MI
30 Q wave ≥ 30 ms in lead II, for inferior MI
30 Q wave ≥ 30 ms in lead aVF, for inferior MI
R40 R wave ≥ 40 ms in lead V_1, for posterior MI
R50 R wave ≥ 50 ms in lead V_2, for posterior MI

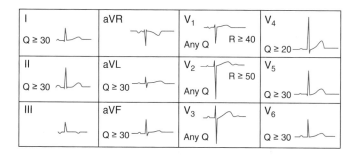

Test Performance Characteristics for Electrocardiographic Criteria in the Diagnosis of Myocardial Infarction

Haisty and coworkers studied 1344 patients with normal hearts documented by coronary arteriography and 837 patients with documented myocardial infarction (366 inferior, 277 anterior, 63 posterior, and 131 inferior and anterior) (Table 7–4). (Patients with LVH, LAFB, LPFB, RVH, LBBB, RBBB, COPD, or WPW patterns were excluded from analysis because these conditions can give false-positive results for myocardial infarction.) Shown below are the sensitivity, specificity, and likelihood ratios for the best-performing infarct criteria. Notice that leads III and aVR are not listed: lead III may normally have a Q wave that is both wide and deep, and lead aVR commonly has a wide Q wave.

TABLE 7–4. DIAGNOSIS OF MYOCARDIAL INFARCTION.

Infarct Location	ECG Lead	Criterion	Sensitivity	Specificity	Likelihood Ratio (+)	Likelihood Ratio (−)
Inferior	II	Q ≥ 30 ms	45	98	22.5	0.6
	aVF	Q ≥ 30 ms	70	94	11.7	0.3
		Q ≥ 40 ms	40	98	20.0	0.6
		R/Q ≤ 1	50	98	25.0	0.5
Anterior	V_1	Any Q	50	97	16.7	0.5
	V_2	Any Q, or R ≤ 0.1 mV and R ≤ 10 ms, or $RV_2 ≤ RV_1$	80	94	13.3	0.2
	V_3	Any Q, or R ≤ 0.2 mV, or R ≤ 20 ms	70	93	10.0	0.3
	V_4	Q ≥ 20 ms	40	92	5.0	0.9
		R/Q ≤ 0.5, or R/S ≤ 0.5	40	97	13.3	0.6
Anterolateral (lateral)						
	I	Q ≥ 30 ms	10	98	5.0	0.9
		R/Q ≤ 1, or R ≤ 2 mm	10	97	3.3	0.9
	aVL	Q ≥ 30 ms	7	97	0.7	1.0
		R/Q ≤ 1	2			
Apical	V_5	Q ≥ 30	5	99	5.0	1.0
		R/Q ≤ 2, or R ≤ 7 mm, or R/S ≤ 2, or notched R	60	91	6.7	0.4
		R/Q ≤ 1, or R/S ≤ 1	25	98	12.5	0.8
	V_6	Q ≤ 30	3	98	1.5	1.0
		R/Q ≤ 3, or R ≤ 6 mm, or R/S ≤ 3, or notched R	40	92	25.0	0.7
		R/Q ≤ 1, or R/S ≤ 1	10	99	10.0	0.9
Posterolateral						
	V_1	R/S ≤ 1	15	97	5.0	0.9
		R ≥ 6 mm, or R ≥ 40 ms	20	93	2.9	0.9
		S ≤ 3 mm	8	97	2.7	0.9
	V_2	R ≥ 15 mm, or R ≥ 50 ms	15	95	3.0	0.9
		R/S ≥ 1.5	10	96	2.5	0.9
		S ≤ 4 mm	2	97	0.7	1.0

Notched R = a notch that begins within the first 40 ms of the R wave; **Q** = Q wave; **R/Q** = ratio of R-wave height to Q-wave depth; **R** = R wave; **R/S ratio** = ratio of R-wave height to S-wave depth; **$RV_2 ≤ RV_1$** = R-wave height in V_2 less than or equal to that in V_1; **S** = S wave. (Reproduced, with permission, from Haisty WK Jr et al. Performance of the automated complete Selvester QRS scoring system in normal subjects and patients with single and multiple myocardial infarctions. J Am Coll Cardiol 1992;19:341.)

TABLE 7–5. MIMICS OF MYOCARDIAL INFARCTION.

Condition	Pseudoinfarct Location
WPW pattern	Any, most commonly inferoposterior or lateral
Hypertrophic cardiomyopathy	Lateral apical (18%), inferior (11%)
LBBB	Anteroseptal, anterolateral, inferior
RBBB	Inferior, posterior (using criteria from leads V_1 and V_2), anterior
LVH	Anterior, inferior
LAFB	Anterior (may cause a tiny Q in V_2)
COPD	Inferior, posterior, anterior
RVH	Inferior, posterior (using criteria from leads V_1 and V_2), anterior, or apical (using criteria for R/S ratios from leads V_{4-6})
Acute cor pulmonale	Inferior, possibly anterior
Cardiomyopathy (nonischemic)	Any, most commonly inferior (with IVCD pattern), less commonly anterior
Chest deformity	Any
Left pneumothorax	Anterior, anterolateral
Hyperkalemia	Any
Normal hearts	Posterior, anterior

COPD = chronic obstructive pulmonary disease; *LAFB* = left anterior fascicular block; *LBBB* = left bundle branch block; *LVH* = left ventricular hypertrophy; *RBBB* = right bundle branch block; *RVH* = right ventricular hypertrophy.

Mimics of Myocardial Infarction

Conditions that can produce pathologic Q waves, ST-segment elevation, or loss of R-wave height in the absence of infarction are set out in Table 7–5.

Step Six

Determine the Age of the Infarction

An **acute infarction** manifests ST-segment elevation in a lead with a pathologic Q wave. The T waves may be either upright or inverted.

An **old** or **age-indeterminate infarction** manifests a pathologic Q wave, with or without slight ST-segment elevation or T-wave abnormalities.

Persistent ST-segment elevation ≥1 mm after a myocardial infarction is a sign of dyskinetic wall motion in the area of infarct. Half of these patients have ventricular aneurysms.

Step Seven

Combine Observations into a Final Diagnosis

There are two possibilities for the major electrocardiographic diagnosis: myocardial infarction or acute injury. If there are pathologic changes in the QRS complex, one should make a diagnosis of myocardial infarction—beginning with the primary area, followed by any contiguous areas—and state the age of the infarction. If there are no pathologic changes in the QRS complex, one should make a diagnosis of acute injury of the affected segments—beginning with the primary area and followed by any contiguous areas.

L. ST Segments

Table 7–6 summarizes major causes of ST-segment elevations. Table 7–7 summarizes major causes of ST-segment depressions or T-wave inversions. The various classes and morphologies of ST–T waves as seen in lead V_2 are shown in Table 7–8.

TABLE 7-6. MAJOR CAUSES OF ST-SEGMENT ELEVATION.

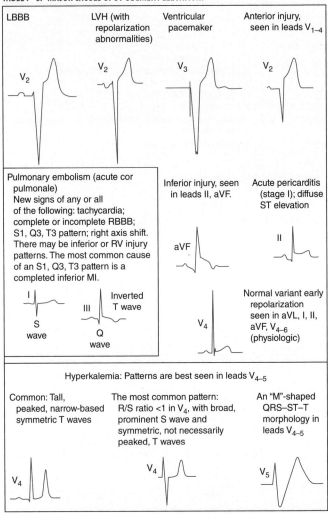

M. U Waves

Normal U Waves

In many normal hearts, low-amplitude positive U waves <1.5 mm tall that range from 160–200 ms in duration are seen in leads V_2 or V_3. Leads V_2 and V_3 are close to the ventricular mass and small-amplitude signals may be best seen in these leads.

Cause: Bradycardias.

TABLE 7–7. MAJOR CAUSES OF ST-SEGMENT DEPRESSION OR T-WAVE INVERSION.

Whenever the ST segment or the T wave is directed counter to an expected repolarization abnormality, consider ischemia, healed MI, or drug or electrolyte effect.	In RBBB, there is an obligatory inverted T wave in right pre-cordial leads with an R′ (usually only in V$_1$) or its equivalent (a qR complex in septal MI). An upright T in these leads suggests completed posterior MI.	Altered depolarization RBBB V$_1$

LBBB	LVH (with repolarization abnormality)	Subarachnoid hemorrhage	RVH
V$_5$	V$_6$	V$_4$	V$_{1-3}$

Inferior subendocardial injury	Posterior subepicardial injury	Anterior subendocardial injury or non-Q wave MI	
II	V$_2$	V$_5$	V$_4$

Hypokalemia	Digitalis	Antiarrhythmics	J point depression secondary to catecholamines
V$_4$	V$_4$	V$_4$	II
When K$^+$ ≤ 2.8, 80% have ECG changes			PR interval and ST segment occupy the same curve

Abnormal U Waves

Abnormal U waves have increased amplitude or merge with abnormal T waves and produce T–U fusion. Criteria include an amplitude ≥1.5 mm or a U wave that is as tall as the T wave that immediately precedes it.

Causes: Hypokalemia, digitalis, antiarrhythmic drugs.

TABLE 7–8. VARIOUS CLASSES AND MORPHOLOGIES OF ST–T WAVES AS SEEN IN LEAD V$_2$.

	Normal ST segment (asymmetric upsloping ST segment with concavity, slight ST-segment elevation)
	Abnormal ST-segment elevation or lack of normal upward concavity in the first part of the ST–T segment (as seen in LVH or acute ischemia or injury)
	ST–T segment typical of acute or recent myocardial infarction, ie, the ST–T segment appears as though a thumb were pushed up into it
	Negative amplitudes in the latter part of the ST–T segment (may be seen in ischemia or old infarction)
	Negative T wave (may be a nonspecific sign, but may be seen in ischemia or old MI)
	Downward sloping in the first part of the ST–T segment (consider ischemia, digitalis, or hypokalemia)
	Flat ST–T segment (a nonspecific sign)

Nonspecific ST-segment or T-wave abnormalities
By definition, nonspecific abnormalities of either the ST segment (ones that are only slightly depressed or abnormal in contour) or T wave (ones that are either 10% the height of the R wave that produced it, or are either flat or slightly inverted) do not conform to the characteristic wave-forms found above or elsewhere.

Inverted U Waves

These are best seen in leads V$_{4-6}$.

Causes: LVH, acute ischemia.

Table 7–9 summarizes various classes and morphologies of ST–T–U abnormalities as seen in lead V$_4$.

N. QT Interval

A prolonged QT interval conveys adverse outcomes. The QT interval is inversely related to the heart rate. QT interval corrections for heart rate often use Bazett's formula, defined as the observed QT interval divided by the square root of the R–R interval in seconds. A corrected QT interval of ≥440 ms is abnormal.

TABLE 7–9. VARIOUS CLASSES AND MORPHOLOGIES OF ST–T–U ABNORMALITIES AS SEEN IN LEAD V$_4$.

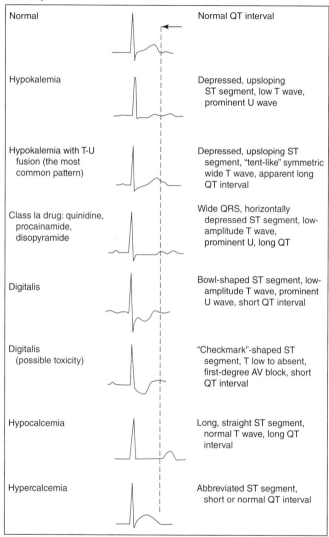

Normal	Normal QT interval
Hypokalemia	Depressed, upsloping ST segment, low T wave, prominent U wave
Hypokalemia with T-U fusion (the most common pattern)	Depressed, upsloping ST segment, "tent-like" symmetric wide T wave, apparent long QT interval
Class Ia drug: quinidine, procainamide, disopyramide	Wide QRS, horizontally depressed ST segment, low-amplitude T wave, prominent U, long QT
Digitalis	Bowl-shaped ST segment, low-amplitude T wave, prominent U wave, short QT interval
Digitalis (possible toxicity)	"Checkmark"-shaped ST segment, T low to absent, first-degree AV block, short QT interval
Hypocalcemia	Long, straight ST segment, normal T wave, long QT interval
Hypercalcemia	Abbreviated ST segment, short or normal QT interval

Use of the QT Nomogram (Hodges Correction)

Measure the QT interval in either lead V$_2$ or V$_3$, where the end of the T wave can usually be clearly distinguished from the beginning of the U wave. If the rate is regular, use the mean rate of the QRS complexes. If the rate is irregular, calculate the rate from the immediately prior R–R cycle, because this cycle determines the subsequent QT interval. Use the numbers you have obtained to classify the QT interval using the nomogram below. Or remember that at heart rates of ≥40 bpm, an observed QT interval ≥480 ms is abnormal.

Prolonged QT Interval

The four major causes of a prolonged QT interval are as follows:

A. Electrolyte Abnormalities: Hypokalemia, hypocalcemia
B. Drugs: Associated with prolonged QT interval and torsades de pointes
Antiarrhythmics:
Class Ia agents: Quinidine, procainamide, disopyramide
Class 1c agent: Flecainide
Class III agents: Amiodarone, N-acetylprocainamide, dofetilide, ibutilide, sotalol
Anticonvulsants: Fosphenytoin, felbamate
Antihistamines: Azelastine, clemastine
Antiinfectives: Amantadine, clarithromycin, chloroquine, foscarnet, erythromycin, itraconazole, halofantrine, ketoconazole, mefloquine, moxifloxacin, pentamidine, quinine, trimethoprim-sulfamethoxazole
Calcium channel blockers: Bepridil, israpidine, nicardipine
Chemotherapeutic agents: Pentamadine, tamoxifen (perhaps anthracyclines)
Diuretics: Indapamide, moexipril/HCTZ
Hormones: Octreotide, vasopressin
Immunosuppressant: Tacrolimus
Migraine serotonin receptor agonists: Naratriptan, sumatriptan, zolmitriptan
Muscle relaxant: Tizanidine
Psychotropic agents: Amitriptyline, chlorpromazine, desipramine, doxepin, fluoxetine, haloperidol, imipramine, lithium pimozide, risperidone, thioridazine, quietiapine, venlafaxine,
Sympathomimetics: Salmeterol
Sedative/hypnotics: Chloral hydrate
Toxins and poisons: Organophosphate insecticides
Miscellaneous: Methadone, prednisone, probucol

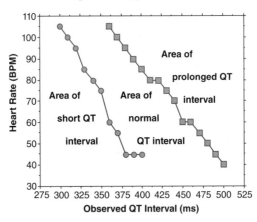

C. Congenital Long QT Syndromes: Though rare, a congenital long QT syndrome should be considered in any young patient who presents with syncope or presyncope.
D. Miscellaneous Causes:
Third-degree and sometimes second-degree AV block
At the cessation of ventricular pacing
LVH (usually minor degrees of lengthening)
Myocardial infarction (in the evolutionary stages where there are marked repolarization abnormalities)
Significant active myocardial ischemia
Cerebrovascular accident (subarachnoid hemorrhage)
Hypothermia

Short QT Interval

The five causes of a short QT interval are hypercalcemia, digitalis, thyrotoxicosis, increased sympathetic tone, and genetic abnormality.

O. Miscellaneous Abnormalities

Right-Left Arm Cable Reversal versus Mirror Image Dextrocardia

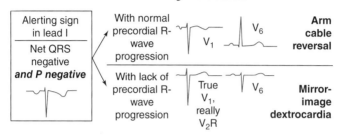

Misplacement of the Right Leg Cable

This error should not occur but it does occur nevertheless. It produces a "far field" signal when one of the bipolar leads (I, II, or III) records the signal between the left and right legs. The lead appears to have no signal except for a tiny deflection representing the QRS complex. There are usually no discernible P waves or T waves. RL–RA cable reversal is shown here.

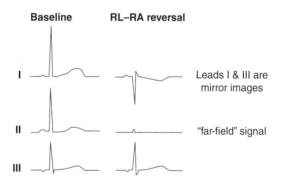

Early Repolarization Normal Variant ST–T Abnormality

Early repolarization normal variant ST–T abnormality

V_4

Tall QRS voltage

Sometimes sharp "fishhook" deformity at the J point, but usually slurring or notching

Prominent T waves

ST-segment elevation, maximal in leads with tallest R waves

Hypothermia

Hypothermia is usually characterized on the ECG by a slow rate, a long QT, and muscle tremor artifact. An Osborn wave is typically present.

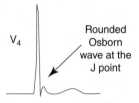

Acute Pericarditis: Stage I (With PR-Segment Abnormalities)

There is usually widespread ST-segment elevation with concomitant PR-segment depression in the same leads. The PR segment in aVR protrudes above the baseline like a knuckle, reflecting atrial injury.

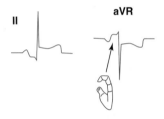

Differentiating Pericarditis From Early Repolarization

Only lead V_6 is used. If the indicated amplitude ratio A/B is ≥25%, suspect pericarditis (shown on left side). If A/B <25%, suspect early repolarization (shown on right side).

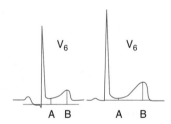

Wolff-Parkinson-White Pattern

The WPW pattern is most commonly manifest as an absent PR segment and initial slurring of the QRS complex in any lead. The lead with the best sensitivity is V_4.

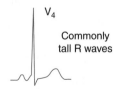

A. Left Lateral Accessory Pathway: This typical WPW pattern mimics lateral or posterior myocardial infarction.

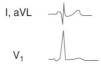

B. Posteroseptal Accessory Pathway: This typical WPW pattern mimics inferoposterior myocardial infarction.

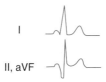

COPD Pattern, Lead II

The P-wave amplitude in the inferior leads is equal to that of the QRS complexes.

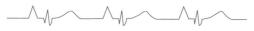

Prominent P waves with low QRS voltage

II. BASIC ECHOCARDIOGRAPHY

Over the last 30 years, echocardiography has arguably transformed cardiology more dramatically than any diagnostic test since the development of the electrocardiogram. With echocardiography, direct visualization of cardiac structures such as the atria, ventricles, valves, great vessels, and pericardium became possible. With the additional application of Doppler principles, besides structural information, echocardiography can now accurately estimate intracardiac blood flow and pressures.

Physical Principles and Standard Views of Echocardiography

In echocardiography, low-intensity, high-frequency signals are produced and, since different tissues have different reflective properties, analysis of the return signals can be collated into a real-time image that can be evaluated by the clinician (Figure 7–6). In addition to providing a two-dimensional image of the heart, application of Doppler principles (named in honor of Christian Johann Doppler, who originally described these principles more than 150 years ago) provides additional information on blood flow. If a sound source is stationary, the wavelength and frequency of the reflected sound are constant, but if the sound source is moving, the wavelength and frequency change. The best everyday example is a siren or train whistle that increases in pitch as it comes toward you and then decreases as it moves away. By evaluating the changes in frequency of the ultrasound sound signal, information on the motion of blood within the cardiac chambers can be obtained.

In transthoracic echocardiography, a hand-held probe that emits and receives the echocardiographic signals is used. Since bone does not allow efficient passage of signals, the heart is best visualized when the transducer is placed between the ribs. As shown in Figure 7–7, two general positions are used: the first, on the anterior chest along the left

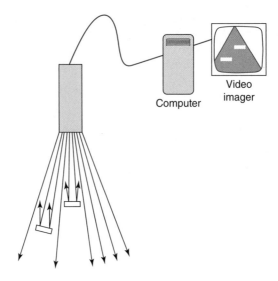

Figure 7–6. Schematic drawing of how echocardiographic images are obtained. A transducer emits sound signals in a pie-slice–shaped pattern. Different types of tissues reflect the signal with varying intensities (eg, blood allows complete transmission of the signal, calcified tissues reflect almost all of the signal, and myocardium has an intermediate value), and the return signal is processed and then displayed on a monitor. (*Adapted, with permission, from Kusumoto FM.* Cardiovascular Pathophysiology. *Hayes Barton Press, 2004.*)

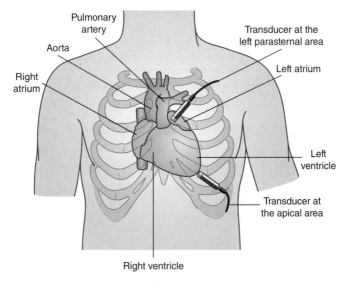

Figure 7–7. For transthoracic echocardiography, two standard transducer positions or windows are used. In the left parasternal view, the transducer is placed just to the left of the sternum in the third or fourth interspace, depending on which interspace provides the best view. In the apical view, the transducer is placed on the anterior left chest below the nipple at the point where the heart can best be palpated (apical impulse). (*Adapted, with permission, from Kusumoto FM.* Cardiovascular Pathophysiology. *Hayes Barton Press, 2004.*)

edge of the sternum (left parasternal view) and the second, lower and more laterally just below the left nipple (called the apical view because when correctly aligned the ventricular apex will be the first cardiac structure visualized). The two views are complementary, since they provide roughly perpendicular imaging planes of the heart.

Figure 7–8 illustrates how a transthoracic echocardiographic image is acquired from the apical position. The probe emits the signal in a pie-slice–shaped plane that is directed to the heart. If the plane is oriented horizontally, the left- and right-sided chambers will be imaged. This view is called the four-chamber view because all four cardiac chambers are observed in the image. The plane can also be oriented vertically (Figure 7–9). In this case, the plane "cuts" the anterior wall and the inferior wall. This view is often called a two-chamber view because the left atrium and the left ventricle are imaged. The right atrium and the right ventricle are no longer in the imaging plane, so they are not seen. Similarly, from the parasternal position, the imaging plane can be oriented to encompass the apex (called the parasternal long-axis view because it follows the axis formed by the mitral valve and the left ventricular apex) or perpendicularly to "cut" the heart like a loaf of bread (short-axis view). In the short-axis view, the left ventricle looks like a doughnut.

An extensive discussion of Doppler flows within the heart is beyond the scope of this introduction to echocardiography, but an example is shown in Figure 7–10. In this example, flow at the mitral valve is evaluated and displayed relative to time. The mitral valve is open

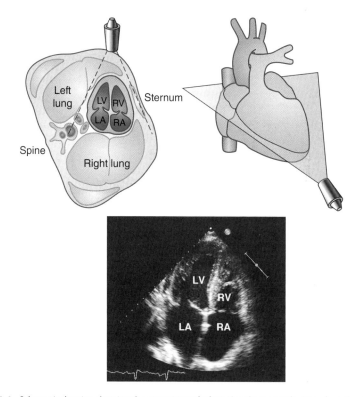

Figure 7–8. Schematic drawing showing the acquisition of a four-chamber view. The transducer is oriented horizontally from the apical position (top right), the imaging plane encompasses all four chambers of the heart (top left) and can be displayed as an echocardiographic image (bottom). ***LA*** = left atrium; ***LV*** = left ventricle; ***RA*** = right atrium; ***RV*** = right ventricle. (Adapted, with permission, from Kusumoto FM. Cardiovascular Pathophysiology. Hayes Barton Press, 2004.)

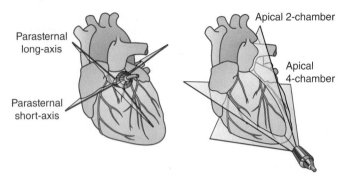

Figure 7–9. From either the parasternal or apical window, the transducer can be oriented with the imaging plane at 90-degree angles. From the parasternal view, the plane can be oriented to simultaneously evaluate the left atrium and the left ventricle (the parasternal long-axis view) or to "cut" the heart like a loaf of bread (the short-axis view). From the apical position, the plane can be horizontal and image all four cardiac chambers simultaneously (also called the four-chamber view) or can be vertical and image only the left ventricle and left atrium (also called the two-chamber view). (*Reproduced, with permission, from Armstrong WF, Ryan T. Feigenbaum's Echocardiography, 7th edition. Lea & Febiger, 2009.*)

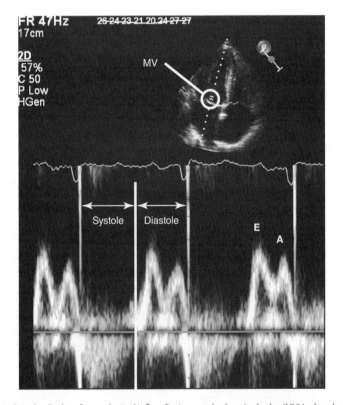

Figure 7–10. Doppler display of normal mitral inflow. During systole, the mitral valve (MV) is closed so that while the left atrium continues to fill from pulmonary venous flow, no blood flows into the left ventricle. During diastole, the mitral valve opens and there is a sudden surge of blood flow into the left ventricle producing the E wave. Filling of the left ventricle slows until left atrial contraction leads to second surge of blood flow and produces an A wave. (*Reproduced with permission of Mayo Foundation for Medical Education and Research.*)

only during diastole, so no signal is recorded during systole. During diastole, mitral flow has two peaks. The first peak is called the E wave (for early filling) and is due to the first rush of blood from the atrium into the left ventricle. (Remember that the left atrium was filling but not emptying during systole.) A second surge of blood flow into the left ventricle is due to left atrial contraction. The second peak is called the A wave because it is due to atrial contraction. The shape and relative size of the E wave and the A wave can be used to evaluate the filling properties of the left ventricle and estimate left atrial pressure.

Normally, the E wave is larger than the A wave, but patients with noncompliant left ventricles and higher left atrial pressures who depend on left atrial filling often have a smaller E wave and a larger A wave. Although only Doppler flow across the mitral valve is described here, it is important to remember that Doppler can be used to evaluate flow across any of the cardiac valves.

Ventricular Anatomy and Function

Transthoracic echocardiography is extremely useful for evaluating left ventricular geometry and function. Figure 7–11 shows parasternal short axis and four-chamber views during systole and diastole in a normal heart. During systole, the left ventricle becomes smaller and the walls thicken. Comparison of systole and diastole provides a visual estimate of overall left ventricular function and also can identify any regional wall motion abnormalities that may be due to coronary artery disease. Overall cardiac function is usually expressed as the ejection fraction—ie, the portion of blood pumped by the left ventricle with each heartbeat. Although methods for quantifying the ejection fraction have been developed, most laboratories estimate the ejection fraction visually by examining the left ventricle in different projections.

In the United States, abnormal left ventricular function is most frequently due to a myocardial infarction from coronary artery disease. In myocardial infarction, reduction

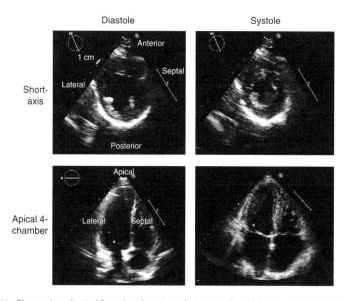

Figure 7–11. Short-axis and apical four-chamber views during systole and diastole in a patient with a normal heart. During systole, the left ventricular cavity shrinks and the left ventricular walls thicken. The four-chamber view during systole shows that the mitral valve (*) is closed and during diastole the mitral valve is open. All echocardiographic displays show 1-cm marks to the side of the image to allow the clinician to estimate ventricular size. (*Reproduced with permission of Mayo Foundation for Medical Education and Research.*)

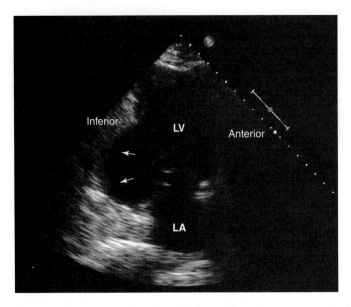

Figure 7-12. A two-chamber view in a patient with an inferior wall left ventricular aneurysm. To obtain a two-chamber view, the imaging plane is vertically oriented (Figure 7-9) so that the anterior wall and inferior wall of the left ventricle are both imaged. The right-sided chambers are not seen because they are out of the imaging plane. In this patient, a prior inferior wall myocardial infarction led to the development of a left ventricular aneurysm (*arrows*). In an aneurysm, development of scar tissue leads to a bulging region in the left ventricle that does not contract. *LA* = *left atrium; LV* = *left ventricle.* (*Reproduced with permission of Mayo Foundation for Medical Education and Research.*)

in blood flow leads to a portion of the heart not receiving enough blood supply, and this in turn leads to decreased muscle function. A regional wall motion abnormality develops, which can be identified as a region of the left ventricle that does not contract and thicken normally.

In some cases, myocardial infarction can lead to a left ventricular aneurysm. Figure 7-12 shows a two-chamber view of a patient with a very large ventricular aneurysm of the inferior wall due to a prior inferior myocardial infarction.

When left ventricular structure or function is abnormal, the term **cardiomyopathy** is usually used. As previously mentioned, myocardial infarction due to coronary artery disease is the most common cause of reduced left ventricular function in the US, and this condition is specifically described as an ischemic cardiomyopathy. In some cases, reduced left ventricular function is due to causes other than coronary artery disease, such as a viral infection or drug toxicity, although most often no specific cause can be identified (this condition is often called **idiopathic dilated cardiomyopathy**). When the heart is enlarged and has reduced function and the patient has no evidence of coronary artery disease, the term **nonischemic cardiomyopathy** is often used. In advanced cases of nonischemic cardiomyopathy, the left ventricle is often enlarged and has a more spherical shape (Figure 7-13).

In hypertrophic cardiomyopathy, a genetic abnormality (usually involving one of the components of the sarcomere) leads to abnormal thickening of the left ventricle (Figure 7-14). Although the ejection fraction is usually normal in patients with hypertrophic cardiomyopathy, abnormal filling of the left ventricle can lead to fluid accumulation in the lungs and shortness of breath. Normally, the left ventricle is less than 1 cm thick. As shown in Figure 7-14, echocardiography is extremely useful for identifying patients with abnormally thick ventricular walls.

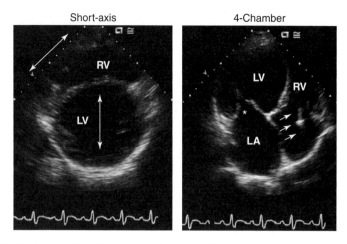

Figure 7–13. Short-axis and four-chamber views of a patient with a nonischemic cardiomyopathy are shown. Double-headed arrows in the short-axis view emphasize the enlarged left ventricular chamber size (almost 6 cm in diameter) and in the four-chamber view, the spherical shape of the left ventricle (LV) can be observed (compare with Figure 7–11). Also in the four-chamber view, a defibrillator lead can be observed in the right ventricle (RV; *arrows*). The (*) marks the mitral valve. **LA** = *left atrium.* (*Reproduced with permission of Mayo Foundation for Medical Education and Research.*)

The echocardiogram also can be used to identify a pericardial effusion, a condition in which fluid accumulates in the pericardial space (Figure 7–15). If the effusion is large enough or accumulates rapidly, the elevated intrapericardial pressure can prevent normal filling of the left and right ventricles. This condition is called **pericardial tamponade**. Even if the ventricles contract normally, inadequate filling can lead to extreme reduction in the amount of blood expelled by the ventricles with each heartbeat (stroke volume), which can lead to profound hypotension. Echocardiography has emerged as the best test for rapidly determining whether a significant pericardial effusion is present.

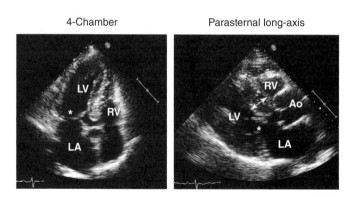

Figure 7–14. An echocardiogram (four-chamber and parasternal long-axis views) from a patient with a hypertrophic cardiomyopathy. The interventricular septum separating the left ventricle (LV) and right ventricle (RV) is abnormally thick (*double headed arrow*). The (*) marks the mitral valve. **LA** = *left atrium; Ao* = *aorta.* (*Reproduced with permission of Mayo Foundation for Medical Education and Research.*)

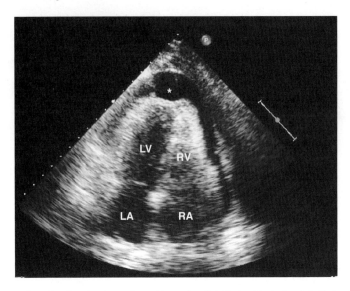

Figure 7–15. A four-chamber view in a patient with a pericardial effusion. The pericardial effusion (*) is identified as a dark echo-free area surrounding the heart due to abnormal fluid accumulation. *LA* = *left atrium;* *LV* = *left ventricle;* *RA* = *right atrium;* *RV* = *right ventricle.* (*Reproduced with permission of Mayo Foundation for Medical Education and Research.*)

Valvular Anatomy and Function

The echocardiogram is an excellent diagnostic test to evaluate the valves of the heart. In general, abnormal valve function can be classified as **stenosis,** in which forward flow of blood through the valve is restricted, or **regurgitation,** in which blood "leaks backward" because the valve leaflets do not come together and close normally. Generally, the severity of valve stenosis or regurgitation is assessed by echocardiography Doppler evaluation. Valvular regurgitation produces a high-velocity jet that can be identified within the chamber into which the blood leaks back. For example, **mitral regurgitation** can be identified by a high-velocity jet within the left atrium and the area of the high-velocity jet correlates roughly with the severity of the valvular abnormality.

Aortic Valve

Narrowing of the aortic valve is one of the most common valvular abnormalities encountered clinically. Normally, the aortic valve has three leaflets, but in some patients only two leaflets are present. During childhood and early adulthood, the valve functions normally, but a harsh murmur due to turbulent blood flow during ventricular contraction (systole) is often heard. However, in the fifth or sixth decade of life, progressive turbulent flow often leads to thickening of the aortic valve leaflets, stenosis of the aortic valve, and reduction in stroke volume.

Aortic stenosis can also develop in patients with trileaflet aortic valves. In this case, progressive calcification of the leaflets presents as aortic stenosis in the seventh or eighth decade. On echocardiography, the aortic valve appears "bright" or echogenic as a result of calcium deposition that almost completely reflects the ultrasound signal (Figure 7–16). Aortic stenosis produces a high-velocity jet across the aortic valve into the aorta (caused by blood being forcefully expelled across the narrow opening), which can be identified by Doppler echocardiography. The velocity of the jet can be used to estimate the severity of the gradient; the normal velocity of blood at the aortic valve is 1 m/s, but in severe aortic

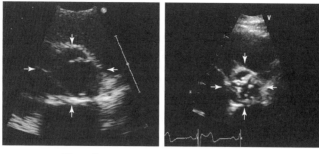

Normal   Aortic stenosis

Figure 7–16. Echocardiographic images of a normal aortic valve and an aortic valve associated with severe aortic stenosis. Although both aortic valves have three leaflets, in the patient with aortic stenosis the leaflets are calcified. In both examples, the aortic valve is outlined by the four arrows. (*Reproduced with permission of Mayo Foundation for Medical Education and Research.*)

stenosis, velocities of 4–5 m/s can be measured at the aortic valve. In general, the higher the velocity recorded across the aortic valve, the larger the pressure gradient between the left ventricle and the aorta and the more severe the aortic stenosis.

If the aortic valve does not close normally, blood from the aorta can leak back into the left ventricle. This condition is called **aortic regurgitation,** in which blood flows backward from the aorta into the left ventricle. Aortic regurgitation can develop with infection of the aortic valve (endocarditis), in the presence of a bicuspid aortic valve, or with any process that causes enlargement of the aortic root (and consequent enlargement of the ring that provides the support for the valve leaflets). The turbulent flow from aortic regurgitation occurs in diastole, and consequently a murmur is heard during diastole. Doppler echocardiography is useful for evaluating the severity of aortic regurgitation. Aortic regurgitation is recorded as a turbulent jet within the left ventricle, emanating from the aortic valve during diastole (Figure 7–17).

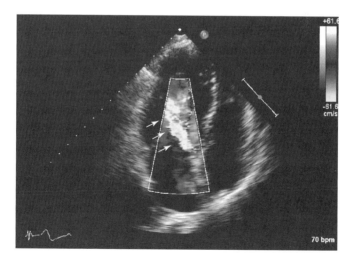

Figure 7–17. A four-chamber view of a patient with severe aortic regurgitation. During diastole, a large turbulent jet is present (*arrows*), emanating from the aortic valve. (*Reproduced with permission of Mayo Foundation for Medical Education and Research.*)

Mitral Valve

The mitral valve can be easily evaluated by transthoracic echocardiography. Abnormal function can be due to either mitral stenosis or mitral regurgitation.

Mitral stenosis is almost always due to rheumatic heart disease related to untreated streptococcal infections (see Chapter 5) and can be identified by restricted opening of the mitral valve leaflets on echocardiography (Figure 7–18). Of all the valvular lesions, mitral stenosis is the least commonly encountered in developed countries but still remains a common problem in many parts of the developing world.

Mitral regurgitation is much more commonly observed than mitral stenosis and can be due to severe mitral valve prolapse, endocarditis of the mitral valve, myocardial ischemia, or rheumatic valvular disease. As with aortic regurgitation, Doppler techniques are used to identify the high-velocity turbulent jet. However, in mitral regurgitation, the high-velocity jet is observed in the left atrium, emanates from the mitral valve, and occurs during ventricular contraction (systole). An example of an echocardiogram from a patient with mitral regurgitation is shown in Figure 7–19. A wide-necked jet that encompasses a larger portion of the left atrium is characteristic of severe mitral regurgitation.

Tricuspid Valve

In tricuspid regurgitation, a regurgitant jet is present in the right atrium, emanating from the tricuspid valve (Figure 7–20). As with mitral regurgitation, the jet is observed during systole. Doppler evaluation of the tricuspid valve is frequently used to assess right-sided cardiac pressures. The relative pressure difference between two chambers can be estimated by using a simplified formula of the Bernoulli equation:

$$\Delta P = 4V^2$$

where ΔP is the pressure difference in mm Hg and V is the velocity between two cardiac chambers in m/s. Figure 7–21 shows a Doppler signal from the tricuspid valve in a patient with severe tricuspid regurgitation. Using the simplified Bernoulli equation, the difference between right atrial pressure and right ventricular pressure reaches 56 mm Hg during systole. Since normal right ventricular peak systolic pressure ranges from 15 to 30 mm Hg, the presence of elevated right-sided cardiac pressure can thus be readily identified.

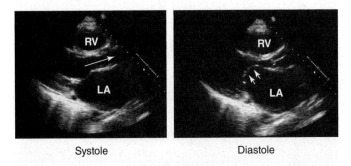

Systole   Diastole

Figure 7–18. A parasternal long-axis view of a patient with severe mitral stenosis due to rheumatic heart disease. During systole, the mitral valve is closed and blood is expelled through the open aortic valve (*single arrow*). During diastole, opening of the mitral valve is restricted, and a characteristic bowing of the mitral valve (*arrows*) is observed. ***LA*** = left atrium; ***RV*** = right ventricle. (*Reproduced with permission of Mayo Foundation for Medical Education and Research.*)

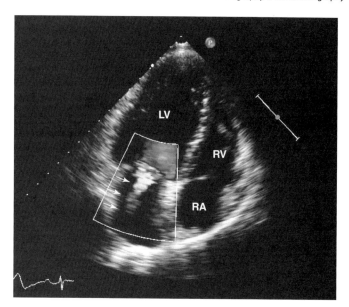

Figure 7–19. A four-chamber view of a patient with mitral regurgitation. A high-velocity jet is observed in the left atrium (*arrows*), emanating from the mitral valve. A wide-necked jet that fills a large portion of the left atrium suggests severe mitral regurgitation. ***LV*** = *left ventricle;* ***RA*** = *right atrium;* ***RV*** = *right ventricle.* (*Reproduced with permission of Mayo Foundation for Medical Education and Research.*)

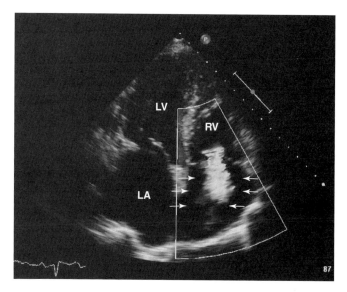

Figure 7–20. A four-chamber view of a patient with severe tricuspid regurgitation. The high-velocity jet (*arrows*) emanates from the tricuspid valve. ***LA*** = *left atrium;* ***LV*** = *left ventricle;* ***RV*** = *right ventricle.* (*Reproduced with permission of Mayo Foundation for Medical Education and Research.*)

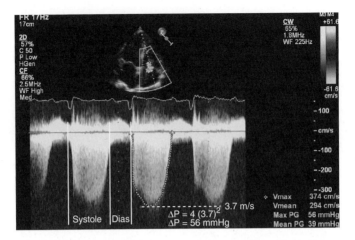

Figure 7–21. A Doppler signal due to the severe tricuspid regurgitation shown in Figure 7–20. In tricuspid regurgitation, the high-velocity flow is recorded during systole and not in diastole (Dias). Since the jet of tricuspid regurgitation is flowing away from the transducer, a negative signal is recorded (contrast this to the normal mitral inflow signal shown in Figure 7–10). The simplified Bernoulli equation can be used to estimate the pressure difference between the right ventricle and right atrium from the peak velocity recorded from the tricuspid regurgitation signal (3.74 m/s or 374 cm/s).

Transesophageal Echocardiography and Intracardiac Echocardiography

In transthoracic echocardiography, the ultrasound transducers are mounted on a hand-held probe that is manipulated on the surface of the chest to obtain the desired images. In transesophageal echocardiography, the transducer can be placed on a probe designed to enter the esophagus (Figure 7–22). In intracardiac echocardiography, the transducer can be placed on a catheter designed to enter the heart itself via one of the central veins (usually the femoral vein) and advanced via the inferior vena cava into the heart. Imaging from a transducer located adjacent to the heart (transesophageal echocardiography) or from inside the heart (intracardiac echocardiography) produces images with exquisite detail and resolution. Figure 7–23 is a transesophageal echocardiogram showing a large clot in the left atrial appendage in a patient with atrial fibrillation.

REFERENCES

Bernath P, Kusumoto FM. *ECG Interpretation for Everyone: An On-The-Spot Guide.* Wiley-Blackwell, 2014.

Boyd AC et al. Principles of transthoracic echocardiographic evaluation. Nat Rev Cardiol 2015;12:426. [PMID: 25917151]

Chan KH et al. Tachycardia, both narrow and broad complex: what are the mechanisms? How to treat? J Cardiovasc Electrophysiol 2015 Apr 29. [Epub ahead of print] [PMID: 25929746]

Collins NA et al. Reconsidering the effectiveness and safety of carotid sinus massage as a therapeutic intervention in patients with supraventricular tachycardia. Am J Emerg Med 2015;33:807. [PMID: 25907500]

Colucci RA et al. Common types of supraventricular tachycardia: diagnosis and management. Am Fam Physician 2010;82:942. [PMID: 20949888]

Couderc JP et al. Short and long QT syndromes: does QT length really matter? J Electrocardiol 2010;43:396. [PMID: 20728018]

deSouza IS et al. Differentiating types of wide-complex tachycardia to determine appropriate treatment in the emergency department. Emerg Med Pract 2015;17:1. [PMID: 26308484]

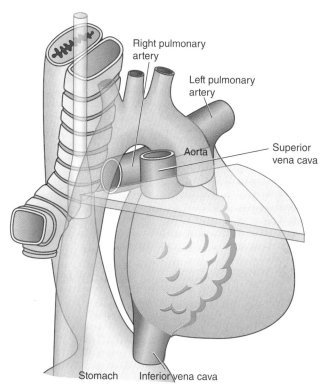

Figure 7–22. Schematic of transesophageal echocardiography. Since the esophagus lies directly behind the left atrium, relatively posterior structures such as the left atrium, right atrium, pulmonary veins, vena cava, and the valves can be clearly seen. (*Reproduced with permission from Kusumoto FM.* Cardiovascular Pathophysiology. *Hayes Barton Press, 1999.*)

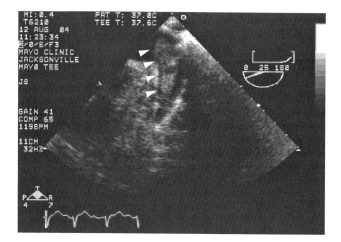

Figure 7–23. Transesophageal echocardiography showing a large clot in the left atrial appendage (arrowheads) in a patient with atrial fibrillation. (*Reproduced with permission of Mayo Foundation for Medical Education and Research.*)

Estes EH Jr et al. The electrocardiogram in left ventricular hypertrophy: past and future. J Electrocardiol 2009;42:589. [PMID: 19643433]

Haqqani HM et al. Using the 12-lead ECG to localize the origin of atrial and ventricular tachycardias: part 2—ventricular tachycardia. J Cardiovasc Electrophysiol 2009;20:825. [PMID: 19302478]

Hudaverdi M et al. Echocardiography for the clinician: a practical update. Intern Med J 2010;40:476. [PMID: 20059600]

Jacobson JT et al. Management of ventricular arrhythmias in structural heart disease. Postgrad Med 2015;127:549. [PMID: 25971427]

Johnson JN et al. QTc: how long is too long? Br J Sports Med 2009;43:657. [PMID: 19734499]

Kumar A et al. Acute coronary syndromes: diagnosis and management, part I. Mayo Clin Proc 2009;84:917. [PMID: 19797781]

Kumar A et al. Acute coronary syndromes: diagnosis and management, part II. Mayo Clin Proc 2009;84:1021. [PMID: 19880693]

Kusumoto FM. *ECG Interpretation: From Pathophysiology to Clinical Application.* Springer Science, 2009.

Littrell R et al. Implications for your practice: important changes in the 2014 guideline for the management of patients with atrial fibrillation. Postgrad Med. 2015;127:535. [PMID: 25812591]

Moukabary T et al. Management of atrial fibrillation. Med Clin North Am 2015;99:781. [PMID: 26042882]

Nikus K et al. Electrocardiographic classification of acute coronary syndromes: a review by a committee of the International Society for Holter and Non-Invasive Electrocardiology. J Electrocardiol 2010;43:91. [PMID: 19913800]

Oh JK, Seward JB, Tajik AJ. *The Echo Manual*, 3rd ed. Wolters Kluwer, 2006.

Sawhney NS et al. Diagnosis and management of typical atrial flutter. Cardiol Clin 2009;27:55. [PMID: 19111764]

Smith GD et al. Effectiveness of the Valsalva manoeuvre for reversion of supraventricular tachycardia. Cochrane Database Syst Rev 2015;2:CD009502. [PMID: 25922864]

8

Diagnostic Tests in Differential Diagnosis

Stephen J. McPhee, MD, Chuanyi Mark Lu, MD, and Diana Nicoll, MD, PhD, MPA

HOW TO USE THIS SECTION

This section shows how diagnostic tests can be used in differential diagnosis and difficult diagnostic challenges. Material is presented in tabular format, and contents are listed in alphabetical order by disease topic.

Abbreviations used throughout this section include the following:

N = Normal
Abn = Abnormal
Pos = Positive
Neg = Negative
↑ = Increased or high
↓ = Decreased or low
Occ = Occasional

Contents (Tables)   *Pages*

TABLE 8–1. ACID–BASE DISTURBANCE: LABORATORY CHARACTERISTICS OF PRIMARY OR SINGLE ACID–BASE DISTURBANCE.

Disturbance	Acute Primary Change	Partial Compensatory Response	Arterial pH	Serum [K$^+$] (meq/L)	Anion Gap[1] (Unmeasured Anions) (meq/L)	Clinical Features
Normal	None	None	7.35–7.45	3.5–5.0	6–12	None
Respiratory acidosis	Pco$_2$ ↑ (co$_2$ retention)	↑ HCO$_3^-$	↓	↑	N	Dyspnea, polypnea, respiratory outflow obstruction, ↑ anterior-posterior chest diameter, rales, wheezes. In severe cases, stupor, disorientation, coma.
Respiratory alkalosis	Pco$_2$ ↓ (co$_2$ depletion)	↓ HCO$_3^-$	↑	↓	N or ↓	Anxiety, occasional complaint of breathlessness, frequent sighing, lungs usually clear to examination, positive Chvostek and Trousseau signs.
Metabolic acidosis	HCO$_3^-$ depletion	↓ Pco$_2$	↓	↑ or ↓	N or ↑	Weakness, air hunger, Kussmaul respiration, dry skin and mucous membranes, poor skin turgor. In severe cases, coma, hypotension, death.
Metabolic alkalosis	HCO$_3^-$ retention	↑ Pco$_2$	↑	↓	N	Weakness, positive Chvostek and Trousseau signs, hyporeflexia.

[1]Anion gap = Na$^+$ − (HCO$_3^-$ + Cl$^-$) = 6–12. Reference ranges for anion gap may vary based on differing laboratory methods. In hypoalbuminemia, a 2 meq/L decrease in anion gap will occur for every 1 g/dL decline in serum albumin.

Reproduced with permission from Papadakis MA, McPhee SJ, Rabow MW. Current Medical Diagnosis & Treatment 2017. 56th ed. McGraw-Hill, 2017.

TABLE 8–2. ANEMIA: DIAGNOSIS OF COMMON ANEMIAS BASED ON RED CELL INDICES.

Type of Anemia	MCV (fL)	MCHC (g/dL)	Common Causes	Common Laboratory Abnormalities	Clinical Findings
Microcytic, hypochromic	<80	<32	Iron deficiency	Hypochromic red cells, elliptocytes, low reticulocyte count, low serum ferritin, low serum iron and absent bone marrow iron, high TIBC, high serum/plasma soluble transferrin receptor (sTfR).	Mucositis, brittle nails, bleeding (eg, positive fecal occult blood, menorrhagia), esophageal webs, pica.
		Variable, but usually <32	Thalassemias	Abnormal red cell morphology, normal to high RBC count, elevated reticulocyte count, normal serum iron parameters, abnormal hemoglobin electrophoresis, high hemoglobin A_2 in β-thalassemia minor.	Asian, African, or Mediterranean descent. Splenomegaly, growth failure, bony deformities.
		<32	Chronic lead poisoning	Basophilic stippling of RBCs, elevated blood lead and free erythrocyte protoporphyrin levels.	Peripheral neuropathy (eg, wrist drop), abdominal pain, learning disorders (in children), headache, history of exposure to lead.
		Variable, but usually < 32	Sideroblastic anemia	High serum iron, high transferrin saturation, erythroid hyperplasia with ring sideroblasts in bone marrow.	Dimorphic red cell population with hypochromic red cells on blood smear, family history.
Normocytic, normochromic	80–100	32–36	Acute blood loss	Fecal occult blood test positive if GI bleeding is the underlying cause. High reticulocyte count, thrombocytosis (variable).	Recent blood loss.
		32–36	Hemolysis	Haptoglobin low or absent, high reticulocyte count, high indirect bilirubin, high serum LDH, spherocytes, schistocytes, or "bite" cells on blood smear.	Hemoglobinuria, splenomegaly.
		32–36	Chronic disease[1]	Low serum iron, TIBC low or low normal, normal sTfR, normal or high ferritin, low reticulocyte count, normal or high bone marrow iron stores with rare or no sideroblasts.	Depends on cause, typically chronic inflammatory conditions.

	MCV	MCHC	Peripheral Smear and Other Laboratory Tests	Associated Conditions
Macrocytic, normochromic	>101[2]			
Vitamin B$_{12}$ deficiency		32–36	Hypersegmented PMNs, macro-ovalocytes, neutropenia and/or thrombocytopenia, low serum or plasma vitamin B$_{12}$ levels, high serum/urine MMA, achlorhydria and high serum gastrin, and high serum LDH.	Peripheral neuropathy, glossitis, anorexia and diarrhea.
Folate deficiency		32–36	Hypersegmented PMNs, macro-ovalocytes, neutropenia and/or thrombocytopenia, low serum and red cell folate levels, high homocysteine level.	Alcoholism, tropical sprue, malnutrition, antifolate agents (eg, trimethoprim-sulfamethoxazole, methotrexate, others).
Liver disease		32–36	Decreased platelets; MCV usually <120 fL; normal serum vitamin B$_{12}$ and folate levels; abnormal liver function tests.	Signs of liver disease, alcohol abuse.
Myelodysplastic syndrome		Usually 32–36	MCV usually <120 fL, low reticulocyte count, may have neutropenia and/or thrombocytopenia, pseudo-Pelgeroid neutrophils, unilineage or multilineage dysplasia in the marrow, blasts in the marrow may increase, abnormal cytogenetics.	Chronic anemia with or without pancytopenia.
Reticulocytosis		32–36 or >36	Marked (>15%) reticulocytosis.	Variable, including acute hemorrhage or hemolysis.

[1]May be microcytic, hypochromic.

[2]If MCV >120–130 fL, vitamin B$_{12}$ or folate deficiency is most likely.

MCV = mean corpuscular volume; **MMA** = methylmalonic acid; **PMN** = polymorphonuclear cell; **TIBC** = total iron-binding capacity, serum.

Modified, with permission, from Stone CK, Humphries RL (editors). Current Diagnosis & Treatment: Emergency Medicine, 7th ed. Copyright © 2011 by The McGraw-Hill Companies, Inc.

TABLE 8–3. ANEMIA: LABORATORY EVALUATION OF MICROCYTIC, HYPOCHROMIC ANEMIAS

Diagnosis	MCV (fL)	Serum Iron (mcg/dL)	Iron-binding Capacity (mcg/dL)	Transferrin Saturation (%)	Serum Ferritin (mcg/L)	Soluble Transferrin Receptor (mg/L)	Bone Marrow Iron Stores
Normal	80–100	50–175	250–460	16–55	30–300	2.0–4.5	Present
Iron deficiency anemia	↓	<30	↑	<16	<45[1]	↑	Absent
Anemia of chronic disease[2]	N or ↓	↓	N or ↓	N or ↓	N or ↑	2.0–4.5	Present
Thalassemia	↓	N	N	N	N	↑	Present

MCV = mean corpuscular volume

[1]*Ferritin levels of 25–45 have a likelihood ratio of 2.0 for iron deficiency anemia.*

[2]*May be normochromic, normocytic*

TABLE 8–4.   ANTICOAGULANTS: MECHANISM OF ACTION, CLINICAL INDICATIONS, AND LABORATORY MONITORING.

Anticoagulant Route of Administration	Mechanism of Action	Route of Elimination	Clinical Indications and Usage	Laboratory Monitoring
Warfarin Oral	Warfarin inhibits vitamin K epoxide reductase (VKOR) (specifically the VKORC1 subunit) and thereby diminishes available vitamin K in the tissues. As a result, warfarin inhibits the vitamin K–dependent synthesis of coagulation factors II, VII, IX and X, as well as the regulatory factors, protein C and protein S. Warfarin is slow-acting and has a long half-life. Its activity is determined partially by genetic factors (eg, polymorphisms in the VKORC1 and CYP2C9 genes).	Metabolized in the liver (CYP2C9); Excreted via the urine and feces T1/2: 20–60 hours (mean 40 hours)	Long-term prophylaxis or treatment of venous thrombosis and systemic embolism in patients with: • Atrial fibrillation or artificial heart valves • Deep venous thrombosis (DVT) and/or pulmonary embolism (PE) • Antiphospholipid antibody syndrome Warfarin is contraindicated in pregnant women.	• PT/INR (most commonly used) • Factor assays (e.g., FVII, FX) • Chromogenic factor Xa assay The chromogenic factor Xa assay is useful if patients have documented lupus anticoagulant (LAC) interference.
Heparin, unfractionated (UFH) Intravenous (infusion); Subcutaneous (injection)	Heparin is a glycosaminoglycan composed of chains of alternating residues of D-glucosamine and iduronic acid. Heparin binds to antithrombin (AT) and enhances its function of inactivating coagulation factors including thrombin and factor Xa. For inhibition of thrombin, heparin must bind to both the coagulation enzyme and AT, whereas binding to the enzyme factor is not required for inhibition of FXa.	Metabolized in the liver; may be partially metabolized in the reticuloendothelial system T1/2: 1–2 hours	Short-term anticoagulation use (prophylaxis and treatment) in hospitalized patients with: • Acute coronary syndrome (eg, unstable angina/non-STEMI) • Venous thromboembolic disorders (DVT and/or PE) • Cardiopulmonary bypass for open heart surgery • Hemodialysis procedure • Atrial fibrillation • Stroke (ischemic) • ECMO circuit for extracorporeal life support • Indwelling central or peripheral venous catheters (to maintain patency)	• aPTT (most commonly used) • Chromogenic anti-Xa assay Institutional aPTT-based heparin therapeutic interval must be used. The chromogenic anti-Xa assay should be used if aPTT is unreliable (eg, LAC interference, FXII deficiency, acute illness with elevated FVIII and/or fibrinogen, liver dysfunction, consumptive coagulopathy).

(Continued)

TABLE 8–4. ANTICOAGULANTS: MECHANISM OF ACTION, CLINICAL INDICATIONS, AND LABORATORY MONITORING (*CONTINUED*).

Anticoagulant Route of Administration	Mechanism of Action	Route of Elimination	Clinical Indications and Usage	Laboratory Monitoring
Heparin, low-molecular weight (LMWH) (eg, Enoxaparin, Dalteparin) Subcutaneous (injection), occasionally intravenous (bolus)	LMWH consists of heparin-derived fragments (about one-third of the size of heparin), which mainly inactivate FXa via AT. It has reduced ability to inactivate thrombin because the smaller fragments cannot bind simultaneously to both AT and thrombin.	Metabolized in the liver (60–90%); excreted via urine (10–40%) T1/2: 4–7 hours	• Prophylaxis of DVT and thromboembolism in hospitalized patients who undergo abdominal surgery, hip or knee replacement surgery and acutely ill patients with severely restricted mobility • Inpatient treatment of acute DVT with or without PE • Outpatient treatment of acute DVT with or without PE • Prophylaxis of ischemic complications in unstable angina and non-Q-wave MI • Treatment of acute STEMI, with or without subsequent percutaneous coronary intervention (PCI)	• Chromogenic anti-Xa assay (4 hours after subcutaneous administration) Monitoring is only required for patients with weight extremes (morbid obesity or cachexia), pregnancy, old age, neonates, renal insufficiency, bleeding, or thrombosis while receiving therapy.
Fondaparinux Subcutaneous (injection)	Fondaparinux is a synthetic pentasaccharide which is identical to a sequence of five monomeric sugar units in heparin. Like LMWH, fondaparinux inactivates FXa via AT. It does not inactivate thrombin.	Excreted unchanged via urine T1/2: 17–21 hours	• Prophylaxis of DVT in patients who have had orthopedic surgery (hip fracture, hip or knee replacement), or abdominal surgery • Treatment of acute DVT and PE when administered in conjunction with warfarin • Treatment of acute heparin-induced thrombocytopenia (HIT) (off label usage) Fondaparinux is contraindicated in patients with severe renal impairment or body weight less than 50 kilograms.	• Chromogenic anti-Xa assay (3 hours after subcutaneous administration) Monitoring is only required for patients with weight extremes (morbid obesity or cachexia), pregnancy, old age, neonates, renal insufficiency, bleeding, or thrombosis while receiving therapy.
Argatroban Intravenous (infusion)	Argatroban is a small molecule direct thrombin inhibitor (DTI). It interacts with the active site of thrombin, but does not make contact with the exosites I or II of thrombin.	Metabolized in the liver T1/2: 40–50 minutes. Because of its hepatic metabolism, it may be used in patients with renal dysfunction	• Prophylaxis and treatment of thrombosis in patients with HIT • Anticoagulation use during PCI in patients who have HIT or are at risk for developing HIT	• aPTT Obtain baseline aPTT, monitor aPTT every 2 hours until therapeutic range of 1.5–3.0 times baseline aPTT achieved.
Bivalirudin Intravenous (injection and infusion)	Bivalirudin is a synthetic hirudin analog, which acts as a specific and reversible DTI. It binds to thrombin via direct interactions with the active site and the exosite of thrombin. It inhibits both circulating and clot-bound thrombin.	Predominantly proteolysis (non-organ elimination), plus renal excretion T1/2: approximately 25 minutes	• Anticoagulation use in patients with unstable angina undergoing percutaneous transluminal coronary angioplasty (PTCA) • Anticoagulation use in patients with or at risk of HIT undergoing PCI • Prophylaxis and treatment of thrombosis in patients with HIT (off-label usage)	• ACT The ACT should be used in patients with renal impairment. ACT >300 seconds indicate adequate anticoagulation.

Drug	Mechanism	Pharmacokinetics	Indications	Monitoring
Dabigatran Oral	Dabigatran is an orally active DTI. Dabigatran etexilate is a prodrug, which needs to be converted in the liver to the active compound that binds directly to thrombin with high affinity and specificity.	Excreted unchanged via kidney T1/2: 12–17 hours. (The drug is not recommended for use in patients with a GFR less than 15 mL/min or in patients who are hemodialysis-dependent.)	• Prophylaxis of stroke in patients with non-valvular atrial fibrillation • Long-term treatment of DVT with or without PE to reduce risk of recurrence • Acute treatment of DVT with or without PE (only after an initial 5-day treatment with a parenteral anticoagulant) • Prophylaxis of thromboembolic disease following hip or knee replacement surgery (European Union and Canada only)	Monitoring is not usually required. If monitoring is indicated, obtain plasma level of the drug. The aPTT is insensitive to dabigatran at higher drug levels. The TT is very sensitive to dabigatran, and a normal TT excludes significant dabigatran effect but is not useful for monitoring or dose adjustment.
Rivaroxaban Oral	Rivaroxaban is an oxazolidinone derivative optimized for inhibiting both free FXa and FXa bound in the prothrombinase complex. It is a highly selective direct FXa inhibitor with oral bioavailability and rapid onset of action. It blocks the active site of FXa and does not require a cofactor.	About two-thirds metabolized in liver and one-third excreted unchanged via kidney T1/2: 5–9 hours	• Prophylaxis of stroke and systemic embolism in non-valvular atrial fibrillation • Treatment of acute DVT with or without PE • Long-term treatment of DVT with or without PE to reduce risk of recurrence • Prophylaxis of DVT following hip or knee replacement surgery	• Chromogenic anti-Xa assay Routine monitoring is not required. Monitoring may be helpful under certain conditions (e.g., renal failure, older age, acute illness, during bleeding or thrombotic episodes, or to verify adherence to therapy).
Apixaban Oral	Apixaban is an oral, reversible, and selective active site inhibitor of FXa. It does not require a cofactor. Apixaban inhibits both free and clot-bound FXa, as well as prothrombinase activity.	Metabolized in the liver. About 75% of metabolites are eliminated in feces (biliary and direct intestinal excretion) and about 25% through urinary excretion. T1/2: 12 hours	• Prophylaxis of stroke and systemic embolism in non-valvular atrial fibrillation • Venous thromboembolism treatment • Prophylaxis of DVT following hip or knee replacement surgery	• Chromogenic anti-Xa assay Routine monitoring is not required.
Edoxaban Oral	Edoxaban is an oral, direct and selective FXa inhibitor. It inhibits free FXa and prothrombinase activity. It also inhibits thrombin-induced platelet aggregation.	Eliminated as unchanged drug in urine. Renal clearance accounts for ~50% of total clearance, and hepatic metabolism and biliary excretion account for the remainder. T1/2: 10–14 hours	• Prophylaxis of stroke and systemic embolism in non-valvular atrial fibrillation • Acute treatment of DVT with or without PE (only after an initial 5-day treatment with a parenteral anticoagulant)	• Chromogenic anti-Xa assay Routine monitoring is not required.

aPTT = activated partial thromboplastin time; **AT** = antithrombin; **DTI** = direct thrombin inhibitor; **DVT** = deep vein thrombosis; **ECMO** = extracorporeal membrane oxygenation; **Fxa** = factor Xa; **GFR** = glomerular filtration rate; **HIT** = heparin-induced thrombocytopenia; **INR** = International Normalized Ratio; **LMWH** = low-molecular-weight heparin; **PCI** = percutaneous coronary intervention; **PE** = pulmonary embolism; **PT** = prothrombin time; **PTCA** = percutaneous transluminal coronary angioplasty; **STEMI** = ST elevation myocardial infarction; **T1/2** = half-life; **TT** = thrombin time; **UFH** = unfractionated heparin. Adapted from respective package inserts.

TABLE 8–5. ARTHRITIS: EXAMINATION AND CLASSIFICATION OF SYNOVIAL (JOINT) FLUID.

Type of Joint Fluid	Volume (mL)	Clarity, Color	WBC (per mcL)	PMNs	Gram Stain and Culture	Fluid Glucose (mg/dL)	Differential Diagnosis	Comments
Normal	<3.5	Transparent, clear	<200	<25%	Neg	Equal to serum glucose		
Non-inflammatory (Group I)	Often >3.5	Transparent, yellow	<2000	<25%	Neg	Equal to serum glucose	Degenerative joint disease, trauma, avascular necrosis, osteochondritis dissecans, osteochondromatosis, neuropathic arthropathy, early or subsiding inflammation, hypertrophic osteoarthropathy, pigmented villonodular synovitis.	
Inflammatory (Group II)	Often >3.5	Translucent to opaque, yellow to opalescent	2000–75,000 (occasionally >75,000 but rarely >100,000)	≥50%	Neg	>25, but lower than serum glucose	Rheumatoid arthritis, acute crystal-induced synovitis (gout, pseudogout), reactive arthritis, ankylosing spondylitis, psoriatic arthritis, sarcoidosis, arthritis accompanying ulcerative colitis and Crohn disease, rheumatic fever, systemic lupus erythematosus, scleroderma; tuberculous, viral, or mycotic infections.	Crystals are diagnostic of gout or pseudogout: gout crystals (urate) are needle-shaped and show negative birefringence; pseudogout crystals (calcium pyrophosphate) are more rectangular and show positive birefringence when red compensator filter is used with polarized light microscopy. Phagocytic inclusions in PMNs suggest rheumatoid arthritis (RA cells).
Purulent (Group III)	Often >3.5	Opaque, yellow to green	>100,000	≥75%	Usually positive (gonococci seen in only about 25% of cases)	<25, much lower than serum glucose	Mostly pyogenic bacterial infections (eg, *Staphylococcus aureus*, *Neisseria gonorrhoeae*).	WBC count and % PMN lower with infections caused by organisms of low virulence (eg, *N. gonorrhoeae*) or if antibiotic therapy already started.
Hemorrhagic (Group IV)	Often >3.5	Cloudy, pink to red	Usually >2000; many RBCs	<30%	Neg	Equal to serum glucose	Trauma with or without fracture, hemophilia or other hemorrhagic diathesis, neuropathic arthropathy, pigmented villonodular synovitis, synovioma, hemangioma and other benign neoplasms.	Fat globules strongly suggest intra-articular fracture.

Modified with permission from Papadakis MA, McPhee SJ, Rabow MW (editors). Current Medical Diagnosis & Treatment 2016, 55th ed. McGraw-Hill, 2016.

TABLE 8–6. ASCITES: ASCITIC FLUID PROFILES IN VARIOUS DISEASE STATES.

Diagnosis	Appearance	Fluid Protein (g/dL)	Serum Albumin-Ascites Gradient (SAAG[1])	Fluid Glucose (mg/dL)	WBC (per mcL); Differential	RBC (per mcL)	Gram Stain and Culture	Cytology	Comments
Normal	Clear	<3.0		Equal to plasma glucose	<250	Few or none	Neg	Neg	
HIGH SAAG[1]									
Cirrhosis	Clear	<3.0	≥1.1	N	<250; MN	Few	Neg	Neg	Occasionally turbid, rarely bloody.
Heart failure	Clear	<2.5	≥1.1	N	<250; MN	Few	Neg	Neg	
LOW SAAG[1]									
Nephrotic syndrome	Clear	<2.5	<1.1	N	<250; MN	Few	Neg	Neg	
Bacterial peritonitis	Cloudy	>3.0	<1.1	<50 with perforated viscus	>500; PMN	Few	Pos	Neg	Blood cultures frequently positive.
Tuberculous peritonitis	Clear, occasionally bloody	>3.0	<1.1	<60	>500; MN	Few, occasionally many	Stain Pos in 25%; culture Pos in 65%	Neg	Occasionally chylous. Peritoneal biopsy positive in 65%.
Malignancy	Clear or bloody	>3.0	<1.1	<60	>500; MN, PMN	Many	Neg	Pos in 60–90%	Occasionally chylous. Peritoneal biopsy diagnostic.
Pancreatitis	Clear or bloody	>2.5	<1.1	N	>500; MN, PMN	Many	Neg	Neg	Occasionally chylous. Fluid amylase >1000 IU/L, sometimes >10,000 IU/L. Fluid amylase > serum amylase.
OTHER									
Chylous ascites	Turbid	Varies, often >2.5		N	Few	Few	Neg	Neg	Fluid TG > 400 mg/dL (turbid). Fluid TG > serum TG.
Pseudomyxoma peritonei	Gelatinous	<2.5		N	<250	Few	Neg	Occ Pos	

[1]**SAAG** = serum–ascites albumin gradient, calculated as serum albumin minus ascitic fluid albumin

IU = international units; **MN** = mononuclear cells; **PMN** = polymorphonuclear cells; **TG** = triglycerides.

TABLE 8–7. AUTOANTIBODIES: FREQUENCY (%) OF AUTOANTIBODIES IN RHEUMATIC DISEASES.[1]

	ANA	Anti-dsDNA	Rheumatoid Factor	Anti-Sm	Anti-SS-A	Anti-SS-B	Anti-SCL-70	Anti-Centromere	Anti-Jo-1	ANCA	Anti-CCP
Rheumatoid arthritis	30–60	0–5	70	0	0–5	0–2	0	0	0	0	70–80
Systemic lupus erythematosus	95–100	60	20	10–25	15–20	5–20	0	0	0	0–1	30–70[2]
Sjögren syndrome	95	0	75	0	65	65	0	0	0	0	0
Diffuse scleroderma	80–95	0	30	0	0	0	33	1	0	0	0
Limited scleroderma (CREST syndrome)	80–95	0	30	0	0	0	20	50	0	0	0
Polymyositis/dermatomyositis	80–95	0	33	0	0	0	0	0	20–30	0	0
Granulomatosis with polyangiitis	0–15	0	50	0	0	0	0	0	0	93–96[1]	0

[1]Frequency for generalized, active disease. [2] Frequency for SLE with deforming erosive arthritis.
Anti-dsDNA = anti-double-stranded DNA antibody; **ANA** = antinuclear antibodies; **ANCA** = antineutrophil cytoplasmic antibody; **Anti-CCP** = antibodies to cyclic citrullinated peptide; **Anti-Jo-1** = antibodies directed against histidyl-tRNA synthetase; **Anti-Sm** = anti-Smith antibody; **Anti-SCL-70** = anti-scleroderma antibody; **Anti-SSA** = antibodies to Ro (SSA) cellular ribonucleoprotein complexes of two types (52 kDa and 60 kDa); **Anti-SSB** = antibodies to La (SSB) cellular ribonucleoprotein complexes; **CREST** = **C**alcinosis cutis, **R**aynaud phenomenon, **E**sophageal motility disorder, **S**clerodactyly, and **T**elangiectasia.
Reproduced with permission from Papadakis MA, McPhee SJ, Rabow MW (editors). Current Medical Diagnosis & Treatment 2016, 55th ed., McGraw-Hill, 2016.

TABLE 8–8. BLEEDING DISORDERS: LABORATORY EVALUATION.

Suspected Diagnosis	Platelet Count	PT	PTT	TT	Further Diagnostic Tests
Idiopathic thrombocytopenic purpura (ITP), drug effect, bone marrow suppression	↓	N	N	N	Platelet antibodies (anti-platelet antibodies), bone marrow examination.
Disseminated intravascular coagulation (DIC)	↓	↑	↑	↑	Fibrinogen (functional), D-dimers (a cut-off of 8.2 mcg/mL has a sensitivity and specificity of 80% for acute DIC).
Platelet function defect, salicylates, or uremia	N	N	N	N	Bleeding time or PFA-100 CT, platelet aggregation, renal function tests (blood urea nitrogen, creatinine, eGFR).
von Willebrand disease	N	N	↑ or N	N	Bleeding time or PFA-100 CT, factor VIII assay, vWF antigen and activity, vWF multimer analysis.
Factor VII deficiency or inhibitor	N	↑	N	N	Factor VII assay, inhibitor screen (mixing study).
Factor V, X, II, I deficiencies, eg, in liver disease or with anticoagulants	N	↑	↑	N or ↑	Liver function tests.
Factor VIII (hemophilia), IX, or XI deficiencies or inhibitor	N	N	↑	N	Inhibitor screen (mixing study), individual factor assays, Bethesda assay.
Factor XIII deficiency	N	N	N	N	5M urea solubility test (screening test), factor XIII activity assay.
Increase in fibrinolytic activity	N	N	N	N	Euglobulin clot lysis time (screening test), α₂-antiplasmin, plasminogen activator inhibitor-1 (PAI-1), thromboelastography, renal function test (eg, blood urea nitrogen, creatinine, eGFR).

Note: *In approaching patients with bleeding disorders, try to distinguish clinically between platelet disorders (eg, patient has petechiae, bruises, gingival bleeding, nosebleeds) and factor deficiency states (eg, patient has deep tissue hematoma and/or hemarthrosis).*

***eGFR** = estimated glomerular filtration rate; **PFA-100 CT** = platelet function analyzer-100 closure time; **PT** = prothrombin time; **PTT** = activated partial thromboplastin time; **TT** = thrombin time.*

TABLE 8–9. CEREBROSPINAL FLUID (CSF): CSF PROFILES IN CENTRAL NERVOUS SYSTEM DISEASES.

Diagnosis	Appearance	Opening Pressure (mm H₂O)	RBC (per mcL)	WBC (per mcL); Differential	CSF Glucose (mg/dL)	CSF Protein (mg/dL)	Smears	Culture	Comments
Normal	Clear, colorless	70–200	0	≤5 MN; 0 PMN	45–85	15–45	Neg	Neg	
Bacterial meningitis	Cloudy	↑↑↑	0	200–20,000; mostly PMN	<45	>50	Gram stain Pos	Pos	PMN predominance may be seen early in course.
Tuberculous meningitis	N or cloudy	↑↑↑	0	100–1000; mostly MN	<45	>50	AFB stain Pos	±	Counterimmunoelectrophoresis or latex agglutination may be diagnostic. CSF and serum cryptococcal antigen positive in cryptococcal meningitis.
Fungal meningitis	N or cloudy	N or ↑	0	100–1000; mostly MN	<45	>50		±	
Viral (aseptic) meningitis	N	N or ↑	0	100–1000; mostly MN	45–85	N or ↑	Neg	Neg	RBC count may be elevated in herpes simplex encephalitis. Glucose may be decreased in herpes simplex or mumps infections. Viral cultures may be helpful.
Parasitic meningitis	N or cloudy	N or ↑	0	100–1000; mostly MN, E	<45	N or ↑	Amebae may be seen on wet smear	±	
Carcinomatous meningitis	N or cloudy	N or ↑	0	N or 100–1000; mostly MN	<45	N or ↑	Cytology Pos	Neg	

									Comments
Cerebral lupus erythematosus	N	N or ↑	0	N or ↑; mostly MN	N	N or ↑	Neg	Neg	
Subarachnoid hemorrhage	Pink-red, supernatant yellow	↑	↑ crenated or fresh	N or 100–1000; mostly PMN	N or ↓	N or ↑	Neg	Neg	Blood in all tubes equally. Pleocytosis and low glucose sometimes seen several days after subarachnoid hemorrhage, reflecting chemical meningitis caused by subarachnoid blood.
"Traumatic" tap	Bloody, supernatant clear	N	↑↑↑ fresh	↑	N	↑	Neg	Neg	Most blood in tube #1; least blood in tube #4.
Spirochetal, early, acute syphilitic meningitis	Clear to turbid	↑	0	25–2000; mostly MN	15–75	>50	Neg	Neg	PMN may predominate early. Positive serum RPR, VDRL, CSF VDRL insensitive. If clinical suspicion is high, institute treatment despite negative CSF VDRL.
Late CNS syphilis	Clear	Usually N	0	N or ↑	N	N or ↑	Neg	Neg	CSF VDRL insensitive. If clinical suspicion is high, institute treatment despite negative CSF VDRL.
"Neighborhood" meningeal reaction	Clear or turbid, often xanthochromic	Variable, usually N	Variable	↑	N	N or ↑	Neg	Usually Neg	May occur in mastoiditis, brain abscess, sinusitis, septic thrombophlebitis, brain tumor, intrathecal drug therapy.
Hepatic encephalopathy	N	N	0	≤5	N	N	Neg	Neg	CSF glutamine >15 mg/dL.
Uremia	N	Usually ↑	0	N or ↑	N or ↑	N or ↑	Neg	Neg	
Diabetic coma	N	Low	0	N or ↑	↑	N	Neg	Neg	

CNS = central nervous system; *E* = eosinophils; *MN* = mononuclear cells (lymphocytes or monocytes); *PMN* = polymorphonuclear cells; *WBC* = white blood cells.

TABLE 8–10. CIRRHOSIS: CHILD-PUGH STAGES AND MODEL FOR END-STAGE LIVER DISEASE (MELD) SCORING SYSTEM.

Parameter	Child-Pugh scoring system		
	1	2	3
Ascites	None	Slight	Moderate to severe
Encephalopathy	None	Slight to moderate	Moderate to severe
Bilirubin, mg/dL (mcmol/L)	<2.0 (<34.2)	2–3 (34.2–51.3)	>3.0 (>51.3)
Albumin, g/dL (g/L)	>3.5 (>35)	2.8–3.5 (28–35)	<2.8 (<28)
Prothrombin time (seconds increased)	1–3	4–6	>6.0

Total Numerical Score and Corresponding Child Class

Score	Class
5–6	A
7–9	B
10–15	C

MELD scoring system

$MELD = 11.2 \times \log_e (INR) + 3.78 \times \log_e (\text{bilirubin [mg/dL]}) + 9.57 \times \log_e (\text{creatinine [mg/dL]}) + 6.43.$ (Range 6–40).

INR = International Normalized Ratio.

Reproduced with permission from Papadakis MA, McPhee SJ, Rabow MW (editors). Current Medical Diagnosis & Treatment 2016, 55th ed. McGraw-Hill, 2016.

TABLE 8–11. GENETIC DISEASES: MOLECULAR DIAGNOSTIC TESTING.

Test/Range/ Collection	Physiologic Basis	Interpretation	Comments and References
Breast cancer *BRCA1* and *BRCA2* mutations DNA sequencing Blood Lavender $$$$	Mutations in two genes, *BRCA1* and *BRCA2*, are the major cause of familial early-onset breast and ovarian cancer. Hundreds of different deleterious germline mutations have been identified in both *BRCA1* and *BRCA2*. A mutation in either gene confers an increased risk of breast and ovarian cancer, as well as prostate and male breast cancer. In the general population, the prevalence of *BRCA1/2* mutations is 1 per 400–800. There is an increased prevalence in certain ethnic groups such as those of Ashkenazi Jewish descent and Icelanders, with a prevalence of 1 per 40 and 1 per 160, respectively. *BRCA1* and *BRCA2* testing may also utilize saliva or buccal mucosa samples for analyses.	For the general population, next-generation DNA sequencing is used to identify mutations in *BRCA1* and *BRCA2*. To assess risk in family members when there is a known familial *BRCA1* or *BRCA2* mutation, a limited mutation detection test should be selected. For Ashkenazi Jews, use first-tier screening test that detects few common mutations (e.g., the 185 del AG and 5382 ins C mutations in *BRCA1* and the 6174 del T mutation in *BRCA2*). If negative, second-tier DNA sequencing is then performed.	Patients who are candidates for genetic testing should be referred to a credentialed provider for pre-test and post-test genetic counseling. Expertise is required to ensure that the most appropriate test is selected and the test is adequately interpreted, and to determine if the results will aid in diagnosis or influence management of the patient or family members at risk for hereditary cancer. Couch FJ et al. Two decades after *BRCA*: setting paradigms in personalized cancer care and prevention. Science 2014;343:1466. [PMID: 24675953] Stuckey AR et al. Hereditary breast cancer: an update on risk assessment and genetic testing in 2015. Am J Obstet Gynecol 2015;213:161. [PMID: 25747548]
Cystic fibrosis mutation PCR, DNA sequencing Blood Lavender $$$$	Cystic fibrosis is caused by a mutation in the cystic fibrosis transmembrane regulator gene (*CFTR*). Over 800 mutations have been found, with the most common being ΔF508, present in 70% of cases. Approximately 90% of people with cystic fibrosis carry at least one ΔF508 mutation. Another mutation, G551D, accounts for 5% of *CFTR* mutations and identifies a select subgroup of patients for treatment with an FDA approved drug (Ivacaftor) that targets the specific mutant protein.	Test specificity approaches 100%, so a positive result should be considered diagnostic of a cystic fibrosis mutation. Because of the wide range of mutations, a limited mutation panel (eg, the standard panel consisting of 23 mutations, or expanded panel offered by various laboratories) is typically done first. If the mutation ΔF508 or R117H is detected, the sample is then tested for certain mutations as part of a second tier reflex test. If indicated, full *CFTR* gene sequencing analysis may also be performed to identify other rare mutations.	Cystic fibrosis is the most common inherited disease in North American Caucasians, affecting 1 in 2500 births. Caucasians have a carrier frequency of 1 in 25. The disease is autosomal recessive. Carrier screening might be offered to individuals and couples in high-risk groups (eg, Ashkenazi Jews, central or northern Europeans), one partner with cystic fibrosis, and individuals with a family history of cystic fibrosis) who seek preconception counseling, infertility care, or prenatal care. Kapoor H et al. Ivacaftor: a novel mutation modulating drug. J Clin Diagn Res 2014;8:SE01. [PMID: 25584290] Tsui LC et al. The cystic fibrosis gene: a molecular genetic perspective. Cold Spring Harb Perspect Med 2013;3:a009472. [PMID: 23378595]

(Continued)

TABLE 8–11. GENETIC DISEASES: MOLECULAR DIAGNOSTIC TESTING (*CONTINUED*).

Test/Range/ Collection	Physiologic Basis	Interpretation	Comments and References
Duchenne muscular dystrophy (DMD) PCR, DNA sequencing Blood (lavender) $$$$	DMD is a rare, X-linked disease. It occurs as a result of mutations (mainly deletions) in the dystrophin gene at locus Xp21.2. Mutations lead to an absence of or defect in dystrophin, causing progressive muscle degeneration and loss of independent ambulation by the age of 13–16 years.	The multiplex PCR-based genetic testing may not detect all mutations, and dystrophin gene sequencing may be necessary. Since the dystrophin gene is a large gene and traditional methods for detection of point mutations and other sequence variants are costly and time-consuming, the use of next-generation sequencing has become a useful tool for confirming the diagnosis.	Testing for a DMD mutation is necessary for confirming the diagnosis even if muscle biopsy demonstrates the absence of dystrophin protein expression. Falzarano MS et al. Duchenne muscular dystrophy: from diagnosis to therapy. Molecules 2015;20:18168. [PMID: 26457695] Theadom A et al. Prevalence of muscular dystrophies: a systematic literature review. Neuroepidemiology 2014;43:259. [PMID: 25532075]
Familial adenomatous polyposis (FAP) PCR, DNA sequencing Lavender $$$$	Familial adenomatous polyposis is an autosomal dominant condition, which predisposes the mutation carrier to colorectal cancer in early adulthood. The condition is characterized by hundreds to thousands of adenomatous polyps in the colon that usually develop in the second to third decade of life. A milder condition, termed Attenuated FAP (AFAP), lacks the classical features of FAP, with patients having fewer polyps and an older age of onset. FAP has been linked to germline mutations of the *APC* gene.	A PCR-based assay is used to amplify all exons of the *APC* gene, and direct sequence analysis of PCR products corresponding to the entire *APC* coding region is performed. The testing is used only to confirm clinical diagnosis of FAP and AFAP, and to identify asymptomatic family members in FAP/AFAP families in which a familial mutation has been identified.	Numerous germline mutations have been located between codons 156 and 2011 of the *APC* gene. Mutations spanning the region between codons 543 and 1309 are strongly associated with congenital hypertrophy of retinal pigment epithelium. Mutations between codons 1310 and 2011 are associated with increased risk of desmoid tumors. Mutations at codon 1309 are associated with early development of colorectal cancer. Mutations between codons 976 and 1067 are associated with increased risk of duodenal adenomas. The cumulative frequency of extracolonic manifestations is highest for mutations between codons 976 and 1067. Leoz ML et al. The genetic basis of familial adenomatous polyposis and its implications for clinical practice and risk management. Appl Clin Genet 2015;8:95. [PMID: 25931827]

Test	Description	Interpretation	Comments
Fragile X syndrome PCR, Southern blot Blood, cultured amniocytes Lavender $$$$	Fragile X syndrome results from a mutation in the familial mental retardation-1 gene (*FMRI*), located at Xq27.3. Fully symptomatic patients have abnormal methylation of the gene (which blocks transcription) during oogenesis. The gene contains a variable number of repeating CGG sequences and, as the number of sequences increases, the probability of abnormal methylation increases. The number of copies increases with subsequent generations so that women who are unaffected carriers may have offspring who are affected.	Normal patients have 6–52 CGG repeat sequences. Patients with 52–200 repeat sequences are asymptomatic carriers (premutation). Patients with more than 200 repeat sequences (full mutation) are very likely to have abnormal methylation and to be symptomatic.	Fragile X syndrome is the most common cause of inherited mental retardation, occurring in 1 in 1000–1500 men and 1 in 2000–2500 women. Full mutations can show variable penetration in females, but most such women will be at least mildly retarded. Carrier screening is usually done in the context of reproductive healthcare whereby test result may inform parents about reproductive options and family planning. Tassone F. Newborn screening for fragile X syndrome. JAMA Neurol 2014;71:355. [PMID: 24395328] Usdin K et al. Repeat-mediated epigenetic dysregulation of the *FMR1* gene in the fragile X-related disorders. Front Genet 2015;6:192. [PMID: 26089834]
Hemochromatosis, hereditary PCR, DNA sequencing Blood Lavender $$$$	Hereditary hemochromatosis is an autosomal recessive disorder of iron metabolism that varies in clinical severity. Three *HFE* gene mutations (C282Y, H63D, and S65C) have been described in most patients with hemochromatosis. Mutations in genes encoding other iron regulation proteins (hepcidin, ferroportin, hemojuvelin (HJV), transferrin receptor 2 (TfR2) account for rare cases of hereditary hemochromatosis.	Homozygosity for the C282Y mutation is responsible for up to 90% of hemochromatosis patients. The estimated penetrance is 80% for men and 35% for women over 40. Compound heterozygosity (C282Y/H63D or C282Y/S65C) may cause hemochromatosis, but the penetrance is very low. Homozygous H63D genotypes (H63D/H63D) rarely show symptoms of hemochromatosis. Heterozygotes for C282Y (C282Y/WT), H63D (H63D/WT), or S65C (S65C/WT) are not significantly associated with hemochromatosis.	Hepcidin deficiency is the pathogenic cause of iron overload in most hereditary hemochromatosis. Hepcidin insufficiency results from the deleterious mutations in the genes encoding hepcidin regulators (HFE, TfR2 and HJV) or hepcidin itself. Ruchala P et al. The pathophysiology and pharmacology of hepcidin. Trends Pharmacol Sci 2014;35:155. [PMID: 24552640] Vujić M. Molecular basis of HFE-hemochromatosis. Front Pharmacol 2014;5:42. [PMID: 24653703]
Hemophilia A Southern blot, PCR Blood, cultured amniocytes Lavender $$$$	Approximately half of severe hemophilia A cases are caused by a recurrent mutation, ie, an inversion mutation within intron 22 of the factor VIII gene. Methods are available for rapid detection of the intron 22 inversions.	Test specificity approaches 100%, so a positive result should be considered diagnostic of a hemophilia A inversion mutation. Because of a variety of mutations, however, test sensitivity for hemophilia A is only about 50%.	Vascular endothelial cells are the principal and possibly exclusive source of plasma factor VIII. Hemophilia A is one of the most common X-linked diseases in humans, affecting 1 in 5000 men. de Brasi C et al. Genetic testing in bleeding disorders. Haemophilia 2014;20(Suppl 4):54. [PMID: 24762276] Gouw SC et al. F8 gene mutation type and inhibitor development in patients with severe hemophilia A: systematic review and meta-analysis. Blood 2012;119:2922. [PMID: 22282501]

(Continued)

TABLE 8–11. GENETIC DISEASES: MOLECULAR DIAGNOSTIC TESTING (*CONTINUED*).

Test/Range/ Collection	Physiologic Basis	Interpretation	Comments and References
Hereditary nonpol-yposis colorectal cancer PCR, DNA sequencing Blood (EDTA) and tumor tissue block $$$$	Hereditary nonpolyposis colorectal cancer (HNPCC) (also called Lynch syndrome) accounts for 3–4% of all colorectal cancers. It is caused by inactivation of DNA mismatch repair (MMR) genes (eg, *MLH1, MSH2, MSH6*), resulting in accumulation of spontaneous mutations in short repetitive DNA sequences, termed microsatellites.	Initial screening includes microsatellite instability (MSI) or immunohistochemistry (IHC) analysis to detect a loss of protein expression in one of the MMR genes. If MSI is scored as high (MSI-H) and/or IHC demonstrates the absence of one of the MMR proteins in tumor tissue, then direct sequencing of *MLH1, MSH2,* or *MSH6* is performed to identify the germline mutation(s).	Testing is used to confirm clinical diagnosis in those with colorectal cancer who meet Amsterdam and/or Bethesda criteria for diagnosis of HNPCC. Once the familial mutation is identified, testing at-risk family members for the specific mutation can be performed. Brosens LA et al. Hereditary colorectal cancer: genetics and screening. Surg Clin North Am 2015;95:1067. [PMID: 26315524] Carethers JM et al. Lynch syndrome and Lynch syndrome mimics: the growing complex landscape of hereditary colon cancer. World J Gastroenterol 2015;21:9253. [PMID: 26309352]
Huntington disease PCR, Southern blot Blood, cultured amniocytes, or buccal cells Lavender $$$$	Huntington disease is an inherited neurodegenerative disorder associated with an autosomal dominant mutation on chromosome 4. The disease is highly penetrant, but symptoms (disordered movements, cognitive decline, and emotional disturbance) are often not expressed until middle age. The mutation results in the expansion of a CAG trinucleotide repeat sequence within the gene that encodes Huntington protein, leading to a mutant Huntington protein.	Normal patients have fewer than 34 CAG repeats, whereas patients with disease usually have more than 37 repeats and may have 80 or more. Occasional affected patients can be seen with "high normal" (32–34) numbers of repeats. Tests showing 34–37 repeats are indeterminate.	Huntington disease is a heritable neurodegenerative disorder that can affect motor, cognitive and psychiatric functioning. Huntington disease testing involves ethical dilemmas for both patients and family members. Genetic counseling is recommended before testing. Agrawal M et al. Molecular diagnostics of neurodegenerative disorders. Front Mol Biosci 2015;2:54. [PMID: 26442283] Dayalu P et al. Huntington disease: pathogenesis and treatment. Neurol Clin 2015;33:101. [PMID: 25437725]
Kennedy disease/ spinal and bulbar muscular atrophy (KD/SBMA) PCR, Southern blot, sequencing Lavender $$$$	The disease is a slowly progressive degenerative neuromuscular disorder. Familial and sporadic cases are caused by expansion of a CAG trinucleotide tandem repeat in exon 1 of the androgen receptor gene on chromosome Xq11-12. The pathogenic CAG expansion mutation confers a toxic gain-of-function to the androgen receptor.	Normal individuals have up to 30 CAG repeats; patients with KD/SBMA have ≥ 40 CAG repeats (sensitivity >99%).	The disease is characterized clinically by progressive atrophy and weakening of the proximal musculature in the limbs and bulbar distribution. Resulting symptoms include dysarthria, dysphagia, fasciculations, tremor, and gait disturbances. Chua JP et al. Pathogenic mechanisms and therapeutic strategies in spinobulbar muscular atrophy. CNS Neurol Disord Drug Targets 2013;12:1146. [PMID: 24040817]

Disease	Description	Notes	References
Myotonic dystrophy (MD) PCR, Southern blot, sequencing Lavender $$$$	The disease is caused by expansions of microsatellite repeats. The most common mutation associated with DM1 is expansion of the trinucleotide repeat CTG in the *DMPK* gene, and for DM2, the expansion of the CCTG repeat in the *ZNF9* gene.	Affected individuals have 50 to 3000 CTG repeats in DMPK and >1000 CCTG repeats in *ZNF9*, respectively.	Caution should be exercised in using CTG/CCTG repeat size to predict future symptoms. Thornton CA. Myotonic dystrophy. Neurol Clin 2014;32:705. [PMID: 25037086] Turner C et al. Myotonic dystrophy: diagnosis, management and new therapies. Curr Opin Neurol 2014;27:599. [PMID: 25121518]
Neurofibromatosis (NF): von Recklinghausen disease (NF1) and bilateral acoustic NF (NF2) PCR, Southern blot, DNA sequencing Lavender $$$$	Neurofibromatosis type I (NF1) is a disease associated with the presence of benign neurofibromas and malignant tumors of the central and peripheral nervous system. The *NF1* gene is located at chromosome region 17q11.2 and codes for the neurofibromin protein. Over 1485 different mutations have been identified in the NF1 gene so far, most of which lead to a synthesis of truncated, non-functional protein. Mutations in the *merlin* gene are responsible for NF2, which is characterized by the development of neoplasms of the nervous system, most notably bilateral vestibular schwannomas. The *NF2/merlin* gene is located on chromosome 22q12.	The mutations tested by the DNA analysis are laboratory-dependent. Clinical correlation is important.	Abramowicz A et al. Neurofibromin in neurofibromatosis type 1—mutations in NF1 gene as a cause of disease. Dev Period Med 2014;18:297. [PMID: 25182393] Hirbe AC et al. Neurofibromatosis type 1: a multidisciplinary approach to care. Lancet Neurol 2014;13:834. [PMID: 25030515] Schroeder RD et al. *NF2/merlin* in hereditary neurofibromatosis 2 versus cancer: biologic mechanisms and clinical associations. Oncotarget 2014;5:67. [PMID: 24393766]
Niemann-Pick disease PCR, DNA sequencing Lavender $$$$	The disease is a rare autosomal recessive lysosomal storage disorder, caused by deficiency of the enzyme, acid sphingomyelinase. Three mutations (c.911T>C, c.996delC, c.1493G>T) in the acid sphingomyelinase (*SMPD1*) gene account for >94% of cases of type A disease that results in severe neurologic impairment in infancy and childhood. Type B has visceral manifestations. For type C disease, mutational analysis (*NPC1* or *NPC2/HE1* gene) is also available.	The combination of DNA and biochemical (sphingomyelinase activity, mass spectroscopy for cholesterol metabolism products) analyses improves the detection rate of the disease.	The disease is more commonly seen in the Ashkenazi Jewish population. McKay Bounford K et al. Genetic and laboratory diagnostic approach in Niemann Pick disease type C. J Neurol 2014;261 (Suppl 2):S569. [PMID: 25145893] Vanier MT. Niemann-Pick diseases. Handb Clin Neurol 2013;113:1717. [PMID: 23622394]

(Continued)

TABLE 8–11. GENETIC DISEASES: MOLECULAR DIAGNOSTIC TESTING (*CONTINUED*).

Test/Range/ Collection	Physiologic Basis	Interpretation	Comments and References
Phenylketonuria (PKU) PCR, DNA sequencing, Southern blot Lavender $$$$	The severity of the disease correlates with extent of mutations of the phenylalanine hydroxylase *(PAH)* gene. Little or no enzyme activity results in the classic PKU. Phenylalanine hydroxylase activity determines the type of replacement therapy.	More than 400 point mutations in the *PAH* gene have been reported, and thus direct sequencing the entire coding regions of the gene may be necessary.	Universal newborn screening for phenylketonuria allows early implementation of the phenylalanine-restricted diet, eliminating the severe neurocognitive and neuromotor impairment associated with untreated phenylketonuria. Berry SA et al. Newborn screening 50 years later: access issues faced by adults with PKU. Genet Med 2013;15:591. [PMID: 23470838] Ney DM et al. Advances in the nutritional and pharmacological management of phenylketonuria. Curr Opin Clin Nutr Metab Care 2014;17:61. [PMID: 24136088]
Prader-Willi syndrome (PWS), Angelman syndrome (AS) FISH, chromosomal analysis Blood Green $$$$	Prader-Willi syndrome and Angelman syndrome are clinically different diseases related at the molecular level. They are caused by loss of function mutations in two chromosomal regions located close to each other on chromosome 15. An interstitial deletion of 15q11–13 is found in about 70% of patients with PWS or AS. PWS results when the deletion affects the paternal chromosome, and AS occurs when it affects the maternal chromosome. A DNA probe from the affected region is used to determine the origin of the deletion by Southern blot analysis. In about 33% of patients with PWS and 20–30% with AS, no deletion can be found. Instead, uniparental disomy (UPD) may be found resulting in either two maternal or two paternal copies of chromosome 15. In 1–2% of patients with PWS and 20% of patients with AS, neither a deletion nor UPD can be found.	This test detects both the deletion and the UPD defects in PWS and AS.	Recombinant human growth hormone treatment should be considered for patients with genetically confirmed PWS in conjunction with dietary, environmental, and lifestyle interventions. Aycan Z et al. Prader-Willi syndrome and growth hormone deficiency. J Clin Res Pediatr Endocrinol 2014;6:62. [PMID: 24932597] Deal CL et al. Growth Hormone Research Society workshop summary: consensus guidelines for recombinant human growth hormone therapy in Prader-Willi syndrome. J Clin Endocrinol Metab 2013;98:E1072. [PMID: 23543664]
Tay-Sachs disease PCR, DNA sequencing Lavender $$$$	Tay-Sachs disease is an autosomal recessive disease caused by a deficiency of β-hexosaminidase A. Mutations in the α-subunit of hexosaminidase A are responsible for the enzyme deficiency. More than 75 mutations of the α-subunit gene have been described.	The mutations tested by the DNA analysis are laboratory-dependent. The combination of DNA and biochemical analyses improves the detection rate of the disease.	Chen H et al. Beyond the cherry-red spot: ocular manifestations of sphingolipid-mediated neurodegenerative and inflammatory disorders. Surv Ophthalmol 2014;59:64. [PMID: 24011710]

Test / Specimen / Cost	Description	Interpretation	Comments
α-Thalassemia PCR, Southern blot Blood, cultured amniocytes, chorionic villi Lavender $$$$	…some 16 due to unequal crossing-over events can lead to defective synthesis of the α-globin subunit of hemoglobin. Normally, there are two copies of the α-globin gene on each chromosome 16, and the severity of disease increases with the number of defective genes.	…ity, however, can vary because detection of different mutations may require the use of different probes. α-Thalassemia due to point mutations may not be detected.	…duced with one defect gene are usually normal or very slightly anemic; patients with two deletions usually have hypochromic microcytic anemia; patients with three deletions have elevated hemoglobin H and moderately severe hemolytic anemia (Hb H disease); patients with four deletions generally die in utero with hydrops fetalis. The most clinically significant situations arise when both parents are carriers for a deletion that encompasses both α-globin genes (*cis* deletion), as seen mostly in Southeast Asian and Filipino populations. Each offspring of such carriers has a 25% risk of hydrops fetalis. Less deleterious effects arise from chromosomes of Mediterranean and black ancestries. These chromosomes usually carry one α-globin gene deletion per chromosome. Offspring of carriers of a two α-globin gene deletion and single α-gene deletion are at risk for Hb H disease. Piel FB et al. The α-thalassemias: N Engl J Med 2014;371:1908. [PMID: 25390741] Vichinsky EP. Clinical manifestations of α-thalassemia. Cold Spring Harb Perspect Med 2013;3:a011742. [PMID: 25543077]
β-Thalassemia PCR, reverse dot blot Blood, chorionic villi, cultured amniocytes Lavender $$$$	β-Thalassemia results from a mutation in the gene encoding the β-globin subunit of hemoglobin A (which is composed of a pair of α chains and a pair of β chains). A relative excess of α-globin chains precipitates within red blood cells, causing hemolysis and anemia. Over 300 different mutations have been described; testing usually covers a panel of the more common mutations. The test can distinguish between heterozygous and homozygous individuals.	Test specificity approaches 100%, so a positive result should be considered diagnostic of a thalassemia mutation. Because of the large number of mutations, sensitivity can be poor. A panel with the 43 most common mutations has a sensitivity that approaches 95%.	β-Thalassemia is very common; about 3% of the world's population are carriers. The incidence is increased in persons of Mediterranean, African, and Asian descent. The mutations may vary from population to population, and different testing panels may be needed for patients of different ethnicities. Mettananda S et al. α-Globin as a molecular target in the treatment of β-thalassemia. Blood 2015;125:3694. [PMID: 25869286] Rivella S. β-thalassemias: paradigmatic diseases for scientific discoveries and development of innovative therapies. Haematologica 2015;100:418. [PMID: 25828088]

PCR (polymerase chain reaction) is a method for amplifying a particular DNA sequence in a specimen, facilitating mutation detection by hybridization-based assay (eg, Southern blot, reverse dot blot, FISH) and direct DNA sequencing; Southern blot is a molecular hybridization technique whereby DNA is extracted from the sample and digested by different restriction enzymes, and the resulting fragments are separated by electrophoresis and identified by labeled probes; Reverse dot blot is a molecular hybridization technique in which a specific oligonucleotide probe is bound to a solid membrane prior to reaction with PCR-amplified DNA. DNA sequencing is the process of determining the precise order of nucleotides within a DNA molecule, using the Sanger sequencing or the next-generation sequencing methods.

TABLE 8–12. HEPATITIS B VIRUS INFECTION: COMMON SEROLOGIC TEST PATTERNS AND THEIR INTERPRETATION.

HBsAg	Anti-HBs	Anti-HBc	HBeAg	Anti-HBe	Interpretation
+	−	IgM	+	−	Acute hepatitis B
+	−	IgG[1]	+	−	Chronic hepatitis B with active viral replication
+	−	IgG	−	+	Inactive HBV carrier state (low HBV DNA level) or HBeAg-negative chronic hepatitis B with active viral replication (high HBV DNA level)
+	+	IgG	+ or −	+ or −	Chronic hepatitis B with heterotypic anti-HBs (about 10% of cases)
−	−	IgM	+ or −	−	Acute hepatitis B
−	+	IgG	−	+ or −	Recovery from hepatitis B (immunity)
−	+	−	−	−	Status-post vaccination (immunity)
−	−	IgG	−	−	False-positive; less commonly, infection in the remote past

[1]Low levels of IgM anti-HBc may also be detected.

Anti-HBc = antibody to hepatitis B core antigen; *Anti-HBe* = antibody to hepatitis B e antigen; *Anti-HBs* = antibody to hepatitis B surface antigen; *HBeAg* = antibody to hepatitis B e antigen; *HBsAg* = hepatitis B surface antigen; *HBV* = hepatitis B virus

Revised with permission from Papadakis MA, McPhee SJ, Rabow MW (editors). Current Medical Diagnosis & Treatment 2016, 55th ed. McGraw-Hill, 2016.

TABLE 8–13. LEUKEMIAS AND LYMPHOMAS: CLASSIFICATION AND IMMUNOPHENOTYPING.

Disease	Typical Immunophenotype	Comments
Acute Myeloid Leukemias (AML)		
AML with t (8;21) (q22;q22), (AML1/ETO)	Blasts express CD34, HLA-DR, CD13, CD33, CD15, MPO, and CD117. CD19 is often expressed.	AML with t (8;21) is usually associated with good response to chemotherapy and high rate of complete remission with long-term disease-free survival.
AML with inv (16) (p13;q22) or t (16;16) (p13;q22), (CBFβ/MYH11)	Blasts express CD13, CD33, MPO, CD117, as well as CD14, CD4, CD11b, CD11c, CD64, and CD36.	AML with inv (16) or t (16;16) typically shows myeloid and monocytic differentiation and the presence of eosinophilia, referred to as AMML-Eo. The disease usually responds well to chemotherapy with high rate of complete remission. Patients with AML and trisomy 22 as the sole karyotype abnormality need to be tested for cryptic inv (16) by PCR or FISH.
AML with t (15;17) (q22;q12), (PML/RARα) and variants	Leukemic cells express CD13, CD33, MPO, and CD117, but not CD34 and HLA-DR.	AML with t (15;17), known as acute promyelocytic leukemia (APL), is sensitive to all-trans retinoic acid (ATRA) treatment. APL is frequently associated with DIC.
AML with t(9;11)(p22;q23), (MLLT3/MLL)	Leukemic cells variably express HLA-DR, CD33, CD117, MPO, and monocytic markers (CD4, CD14, CD11b, CD11c, CD64, and lysozyme). CD34 is often absent.	AML with 11q23 (MLL) abnormalities is usually associated with monocytic features. AML with 11q23 abnormalities has an intermediate survival.
AML with t(6;9)(p23;q34) (DEK/NUP214)	Blasts often express MPO, CD13, CD33, HLA-DR, CD117, CD34, and CD15. Some cases also express CD64 or TdT.	AML with t(6;9) may have monocytic features, and is often associated with basophilia and multilineage dysplasia. Disease in both adults and children has a poor prognosis.
AML with inv(3)(q21q26) or t(3;3)(q21;q26), (RPN1/EVI1)	Blasts often express CD13, CD33, HLA-DR, CD34. Some cases may also express CD7 (aberrant), CD41 or CD61.	AML with inv(3) or t(3;3) is an aggressive disease with poor prognosis.
AML with t(1;22)(p13;q13) (RBM15/MKL1) (megakaryocytic)	Blasts often express CD41, CD61, CD36, and may also express CD13 and CD33.	Disease most commonly occurs in infants without Down syndrome. Outcome is generally poor, but may respond to intensive chemotherapy with long survival.
AML with myelodysplasia-related changes	Blasts often express CD34, HLA-DR, CD13, CD33, MPO, CD117. Aberrant expression of CD7 and/or CD56 may occur.	AML with myelodysplasia-related changes including AML arising from prior MDS or MDS/MPN, AML with an MDS-related cytogenetic abnormality, and AML with multilineage dysplasia. The disease has poor prognosis with low rate of achieving remission.

(Continued)

TABLE 8–13.   LEUKEMIAS AND LYMPHOMAS: CLASSIFICATION AND IMMUNOPHENOTYPING (*CONTINUED*).

Disease	Typical Immunophenotype	Comments
AML, therapy-related (t-AML)	Alkylating agent/radiation related: Blasts express CD34, HLA-DR, CD13, CD33, MPO, and CD117. Topoisomerase II inhibitor related: Same as AML with 11q23 abnormalities.	Alkylating agent/radiation related AML is generally refractory to chemotherapy and is associated with short survival. Topoisomerase II inhibitor-related AML often show monocytic differentiation. Therapy-related myelodysplastic syndrome (t-MDS) has similar prognosis as t-AML. Together, they are called therapy-related myeloid neoplasms.
AML, minimally differentiated (also known as AML-M0)	Blasts express CD13, CD33, CD117, CD34, HLA-DR, but not MPO.	Flow cytometric immunophenotyping is required for the confirmation of myeloid differentiation.
AML without maturation (also known as AML-M1)	Blasts express CD13, CD33, CD117, and MPO. CD34 is often positive.	Blasts constitute >90% of the nonerythroid nucleated cells in the marrow, and at least 3% of the blasts are positive for MPO.
AML with maturation (also known as AML-M2)	Blasts express CD13, CD33, CD15, CD117, and MPO. CD34 and HLA-DR are often positive.	Blasts constitute 20–89% of nonerythroid cells, and monocytes comprise <20% of the bone marrow cells.
Acute myelomonocytic leukemia (also known as AML-M4)	Leukemic cells variably express CD13, CD33, CD117, HLA-DR, CD4, CD11b, CD11c, and CD64. CD34 may be positive.	Monocytic component (monoblasts to monocytes) comprises 20–79% of bone marrow cells. Neutrophils and their precursors and monocytes and their precursors each comprise at least 20% of the nucleated bone marrow cells.
Acute monoblastic/monocytic leukemia (also known as AML-M5)	Leukemic cells variably express CD13, CD33, CD117, HLA-DR, CD14, CD4, CD11b, CD11c, CD64, and CD68. CD34 is typically negative.	Monocytic component (monoblasts to monocytes) comprises >80% of nucleated bone marrow cells.
Acute erythroid leukemia (also known as AML-M6) and pure erythroid leukemia	Erythroblasts generally lack myeloid markers, but are positive for CD36 and glycophorin A (CD235). Myeloblasts express CD13, CD33, CD117, and MPO with or without CD34 and HLA-DR. The erythroid cells in pure erythroid leukemia express CD36 and glycophorin A with the more immature forms expressing CD34 and HLA-DR.	The diagnostic criteria for acute erythroid leukemia: erythroblasts constitute >50% of the marrow cells, and myeloblasts comprise >20% of the nonerythroid cells. Pure erythroid leukemia is a neoplastic proliferation of erythroid precursors (>80% of nucleated marrow cells) without a significant myeloblastic component.
Acute megakaryocytic leukemia (known as AML-M7)	Blasts express one or more of the platelet glycoproteins (CD41, CD61, CD42), and variably express HLA-DR, CD34, CD117, CD13, and CD33.	Flow cytometric immunophenotyping is required for confirmation of megakaryocytic differentiation.
Blastic plasmacytoid dendritic cell neoplasm (formerly known as blastic NK-cell lymphoma)	Neoplastic cells express CD4, CD43, CD45RA, CD56, and plasmacytoid dendritic cell-associated antigens CD123, CD303, TCL1. May also express CD68 and TdT.	The disease is also called agranular CD4+/CD56+ hematodermic tumor. Besides marrow involvement, skin lesions are present. The disease is aggressive with short survival.

Acute leukemia of ambiguous lineage	Undifferentiated acute leukemia: Blasts express HLA-DR, CD34, CD38, and may express TdT, but lack lineage-specific markers such as CD79a, CD22, strong CD19, IgM, CD3, and MPO. Bilineal acute leukemia: There is a dual population of blasts with each population expressing markers of a distinct lineage, such as myeloid and lymphoid, or B and T. Biphenotypic acute leukemia: The blasts co-express myeloid and T or B lineage-specific antigens, or concurrent B and T antigens.	Cases of bilineal and biphenotypic acute leukemia usually present with cytogenetic abnormalities. The common abnormalities include Philadelphia chromosome, t (4;11)(q21;q23) or other 11q23 abnormalities. The prognosis of acute leukemia of ambiguous lineage is poor.
Acute Lymphoblastic Leukemias/Lymphomas (ALL/LBL)		
Precursor B-lymphoblastic leukemia/lymphoblastic lymphoma (B-ALL/LBL) (also known as B-cell acute lymphoblastic leukemia)	Early precursor B-ALL/LBL: TdT+, HLA-DR+, CD34(-/+), CD10−, CD45(-/+), CD19+, cCD22+, CD20−, CD15+, cIg−, sIg−. Common B-ALL/LBL: TdT+, HLA-DR+, CD34+, CD10+, CD45+(weak), CD19+, CD20+, cIg−, sIg−. Pre−B-ALL/LBL: TdT(-/+), CD34(-/+), HLA-DR+, CD45+(weak), CD19+, CD20+, cIgM+, sIg−.	Cytogenetic abnormalities in B-ALL/LBL include several groups: hypodiploid, low hyperdiploid (<50), high hyperdiploid (>50), translocations, and pseudodiploid. The commonly seen translocations include t (9;22), t (12;21), t (5;14), t (1;19), t (17;19), t (4;11), and other translocations involving 11q23. The cytogenetic findings are prognostically important.
Precursor T-lymphoblastic leukemia/lymphoblastic lymphoma (T-ALL/LBL)	T-ALL/LBL often has an immunophenotype that corresponds to the common thymocyte stage of differentiation. The blasts are positive for TdT and often CD10, and variably express CD1a, CD2, CD3, CD4, CD5, CD7, and CD8. CD4 and CD8 are frequently co-expressed on the blasts. Some T-ALL/LBL have an immunophenotype that corresponds to prothymocyte stage of differentiation. The blasts are negative for both CD4 and CD8.	In about one-third of T-ALL/LBL, translocations have been detected involving the α and δ T-cell receptor (TCR) loci at 14q11.2, the β locus at 7q35, and the γ locus at 7p14-15, with a variety of partner genes. T-ALL/LBL can be part of a unique disease entity known as the 8p11 myeloproliferative syndrome caused by constitutive activation of FGFR1. The most commonly seen karyotype abnormality is t(8;13)(p11;q12). The disease is characterized by chronic myeloproliferative disorder that frequently presents with eosinophilia and associated T-cell lymphoblastic lymphoma.
Mature B-cell Neoplasms		
Chronic lymphocytic leukemia/small lymphocytic lymphoma (CLL/SLL)	Lymphoma cells are light chain restricted and express CD5, CD19, CD20 (weak), CD22 (weak), CD79a, CD23, CD43, and are negative for CD10, Bcl-1 (cyclin D1), and FMC-7. A subset of cases expresses CD11c (weak). Cases with unmutated Ig variable region genes have been reported to be positive for CD38 and ZAP-70.	The clinical course is often indolent but incurable. The disease may progress/transform to prolymphocytic leukemia (PLL) or large B-cell lymphoma (Richter syndrome). CD38 and/or ZAP-70 positivity is associated with worse prognosis, and both have been used as prognostic markers for the disease. Trisomy 12 is reported in ~20% of cases, and deletions at 13q14 in up to 50% of cases. Trisomy 12 in CLL/SLL correlates with a worse prognosis.

(Continued)

TABLE 8–13.   LEUKEMIAS AND LYMPHOMAS: CLASSIFICATION AND IMMUNOPHENOTYPING (*CONTINUED*).

Disease	Typical Immunophenotype	Comments
B-cell prolymphocytic leukemia (B-PLL)	The cells of B-PLL strongly express surface IgM and B-cell antigens CD19, CD20, CD22, CD79a, CD79b, and FMC-7. CD5 is present in about one-third of cases and CD23 is typically negative.	B-PLL can be divided into CD5+ B-PLL (arising in CLL/SLL) and CD5− B-PLL (de novo PLL). CD5+ B-PLL has a longer median survival than CD5− B-PLL.
Lymphoplasmacytic lymphoma/Waldenström macroglobulinemia (LPL)	The cells express strong surface immunoglobulin, usually of IgM type, and express B-cell antigens (CD19, CD20, CD22, CD79a) and are CD5−, CD10−, CD23−, CD43±, and CD38+. Lack of CD5 and strong immunoglobulin expression are useful in distinction from CLL/SLL.	Characteristic features include IgM monoclonal gammopathy; spectrum of small lymphocytes, plasmacytoid lymphocytes, and plasma cells; interstitial, nodular, or diffuse pattern of bone marrow involvement; and typical immunophenotype (sIgM+, CD19+, CD20+, CD5−, CD23−, CD10−). MYD88 L265P mutation is present in >90% of LPL cases.
Splenic marginal zone lymphoma (SMZL)	The tumor cells express surface IgM, and are positive for CD19, CD20, CD79a, and negative for CD5, CD10, CD23, CD25, CD43, CD103, and Bcl-1 (cyclin D1).	Circulating lymphoma cells are usually characterized by the presence of short polar villi (villous lymphocytes). The clinical course is indolent, but the disease is incurable.
Hairy cell leukemia (HCL)	Leukemic cells express surface immunoglobulin, B-cell markers (CD19, CD20, CD22, CD79a), and are often positive for CD11c, CD25, FMC-7, and CD103, but negative for CD5, CD10, and CD23.	Patients often present with splenomegaly, pancytopenia (monocytopenia is characteristic), and may have circulating hairy leukemic cells. Bone marrow reticulin fibers are characteristically increased, resulting in "dry tap" during aspirate procedure. *BRAF* V600E mutation is present in all cases. Interferon-alpha, deoxycoformycin (pentostatin), or 2–chlorodeoxyadenosine (2-CdA, cladribine) can induce long-term remissions.
Plasma cell myeloma/plasmacytoma	The malignant cells express monoclonal cytoplasmic immunoglobulin, lack CD45 and pan-B cell antigens (CD19, CD20, CD22), but CD79 is often positive. The cells are typically positive for CD38, CD138, and often express CD56, CD43, and rarely CD10. The phenotype of plasma cell leukemia is similar to that of myeloma, but CD56 is negative.	Plasma cells do not express surface immunoglobulin. For clonality (or light chain restriction) determination by flow cytometry analysis, the cell permeabilization procedure is necessary. The procedure gives antibodies access to intracellular structures/molecules. Unfavorable karyotype abnormalities include del(17p), t(4;14), t(14;16), t(14;20), and complex abnormalities. The presence of t(11;14) is associated with a lymphoplasmacytic morphologic appearance and a more favorable prognosis.
Extranodal marginal zone B-cell lymphoma of mucosa-associated lymphoid tissue (MALT lymphoma)	Lymphoma cells typically express surface immunoglobulin with light chain restriction. The cells are positive for CD19, CD20, CD79a, CD43, and negative for CD5, CD10, CD23, and Bcl-1.	Trisomy 3 is found in ~60% and t (11;18) (q21;q21) has been detected in 25–50% of MALT lymphoma cases. Neither t(14;18) nor t (11;14) is present. Cases with t (11;18) appear to be resistant to *H. pylori* eradication therapy.
Nodal marginal zone B-cell lymphoma (NMZL)	The immunophenotype of most cases is similar to that of extranodal MALT lymphoma.	NMZL is a primary nodal B-cell neoplasm that morphologically resembles lymph nodes involved by marginal zone lymphomas of extranodal or splenic types, but without evidence of extranodal or splenic disease.

Follicular lymphoma (FL)	Lymphoma cells are usually positive for pan–B-cell antigens (CD19, CD20), surface immunoglobulin, CD10, Bcl-2, Bcl-6, and negative for CD5. Bcl-2 is expressed in the majority of cases, ranging from nearly 100% in grade 1 to 75% in grade 3 FL.	All cases have cytogenetic abnormalities. The t (14;18) (q32;q21) translocation, involving rearrangement of the Bcl-2 gene and IgH gene, is present in 80–95% of FL. FL may transform into high-grade B-cell lymphoma with features intermediate between DLBCL and Burkitt lymphoma, and c-myc (8q24) rearrangement is often involved. Bcl-2 is useful in distinguishing reactive follicular hyperplasia (Bcl-2 negative) and FL (Bcl-2-positive).
Mantle cell lymphoma (MCL)	Lymphoma cells express surface immunoglobulin, pan–B-cell antigens (CD19, CD20), Bcl-1, FMC-7, CD5, CD43, and are typically negative for CD10, CD23, and Bcl-6. Expression of Bcl-1 (cyclin D1) is required for diagnosis.	MCL and CLL/SLL are the two common CD5-positive B-cell lymphoproliferative disorders. But unlike CLL/SLL, MCL cells express bright surface immunoglobulin, bright CD20 and FMC-7, and are CD23 negative. Virtually all cases express Bcl-1 (cyclin D1) due to gene rearrangement.
Diffuse large B-cell lymphoma (DLBCL)	DLBCL cells typically express various pan–B-cell antigens (CD19, CD20, CD22, CD79a), surface and/or cytoplasmic immunoglobulin with light chain restriction, Bcl-6, and CD10. Bcl-2 is positive in 30–50% of cases.	Morphologic variants of DLBCL include centroblastic, immunoblastic, T-cell/histiocyte rich, anaplastic, and plasmablastic DLBCL. Bcl-2 expression has been reported to be associated with an adverse disease-free survival, while expression of Bcl-6 appears to be associated with a better prognosis. Unclassifiable large B-cell lymphomas with features intermediate between DLBCL and Burkitt lymphoma (eg, "double-hit" or "double-expressor" large B-cell lymphomas) require more intensive therapy.
Mediastinal (thymic) large B-cell lymphoma (Med-DLBCL)	Lymphoma cells express CD45 and B-cell antigen (CD19, CD20). Immunoglobulin and HLA-DR are often absent. The cells do not express CD5 and CD10, and lack Bcl-2, Bcl-6, and c-myc rearrangements.	Med-DLBCL is a subtype of DLBCL arising in the mediastinum of putative thymic B-cell origin with distinct clinical, immunophenotypic, and genotypic features. Tissue sections usually show diffuse lymphoid proliferation, compartmentalized into groups by fine/delicate fibrotic bands.
Intravascular large B-cell lymphoma	Lymphoma cells express pan–B-cell antigens (CD19, CD20).	The disease is a rare subtype of extranodal DLBCL characterized by the presence of lymphoma cells only in the lumina of small vessels, particularly capillaries. Brain and skin are the common sites of involvement.
Primary effusion lymphoma (PEL)	Lymphoma cells express CD45, but are usually negative for pan–B-cell markers (CD19, CD20). Surface and cytoplasmic immunoglobulin is often absent. Activation and plasma cell-related markers such as CD30, CD38, and CD138 are usually positive.	PEL is a neoplasm of large B cells usually presenting as serous effusions without detectable tumor masses. It is universally associated with human herpes virus 8 (HHV-8), most often occurring in the setting of immunodeficiency (eg, HIV/AIDS).

(Continued)

TABLE 8–13. LEUKEMIAS AND LYMPHOMAS: CLASSIFICATION AND IMMUNOPHENOTYPING (*CONTINUED*).

Disease	Typical Immunophenotype	Comments
Lymphomatoid granulomatosis (LYG)	Lymphoma cells express CD20, and are variably positive for CD30, but negative for CD15. The cells lack immunoglobulin expression. The background small lymphocytes are CD3–positive T cells.	LYG is an angiocentric and angiodestructive lymphoproliferative disease involving extranodal sites, composed of Epstein-Barr virus (EBV)-positive B cells admixed with reactive T cells, which usually numerically predominate. LYG may progress to an EBV-positive DLBCL. The common sites of involvement are lung, kidney, brain, liver, and skin.
Burkitt lymphoma (BL)	Lymphoma cells express surface immunoglobulin with light chain restriction, pan–B-cell antigens (CD19, CD20), CD10, and Bcl-6. The cells are negative for CD5, CD23, CD34, and TdT. Nearly 100% of the cells are positive for Ki-67, a proliferation marker.	All BL cases show a translocation of *c-myc* gene at chromosome 8q24 to the *Igh* gene at 14q32 or less commonly to light chain loci at 2p12 or 22q11. Genetic abnormalities involving the *c-myc* gene play an essential role in BL pathogenesis. The expression of CD10 and Bcl-6 indicates a germinal center origin of the tumor cells. BL is highly aggressive but potentially curable.
Mature T-cell and NK-cell Neoplasms		
T-cell prolymphocytic leukemia (T-PLL)	Leukemic cells express CD2, CD3, CD7, but not TdT and CD1a. The cells can be CD4+/CD8-(60%), CD4+/CD8+ (25%), or CD4–/CD8+ (15%).	T-PLL is an aggressive T-cell leukemia characterized by the proliferation of small to medium sized prolymphocytes with a mature post-thymic T-cell phenotype involving the blood, bone marrow, lymph nodes, spleen, and skin.
T-cell large granular lymphocyte leukemia (T-LGL)	T-LGL cells have a mature T-cell immunophenotype. Approximately 80% of cases are CD3+, TCR α β+, CD4–, and CD8+.	T-LGL is a heterogeneous disorder characterized by a persistent (>6 months) increase in peripheral blood large granular lymphocytes (LGLs), without a clearly identified cause. Severe neutropenia with or without anemia is a characteristic clinical feature. Pure red cell hypoplasia has been reported in association with T-LGL leukemia. Splenomegaly, rheumatoid arthritis, and the presence of autoantibodies are commonly seen in patients with T-LGL.
Aggressive NK-cell leukemia	Leukemic cells are CD2+, surface CD3–, cytoplasmic CD3ε+, CD56+, and positive for cytotoxic molecules (TIA-1, granzyme B, and/or perforin). This immunophenotype is identical to that of extranodal NK/T-cell lymphoma, nasal type.	Aggressive NK-cell leukemia is characterized by a systemic proliferation of NK cells. The disease has an aggressive clinical course. T-cell receptor (TCR) genes are in germline configuration.
Adult T-cell leukemia/lymphoma (ATLL)	Tumor cells express T-cell antigens (CD2, CD3, CD5), but usually lack CD7. Most cases are CD4+, CD8–. Rare cases are CD4–, CD8+, or double negative for CD4 and CD8. CD25 is expressed in virtually all cases.	ATLL is a peripheral T-cell neoplasm most often composed of highly pleomorphic lymphoid cells. The disease is usually widely disseminated, and is caused by the human T-cell leukemia virus type 1 (HTLV-1). ATLL is endemic in Japan, the Caribbean basin, and parts of Central Africa.

Extranodal NK/T-cell lymphoma, nasal type	The typical immunophenotype is CD2+, CD56+, surface CD3−, and cytoplasmic CD3 ε+. Most cases are positive for cytotoxic molecules (TIA-1, granzyme B, perforin).	The disease entity is designated NK/T (rather than NK) cell lymphoma because while most cases appear to be NK-cell neoplasms (EBV+, CD56+), rare cases show an EBV+, CD56− cytotoxic T-cell phenotype. T-cell receptor and immunoglobulin genes are in germline configuration in a majority of cases. EBV can be demonstrated in the tumor cells in nearly all cases. The prognosis is variable.
Enteropathy-type T-cell lymphoma	Tumor cells are CD3+, CD5−, CD7+, CD8±, CD4−, CD103+, and contain cytotoxic molecules.	The tumor occurs most commonly in the jejunum or ileum, and there is a clear association with celiac disease (gluten enteropathy). The prognosis is usually poor.
Hepatosplenic T-cell lymphoma	Tumor cells are CD3+, CD4−, CD8−, CD5−, CD56±. The cells are usually TCR γδ + and TCR αβ−.	Hepatosplenic T-cell lymphoma is an extranodal and systemic neoplasm derived from cytotoxic T cells usually of γδ T-cell receptor type, demonstrating marked sinusoidal infiltration of spleen, liver, and bone marrow. The clinical course is aggressive.
Subcutaneous panniculitis-like T-cell lymphoma (SPTCL)	Tumor cells are usually CD3+, TCR αβ +, CD5−, CD4−, CD8−, and express cytotoxic molecules.	SPTCL is a cytotoxic T-cell lymphoma, which preferentially infiltrates subcutaneous tissue. Some patients may present with a hemophagocytic syndrome with pancytopenia. The clinical course is aggressive.
Mycosis fungoides and Sézary syndrome (MF/SS)	The typical phenotype is CD2+, CD3+, TCR β +, CD5+, CD4+/CD8− (rarely CD4−/CD8+). Virtually all cases are negative for CD26 (a marker for treatment monitoring). CD7 is usually negative.	MF is a mature T-cell lymphoma, presenting in the skin with patches/plaques and characterized by epidermal and dermal infiltration of small to medium-sized T cells with cerebriform nuclei. SS is a generalized mature T-cell lymphoma characterized by the presence of erythroderma, lymphadenopathy, and neoplastic T lymphocytes in the blood.
Primary cutaneous CD30−positive T-cell lymphoproliferative disorders	Primary cutaneous anaplastic large cell lymphoma (C-ALCL): Tumor cells express T-cell antigens (CD2, CD3, CD5, CD7) and are usually positive for CD4. CD30 is expressed in >75% of the cells. Aberrant T-cell phenotype with loss of one or more T-cell antigens is common. Lymphomatoid papulosis (LyP): The atypical T cells are CD4+, CD8−. The cells often express aberrant phenotypes with variable loss of pan−T-cell antigens (eg, CD2, CD5, or CD7). CD30 is positive in a LyP subtype (type A).	LyP and C-ALCL constitute a spectrum of related conditions originating from transformed or activated CD30-positive T lymphocytes. They may coexist in individual patients, they can be clonally related and they often show overlapping clinical and/or histologic features.

(Continued)

TABLE 8–13. LEUKEMIAS AND LYMPHOMAS: CLASSIFICATION AND IMMUNOPHENOTYPING (*CONTINUED*).

Disease	Typical Immunophenotype	Comments
Angioimmunoblastic T-cell lymphoma (AITL)	Neoplastic cells express T cell antigens (CD2, CD3, CD5, CD7), usually without aberrant antigen loss, and are CD4+ and CD8–. The neoplastic T cells are positive for CD10 and/or Bcl-6. CD21 stain highlights the intact or disrupted follicular dendritic meshwork.	AITL is a T-cell lymphoma characterized by systemic disease and a polymorphous infiltrate involving lymph nodes. TCR genes are rearranged in the majority (>75%) of cases. Secondary EBV-related B-cell lymphoma may occur. Almost all cases are positive for CD10 and/or Bcl-6, suggesting a germinal center derivation of the tumor cells. The clinical course is very aggressive.
Peripheral T-cell lymphoma, unspecified	Neoplastic cells express T cell antigens (CD2, CD3, CD5, CD7), but aberrant T-cell phenotypes with antigen loss are frequent. Most nodal cases are CD4+, CD8–, CD30, and CD56 may be positive.	These cases are among the most aggressive of the non-Hodgkin lymphomas.
Anaplastic large cell lymphoma (ALCL)	The tumor cells express one or more T-cell antigens (CD2, CD3, CD5, CD7). The cells usually express CD30 (membrane and in the Golgi region), ALK (cytoplasmic and/or nuclear), EMA, cytotoxic molecules, CD43, and CD45.	Expression of ALK in ALCL is due to genetic alteration of the ALK locus on chromosome 2. The most common alteration is t(2;5)(p23;q35), resulting in fusion of the ALK gene and nucleophosmin (NPM) gene on 5q35. ALK-positive ALCL has a favorable prognosis.

For details, see Swerdlow SH, et al (editors). *WHO Classification of Tumours of Haematopoietic and Lymphoid Tissues*. IARC Press: Lyon 2008.
ALK = *anaplastic large cell lymphoma kinase;* **CD** = *cluster of differentiation;* **EMA** = *epithelial membrane antigen;* **FISH** = *fluorescence in-situ hybridization;* **MPO** = *myeloperoxidase;* **PCR** = *polymerase chain reaction.*

TABLE 8–14. OSMOL GAP: CALCULATION AND APPLICATION IN CLINICAL TOXICOLOGY.

The osmol gap (Δ osm) is determined by subtracting the calculated serum osmolality from the measured serum osmolality.

$$\text{Calculated osmolality (oms)} = 2(Na^+ [meq/L]) + \frac{\text{Glucose (mg/dL)}}{18} + \frac{\text{BUN (mg/dL)}}{2.8}$$

$$\text{osmol gap } (\Delta\ osm) = \text{Measured osmolality} - \text{Calculated osmolality}$$

Serum osmolality may be increased by contributions of circulating alcohols and other low-molecular-weight substances. Since these substances are not included in the calculated osmolality, there will be a gap proportionate to their serum concentration and inversely proportionate to their molecular weight:

$$\text{Serum concentration (mg/dL)} = \Delta\ osm \times \frac{\text{Molecular weight of toxin}}{10}$$

For ethanol (the most common cause of Δ osm), a gap of 30 mosm/L indicates an ethanol level of:

$$30 \times \frac{46}{10} = 138\,mg/dL$$

See the following for toxic concentrations of alcohols and their corresponding osmol gaps.

TOXIC CONCENTRATIONS OF ALCOHOLS AND THEIR CORRESPONDING OSMOL GAPS			
	Molecular Weight	**Toxic Concentration (mg/dL)**	**Approximate Corresponding Δ osm (mosm/L)**
Ethanol	46	300	65
Methanol	32	100	16
Ethylene glycol	60	100	16
Isopropanol	60	150	25

Note: The normal osmol gap may vary by as much as ± 10 mosm/L; thus, small osmol gaps may be unreliable in the diagnosis of poisoning. **BUN** = blood urea nitrogen; **Na** ⁺ = sodium.
Modified with permission from Stone CK, Humphries RL (editors): Current Emergency Diagnosis & Treatment, 7th ed. McGraw-Hill, 2011; and Tintinalli J, Stapczynski J: Tintinalli's Emergency Medicine: A Comprehensive Study Guide, 8th ed. McGraw-Hill, 2015.

TABLE 8–15. RANSON CRITERIA FOR ASSESSING SEVERITY OF ACUTE PANCREATITIS.

Three or more of the following predict a severe course complicated by pancreatic necrosis with a sensitivity of 60–80%: Age >55 years White blood cell count > 16×10^3/mcL (16×10^9/L) Blood glucose > 200 mg/dL (11 mmol/L) Serum lactic dehydrogenase >350 units/L (7 mkat/L) Serum aspartate aminotransferase >250 units/L (5 mkat/L)
Development of the following in the first 48 hours indicates a worsening prognosis: Hematocrit drop of >10 percentage points Blood urea nitrogen rise of >5 mg/dL (1.8 mmol/L) Arterial PO_2 <60 mm Hg (7.8 kPa) Serum calcium <8 mg/dL (0.2 mmol/L) Base deficit >4 meq/L Estimated fluid sequestration of >6 L

Mortality rates correlate with the number of criteria present[1]:

Number of Criteria	Mortality Rate
0–2	1%
3–4	16%
5–6	40%
7–8	100%

[1]An Acute Physiology and Chronic Health Evaluation (APACHE) II score ≥ 8 also correlates with mortality.

TABLE 8–16. PLEURAL EFFUSION: PLEURAL FLUID PROFILES IN VARIOUS DISEASE STATES.

Diagnosis	Gross Appearance	Protein (g/dL)	Glucose[1] (mg/dL)	WBC (per mcL); Differential	RBC (per mcL)	Microscopic Exam	Culture	Comments
Normal	Clear	1.0–1.5	Equal to serum	≤1000; mostly MN	0 or Few	Neg	Neg	
TRANSUDATES[2]								
Heart failure	Serous	<3: sometimes ≥3	Equal to serum	<1000	<10,000	Neg	Neg	Most common cause of pleural effusion. Effusion right-sided in 55–70% of patients.
Nephrotic syndrome	Serous	<3	Equal to serum	<1000	<1000	Neg	Neg	Occurs in 20% of patients. Cause is low protein osmotic pressure.
Cirrhosis with ascites	Serous	<3	Equal to serum	<1000	<1000	Neg	Neg	From movement of ascites across diaphragm. Treatment of underlying ascites usually sufficient.
EXUDATES[3,4]								
Tuberculosis	Serous to serosanguineous	>3 (in 90%); may exceed 5 g/dL	<60 (in 60%)	1000–10,000; mostly MN	<10,000	Concentrate Pos for AFB in <50%; cholesterol crystals	May yield MTb	Quantiferon positive; PPD usually positive; pleural biopsy positive; eosinophils (>10%) or mesothelial cells (>5%) make diagnosis unlikely.
Malignancy	Turbid to bloody; Occ serous	≥3 in 90%	Equal to serum; <60 in 15% of cases	1000 to <100,000; mostly MN	100 – >100,000	Pos cytology in >50%	Neg	Eosinophils uncommon; fluid tends to reaccumulate after removal.
Empyema	Turbid to purulent	≥3	Less than serum; often <20	25,000–100,000; mostly PMN	<5000	Pos	Pos	Drainage necessary; putrid odor suggests anaerobic infection.
Parapneumonic effusion, uncomplicated	Clear to turbid	≥3	Equal to serum; Occ <60	5000–25,000; mostly PMN	<5000	Neg	Neg	Tube thoracostomy unnecessary; associated infiltrate on chest x-ray; fluid pH ≥7.2.

(Continued)

TABLE 8–16. PLEURAL EFFUSION: PLEURAL FLUID PROFILES IN VARIOUS DISEASE STATES (*CONTINUED*).

Diagnosis	Gross Appearance	Protein (g/dL)	Glucose[1] (mg/dL)	WBC (per mcL); Differential	RBC (per mcL)	Microscopic Exam	Culture	Comments
Pulmonary embolism, infarction	Serous to grossly bloody	≥3	Equal to serum	1000–50,000; MN or PMN	100–>100,000	Neg	Neg	Variable findings; no pathognomonic features; 25% are transudates.
Rheumatoid arthritis, other collagen vascular diseases	Turbid or yellow-green	≥3	Very low (<40 in most)	1000–20,000; mostly MN	<1000	Neg	Neg	Secondary empyema common; high LDH, low complement, high rheumatoid factor, cholesterol crystals are characteristic.
Pancreatitis	Turbid to serosanguineous	≥3	Equal to serum	1000–50,000; mostly PMN	1000–10,000	Neg	Neg	Effusion usually left-sided; high amylase level.
Esophageal rupture	Turbid to purulent; red-brown	≥3	Equal to serum	<5000–>50,000; mostly PMN	1000–10,000	Pos	Pos	Usually left-sided; high fluid amylase level (salivary); pneumothorax in 25% of cases; pH <6.0 strongly suggests diagnosis.

[1]Glucose of pleural fluid in comparison to serum glucose.

[2]Transudative effusions also occur in peritoneal dialysis; myxedema; acute atelectasis; constrictive pericarditis; SVC obstruction; and pulmonary embolism (some).

[3]Exudative pleural effusions meet at least one of the following criteria: (1) pleural fluid protein/serum protein ratio >0.5; (2) pleural fluid LDH/serum LDH ratio >0.6; and (3) pleural fluid LDH >2/3 upper normal limit for serum LDH. Transudative pleural effusions meet none of these criteria.

[4]Exudative pleural effusions also occur in viral, fungal, rickettsial, parasitic infections; asbestos; Meigs syndrome; uremia; chronic atelectasis; trapped lung; chylothorax; sarcoidosis; post-MI injury syndrome; and drug reaction.

AFB = acid-fast bacilli; **LDH** = lactate dehydrogenase; **MN** = mononuclear cells (lymphocytes or monocytes); **MTb** = Mycobacterium tuberculosis; **PMN** = polymorphonuclear cells.

Data from Therapy of pleural effusion. A statement by the Committee on Therapy. Am Rev Respir Dis 1968;97:479; Doherty GM (editor). Current Diagnosis & Treatment: Surgery. 14th ed. McGraw-Hill 2015; and Papadakis MA, McPhee SJ, Rabow MW (editors). Current Medical Diagnosis & Treatment 2016, 55th ed. McGraw-Hill, 2016.

TABLE 8–17.   PRENATAL DIAGNOSTIC METHODS: AMNIOCENTESIS, CHORIONIC VILLUS SAMPLING, AND CORDOCENTESIS.

Method	Procedure	Laboratory Analyses	Waiting Time for Results	Advantages	Disadvantages
Amniocentesis	Between the 15th and 20th weeks, and by the transabdominal approach, 20–30 mL of amniotic fluid is removed for analysis. Preceding ultrasound locates the placenta and identifies twinning and missed abortion.	1. **Amniotic fluid** • α-Fetoprotein, acetylcholinesterase • Biochemical analysis (metabolic diseases) • Virus isolation studies 2. **Amniotic cell culture** • Chromosomal analysis (cytogenetic [karyotyping], molecular, certain gene mutation analyses)	7–10 days	Over 55 years of experience.	Therapeutic abortion, if indicated, must be done in the 2nd trimester. (RhoGam should be given to Rh-negative mothers to prevent sensitization.) Risks: • Fetal: abortion (0.06–0.3%). • Maternal: transient vaginal spotting or amniotic fluid leakage (1.2%) or chorioamnionitis (<0.1%). Risks are somewhat higher if amniocentesis is performed earlier (11th to 14th weeks).
Chorionic villus sampling (CVS)	Between the 9th and 13th week, and with constant ultrasound guidance, the trophoblastic cells of the chorionic villi are obtained by transcervical or transabdominal endoscopic needle biopsy or aspiration.	1. **Direct cell analysis** • Chromosomal and DNA analysis (cytogenetic, certain gene mutations) 2. **Cell culture** • Biochemical analyses (as above)	7–10 days	Over 45 years of experience. Therapeutic abortion, if indicated, can be done in the 1st trimester.	Chromosomal abnormalities detected by this technique may be confined to the placenta (confined placental mosaicism) and thus CVS may be less informative than amniocentesis. Does not allow diagnosis of neural tube defects. Risks • Fetal: abortion (0.06–0.3%). • Maternal: spotting or infection (<0.5%).
Cordocentesis (percutaneous umbilical blood [fetal blood] sampling, PUBS)	PUBS can be performed in 2nd and 3rd trimesters (after 17 weeks). It is usually done when diagnostic information cannot be obtained through amniocentesis, CVS or ultrasound, or if the results of these tests are inconclusive.	1. **Direct cell analysis** • Chromosomal analysis (cytogenetics) 2. **Cell culture** • Biochemical analyses (metabolic diseases) 3. **Blood analyses** • Rh sensitization • Alloimmune thrombocytopenia • Fetal anemia assessment	<1 day (1–2 days for karyotyping)	Rapid turnaround	Done in 2nd and 3rd trimesters; therapeutic abortion, if indicated, must be done in the 2nd trimester. Risks • Fetal: abortion (1.4–2%), can vary with fetal condition; bradycardia (5%). • Maternal: cord vessel bleeding (20–30%). • Fetal-maternal: bleeding (40%) if placenta is traversed.

TABLE 8–18 PULMONARY FUNCTION TESTS: INTERPRETATION IN OBSTRUCTIVE AND RESTRICTIVE PULMONARY DISEASES.

Tests	Units	Definition	Obstructive Disease	Restrictive Disease
SPIROMETRY				
Forced vital capacity (FVC)	L	The volume that can be forcefully expelled from the lungs after maximal inspiration.	N or ↓	↓
Forced expiratory volume in 1 second (FEV$_1$)	L	The volume expelled in the first second of the FVC maneuver.	↓	N or ↓
FEV$_1$/FVC [1]	%		↓	N or ↑
Forced expiratory flow from 25% to 75% of the forced vital capacity (FEF 25–75%)	L/sec	The maximal midexpiratory airflow rate.	↓	N or ↓
Peak expiratory flow rate (PEFR)	L/sec	The maximal airflow rate achieved in the FVC maneuver.	↓	N or ↑
Maximum voluntary ventilation (MVV)	L/min	The maximum volume that can be breathed in 1 minute (usually measured for 15 seconds and multiplied by 4).	↓	N or ↓
LUNG VOLUMES				
Slow vital capacity (SVC)	L	The volume that can be slowly exhaled after maximal inspiration.	N or ↓	↓
Total lung capacity (TLC)	L	The volume in the lungs after a maximal inspiration.	N or ↑	↓
Functional residual capacity (FRC)	L	The volume in the lungs at the end of a normal tidal expiration.	↑	N or ↑
Expiratory reserve volume (ERV)	L	The volume representing the difference between FRC and RV.	N or ↓	N or ↓
Residual volume (RV)	L	The volume remaining in the lungs after maximal expiration.	↑	N or ↑
RV/TLC ratio			↑	N or ↑

N = *normal;* ↓ = *less than predicted;* ↑ = *greater than predicted. Normal values vary according to subject sex, age, body size, and ethnicity.*
[1]*Perhaps the most useful single parameter for differentiating obstructive from restrictive lung disease.*
Modified with permission from Tierney LM Jr, McPhee SJ, Papadakis MA (editors). Current Medical Diagnosis & Treatment 2001, 40th ed. McGraw-Hill, 2001.

TABLE 8–19. RENAL FAILURE: CLASSIFICATION AND DIFFERENTIAL DIAGNOSIS.

	Prerenal Azotemia	Postrenal Azotemia	Acute Tubular Necrosis (Oliguric or Polyuric)	Intrinsic Renal Disease	
				Acute Glomerulonephritis	Acute Interstitial Nephritis
Etiology	Poor renal perfusion (eg, hypovolemia [vomiting, diarrhea]; hypotension; severe heart failure)	Obstruction of the urinary tract	Ischemia; nephrotoxins	Immune complex-mediated; pauci-immune; anti-GBM related	Allergic reaction; drug reaction; infection; collagen vascular disease
BUN: Cr ratio	>20:1	>20:1	<20:1	>20:1	<20:1
Urinary indices					
U_{Na+} (meq/L)	<20	Variable	>20	<20	Variable
FE_{Na+} (%)	<1	Variable	>1 (when oliguric)	<1	<1; >1
Urine osmolality (mosm/kg)	>500	<400	250–300	Variable	Variable
Urinary sediment	Benign, or hyaline casts	Normal or red cells, white cells, or crystals	Granular (muddy brown) casts, renal tubular casts	Red cells, dysmorphic red cells, and red cell casts	White cells, white cell casts, with or without eosinophils

BUN:Cr = blood urea nitrogen:creatinine

$$FE_{Na^+} = \left(\dfrac{\dfrac{Urine\ Na^+}{Plasma\ Na^+}}{\dfrac{Urine\ creatinine}{Plasma\ creatinine}} \right) \times 100$$

U_{Na^+} = urine sodium.

Reproduced with permission from Papadakis MA, McPhee SJ, Rabow MW (editors), Current Medical Diagnosis & Treatment 2016, 55th ed. McGraw-Hill 2016.

TABLE 8–20. RENAL TUBULAR ACIDOSIS (RTA): LABORATORY DIAGNOSIS.

Clinical Condition	Mechanism	GFR	Serum HCO_3^- (meq/L)	Minimal Urine pH	Serum K^+ (meq/L)	Calcium Excretion	Associated Disease States	Treatment
Normal	None	N	24–28	4.8–5.2	3.5–5	100–300 mg/24h	None	None
Distal (Type I) RTA	Defective collecting duct H^+ secretion	N	20–23	>5.5	→	↑	Various genetic disorders, autoimmune diseases, paraproteinemias, nephrocalcinosis, nephrolithiasis, drugs [amphotericin], toxins, tubulointerstitial diseases.	$NaHCO_3$ (1–3 meq/kg/d).
Proximal (Type II) RTA	Defective proximal tubule HCO_3^- absorption	N	15–18	<5.5	→	↑	Drugs, Fanconi syndrome, various genetic disorders, dysproteinemic states, secondary hyperparathyroidism, toxins (heavy metals), tubulointerstitial diseases, nephrotic syndrome, paroxysmal nocturnal hemoglobinuria.	$NaHCO_3$ or $KHCO_3$ (10–15 meq/kg/d), thiazides.
Hyporeninemic hypoaldosteronemic (Type IV) RTA	Defective collecting duct K^+ secretion, Na^+ reabsorption	↓	24–28	<5.5	↑	N	Hyporeninemic hypoaldosteronism (diabetes mellitus, tubulointerstitial diseases, hypertensive nephrosclerosis, AIDS, drugs [ACE inhibitors, spironolactone, NSAIDs]), primary mineralocorticoid deficiency (eg, Addison disease), salt-wasting mineralocorticoid-resistant hyperkalemia.	Fludrocortisone (0.1–0.5 mg/d), dietary K^+ restriction, furosemide (40–160 mg/d), $NaHCO_3$ (1–3 meq/kg/d).

GFR = glomerular filtration rate.
Modified with permission from Lerma EV et al. Current Diagnosis & Treatment: Nephrology & Hypertension. McGraw-Hill, 2009.

TABLE 8–21. SYPHILIS: CLINICAL AND LABORATORY DIAGNOSIS IN UNTREATED PATIENTS.

	Primary Stage	Secondary Stage	Latent Stage	Late (Tertiary) Stage	Test Specificity, % (range)
CLINICAL					
Onset After Exposure	21 days (range 10–90)	6 wk–6 mo	Early: <1 yr Late: >1 yr	1 yr until death	
Persistence	2–12 wk	1–3 mo	Early: Up to 1 year Late: Lifelong unless late (tertiary) syphilis appears	Until death	
Clinical Findings	Chancre	Rash, condylomata lata, mucous patches, fever, lymphadenopathy, patchy alopecia	Early: Relapses of secondary syphilis Late: Clinically silent	Dementia, tabes dorsalis, aortitis, aortic aneurysm, gummas	
LABORATORY		**Test Sensitivity** by stage of infection, % (range)			**Test Specificity**, % (range)
Nontreponemal tests					
VDRL	78 (74–87)	100	96 (88–100)	71 (37–94)	98 (96–99)
RPR	86 (77–99)	100	98 (95–100)	73	98 (93–99)
Early treponemal tests					
TP-PA	88 (86–100)	100	100	NA	96 (95–100)
FTA-ABS	84 (70–100)	100	100	96	97 (94–100)
Enzyme immunoassays					
IgG-ELISA	100	100	100	NA	100
IgM-EIA	93	85	64	NA	NA
ICE	77	100	100	100	99
Immunochemiluminescence assays					
CLIA	98	100	100	100	99

CLIA = chemiluminescence assay; ***EIA*** = enzyme immunoassay; ***ELISA*** = enzyme-linked immunosorbent assay; ***FTA-ABS*** = fluorescent treponemal antibody absorption test; ***ICE*** = immune-capture EIA; ***IgG*** = immunoglobulin G; ***IgM*** = immunoglobulin M; ***NA*** = not available; ***RPR*** = rapid plasma reagin test; ***TPPA*** = Treponema pallidum particle agglutination; ***VDRL*** = Venereal Disease Research Laboratories test.
Data from Sena AC et al. Novel Treponema pallidum serologic tests: a paradigm shift in syphilis screening for the 21st century. Clin Infect Dis 2010;51:700.

TABLE 8–22. THALASSEMIA SYNDROMES: GENETICS AND LABORATORY CHARACTERISTICS.

α-Thalassemia[1]

Syndrome	α-Globin Genes (functional)	Hematocrit	MCV (fL)
Normal	4	N	N
Silent carrier	3	N	N
Thalassemia minor (or trait)	2	28–40%	60–75
Hemoglobin H disease	1	22–32%	60–70
Hydrops fetalis	0	18%; fetal death occurs in utero	<60

MCV = mean corpuscular volume
[1]*Alpha thalassemias are due primarily to functional deletion of the α-globin genes on chromosome 16.*

β-Thalassemia[1]

Syndrome	β-Globin Genes (functional)	Hb A[2]	Hb A$_2$[3]	Hb F[4]	Transfusion Requirement
Normal	Homozygous β	97–99%	1–3%	<1%	None
Thalassemia minor	Heterozygous β[0][5]	80–95%	4–8%	1–5%	None
	Heterozygous β[+][6]	80–95%	4–8%	1–5%	None
Thalassemia intermedia	Homozygous β[+] (mild)	0–30%	0–10%	6–100%	Occasional
Thalassemia major	Homozygous β[0]	0%	4–10%	90–96%	Dependent
	Homozygous β[+]	0–10%	4–10%	90–96%	Dependent

Hb = hemoglobin; *MCV* = mean corpuscular volume.
[1] *β-Thalassemias are usually caused by point mutations in the β-globin gene on chromosome 11 that result in premature chain termina-tions or defective RNA transcription, leading to reduced or absent β-globin-chain synthesis.*
[2]*Hb A is composed of two α chains and two β chains: $α_2β_2$.*
[3]*Hb A$_2$ is composed of two α chains and two δ chains: $α_2δ_2$.*
[4]*Hb F is composed of two α chains and two γ chains: $α_2γ_2$.*
[5] *β[0] refers to defects that result in absent globin-chain synthesis.*
[6] *β[+] refers to defects that cause reduced but not absent globin-chain synthesis.*
Modified with permission from Papadakis MA, McPhee SJ, Rabow MW (editors). Current Medical Diagnosis & Treatment 2016, 55th ed. McGraw-Hill, 2016.

TABLE 8–23. TRANSFUSION: SUMMARY CHART OF BLOOD COMPONENT THERAPY.[1]

Component	Major Indications	Action/Benefit	Not Indicated For	Special Precautions	Hazards[1]	Rate/Time of Infusion
Whole blood	Symptomatic anemia with large volume deficit	Increases oxygen-carrying capacity. Increases blood volume.	Condition responsive to specific component. Treatment of coagulopathy.	Must be ABO-identical	Infectious diseases; hemolytic, septic/toxic, allergic, febrile reactions; TACO, TRALI, TA-GVHD	As fast as patient can tolerate but less than 4 hours
Red blood cells; Red blood cells, low volume; Apheresis red blood cells	Symptomatic anemia	Increases oxygen-carrying capacity.	Pharmacologically treatable anemia. Coagulation deficiency. Volume expansion.	Must be ABO-compatible	Infectious diseases; Hemolytic, septic/toxic, allergic, febrile reactions; TACO, TRALI, TA-GVHD	As fast as patient can tolerate but less than 4 hours
Red blood cells, leukocyte-reduced[4]	Symptomatic anemia; Reduction of febrile reactions	Increases oxygen-carrying capacity. Reduction of risks of febrile reactions, HLA alloimmunization and CMV infection (equivalent to CMV-negative component).	Pharmacologically treatable anemia. Coagulation deficiency. Volume expansion. Prevention of TA-GVHD.	Must be ABO-compatible	Infectious diseases; Hemolytic, septic/toxic, allergic, febrile reactions; TACO, TRALI, TA-GVHD. Hypotensive reaction may occur if bedside leukocyte reduction filter is used.	As fast as patient can tolerate but less than 4 hours
Red blood cells, washed	Symptomatic anemia; IgA deficiency with anaphylactoid reaction; Recurrent severe allergic reactions to unwashed red cell products; Paroxysmal nocturnal hemoglobinuria	Increases oxygen carrying capacity. Washing reduces plasma proteins. Risk of allergic reactions may be reduced.	Pharmacologically treatable anemia. Coagulation deficiency. Volume expansion.	Must be ABO-compatible	Infectious diseases; Hemolytic, septic/toxic, allergic, febrile reactions; TACO, TRALI, TA-GVHD	As fast as patient can tolerate but less than 4 hours
Fresh-frozen plasma (FFP)[2]	Clinically significant plasma protein deficiencies when no specific coagulation factors are available; TTP	Source of plasma proteins, including all coagulation factors.	Volume expansion. Coagulopathy that can be more effectively treated with specific therapy.	Must be ABO-compatible	Infectious diseases; allergic reactions; TACO, TRALI	Less than 4 hours
Cryoprecipitated AHF; Pooled cryoprecipitated AHF	Hemophilia A[3]; von Willebrand disease[3]; hypofibrinogenemia; factor XIII deficiency	Provides factor VIII, fibrinogen, von Willebrand factor, factor XIII.	Deficit of any plasma protein other than those enriched in cryoprecipitated AHF.		Infectious diseases; allergic reactions	Less than 4 hours

(Continued)

TABLE 8–23. TRANSFUSION: SUMMARY CHART OF BLOOD COMPONENT THERAPY (*CONTINUED*).[1]

Component	Major Indications	Action/Benefit	Not Indicated For	Special Precautions	Hazards[1]	Rate/Time of Infusion
Apheresis platelets[4]; Pooled platelet concentrates	Bleeding due to thrombocytopenia or platelet function abnormality; prevention of bleeding from marrow hypoplasia	Improves hemostasis. May be HLA (or other antigen) selected.	Plasma coagulation deficits, some conditions with rapid platelet destruction (eg, ITP, TTP) unless life-threatening hemorrhage.	Should not use some filters (check manufacturer's instructions)	Infectious diseases; Septic/toxic, allergic, febrile reactions; TACO, TA-GVHD, TRALI	Less than 4 hours
Apheresis granulocytes	Neutropenia with infection, unresponsive to appropriate antibiotics	Provides granulocytes with or without platelets.	Infection responsive to antibiotics, eventual marrow recovery not expected.	Must be ABO-compatible. Should not use filters (check manufacturer's instructions)	Infectious diseases; Hemolytic, allergic, febrile reactions; TACO, TRALI, TA-GVHD	One unit over 2–4 hours. Observe closely for reactions.
Irradiated components (eg, leukocyte-reduced red blood cells, apheresis platelets)	Increased risk of TA-GVHD (eg, stem cell transplant, IUT, and selected immunodeficiencies, HLA-matched platelets or transfusions from blood relatives)	Donor lymphocytes are inactivated, reducing risk of TA-GVHD.	See relevant component (eg, leukocyte-reduced red blood cells, apheresis platelets).	See relevant component (eg, leukocyte-reduced red blood cells, apheresis platelets).	See relevant component (eg, leukocyte-reduced red blood cells, apheresis platelets).	See relevant component (eg, leukocyte-reduced red blood cells, apheresis platelets).

[1]For all cellular components, there is a risk that the recipient may become alloimmunized and experience rapid destruction of certain types of blood products. Red cell to containing components and thawed plasma should be stored at 1–6°C. Platelets, granulocytes, and thawed cryoprecipitate should be stored at 20–24°C.

[2]Solvent detergent pooled plasma is an alternative in which some viruses are inactivated, but clotting factor composition is changed.

[3]When virus-inactivated concentrates are not available.

[4]Red blood cells and platelets may be processed in a manner that yields leukocyte-reduced components. The main indications for leukocyte-reduced components are prevention of febrile, nonhemolytic transfusion reactions and prevention of leukocyte alloimmunization, HLA alloimmunization and CMV infection. One unit of apheresis platelet, is equivalent to 68 units of platelet concentrates.

AHF = antihemophilic factor; **ITP** = idiopathic thrombocytopenic purpura; **IUT** = intrauterine transfusion; **TACO** = transfusion–associated circulatory overload; **TA-GVHD** = transfusion-associated graft-versus-host disease; **TRALI** = transfusion-related acute lung injury; **TTP** = thrombotic thrombocytopenic purpura.

Data adapted from American Association of Blood Banks, American Red Cross, America's Blood Centers. Circulars of information for the use of human blood and blood components. Revised November 2013 (available at http://www.aabb.org).

TABLE 8–24. VALVULAR HEART DISEASE: DIAGNOSTIC EVALUATION.

	Mitral Stenosis	Mitral Regurgitation	Aortic Stenosis	Aortic Regurgitation	Tricuspid Stenosis	Tricuspid Regurgitation
Inspection	Malar flush, precordial bulge, and diffuse pulsation in young patients.	Usually prominent and hyperdynamic apical impulse to left of MCL.	Sustained PMI, prominent atrial filling wave.	Hyperdynamic PMI to left of MCL and downward. Pulsating carotid pulsations. Pulsating nailbeds (Quincke), head bob (de Musset).	Giant a wave in jugular pulse with sinus rhythm. Peripheral edema or ascites, or both.	Large v wave in jugular pulse; time with carotid pulsation. Peripheral edema or ascites, or both.
Palpation	"Tapping" sensation over area of expected PMI. Right ventricular pulsation left third to fifth ICS parasternally when pulmonary hypertension is present. P₂ may be palpable.	Forceful, brisk PMI; systolic thrill over PMI. Pulse normal, small, or slightly collapsing.	Powerful, heaving PMI to left and slightly below MCL. Systolic thrill over aortic area, sternal notch, or carotid arteries in severe disease. Small and slowly rising carotid pulse. If bicuspid AS check for delay at femoral artery to exclude coarctation.	Apical impulse forceful and displaced significantly to left and downward. Prominent carotid pulses. Rapidly rising and collapsing pulse (Corrigan pulse).	Pulsating, enlarged liver in ventricular systole.	Right ventricular pulsation. Systolic pulsation of liver.
Heart sounds, rhythm, and blood pressure	S₁ loud if valve mobile. Opening snap following S₂. The worse the disease, the closer the S₂–opening snap interval.	S₁ normal or buried in early part of murmur (exception in mitral prolapse where murmur may be late). Prominent third heart sound when severe MR. Atrial fibrillation common. Blood pressure normal. Midsystolic clicks may be present and may be multiple.	A₂ normal, soft, or absent. Prominent S₄. Blood pressure normal, or systolic pressure normal with high diastolic pressure.	S₁ normal or reduced, A₂ loud. Wide pulse pressure with diastolic pressure <60 mm Hg. When severe, gentle compression of femoral artery with diaphragm of stethoscope may reveal diastolic flow (Duroziez) and pressure in leg on palpation >40 mm Hg than arm (Hill).	S₁ often loud.	Atrial fibrillation may be present.

(Continued)

TABLE 8–24. VALVULAR HEART DISEASE: DIAGNOSTIC EVALUATION (*CONTINUED*).

	Mitral Stenosis	Mitral Regurgitation	Aortic Stenosis	Aortic Regurgitation	Tricuspid Stenosis	Tricuspid Regurgitation
Murmurs						
Location and transmission	Localized at or near apex. Diastolic rumble best heard in left lateral position; may be accentuated by having patient do sit-ups. Rarely, short diastolic murmur along lower left sternal border (Graham-Steell) in severe pulmonary hypertension.	Loudest over PMI; posteriorly directed jets (ie, anterior mitral prolapse) transmitted to left axilla, left infrascapular area; anteriorly directed jets (ie, posterior mitral prolapse) heard over anterior precordium. Murmur unchanged after premature beat.	Right second ICS parasternally or at apex, heard in carotid arteries and occasionally in upper interscapular area. May sound like MR at apex (Gallaverdin phenomenon), but murmur occurs after S₁ and stops before S₂. The later the peak in the murmur, the more severe the AS.	Diastolic: louder along left sternal border in third to fourth interspace. Heard over aortic area and apex. May be associated with low-pitched mid diastolic murmur at apex (Austin Flint) due to functional mitral stenosis. If due to an enlarged aorta, murmur may radiate to right sternal border.	Third to fifth ICS along left sternal border out to apex. Murmur increases with inspiration.	Third to fifth ICS along left sternal border. Murmur hard to hear but increases with inspiration. Sit-ups can increase cardiac output and accentuate.
Timing	Relation of opening snap to A₂ important. The higher the LA pressure, the earlier the opening snap. Presystolic murmur begins before S₁ if in sinus rhythm. Graham-Steell begins with P₂ (early diastole) if associated pulmonary hypertension.	Pansystolic: begins with S₁ and ends at or after A₂. May be late systolic in mitral valve prolapse.	Begins after S₁, ends before A₂. The more severe the stenosis, the later the murmur peaks.	Begins immediately after aortic second sound and ends before first sound (blurring both); helps distinguish from MR.	Rumble often follows audible opening snap.	At times, hard to hear. Begins with S₁ and fills systole. Increases with inspiration.
Character	Low-pitched, rumbling; presystolic murmur merges with loud S₁.	Blowing, high-pitched; occasionally harsh or musical.	Harsh, rough.	Blowing, often faint.	As for mitral stenosis.	Blowing, coarse, or musical.

Optimum auscultatory conditions	After exercise, left lateral recumbence. Bell chest piece lightly applied.	After exercise; use diaphragm chest piece. In prolapse, findings may be more evident while standing.	Use stethoscope diaphragm. Patient resting, leaning forward, breath held in full expiration.	Use stethoscope diaphragm. Patient leaning forward, breath held in expiration.	Use stethoscope bell. Murmur usually louder and at peak during inspiration. Patient recumbent.	Use stethoscope diaphragm. Murmur usually becomes louder during inspiration.
Radiography	Straight left heart border from enlarged LA appendage. Elevation of left mainstem bronchus. Large right ventricle and pulmonary artery if pulmonary hypertension is present. Calcification in mitral valve in rheumatic mitral stenosis or in annulus in calcific mitral stenosis.	Enlarged left ventricle and LA.	Concentric left ventricular hypertrophy. Prominent ascending aorta. Calcified aortic valve common.	Moderate to severe left ventricular enlargement. Aortic root often dilated.	Enlarged right atrium with prominent SVC and azygous shadow.	Enlarged right atrium and right ventricle.
ECG	Broad P waves in standard leads; broad negative phase of diphasic P in V_1. If pulmonary hypertension is present, tall peaked P waves, right axis deviation, or right ventricular hypertrophy appears.	Left axis deviation or frank left ventricular hypertrophy. P waves broad, tall, or notched in standard leads. Broad negative phase of diphasic P in V_1.	Left ventricular hypertrophy.	Left ventricular hypertrophy.	Tall, peaked P waves. Possible right ventricular hypertrophy.	Right axis usual.

(Continued)

TABLE 8–24. VALVULAR HEART DISEASE: DIAGNOSTIC EVALUATION (*CONTINUED*).

	Mitral Stenosis	Mitral Regurgitation	Aortic Stenosis	Aortic Regurgitation	Tricuspid Stenosis	Tricuspid Regurgitation
Echocardiography						
Two-dimensional echocardiography	Thickened, immobile mitral valve with anterior and posterior leaflets moving together. "Hockey stick" shape to opened anterior leaflet in rheumatic mitral stenosis. Annular calcium with thin leaflets in calcific mitral stenosis. LA enlargement, normal to small left ventricle. Orifice can be traced to approximate mitral valve orifice area.	Thickened mitral valve in rheumatic disease; mitral valve prolapse; flail leaflet or vegetations may be seen. Dilated left ventricle in volume overload. Operate for left ventricular end-systolic dimension >4.5 cm.	Dense persistent echoes from the aortic valve with poor leaflet excursion. Left ventricular hypertrophy late in the disease. Bicuspid valve in younger patients.	Abnormal aortic valve or dilated aortic root. Diastolic vibrations of the anterior leaflet of the mitral valve and septum. In acute aortic regurgitation, premature closure of the mitral valve before the QRS. When severe, dilated left ventricle with normal or decreased contractility. Operate when left ventricular end-systolic dimension >5.0 cm.	In rheumatic disease, tricuspid valve thickening, decreased early diastolic filling slope of the tricuspid valve. In carcinoid, leaflets fixed, but no significant thickening.	Enlarged right ventricle with paradoxical septal motion. Tricuspid valve often pulled open by displaced chordae.
Continuous and color flow Doppler and TEE	Prolonged pressure half-time across mitral valve allows estimation of gradient. MVA estimated from pressure half-time. Indirect evidence of pulmonary hypertension by noting elevated right ventricular systolic pressure measured from the tricuspid regurgitation jet.	Regurgitant flow mapped into LA. Use of PISA helps assess MR severity. TEE important in prosthetic mitral valve regurgitation.	Increased transvalvular flow velocity; severe AS when peak jet >4 m/sec (64 mm Hg). Valve area estimate using continuity equation is poorly reproducible.	Demonstrates regurgitation and qualitatively estimates severity based on percentage of left ventricular outflow filled with jet and distance jet penetrates into left ventricle. TEE important in aortic valve endocarditis to exclude abscess. Mitral inflow pattern describes diastolic dysfunction.	Prolonged pressure half-time across tricuspid valve can be used to estimate mean gradient. Severe tricuspid stenosis present when mean gradient >5 mm Hg.	Regurgitant flow mapped into right atrium and venae cavae. Right ventricular systolic pressure estimated by tricuspid regurgitation jet velocity.

A_2 = aortic second sound; **AS** = aortic stenosis; **ICS** = interspace; **LA** = left atrial; **MCL** = midclavicular line; **MR** = mitral regurgitation; **MVA** = measured valve area; P_2 = pulmonary second sound; **PISA** = proximal isovelocity surface area; **PMI** = point of maximal impulse; S_1 = first heart sound; S_2 = second heart sound; S_3 = fourth heart sound; **SVC** = superior vena cava; **TEE** = transesophageal echocardiography; V_1 = chest ECG lead 1.
Reproduced with permission from Papadakis MA, McPhee SJ, Rabow MW (editors). Current Medical Diagnosis & Treatment 2016, 55th ed. McGraw-Hill, 2016.

9

Diagnostic Algorithms

Chuanyi Mark Lu, MD, Stephen J. McPhee, MD, and
Diana Nicoll, MD, PhD, MPA

HOW TO USE THIS SECTION

This section shows how diagnostic tests can be used in differential diagnosis and difficult diagnostic challenges. Material is presented in algorithmic forms, and contents are listed in alphabetical order by condition.

Abbreviations used throughout this section include the following: N = Normal; ↑ = Increased or high; ↓ = Decreased or low.

Each algorithm uses the following conventions:

SUSPECTED DIAGNOSIS/CLINICAL SITUATION

↓

Diagnostic test

Test abnormal   Test normal

↓   ↓

Diagnosis   ***Diagnosis***

↓

Treatment

Contents (Figures)   **Pages**

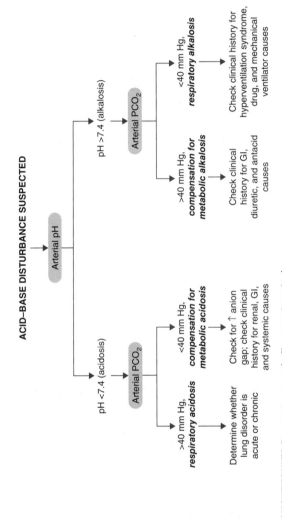

Figure 9–1. ACID–BASE DISTURBANCES: Diagnostic approach. **GI** = gastrointestinal.

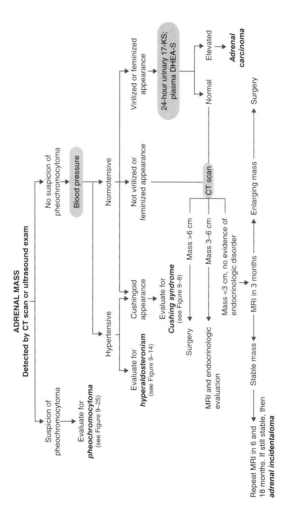

Figure 9–2. ADRENAL MASS: Diagnostic evaluation. *CT = computed tomography; DHEA-S = dehydroepiandrosterone sulfate; 17-KS = 17-ketosteroids; MRI = magnetic resonance imaging.*

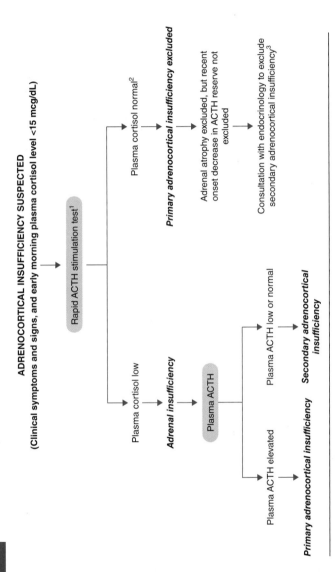

Figure 9–3. ADRENOCORTICAL INSUFFICIENCY (HYPOCORTISOLISM): Laboratory evaluation of suspected adrenocortical insufficiency (hypocortisolism). *ACTH* = adrenocorticotropic hormone.

ADRENOCORTICAL INSUFFICIENCY SUSPECTED

(Clinical symptoms and signs, and early morning plasma cortisol level <15 mcg/dL)

Rapid ACTH stimulation test[1]

Plasma cortisol low → *Adrenal insufficiency*

Plasma ACTH

- Plasma ACTH elevated → *Primary adrenocortical insufficiency*
- Plasma ACTH low or normal → *Secondary adrenocortical insufficiency*

Plasma cortisol normal[2] → *Primary adrenocortical insufficiency excluded*

Adrenal atrophy excluded, but recent onset decrease in ACTH reserve not excluded

Consultation with endocrinology to exclude secondary adrenocortical insufficiency[3]

[1]In the rapid ACTH stimulation test, a baseline cortisol sample is obtained; Cosyntropin (a synthetic peptide analog of ACTH, also called Cortrosyn), 10–25 mcg, is given IM or IV; and plasma cortisol samples are obtained 30 or 60 minutes later.

[2]The normal response is a cortisol increment >7 mcg/dL. If a cortisol level of >18 mcg/dL is obtained, the response is normal regardless of the increment.

[3]Previously performed tests to exclude secondary adrenocortical insufficiency are not often done: metyrapone is no longer available in the U.S. and many other countries, and the insulin tolerance test involves induction of hypoglycemia and thus can be risky.

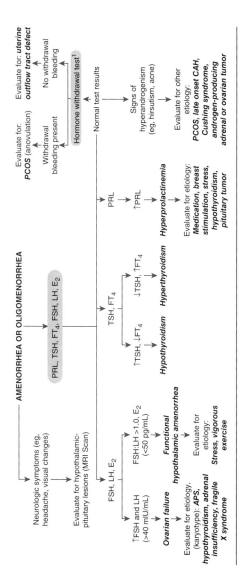

Figure 9–4. AMENORRHEA OR OLIGOMENORRHEA: Diagnostic laboratory evaluation for amenorrhea or oligomenorrhea. Primary amenorrhea is defined as the failure of menses to appear by age 16. Secondary amenorrhea is defined as occurring in women who have secondary sexual characteristics, have experienced menarche, and are presenting with consistently absent menses (more than 3 consecutive months). Oligomenorrhea is defined as scanty menses, or menses occurring at intervals of >35 days with only 4–9 menstrual periods in 1 year. Pregnancy must be ruled out before pursuing the testing outlined in the algorithm. **APS** = *autoimmune polyglandular syndrome;* **CAH** = *congenital adrenal hyperplasia;* **E₂** = *estradiol;* **FSH** = *follicle-stimulating hormone;* **FT₄** = *free thyroxine;* **LH** = *luteinizing hormone;* **MRI** = *magnetic resonance imaging;* **PCOS** = *polycystic ovarian syndrome;* **PRL** = *prolactin;* **TSH** = *thyroid-stimulating hormone.* (Modified with permission from Gardner DG, Shoback D [editors]: Greenspan's Basic & Clinical Endocrinology, 9th ed. McGraw-Hill, 2011.)

¹Give medroxyprogesterone 5–10 mg orally daily for 5 days. If withdrawal bleeding ensues, endogenous estrogen is adequate (eg, anovulation is occurring).

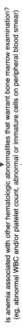
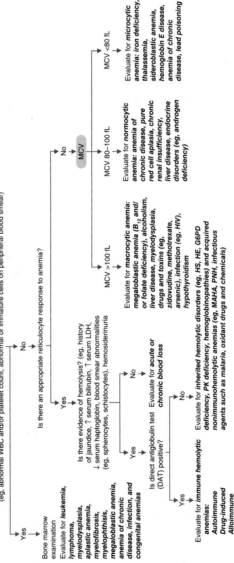

Figure 9–5. **ANEMIA:** General considerations and initial evaluation. The initial evaluation of anemia should include complete blood cell count, reticulocyte count and review of peripheral blood smear. *G6PD* = glucose-6-phosphate dehydrogenase; *HE* = hereditary elliptocytosis; *HS* = hereditary spherocytosis; *LDH* = lactate dehydrogenase; *MAHA* = microangiopathic hemolytic anemia; *MCV* = mean corpuscular volume; *PK* = pyruvate kinase; *PNH* = paroxysmal nocturnal hemoglobinuria.

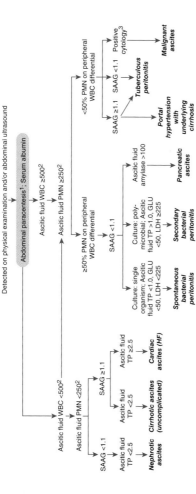

ASCITES
Detected on physical examination and/or abdominal ultrasound

Abdominal paracentesis [1]: Serum albumin

[Algorithm content:]

Ascitic fluid WBC ≥500 [2]
Ascitic fluid PMN ≥250 [2]

≥50% PMN on peripheral WBC differential
SAAG <1.1

Culture: single organism; Ascitic fluid TP <1.0, GLU <50, LDH <225 — **Spontaneous bacterial peritonitis**

Culture: poly-microbial; Ascitic fluid TP >1.0, GLU <50, LDH ≥225 — **Secondary bacterial peritonitis**

Ascitic fluid amylase >100 — **Pancreatic ascites**

<50% PMN on peripheral WBC differential
SAAG ≥1.1 — **Portal hypertension with underlying cirrhosis**
SAAG <1.1 — **Tuberculous peritonitis**
Positive cytology [3] — **Malignant ascites**

Ascitic fluid WBC <500 [2]
Ascitic fluid PMN <250 [2]

SAAG <1.1
Ascitic fluid TP <2.5 — **Nephrotic ascites**
Ascitic fluid TP <2.5 — **Cirrhotic ascites (uncomplicated)**

SAAG ≥1.1
Ascitic fluid TP ≥2.5 — **Cardiac ascites (HF)**

[1]Note the gross appearance of fluid (crystal clear, transparent or cloudy yellow, bloody, milky, or dark brown), and send ascitic fluid for cell count and differential, total protein, albumin, glucose, LDH, amylase, Gram stain, AFB stain, bacterial and other cultures and cytology as indicated. Also send triglyceride for milky fluid, bilirubin for dark-brown fluid. (See Table 8–6.)
[2]For bloody fluid, subtract 1 WBC per 750 RBC and subtract 1 PMN per 250 RBC (cells/mm³).
[3]Malignant cells present.

Figure 9–6. ASCITES: Diagnostic evaluation. *GLU* = glucose (mg/dL); *HF* = heart failure; *LDH* = lactate dehydrogenase (IU/L); *PMN* = polymorphonuclear neutrophil (cells/mm³); *RBC* = red blood cell count (cells/mm³); *SAAG* = serum-ascites albumin gradient (g/dL); *TP* = total protein (g/dL); *WBC* = white blood cell count (cells/mm³). (Modified, with permission, from Feldman M, Friedman LS, Brandt LJ [editors]. Sleisenger and Fordtran's Gastrointestinal and Liver Disease: Pathophysiology, Diagnosis, Management. 9th ed. Saunders, 2010.)

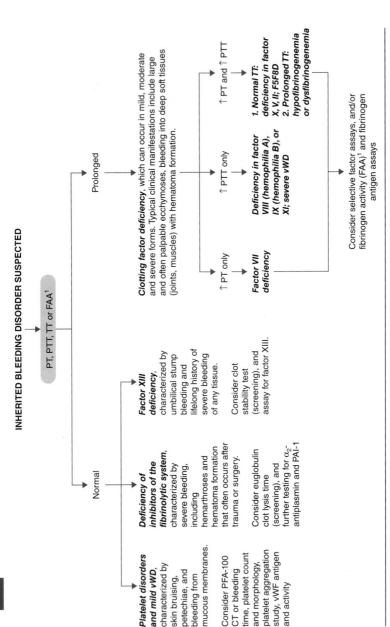

INHERITED BLEEDING DISORDER SUSPECTED

PT, PTT, TT or FAA[1]

Normal

Platelet disorders and mild vWD, characterized by skin bruising, petechiae, and bleeding from mucous membranes.

Consider PFA-100 CT or bleeding time, platelet count and morphology, platelet aggregation study, vWF antigen and activity

Deficiency of inhibitors of the fibrinolytic system, characterized by severe bleeding, including hemarthroses and hematoma formation that often occurs after trauma or surgery.

Consider euglobulin clot lysis time (screening), and further testing for α_2-antiplasmin and PAI-1

Factor XIII deficiency, characterized by umbilical stump bleeding and lifelong history of severe bleeding of any tissue.

Consider clot stability test (screening), and assay for factor XIII.

Prolonged

Clotting factor deficiency, which can occur in mild, moderate and severe forms. Typical clinical manifestations include large and often palpable ecchymoses, bleeding into deep soft tissues (joints, muscles) with hematoma formation.

↑ PT only

Factor VII deficiency

↑ PTT only

Deficiency in factor VIII (hemophilia A), IX (hemophilia B), or XI; severe vWD

↑ PT and ↑ PTT

1. Normal TT: deficiency in factor X, V, II; F5F8D

2. Prolonged TT: hypofibrinogenemia or dysfibrinogenemia

Consider selective factor assays, and/or fibrinogen activity (FAA)[1] and fibrinogen antigen assays

[1]FAA (fibrinogen activity assay) is now routinely available in clinical laboratories, and has largely replaced the need for TT for evaluation of fibrinogen activity (function).

Figure 9–7. BLEEDING DISORDERS, INHERITED: Evaluation of suspected inherited bleeding disorders. **F5F8D** = combined deficiency of factor V and factor VIII; **PAI-1** = plasminogen activator inhibitor 1; **PFA-100 CT** = platelet function analyzer-100 closure time; **PT** = prothrombin time; **PTT** = partial thromboplastin time; **TT** = thrombin time; **vWD** = von

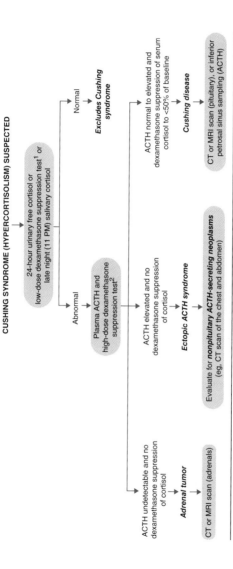

CUSHING SYNDROME (HYPERCORTISOLISM) SUSPECTED

24-hour urinary free cortisol or low-dose dexamethasone suppression test[1] or late night (11 PM) salivary cortisol

→ Normal → **Excludes Cushing syndrome**

→ Abnormal

Plasma ACTH and high-dose dexamethasone suppression test[2]

ACTH undetectable and no dexamethasone suppression of cortisol

Adrenal tumor

CT or MRI scan (adrenals)

ACTH elevated and no dexamethasone suppression of cortisol

Ectopic ACTH syndrome

Evaluate for **nonpituitary ACTH-secreting neoplasms** (eg, CT scan of the chest and abdomen)

ACTH normal to elevated and dexamethasone suppression of serum cortisol to <50% of baseline

Cushing disease

CT or MRI scan (pituitary), or inferior petrosal sinus sampling (ACTH)

[1]Low dose: Give 1 mg dexamethasone at 11 PM; draw serum cortisol at 8 AM. Normally, AM cortisol is <1.8 mcg/dL (50 nmol/L).
[2]High dose: Give 8 mg dexamethasone at 11 PM; draw serum cortisol at 8 AM or collect 24-hour urinary free cortisol. Normally, AM cortisol is <5 mcg/dL (<135 nmol/L) or 24-hour urinary free cortisol is <20 mcg.

Figure 9–8. CUSHING SYNDROME (HYPERCORTISOLISM): Diagnostic evaluation of suspected Cushing syndrome (hypercortisolism). **ACTH** = adrenocorticotropic hormone; **CT** = computed tomography; **HPLC** = high-performance liquid chromatography; **MRI** = magnetic resonance imaging.

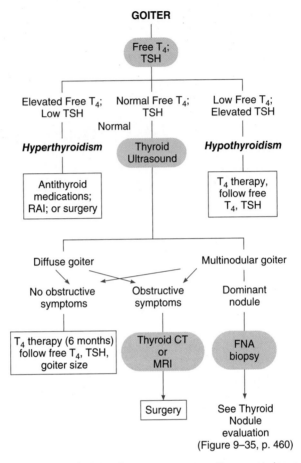

GOITER

Free T$_4$; TSH

| Elevated Free T$_4$; Low TSH | Normal Free T$_4$; TSH | Low Free T$_4$; Elevated TSH |

Normal

Hyperthyroidism

Thyroid Ultrasound

Hypothyroidism

Antithyroid medications; RAI; or surgery

T$_4$ therapy, follow free T$_4$, TSH

Diffuse goiter   Multinodular goiter

No obstructive symptoms   Obstructive symptoms   Dominant nodule

T$_4$ therapy (6 months) follow free T$_4$, TSH, goiter size

Thyroid CT or MRI

FNA biopsy

Surgery

See Thyroid Nodule evaluation (Figure 9–35, p. 460)

Figure 9–9. **GOITER:** Diagnostic evaluation and management strategy. ***CT*** = *computed tomography;* ***FNA*** = *fine-needle aspiration;* ***MRI*** = *magnetic resonance imaging;* ***RAI*** = *radioactive iodine;* ***T$_4$*** = *L-thyroxine;* ***TSH*** = *thyroid-stimulating hormone.* (*Modified, with permission, from Goldman L, Bennett JC [editors]. Cecil's Textbook of Medicine, 22nd ed. Saunders, 2004.*)

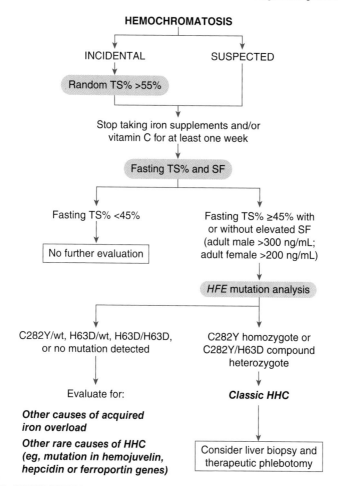

Figure 9–10. **HEMOCHROMATOSIS:** Diagnostic evaluation of suspected hemochromatosis. **HHC** = hereditary hemochromatosis; **SF** = serum ferritin; **TS%** = transferrin-iron saturation percentage (serum iron/total iron binding capacity × 100%).

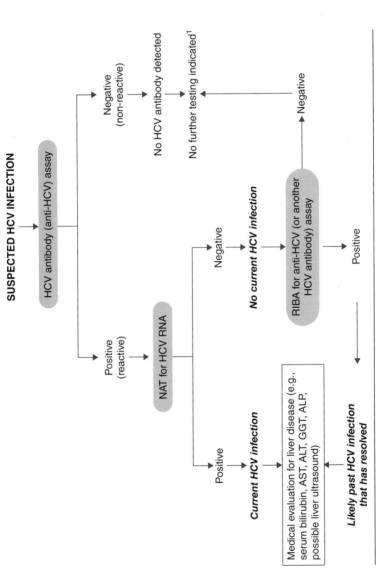

Figure 9-11. HCV INFECTION: Diagnostic strategy for patients with suspected HCV infection. ***Anti-HCV*** = *antibody to HCV;* ***ALP*** = *alkaline phosphatase;* ***ALT*** = *alanine transaminase;* ***AST*** = *aspartate aminotransferase;* ***GGT*** = *gamma-glutamyl transpeptidase;* ***HCV*** = *hepatitis C virus;* ***NAT*** = *nucleic acid testing;* ***RIBA*** = *recombinant immunoblot assay;* ***RNA*** = *ribonucleic acid.* (http://www.cdc.gov/mmwr/preview/mmwrhtml/mm6218a5.htm)

The following text appears within the figure:

SUSPECTED HCV INFECTION

HCV antibody (anti-HCV) assay

Positive (reactive) → NAT for HCV RNA

Negative (non-reactive) → No HCV antibody detected → No further testing indicated[1]

NAT for HCV RNA:
- Positive → **Current HCV infection** → Medical evaluation for liver disease (e.g., serum bilirubin, AST, ALT, GGT, ALP, possible liver ultrasound)
- Negative → **No current HCV infection** → RIBA for anti-HCV (or another HCV antibody) assay
  - Positive → **Likely past HCV infection that has resolved**
  - Negative → No further testing indicated[1]

[1]For persons who are suspected to have had HCV exposure within the past 6 months or have clinical evidence of HCV disease, HCV RNA testing (or repeat HCV RNA testing) is recommended.

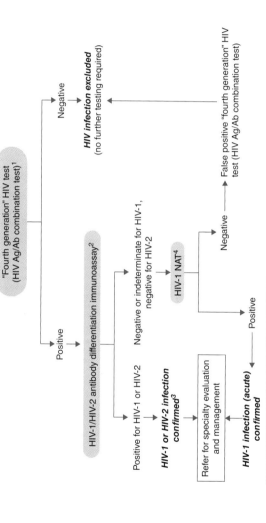

Figure 9-12. HIV INFECTION: Diagnostic strategy for patients with suspected HIV infection. This new testing algorithm, recommended in 2015 by the Centers for Disease Control & Prevention, capitalizes on the latest technologies available. It can help to diagnose HIV infection earlier in its course (as much as 3–4 weeks earlier than older HIV antibody-based approaches), potentially preventing transmission of new infections by patients in the earliest ("acute") stage of infection. **Ab = antibody; Ag = antigen; HIV = human immunodeficiency virus; NAT = nucleic acid test.** (Algorithm modified from: http://www.cdc.gov/hiv/pdf/HIVtestingAlgorithmRecommendation-Final.pdf. See also: http://www.cdc.gov/hiv/testing/index.html)

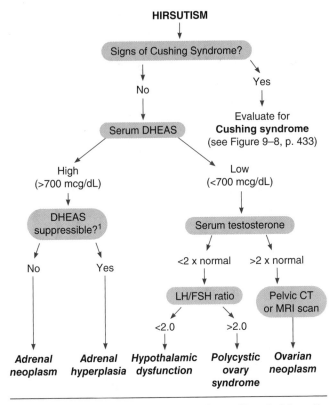

HIRSUTISM

Signs of Cushing Syndrome?

No

Yes

Evaluate for
Cushing syndrome
(see Figure 9–8, p. 433)

Serum DHEAS

High
(>700 mcg/dL)

Low
(<700 mcg/dL)

DHEAS
suppressible?[1]

Serum testosterone

No

Yes

<2 x normal

>2 x normal

LH/FSH ratio

Pelvic CT
or MRI scan

<2.0

>2.0

*Adrenal
neoplasm*

*Adrenal
hyperplasia*

*Hypothalamic
dysfunction*

*Polycystic
ovary
syndrome*

*Ovarian
neoplasm*

[1]DHEAS < 170 mcg/dL after dexamethasone 0.5 mg orally every 6 hours for 5 days, with
DHEAS repeated on the fifth day.

Figure 9–13. HIRSUTISM: Evaluation of hirsutism in females. Exceptions occur that do not fit this algorithm.
CT = *computed tomography;* **DHEAS** = *dehydroepiandrosterone sulfate;* **FSH** = *follicle-stimulating
hormone;* **LH** = *luteinizing hormone.* (*Reproduced with permission from Fitzgerald PA [editor].*
Handbook of Clinical Endocrinology, *2nd ed. McGraw-Hill, 1992.*)

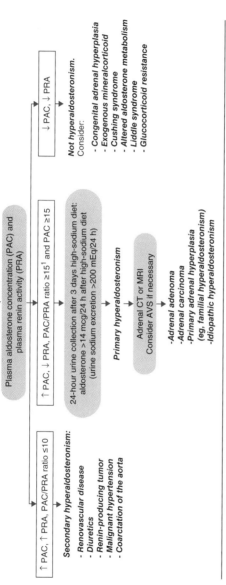

HYPERALDOSTERONISM SUSPECTED (eg. hypertension with hypokalemia)

Plasma aldosterone concentration (PAC) and plasma renin activity (PRA)

↑ PAC, ↑ PRA, PAC/PRA ratio ≤10

Secondary hyperaldosteronism:
- *Renovascular disease*
- *Diuretics*
- *Renin-producing tumor*
- *Malignant hypertension*
- *Coarctation of the aorta*

↑ PAC, ↓ PRA, PAC/PRA ratio ≥15[1] and PAC ≥15

24-hour urine collection after 3 days high-sodium diet: aldosterone >14 mcg/24 h after high-sodium diet (urine sodium excretion >200 mEq/24 h)

Primary hyperaldosteronism

Adrenal CT or MRI
Consider AVS if necessary

-*Adrenal adenoma*
-*Adrenal carcinoma*
-*Primary adrenal hyperplasia (eg, familial hyperaldosteronism)*
-*Idiopathic hyperaldosteronism*

↓ PAC, ↓ PRA

Not hyperaldosteronism.
Consider:

- *Congenital adrenal hyperplasia*
- *Exogenous mineralcorticoid*
- *Cushing syndrome*
- *Altered aldosterone metabolism*
- *Liddle syndrome*
- *Glucocorticoid resistance*

[1]The cutoff for a "high" PAC/PRA ratio is laboratory-dependent and, more specifically, PRA assay-dependent, and therefore an increased PAC is required for the diagnosis.

Figure 9–14. HYPERALDOSTERONISM: Laboratory evaluation of suspected hyperaldosteronism. *AVS* = *adrenal venous sampling; CT = computed tomography; MRI = magnetic resonance imaging; PAC = plasma aldosterone concentration (ng/dL); PRA = plasma renin activity (ng/mL/hr); PAC/PRA ratio = plasma aldosterone concentration to plasma renin activity ratio.*

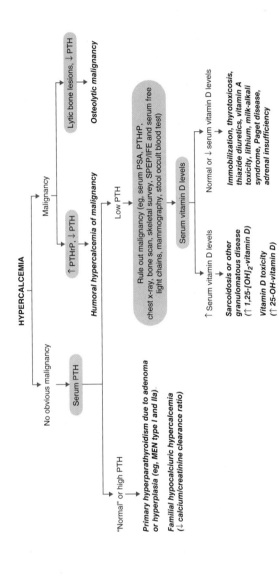

Figure 9–15. HYPERCALCEMIA: Diagnostic approach to hypercalcemia; *IF* = immunofixation electrophoresis; *PTH* = parathyroid hormone (measured by intact PTH assay); *PThrP* = PTH related protein; *PSA* = prostate specific antigen; *SPEP* = serum protein electrophoresis; ↑ = increase; ↓ = decrease.

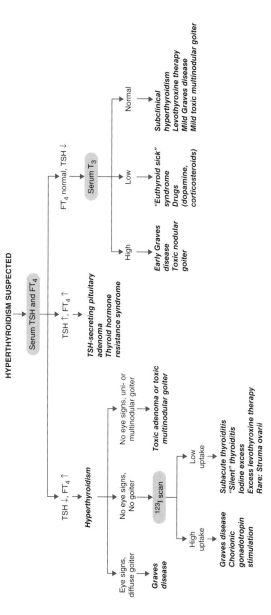

Figure 9–16. HYPERTHYROIDISM: Laboratory evaluation. **FT₄** = free thyroxine; **T₃** = 3,5,3′-triiodothyronine; **TSH** = thyroid-stimulating hormone. (Modified with permission from Gardner DG, Shoback D [editors]: Greenspan's Basic & Clinical Endocrinology, 9th ed. McGraw-Hill, 2011.)

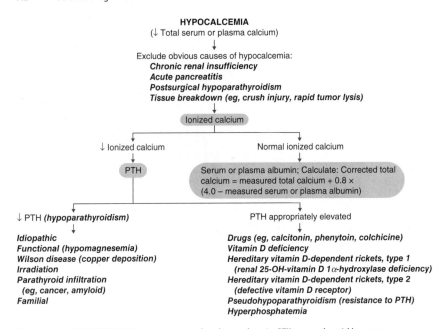

HYPOCALCEMIA
(↓ Total serum or plasma calcium)
↓
Exclude obvious causes of hypocalcemia:
Chronic renal insufficiency
Acute pancreatitis
Postsurgical hypoparathyroidism
Tissue breakdown (eg, crush injury, rapid tumor lysis)
↓

Ionized calcium

↓ Ionized calcium   Normal ionized calcium

PTH   Serum or plasma albumin; Calculate: Corrected total calcium = measured total calcium + 0.8 × (4.0 − measured serum or plasma albumin)

↓ PTH *(hypoparathyroidism)*   PTH appropriately elevated

Idiopathic   *Drugs (eg, calcitonin, phenytoin, colchicine)*
Functional (hypomagnesemia)   *Vitamin D deficiency*
Wilson disease (copper deposition)   *Hereditary vitamin D-dependent rickets, type 1*
Irradiation   *(renal 25-OH-vitamin D 1α-hydroxylase deficiency)*
Parathyroid infiltration   *Hereditary vitamin D-dependent rickets, type 2*
  (eg, cancer, amyloid)   *(defective vitamin D receptor)*
Familial   *Pseudohypoparathyroidism (resistance to PTH)*
                                                    Hyperphosphatemia

Figure 9–17. HYPOCALCEMIA: Diagnostic approach to hypocalcemia. *PTH* = *parathyroid hormone.*

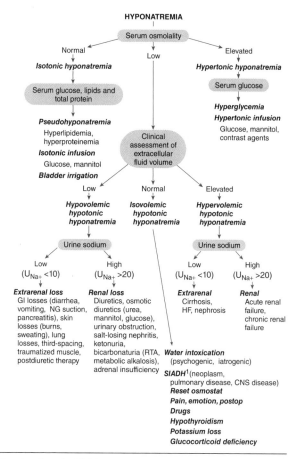

Figure 9–18. HYPONATREMIA: Evaluation of hyponatremia. *CNS* = *central nervous system;* *GI* = *gastrointestinal;* *HF* = *heart failure;* *NG* = *nasogastric;* *RTA* = *renal tubular acidosis;* *SIADH* = *syndrome of inappropriate antidiuretic hormone;* U_{Na+} = *urinary sodium (mg/dL). (Adapted with permission from Narins RG et al. Diagnostic strategies in disorders of fluid, electrolyte, and acid-base homeostasis.* Am J Med *1982;72:496. [PMID: 7036739])*

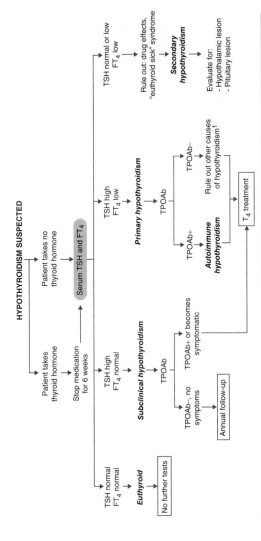

HYPOTHYROIDISM SUSPECTED

Figure 9–19. HYPOTHYROIDISM: Diagnostic approach. FT_4 = free thyroxine; $TPOAb$– = thyroid peroxidase antibodies negative; $TPOAb$+ = thyroid peroxidase antibodies positive; TSH = thyroid-stimulating hormone.

[1]Other causes of hypothyroidism include iatrogenic (eg, irradiation, thyroidectomy), drugs (eg, lithium, antithyroid drugs), congenital, iodine deficiency, and infiltrative disorders involving thyroid gland.

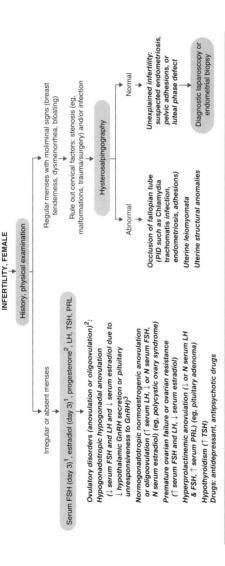

INFERTILITY, FEMALE

History, physical examination

Irregular or absent menses

Serum FSH (day 3)[1], estradiol (day 3)[1], progesterone[2], LH, TSH, PRL

Ovulatory disorders (anovulation or oligoovulation)[2]:

Hypogonadotropic hypogonadal anovulation (↓ serum FSH and LH and ↓ serum estradiol due to ↓ hypothalamic GnRH secretion or pituitary unresponsiveness to GnRH)[3]

Normogonadotropic normoestrogenic anovulation or oligoovulation (↑ serum LH, ↓ or N serum FSH, N serum estradiol) (eg, polycystic ovary syndrome)

Premature ovarian failure or ovarian resistance (↑ serum FSH and LH, ↓ serum estradiol)

Hyperprolactinemic anovulation (↓ or N serum LH & FSH, ↑ serum PRL) (eg, pituitary adenoma)

Hypothyroidism (↑ TSH)

Drugs: antidepressant, antipsychotic drugs

Regular menses with moliminal signs (breast tenderness, dysmenorrhea, bloating)

Rule out cervical factors: stenosis (eg, malformations, trauma/surgery) and/or infection

Hysterosalpingography

Abnormal

Occlusion of fallopian tube *(PID such as Chlamydia trachomatis infection, endometriosis, adhesions)*

Uterine leiomyomata

Uterine structural anomalies

Normal

Unexplained infertility: *suspected endometriosis, pelvic adhesions, or luteal phase defect*

Diagnostic laparoscopy or endometrial biopsy

---

[1]Day 1 is the first day of full menstrual flow.

[2]A mid-luteal phase serum progesterone level <3 ng/mL suggests anovulation.

[3]Hypogonadotropic hypogonadal anovulation (hypothalamic-pituitary amenorrhea) can be caused by Kallman syndrome, Sheehan syndrome, empty sella syndrome, autoimmune diseases (eg, lymphocytic hypophysitis), tumors/trauma/radiation of the hypothalamic or pituitary area, stress, eating disorders, and intense exercise.

Figure 9–20. INFERTILITY, FEMALE: Evaluation of female infertility. *FSH* = follicle-stimulating hormone; *GnRH* = gonadotropin-releasing hormone; *LH* = luteinizing hormone; *PID* = pelvic inflammatory disease; *PRL* = prolactin; *TSH* = thyroid stimulating hormone.

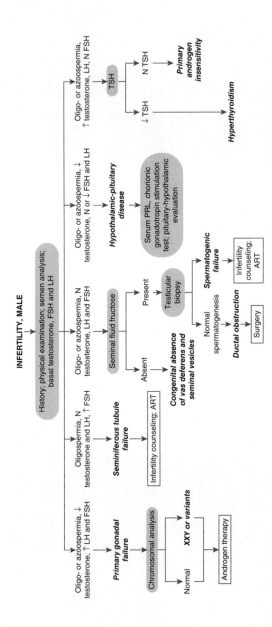

Figure 9–21. INFERTILITY, MALE: Evaluation of male factor infertility. **ART** = assisted reproductive technologies; **FSH** = follicle-stimulating hormone; **LH** = luteinizing hormone; **PRL** = prolactin; **TSH** = thyroid-stimulating hormone. (Adapted, with permission, from Gardner DG, Shoback D [editors]. Greenspan's Basic and Clinical Endocrinology, 9th ed. McGraw-Hill, 2011.)

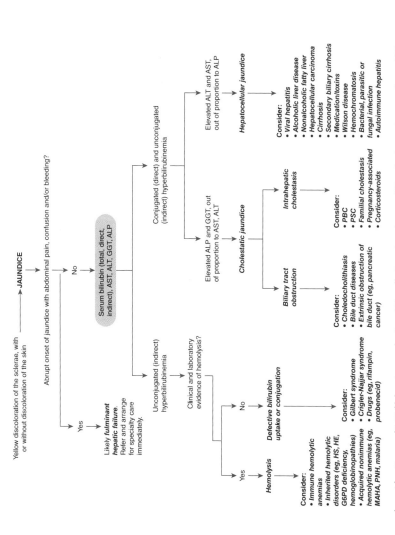

Figure 9–22. JAUNDICE: General considerations and initial laboratory evaluation. ***ALP*** = alkaline phosphatase; ***ALT*** = alanine aminotransferase; ***AST*** = aspartate aminotransferase; ***G6PD*** = glucose-6-phosphate dehydrogenase; ***GGT*** = gamma-glutamyl transpeptidase; ***HE*** = hereditary elliptocytosis; ***HS*** = hereditary spherocytosis; ***MAHA*** = microangiopathic hemolytic anemia; ***PBC*** = primary biliary cirrhosis; ***PNH*** = paroxysmal nocturnal hemoglobinuria; ***PSC*** = primary sclerosing cholangitis.

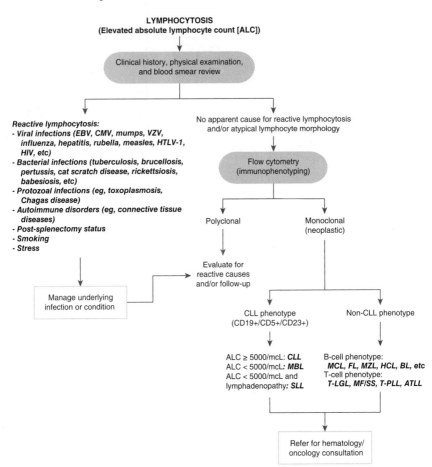

Figure 9–23. LYMPHOCYTOSIS: General approach to established lymphocytosis. *ALC = absolute lymphocyte count; ATLL = adult T-cell leukemia/lymphoma; BL = Burkitt lymphoma/leukemia; CLL = chronic lymphocytic leukemia; CMV = cytomegalovirus; EBV = Epstein-Barr virus; FL = follicular lymphoma; HCL = hairy cell leukemia; HIV = human immunodeficiency virus; HTLV-1 = human T-cell leukemia virus-1; MBL = monoclonal B-cell lymphocytosis; MCL = mantle cell lymphoma; MF/SS = mycosis fungoides/Sézary syndrome; MZL = marginal zone (B-cell) lymphoma; SLL = small lymphocytic lymphoma; T-LGL = T-cell large granular lymphocytic leukemia; T-PLL = T-cell prolymphocytic leukemia; VZV = varicella zoster virus.*

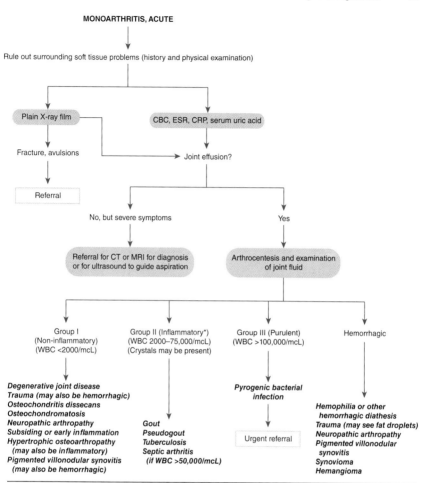

Figure 9–24. MONOARTHRITIS, ACUTE: Evaluation of acute monoarthritis. **CBC** = *complete blood count;* **CT** = *computed tomography;* **ESR** = *erythrocyte sedimentation rate;* **MRI** = *magnetic resonance imaging;* **WBC** = *white blood cell count (total).*

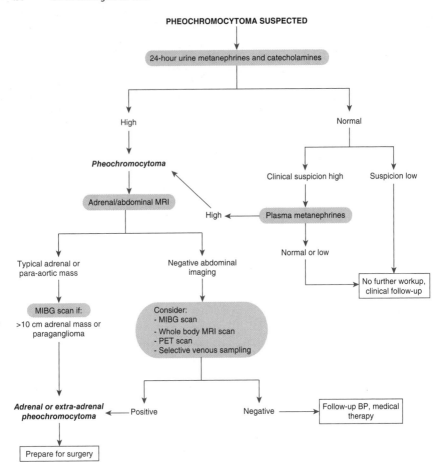

Figure 9–25. PHEOCHROMOCYTOMA: Evaluation and localization of a possible pheochromocytoma. Clinical suspicion is triggered by paroxysmal symptoms (especially hypertension); hypertension that is intermittent, unusually labile, or resistant to treatment; family history of pheochromocytoma or associated conditions; or an incidentally discovered adrenal mass. **BP** = *blood pressure;* **MIBG** = [131]I- or [123]I-*labeled metaiodobenzylguanidine;* **MRI** = *magnetic resonance imaging;* **PET** = *positron emission tomography.*

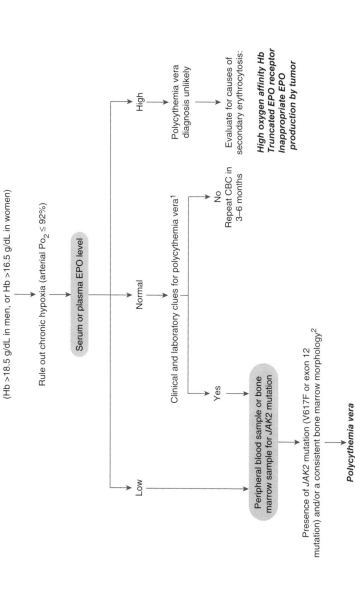

POLYCYTHEMIA
(Hb >18.5 g/dL in men, or Hb >16.5 g/dL in women)

Rule out chronic hypoxia (arterial $Po_2 \leq 92\%$)

Serum or plasma EPO level

Low

Normal

High

Peripheral blood sample or bone marrow sample for *JAK2* mutation

Clinical and laboratory clues for polycythemia vera[1]

Polycythemia vera diagnosis unlikely

Presence of *JAK2* mutation (V617F or exon 12 mutation) and/or a consistent bone marrow morphology[2]

Yes

No
Repeat CBC in 3–6 months

Evaluate for causes of secondary erythrocytosis:

High oxygen affinity Hb
Truncated EPO receptor
Inappropriate EPO
production by tumor

Polycythemia vera

[1]Clinical and laboratory clues for polycythemia vera include splenomegaly, platelet count >400,000/mcL, WBC >12,000/mcL, increased serum vitamin B_{12} or vitamin B_{12} binding capacity, and no history of familial erythrocytosis.
[2]*JAK2*[V617F] mutation has been found to be present in >95% of patients with polycythemia vera; mutation in exon 12 of *JAK2* has also been reported. Bone marrow biopsy shows panmyelosis with prominent erythroid and megakaryocytic proliferation.

Figure 9–26. POLYCYTHEMIA: Diagnostic evaluation. *CBC* = complete blood cell count; *EPO* = erythropoietin; *Hb* = hemoglobin; *JAK2* = Janus kinase 2 gene.

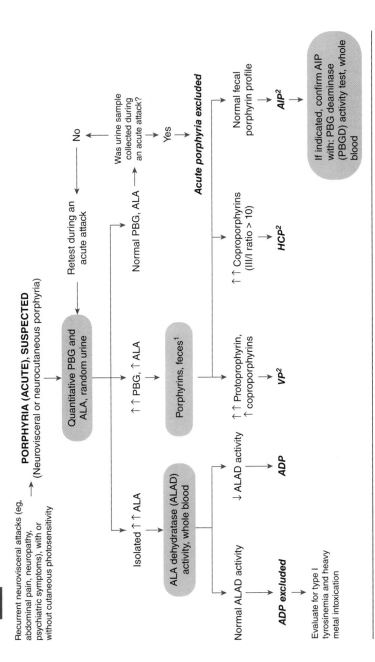

Figure 9–27. PORPHYRIA, ACUTE: Laboratory evaluation of suspected acute neurovisceral or neurocutaneous porphyria. **ADP** = aminolevulinic acid dehydratase deficiency porphyria (olumbonorphria; neurovisceral); **AIP** = acute intermittent porphyria (neurovisceral); **ALA** = aminolevulinic acid; **ALAD** = aminolevulinic acid dehydratase;

[1] Expert interpretation of test results is necessary.

[2] Autosomal dominant disorder. If clinically indicated, evaluate family members for acute porphyria. Gene analysis by DNA sequencing may be needed to confirm the diagnosis (rarely necessary).

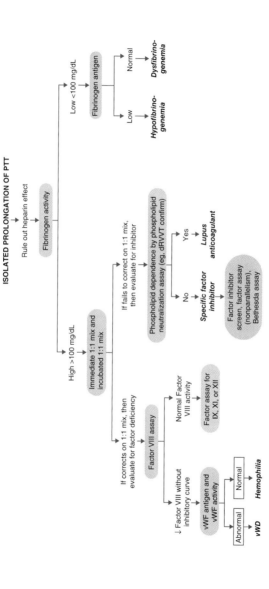

Figure 9–28. ISOLATED PROLONGATION OF PTT: Laboratory evaluation. ***dRVVT*** = *dilute Russell viper venom time*; ***PTT*** = *activated partial thromboplastin time*; ***vWF*** = *von Willebrand factor*; ***vWD*** = *von Willebrand disease.*

PULMONARY EMBOLISM SUSPECTED

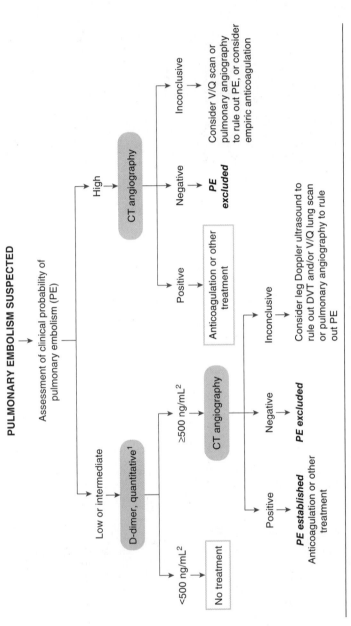

Figure 9–29. PULMONARY EMBOLISM: Diagnostic strategy for patients with suspected pulmonary embolism. *CT* = computed tomography; *DVT* = deep venous thrombosis; *PE* = pulmonary embolism; *V/Q scan* = ventilation-perfusion scan. (Modified from Le Gal et al. Prediction of pulmonary embolism in the emergency department: the revised Geneva score. Ann Intern Med 2006;144:165. [PMID: 16461960])

[1]D-dimer testing is typically used in the outpatient setting (eg, emergency department) to rule out PE.

[2]The cut-off value is method-dependent, but 500 ng/mL (fibrinogen equivalent units or FEU) is the most commonly used. A D-dimer level below the cut-off value of 500 ng/mL [or (age × 10) ng/mL in patients 50 years or older] rules out PE.

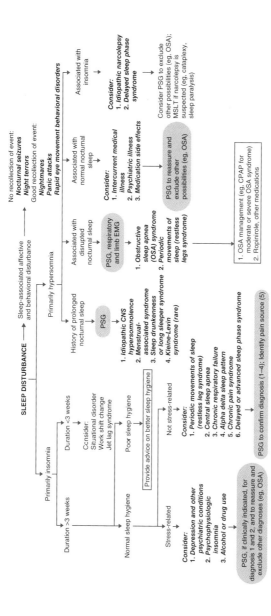

Figure 9–30. SLEEP DISTURBANCE: Diagnostic evaluation. Poor sleep hygiene refers to ingestion of products (such as caffeine, alcohol, and tobacco) or to behaviors that can interfere with sleep (such as intense exercise in the evening and irregular sleeping schedule). *CNS* = central nervous system; *CPAP* = continuous positive airway pressure; *EMG* = electromyelogram; *MSLTs* = multiple sleep latency tests (note: patient must be off antidepressants and stimulants to undergo an MSLT); *PSG* = polysomnography.

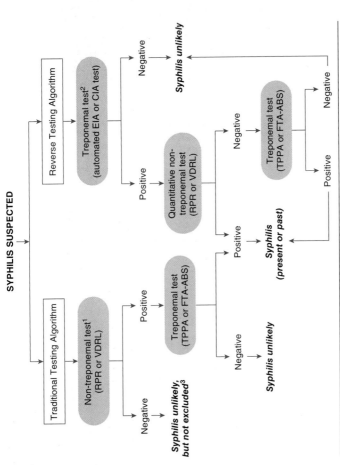

SYPHILIS SUSPECTED

[1]Non-treponemal tests measure levels of IgG and IgM antibodies produced by the host in response to lipids (mostly cardiolipin) released from damaged host cells associated with *T pallidum* infection.

[2]Treponemal tests detect either IgG or IgM antibodies produced by the host in response to specific *T pallidum* antigens; the tests use either whole cells or antigens derived from cells of *T pallidum*.

[3]RPR- or VDRL-based screening may miss some cases of early untreated, previously treated, and late latent syphilis. If clinically indicated, a treponemal test should be performed.

Figure 9–31. SYPHILIS SEROLOGIC TESTING: Two commonly used approaches to the serological diagnosis of syphilis. *CIA* = chemiluminescence immunoassay; *EIA* = enzyme immunoassay; *FTA-ABS* = fluorescent treponemal antibody absorption assay; *RPR* = rapid plasma reagin test; *TPPA* = Treponema pallidum particle

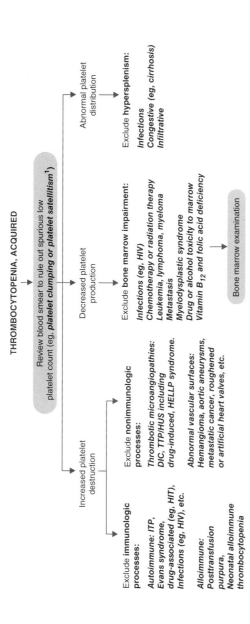

THROMBOCYTOPENIA, ACQUIRED

Review blood smear to rule out spurious low platelet count (eg, *platelet clumping or platelet satellitism*[1])

Increased platelet destruction

Exclude **immunologic processes:**

Autoimmune: ITP, Evans syndrome, drug-associated (eg, HIT), Infections (eg, HIV), etc.

Alloimmune: Posttransfusion purpura, Neonatal alloimmune thrombocytopenia

Exclude **nonimmunologic processes:**

Thrombotic microangiopathies: DIC, TTP/HUS including drug-induced, HELLP syndrome.

Abnormal vascular surfaces: Hemangioma, aortic aneurysms, metastatic cancer, roughened or artificial heart valves, etc.

Decreased platelet production

Exclude **bone marrow impairment:**

Infections (eg, HIV)
Chemotherapy or radiation therapy
Leukemia, lymphoma, myeloma
Metastasis
Myelodysplastic syndrome
Drug or alcohol toxicity to marrow
Vitamin B_{12} and folic acid deficiency

Bone marrow examination

Abnormal platelet distribution

Exclude **hypersplenism:**

Infections
Congestive (eg, cirrhosis)
Infiltrative

---

[1]Platelet satellitism, a rare peripheral blood finding, is adherence of 4 or more platelets to the surface of a neutrophil or monocyte. Similar to platelet clumping, it is an *in vitro* phenomenon often seen in EDTA-anticoagulated (lavender tube) whole blood. It may cause false thrombocytopenia with automated cell counters.

Figure 9–32. THROMBOCYTOPENIA, ACQUIRED: Diagnostic approach to acquired thrombocytopenia. *DIC* = *disseminated intravascular coagulation; HELLP syndrome* = *hemolytic anemia, elevated liver enzymes, and low platelet count; HIT* = *heparin-induced thrombocytopenia; HIV* = *human immunodeficiency virus; HUS* = *hemolytic uremic syndrome; ITP* = *idiopathic thrombocytopenic purpura; TTP* = *thrombotic thrombocytopenic purpura.*

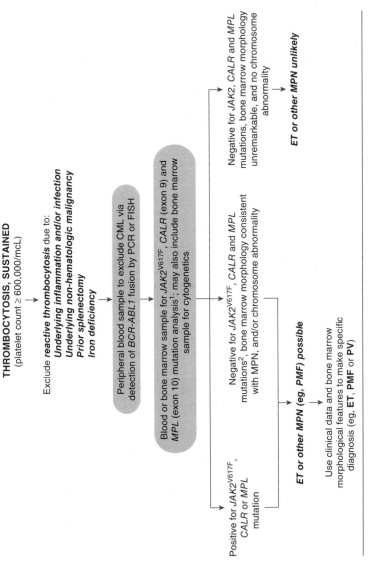

THROMBOCYTOSIS, SUSTAINED
(platelet count ≥ 600,000/mcL)

Exclude *reactive thrombocytosis* due to:
Underlying inflammation and/or infection
Underlying non-hematologic malignancy
Prior splenectomy
Iron deficiency

Peripheral blood sample to exclude CML via detection of *BCR-ABL1* fusion by PCR or FISH

Blood or bone marrow sample for $JAK2^{V617F}$, *CALR* (exon 9) and *MPL* (exon 10) mutation analysis[1]; may also include bone marrow sample for cytogenetics

Positive for $JAK2^{V617F}$, *CALR* or *MPL* mutation

ET or other MPN (eg, PMF) possible

Use clinical data and bone marrow morphological features to make specific diagnosis (eg, **ET**, **PMF** or **PV**)

Negative for $JAK2^{V617F}$, *CALR* and *MPL* mutations[2], bone marrow morphology consistent with MPN, and/or chromosome abnormality

Negative for *JAK2*, *CALR* and *MPL* mutations, bone marrow morphology unremarkable, and no chromosome abnormality

ET or other MPN unlikely

[1] *JAK2* mutation analysis should be performed first, then *CALR* mutation analysis, followed by *MPL* mutation analysis.

[2] ET and PMF that are negative for $JAK2^{V617F}$, *CALR* (exon 9) and *MPL* (exon 10) mutations are defined as "triple negative" cases; novel mutations in *MPL* and *JAK2* genes have been reported in such cases.

Figure 9–33. THROMBOCYTOSIS: Diagnostic evaluation of sustained thrombocytosis. *CALR* = calreticulin gene; *CML* = chronic myeloid leukemia; *ET* = essential thrombocythemia; *FISH* = fluorescence in-situ hybridization; *JAK2* = Janus kinase 2 gene; *MPL* = myeloproliferative leukemia gene (encodes thrombopoietin receptor); *MPN* = myeloproliferative

VENOUS THROMBOSIS, ESTABLISHED

Exclude *acquired thrombosis (eg, malignancy, orthopedic surgery, trauma, immobilization, HF, CMPD, nephrotic syndrome, hyperviscosity, PNH[1])*

If none present, and:

First episode of idiopathic venous thrombosis at age <50 years OR
History of recurrent thrombotic episodes OR
First-degree relative(s) with documented thromboembolism
at age <50 years

Evaluate for:

Factor V Leiden mutation by PCR
Prothrombin gene G20210A mutation by PCR
Presence of lupus anticoagulant (eg, dRVVT)
Hyperhomocysteinemia
Protein C deficiency
Protein S deficiency
Antithrombin deficiency
MTHFR mutation by PCR

First episodes of idiopathic venous thromboembolism
at age ≥50 years AND
Negative family history of thromboembolism

Evaluate for:

Factor V Leiden mutation by PCR
Prothrombin gene G20210A mutation by PCR
Presence of lupus anticoagulant (eg, dRVVT)
Hyperhomocysteinemia

[1]Thrombosis occurs in 40–45% of patients with PNH, often at unusual sites, including hepatic veins (Budd-Chiari syndrome), other intra-abdominal veins (portal, splenic, splanchnic), cerebral sinuses, and dermal veins.

Figure 9–34. THROMBOSIS, VENOUS: Evaluation for possible hypercoagulability (thrombophilia) causing venous thrombosis. **CMPD** = *chronic myeloproliferative disorder;* **dRVVT** = *dilute Russell viper venom clotting time;* **HF** = *heart failure;* **MTHFR** = *methylene tetrahydrofolate reductase;* **PCR** = *polymerase chain reaction;* **PNH** = *paroxysmal nocturnal hemoglobinuria.*

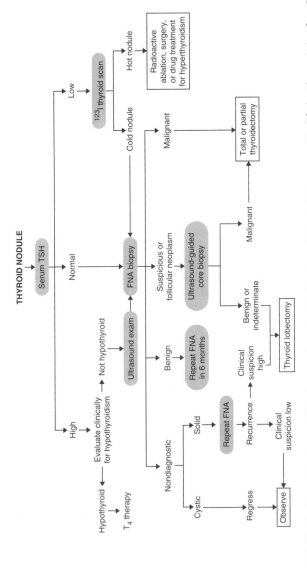

Figure 9–35. THYROID NODULE: Diagnostic evaluation. **FNA** = fine-needle aspiration; **TSH** = thyroid-stimulating hormone. (Modified, with permission, from Burch HB. Evaluation and management of the solid thyroid nodule. Endocrinol Metab Clin North Am 1995;24:663.)

TRANSFUSION

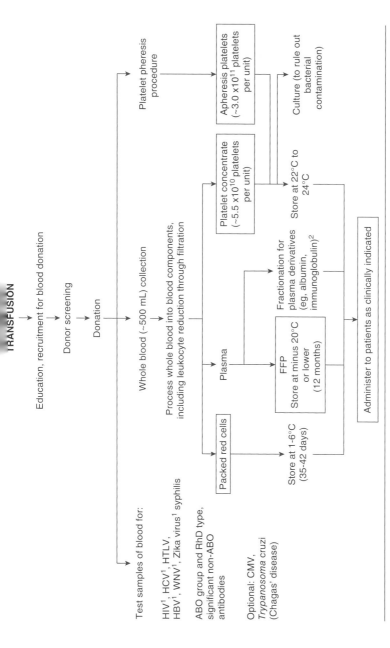

Education, recruitment for blood donation

Donor screening

Donation

Whole blood (~500 mL) collection

Test samples of blood for:

HIV[1], HCV[1], HTLV,
HBV[1], WNV[1], Zika virus[1] syphilis

ABO group and RhD type,
significant non-ABO
antibodies

Optional: CMV,
Trypanosoma cruzi
(Chagas' disease)

Process whole blood into blood components,
including leukocyte reduction through filtration

Packed red cells

Store at 1-6°C
(35-42 days)

Plasma

FFP
Store at minus 20°C
or lower
(12 months)

Fractionation for
plasma derivatives
(eg, albumin,
immunoglobulin)[2]

Platelet concentrate
(~5.5 x10^{10} platelets
per unit)

Store at 22°C to
24°C

Platelet pheresis
procedure

Apheresis platelets
(~3.0 x10^{11} platelets
per unit)

Culture (to rule out
bacterial
contamination)

Administer to patients as clinically indicated

[1]Nucleic acid testing (NAT) to screen for HIV, HBV, HCV, WNV and Zika virus.

[2]Plasma derivatives are also prepared through plasmapheresis.

Figure 9–36. TRANSFUSION: Blood donation and preparation of blood components. *CMV = cytomegalovirus; FFP = fresh frozen plasma; HBV = hepatitis B virus; HCV = hepatitis C virus; HIV = human immunodeficiency virus; HTLV = human T-cell leukemia virus; WNV = West Nile virus.*

10

Nomograms & Reference Material

Stephen J. McPhee, MD, Chuanyi Mark Lu, MD,
and Diana Nicoll, MD, PhD, MPA

HOW TO USE THIS SECTION

This section contains useful nomograms and reference material. Material is presented in alphabetical order by subject.

Contents (Figures)   *Pages*

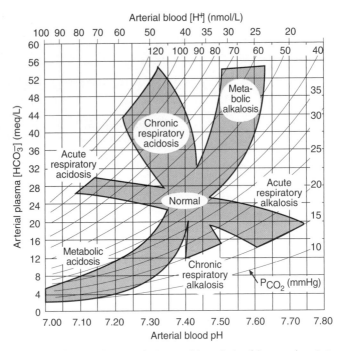

Figure 10-1. ACID-BASE NOMOGRAM: Shown are the 95% confidence limits of the normal respiratory and metabolic compensations for primary acid-base disturbances. (*Reproduced with permission from Brenner BM, Rector FC [editors]. Brenner & Rector's The Kidney, 8th ed. Saunders/Elsevier, 2008.*)

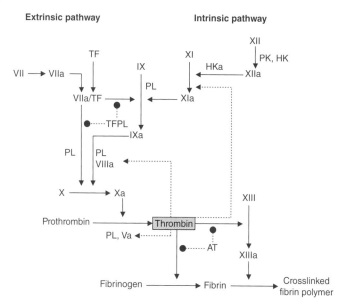

Figure 10–2. COAGULATION CASCADE: Schematic representation of the coagulation pathways. The central precipitating event is considered to involve tissue factor (TF), which, under physiologic conditions, is not exposed to the blood. With vascular or endothelial cell injury, TF acts together with Factor VIIa and phospholipids (PL) to convert Factor IX to IXa and Factor X to Xa. The "intrinsic pathway" includes "contact" activation of Factor XI by XIIa-activated high molecular-weight kininogen complex (XIIa-HKa). Factor XIa converts Factor IX to IXa, which, in turn, converts Factor X to Xa, in concert with Factor VIIIa and PL. Factor Xa is the active ingredient of the "prothrombinase" complex, which includes Factor Va and PL, and converts prothrombin to thrombin (TH). TH cleaves fibrinopeptides from fibrinogen, allowing the resultant fibrin monomers to polymerize, and converts Factor XIII to XIIIa, which cross-links the fibrin clot. TH also accelerates and augments the process (in dashed lines) by activating Factor V and VIII, but continued proteolytic action also dampens the process by activating protein C, which degrades Factor Va and VIIIa. TH activation of Factor XI to XIa is a proposed pathway. There are natural plasma inhibitors of the cascade: tissue factor pathway inhibitor (TFPI) blocks VIIa/TF and thus inactivates the "extrinsic pathway" after the clotting process is initiated; antithrombin (AT) blocks IXa, and Xa, and thrombin. Arrows = active enzymes; dashed lines with arrows = positive feedback reactions, which are considered important to maintain the process after the "extrinsic pathway" is shut down by TFPI; dashed lines with solid dots = inhibitory effects; *PK* = *prekallikrein*. Note that the contact system (PK, HK, and XII) actually contributes to fibrinolysis and bradykinin formation in vivo, and its role in initiation of the intrinsic pathway in vivo is questionable.

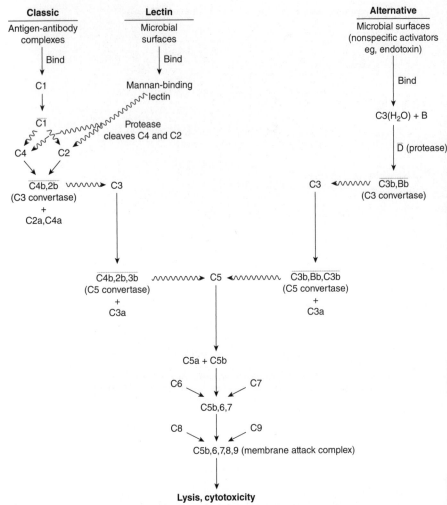

Figure 10-3. COMPLEMENT SYSTEM: The classic (antigen-antibody complexes), alternative (microbial surfaces) and lectin (microbial surfaces) pathways of activation of the complement system. Each wavy line with arrow ∿∿➤ indicates that there has been proteolytic cleavage of the molecule at the tip of the arrow; a complex with a line over it indicates that it is now enzymatically active. Note that, following cleavage, all smaller fragments are labeled with an "a," and all larger fragments are labeled with a "b." Hence, the C3 convertase is depicted as C4b,2b with a line over it. Note that, for the lectin pathway, proteases associated with the mannan-binding lectin cleave both C4 and C2. *(Reproduced with permission from Levinson W. Complement, Figure 63-1. in* Review of Medical Microbiology and Immunology, *13th ed. McGraw-Hill, 2014.)*

In addition, a useful animated video demonstration of the activation of the complement system classic and alternative pathways is available at: http://highered.mheducation.com/sites/0072507470/student_view0/chapter22/animation__activation_of_complement.html

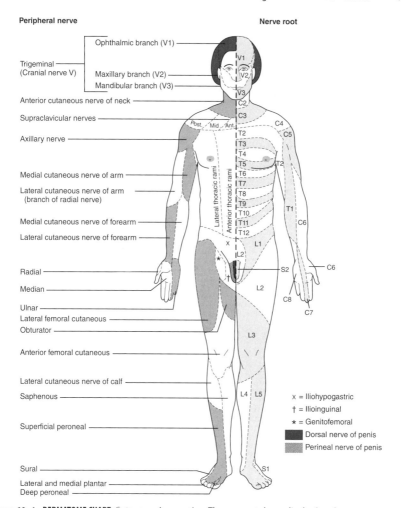

Peripheral nerve

Trigeminal (Cranial nerve V)
- Ophthalmic branch (V1)
- Maxillary branch (V2)
- Mandibular branch (V3)

Anterior cutaneous nerve of neck
Supraclavicular nerves
Axillary nerve
Medial cutaneous nerve of arm
Lateral cutaneous nerve of arm (branch of radial nerve)
Medial cutaneous nerve of forearm
Lateral cutaneous nerve of forearm
Radial
Median
Ulnar
Lateral femoral cutaneous
Obturator
Anterior femoral cutaneous
Lateral cutaneous nerve of calf
Saphenous
Superficial peroneal
Sural
Lateral and medial plantar
Deep peroneal

Nerve root

x = Iliohypogastric
† = Ilioinguinal
★ = Genitofemoral
Dorsal nerve of penis
Perineal nerve of penis

Figure 10–4. DERMATOME CHART: Cutaneous innervation. The segmental or radicular (root) distribution is shown on the right side of the body, and the peripheral nerve distribution on the left side. **Above:** anterior view; **next page:** posterior view. (*Adapted with permission from Simon R et al [editors].* Clinical Neurology, *7th ed. McGraw-Hill, 2009.*)

Nerve root

Peripheral nerve

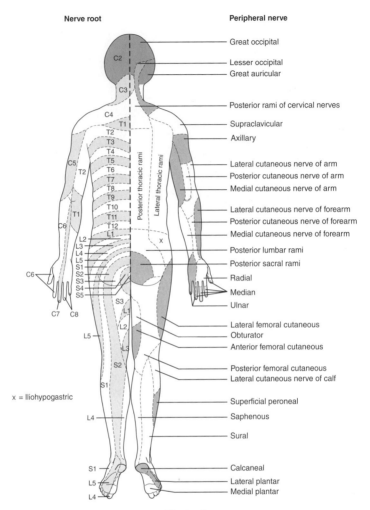

- Great occipital
- Lesser occipital
- Great auricular

- Posterior rami of cervical nerves

- Supraclavicular
- Axillary

- Lateral cutaneous nerve of arm
- Posterior cutaneous nerve of arm
- Medial cutaneous nerve of arm

- Lateral cutaneous nerve of forearm
- Posterior cutaneous nerve of forearm
- Medial cutaneous nerve of forearm

- Posterior lumbar rami
- Posterior sacral rami
- Radial
- Median
- Ulnar

- Lateral femoral cutaneous
- Obturator
- Anterior femoral cutaneous

- Posterior femoral cutaneous
- Lateral cutaneous nerve of calf

- Superficial peroneal
- Saphenous

- Sural

- Calcaneal
- Lateral plantar
- Medial plantar

x = Iliohypogastric

Figure 10–4. (*Continued*)

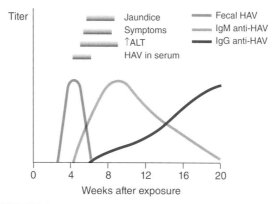

Figure 10–5. HEPATITIS A SEROLOGIC CHANGES: Usual pattern of serologic changes in hepatitis A. *ALT* = *alanine aminotransferase; **Anti-HAV** = hepatitis A virus antibody; **HAV** = hepatitis A virus; **IgM** =immunoglobulin M; **IgG** = immunoglobulin G. (Reproduced with permission from Koff RS: Acute viral hepatitis. In: Handbook of Liver Disease. Friedman LS, Keeffe EB [editors], 2nd ed. © Elsevier, 2004.)*

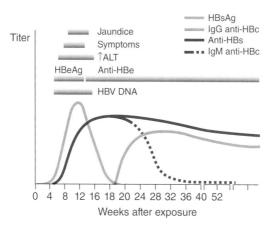

Figure 10–6. HEPATITIS B SEROLOGIC CHANGES: Usual pattern of serologic changes in hepatitis B. *ALT* = *alanine aminotransferase; **Anti-HBc** = hepatitis B core antibody; **Anti-HBe** = antibody to hepatitis B e antigen; **Anti-HBs** = hepatitis B surface antibody; **HBeAg** = hepatitis B e antigen; **HBsAg** = hepatitis B surface antigen; **HBV** = hepatitis B virus; **HBV DNA** = hepatitis B viral DNA; **IgG** = immunoglobulin G; **IgM** = immunoglobulin M. (Reproduced with permission from Koff RS: Acute viral hepatitis. In: Handbook of Liver Disease. Friedman LS, Keeffe EB [editors], 2nd ed. © Elsevier, 2004.)*

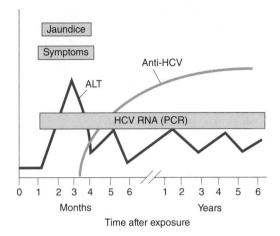

Figure 10–7. HEPATITIS C SEROLOGY AND VIRAL LOAD: The typical course of chronic hepatitis C. *ALT* = alanine aminotransferase. *Anti-HCV* = antibody to hepatitis C virus by enzyme immunoassay; *HCV RNA [PCR]* = hepatitis C viral RNA by polymerase chain reaction. (*Reproduced with permission from McPhee SJ, Papadakis MA, Rabow MW [editors].* Current Medical Diagnosis & Treatment 2012. *McGraw-Hill, 2012.*)

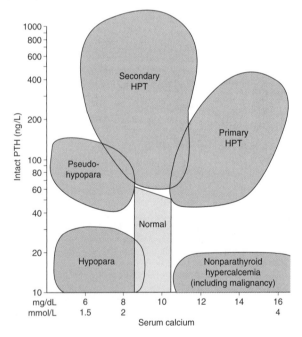

Figure 10–8. PARATHYROID HORMONE AND CALCIUM NOMOGRAM. Relation between serum intact parathyroid hormone (PTH) and serum calcium levels in patients with hypoparathyroidism, pseudohypoparathyroidism, nonparathyroid hypercalcemia (eg, malignancy), primary hyperparathyroidism, and secondary hyperparathyroidism. *HPT* = hyperparathyroidism. (*Used with permission from Gordon Strewler, MD.*)

Note: A multivariate analysis suggests that a model that adds clinical and demographic information may perform better than the nomogram alone. (*See O'Neill SS et al. Multivariate analysis of clinical, demographic, and laboratory data for classification of disorders of calcium homeostasis.* Am J Clin Pathol *2011;135:100. [PMID: 21173131]*)

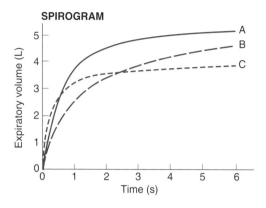

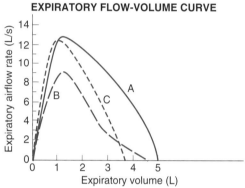

Figure 10–9. PULMONARY FUNCTION TESTS: SPIROMETRY. Representative spirograms (upper panel) and expiratory flow-volume curves (lower panel) for normal (A), obstructive (B), and restrictive (C) patterns. (*Reproduced with permission from Tierney LM Jr, McPhee SJ, Papadakis MA [editors]. Current Medical Diagnosis & Treatment 2005, 44th ed. McGraw-Hill, 2005.*)

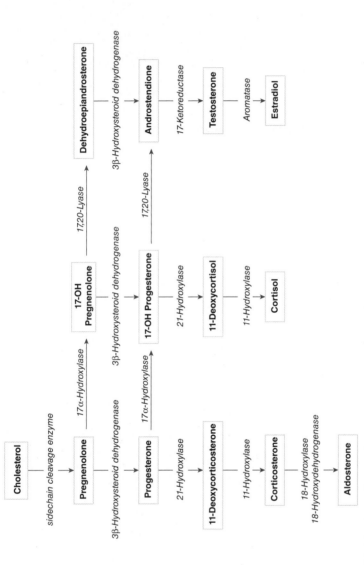

Figure 10–10. STEROIDOGENESIS PATHWAY. Steroidogenesis is the biosynthetic process by which the various types of steroids (in bold) are generated from cholesterol by various enzymes (in italics) and then transformed enzymatically into other steroids. This diagram is a simplified overview of the hormone synthetic pathways for the three main types of steroids produced: the mineralocorticoids (chiefly aldosterone), glucocorticoids (chiefly cortisol), and sex hormones (testosterone and estradiol). The pathways shown are present in differing amounts in the body's various steroid-producing tissues, namely, the adrenal glands, and the ovaries in women, and the testes in men. In the adrenal glands, the mineralocorticoids derive mainly from the zona glomerulosa, the glucocorticoids from the zona fasciculata, and the androgens (and estrogens) from the zona reticularis. The major adrenal androgen is androstenedione, because 17-ketoreductase activity is relatively low. In the gonads, the pathways leading to the synthesis of mineralocorticoids and glucocorticoids are not present to any significant degree; however, the ovaries and testes each do produce both androgens and estrogens. Further metabolism of testosterone occurs in target tissues by action of the enzyme 5α-reductase (not shown).

Index

Note: Page numbers followed by *f* or *t* refer to the page location of figures or tables, respectively.

interpretation and uses of, 194*t*
1:1 mix (inhibitor screen) and, 137*t*
ds-DNA Ab (double-stranded DNA
   antibody), 90*t*, 386*t*
Duchenne muscular dystrophy,
   392*t*
DVT (deep venous thrombosis)
   AT (antithrombin), 50*t*
   algorithm of venous thrombosis,
      459*f*
   anticoagulation therapy, 381–383*t*
   D-dimer, 87*t*
   dRVVT (dilute Russell's viper venom
      time), 194*t*
   factor II (prothrombin) G20210A
      mutation, 95*t*
   factor V Leiden mutation, 96*t*
   US (ultrasound), 322*t*
Dysentery, 259*t*
Dysfibrinogenemia, 101*t*
Dystrophin gene mutation, 392*t*

E

E2 (estradiol), 93*t*
EAEC (enteroaggregative *E. coli*), 280*t*
Ear infections, 247*t*
Ebola virus, 279*t*
EBOV (Zaire Ebola virus), 279*t*
EBV Ab (Epstein Barr virus antibodies),
   91*t*, 126*t*
ECG (electrocardiography), 325–361
   hexaxial reference system, 342
   for morphologic diagnosis
      approach to, 325
      atrial abnormalities, 339
      bundle branch block.
         See Bundle branch blocks
      early repolarization normal variant
         ST–T abnormality, 359*f*
      fascicular blocks (hemiblocks),
         341–342
      low-voltage QRS complex, 345
      mean QRS axis determination,
         342–343
      mirror-image dextrocardia, 359*f*
      myocardial injury, ischemia, and
         infarction, 346. *See also* MI
         (myocardial infarction)

normal QRST patterns, 339
QT interval. *See* QT interval
right-left arm cable reversal, 359*f*
right leg cable misplacement, 359,
   359*f*
R wave progression in precordial
   leads, 345
ST segments, 353, 354*t*, 355*t*
ST–T waves, 356*t*
tall R waves in right precordial
   leads, 345–346
U waves, 354–356, 357*t*
ventricular hypertrophy, 343–345
for rhythm diagnosis
   approach to, 325, 326
   atrial flutter. *See* Atrial flutter
   bradycardia, 337–339
   ectopic atrial rhythm, 327
   premature QRS activity, 327–328
   sinus rhythm, 326–327
   sustained irregular rhythms, 327*t*
   sustained regular rhythms, 326,
      326*t*
   tachycardia. *See* Tachycardia
in valvular heart disease, 421*t*
Echocardiography
   of aortic valve, 368–369, 369*f*, 422*t*
   intracardiac, 372
   of mitral valve, 364*f*, 370, 370*f*, 372,
      422*t*
   normal, 365, 365*f*
   physical principles and standard
      views, 361, 362*f*, 363, 363*f*,
      364*f*, 365
   transesophageal. *See* TEE
      (transesophageal
      echocardiography)
   of tricuspid valve, 370, 370*f*, 422*t*
   of ventricular anatomy and function,
      365–367, 365*f*, 366*f*, 367*f*, 368*f*
Ectopic atrial rhythm, 327
Ectopic pregnancy, 55*t*
Edoxaban, 383*t*
eGFR (estimated glomerular filtration
   rate), 105*t*
eGFRcys (CyC-based eGFR), 86*t*, 105*t*
EHEC/STEC (enterohemorrhagic/
   Shiga-toxin-producing *E. coli*),
   281*t*